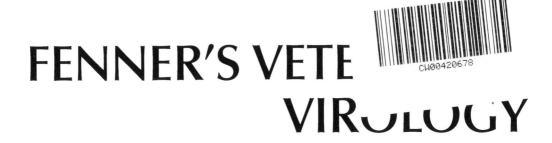

FENNER'S VETE VIROLOGY

Fourth Edition

Edited by
N. James MacLachlan
Distinguished Professor, Department of Pathology,
Microbiology and Immunology
School of Veterinary Medicine
University of California,
Davis, California, USA

and

Extraordinary Professor, Department of
Veterinary Tropical Diseases
Faculty of Veterinary Science
University of Pretoria
Onderstepoort, Republic of South Africa

Edward J. Dubovi
Director, Virology Section
Animal Health Diagnostic Center
Department of Population Medicine and
Diagnostic Sciences
College of Veterinary Medicine
Cornell University
Ithaca, New York, USA

AMSTERDAM • BOSTON • HEIDELBERG • LONDON • NEW YORK • OXFORD
PARIS • SAN DIEGO • SAN FRANCISCO • SINGAPORE • SYDNEY • TOKYO
Academic Press is an imprint of Elsevier

Academic Press is an imprint of Elsevier
32 Jamestown Road, London NW1 7BY, UK
30 Corporate Drive, Suite 400, Burlington, MA 01803, USA
525 B Street, Suite 1800, San Diego, CA 92101-4495, USA

Fourth Edition, 2011

Notice
No responsibility is assumed by the publisher for any injury and/or damage to persons
or property as a matter of products liability, negligence or otherwise, or from any use or
operation of any methods, products, instructions or ideas contained in the material herein.
Because of rapid advances in the medical sciences, in particular, independent verification of
diagnoses and drug dosages should be made

British Library Cataloguing-in-Publication Data
A catalogue record for this book is available from the British Library

Library of Congress Cataloging-in-Publication Data
A catalog record for this book is available from the Library of Congress

ISBN : 978-0-12-375158-4

For information on all Academic Press publications
visit our website at www.elsevierdirect.com

Typeset by MPS Limited, a Macmillan Company, Chennai, India
www.macmillansolutions.com

Printed and bound in the United States of America

Transferred to Digital Printing in 2013

Fenner's Veterinary Virology

Fourth Edition

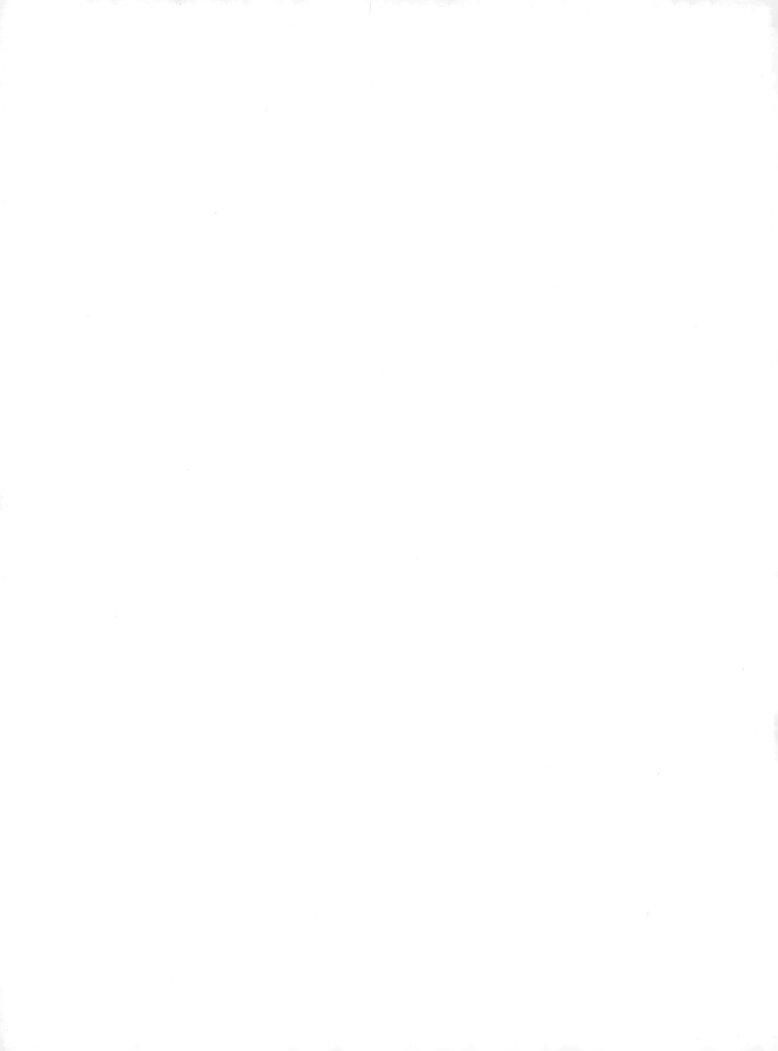

Dedication

This book is dedicated to those who laid the foundation for this text, specifically Frank J. Fenner and the late David O. White who first documented so many of the principles of animal virology in the original versions of this book, and Fred Murphy, Paul Gibbs, Marian Horzinek and Michael Studdert who so eloquently engineered the third edition. This fourth revision was undertaken with a great deal of trepidation, thus our overriding rule was not to alter the easy readability and wonderfully global presentation of the third edition. Rather, our intent was to retain the enthusiasm experienced by of all of us who have the remarkable privilege to enjoy careers that allow us to study veterinary and zoonotic virus diseases, but to also bring all aspects of veterinary virology under the umbrella of this fourth edition. Virus diseases of laboratory animals, fish and other aquatic species, and birds are increasingly important, and we are indebted to the remarkable individuals who contributed their specialist expertise to this endeavor. Similarly, we are indebted to the small group of altruistic individuals who accepted the onerous task of updating the various chapters in a classic text, and to those who, without recognition, agreed to proof the various chapters and sections thereof.

Like the authors of the third edition, we also acknowledge our families, teachers, mentors, and students for their inspiration and direction.

Contents

Contents

Diagnosis 319
Immunity, Prevention, and Control 320
Marine (Phocine and Cetacean)
Morbilliviruses 320
Measles Virus 321
Members of the Subfamily
Paramyxovirinae, Genus *Henipavirus* 321
Hendra Virus 321
Clinical Features and Epidemiology 321
Pathogenesis and Pathology 322
Diagnosis 322
Immunity, Prevention, and Control 322
Nipah Virus 322
Other Henipaviruses 323
Members of the Subfamily *Pneumovirinae*,
Genus *Pneumovirus* 323
Bovine Respiratory Syncytial Virus 323
Clinical Features and Epidemiology 323
Pathogenesis and Pathology 323
Diagnosis 324
Immunity, Prevention, and Control 324
Pneumonia Virus of Mice 324
Members of the Subfamily *Pneumovirinae*,
Genus *Metapneumovirus* 324
Avian Rhinotracheitis Virus
(Metapneumovirus) 324
Unclassified Members of Family
Paramyxoviridae 325
Bottlenose Dolphin (*Tursiops Truncates*)
Parainfluenza Virus 325
Fer-de-Lance and other Ophidian
Paramyxoviruses 325
Salem Virus 325
Atlantic Salmon Paramyxovirus 325

18. *Rhabdoviridae* 327
Properties of Rhabdoviruses 327
Classification 327
Virion Properties 328
Virus Replication 330
Members of the Genus *Lyssavirus* 331
Rabies Virus 331
Clinical Features and Epidemiology 332
Pathogenesis and Pathology 333
Diagnosis 334
Immunity, Prevention, and Control 334
Rabies-Free Countries 334
Rabies-Enzootic Countries 335
Human Disease 335
Rabies-Like Viruses and Bat
Lyssaviruses 336
Members of the Genus *Vesiculovirus* 336
Vesicular Stomatitis Virus 336
Clinical Features and Epidemiology 337

Pathogenesis and Pathology 337
Diagnosis 337
Immunity, Prevention, and Control 338
Human Disease 338
Members of the Genus *Ephemerovirus* 338
Bovine Ephemeral Fever Virus 338
Clinical Features and Epidemiology 338
Pathogenesis and Pathology 339
Diagnosis 339
Immunity, Prevention, and Control 339
Rhabdovirus Diseases of Fish: Genera
Vesiculovirus and *Novirhabdovirus* 339
Viral Hemorrhagic Septicemia Virus 339
Infectious Hematopoietic Necrosis
Virus 340
Spring Viremia of Carp Virus 340
Other Rhabdoviruses of Fish 341

19. *Filoviridae* 343
Properties of Filoviruses 343
Classification 343
Virion Properties 344
Virus Replication 345
Marburg and Ebola Hemorrhagic Fever Viruses 345
Clinical Features and Epidemiology 345
Pathogenesis and Pathology 347
Diagnosis 348
Immunity, Prevention, and Control 348

20. *Bornaviridae* 349
Properties of Borna Disease Virus 349
Classification 349
Virion Properties 349
Virus Replication 350
Borna Disease Virus 350
Clinical Features and Epidemiology 350
Pathogenesis and Pathology 351
Diagnosis 351
Immunity, Prevention, and Control 351
Avian Bornavirus 352

21. *Orthomyxoviridae* 353
Properties of Orthomyxoviruses 356
Classification 356
Virion Properties 357
Virus Replication 358
Molecular Determinants of
Pathogenesis 360
Members of the Genus *Influenzavirus A* 361
Equine Influenza Viruses 361
Clinical Features and Epidemiology 362
Pathogenesis and Pathology 362
Diagnosis 363

Stephen W. Barthold, DVM, PhD, Dip ACVP

Director, Center for Comparative Medicine
Distinguished Professor, Department of Pathology,
Microbiology and Immunology
School of Veterinary Medicine
University of California,
Davis, California, USA
Virus infections of laboratory animals

Richard A. Bowen, DVM, PhD

Professor, Department of Biomedical Sciences
College of Veterinary Medicine and Biomedical
Sciences
Colorado State University
Fort Collins, Colorado, USA
*Rhabdoviridae, Filoviridae, Bornaviridae, Bunyaviridae,
Arenaviridae, Flaviviridae*

Ronald P. Hedrick, PhD

Professor, Department of Medicine and Epidemiology
School of Veterinary Medicine
University of California,
Davis, California, USA
Virus infections of fish

Donald P. Knowles, DVM, PhD, Dip ACVP

Research Leader, USDA/Agricultural Research Services,
Animal Diseases Research Unit
Professor, Department of Veterinary Microbiology and
Pathology
College of Veterinary Medicine
Washington State University
Pullman, Washington, USA
*Poxviridae, Asfarviridae and Iridoviridae, Herpesvirales,
Adenoviridae, Prion Diseases*

**Michael D. Lairmore, DVM, PhD, Dip
ACVP, Dip ACVM**

Professor of Veterinary Biosciences and Associate Dean
for Research and Graduate Studies, College of Veterinary
Medicine
Associate Director for Basic Sciences, Comprehensive
Cancer Center
The Ohio State University
Columbus, Ohio, USA
Retroviridae

Colin R. Parrish, PhD

Professor of Virology
Baker Institute for Animal Health
Department of Microbiology and Immunology
College of Veterinary Medicine
Cornell University
Ithaca, New York, USA
*Papillomaviridae and Polyomaviridae, Parvoviridae,
Circoviridae*

Linda J. Saif, PhD, Dip ACVM

Distinguished University Professor
Food Animal Health Research Program
Department of Veterinary Preventive Medicine
Ohio Agricultural Research and Development Center
The Ohio State University
Wooster, Ohio, USA
Reoviridae, Coronaviridae

David E. Swayne, DVM, PhD, Dip ACVP

Center Director
USDA/Agricultural Research Services
Southeast Poultry Research Laboratory
Athens, Georgia, USA
Virus infections of birds

Acknowledgments

We gratefully acknowledge the following individuals who reviewed specific topics in this text: Drs John Cullen (hepadnaviruses), Patricia Pesavento (feline caliciviruses), Robert Higgins (canine distemper), Aaron Brault (Flaviviridae), William Reisen (Togaviridae and Flaviviridae), Udeni Balasuriya (Arteriviridae), Peter Mertens (Reoviridae), Brian Bird (Filoviridae and Bunyaviridae), Jennifer Luff (Papillomaviridae), Dan Rock (Asfarviridae and Iridoviridae), John Ellis and Daniel Todd (Circoviridae), James Gilkerson and Peter Barry (Herpesvirales), Brian Murphy (Retroviridae), Peter Kirkland (diagnostics), Katherine O'Rourke (prions and transmissible spongiform encephalopathies), Ronald Schultz (antiviral resistance and prophylaxis), Ian Gardner (epidemiology and control), and Jim Winton, Paul Bowser, and Mark Okihiro (diseases of fish).

Part I

The Principles of Veterinary and Zoonotic Virology

Chapter 1

The Nature of Viruses

Chapter Contents

INTRODUCTION: A BRIEF HISTORY OF ANIMAL VIROLOGY

The history of human development has been shaped by at least three major recurring elements: (1) environmental changes; (2) human conflicts; (3) infectious diseases. With regard to infectious diseases, the impact has been not only directly on the human population, but also on the food supply. The origins of veterinary medicine are rooted in efforts to maintain the health of animals for food and fiber production, and animals essential for work-related activities. Control of animal disease outbreaks was not possible until the pioneering work of the late 19th century that linked microbes to specific diseases of plants and animals. Many attribute the beginning of virology with the work of Ivanofsky and Beijerinck (1892–1898) on the transmission of tobacco mosaic virus. Both scientists were able to show the transmission of the agent causing disease in tobacco plants using fluids that passed through filters that retained bacteria. Beijerinck also noted that the filterable agent could regain its "strength" from diluted material, but only if it were put back into the tobacco plants. The concept of a replicating entity rather than a chemical or toxin had its genesis with these astute observations. The era of veterinary virology had its beginning virtually at the same time as Beijerinck was characterizing tobacco mosaic virus transmission. Loeffler and Frosch (1898) applied the filtration criteria to a disease in cattle that later would be known as foot and mouth disease. Repeated passage of the filtrate into susceptible animals with the reproduction of acute disease firmly established the "contagious" nature of the filtrate and provided more evidence for a process that was inconsistent with toxic substances. These early studies provided the essential operational definition of viruses as filterable agents until chemical and physical studies revealed the structural basis of viruses nearly 40 years later.

In the early 20th century, use of the filtration criteria saw the association of many acute animal diseases with what were to be defined as viral infections: African horse sickness, fowl plague (high pathogenicity avian influenza), rabies, canine distemper, equine infectious anemia, rinderpest, and classical swine fever (hog cholera) (Table 1.1). In 1911, Rous discovered the first virus that could produce neoplasia (tumors), and for this discovery he was awarded a Nobel Prize. This early phase of virology was one of skepticism and uncertainty because of the limited tools available to define the filterable agents. Even with filtration, there were differences among the agents as to their size as defined by filter retention. Some agents were inactivated with organic solvents, whereas others were resistant. For equine infectious anemia, the acute and chronic forms of the disease were perplexing and an unresolved conundrum. These types of apparent inconsistencies made it difficult to establish a unifying concept for the filterable agents. For research on animal diseases, early workers were restricted to using animal inoculation in order to assess the impact of any treatment on any putative disease causing agent. For equine and bovine disease work, the logistics could be daunting. Help in providing definition to filterable agents came from the discovery of viruses that infected bacteria. Twort in 1915 detected the existence of a filterable agent that could kill bacteria. Like its plant and animal counterparts, the strength of a dilute solution of the bacterial virus could be regained by inoculating new cultures of bacteria. Felix d'Herelle also noted the killing of bacteria by an agent that he called "bacteriophage." He defined the plaque assay for quantitating

Fenner's Veterinary Virology. DOI: 10.1016/B978-0-12-375158-4.00001-8

TABLE 1.1 Selected Moments in the History of Virology

Year	Investigator(s)	Event	Year	Investigator(s)	Event
1892	Ivanofsky	Identification of tobacco mosaic virus as filterable agent	1935	Stanley	Tobacco mosaic virus (TMV) crystallized; protein nature of viruses confirmed
1898	Loeffler, Frosch	Foot-and-mouth disease caused by filterable agent	1938	Kausche, Ankuch, Ruska	First electron microscopy pictures—TMV
1898	Sanarelli	Myxoma virus	1939	Ellis, Delbruck	One step growth curve— bacteriophage
1900	Reed	Yellow fever virus			
1900	Mcfadyean, Theiler	African horse sickness virus	1946	Olafson, MacCallum, Fox	Bovine viral diarrhea virus
1901	Centanni, Lode, Gruber	Fowl plague virus (avian influenza virus)	1948	Sanford, Earle, Likely	Culture of isolated mammalian cells
1902	Nicolle, Adil-Bey	Rinderpest virus	1952	Dulbecco, Vogt	Plaque assay for first animal virus—poliovirus
1902	Spruell, Theiler	Bluetongue virus	1956	Madin, York, McKercher	Isolation of bovine herpesvirus 1
1902	Aujeszky	Pseudorabies virus	1957	Isaacs, Lindemann	Discovery of interferon
1903	Remlinger, Riffat-Bay	Rabies virus	1958	Horne, Brenner	Development of negative-stain electron microscopy
1903	DeSchweinitz, Dorset	Hog cholera virus (classical swine fever virus)	1961	Becker	First isolation of avian influenza virus from wild bird reservoir
1904	Carré, Vallée	Equine infectious anemia virus	1963	Plummer, Waterson	Equine abortion virus = herpesvirus
1905	Spreull	Insect transmission of bluetongue virus	1970	Temin, Baltimore	Discovery of reverse transcriptase
1905	Carré	Canine distemper virus	1978	Carmichael, Appel, Scott	Canine parvovirus 2
1908	Ellermann, Bang	Avian leukemia virus	1979	World Health Organization	WHO declares smallpox eradicated
1909	Landsteiner, Popper	Poliovirus			
1911	Rous	Rous sarcoma virus—first tumor virus	1981	Pedersen	Feline coronavirus
1915	Twort, d'Herelle	Bacterial viruses	1981	Baltimore	First infectious clone of an RNA virus
1917	d'Herelle	Development of the plaque assay	1983	Montagnier, Barre-Sinoussi, Gallo	Discovery of human immunodeficiency virus
1927	Doyle	Newcastle disease virus	1987	Pedersen	Feline immunodeficiency virus
1928	Verge, Christofornoni Seifried, Krembs	Feline parvovirus (feline panleukopenia virus)	1991	Wensvoort, Terpstra	Isolation of porcine reproductive and respiratory syndrome virus (PRRSV)
1930	Green	Fox encephalitis (canine adenovirus 1)	1994	Murray	Hendra virus isolated
1931	Shope	Swine influenza virus	1999		West Nile virus enters North America
1931	Woodruff, Goodpasture	Embryonated eggs for virus propagation	2002		SARS outbreak
1933	Dimmock, Edwards	Viral etiology for equine abortions	2005	Palase, Garcia-Sastre, Tumpey, Taubenberger	Reconstruction of the 1918 pandemic influenza virus
1933	Andrewes, Laidlaw, Smith	First isolation of human influenza virus	2007		End of vaccination program for rinderpest
1933	Shope	Swine natural host of pseudorabies	2011?		Declaration of the eradication of rinderpest
1933	Bushnell, Brandly	Avian bronchitis virus			

bacteriophage, a technique that became a keystone for defining the properties of viruses and for the studies that became the basis of virus genetics.

The initial studies on tobacco mosaic virus led to further understanding of "filterable agents"—namely viruses. Specifically, the high concentration of virus produced in infected tobacco plants permitted the chemical and physical characterization of the infectious material. By the early 1930s, there was evidence that the agent infecting tobacco plants was composed of protein, and that antibodies produced in rabbits could neutralize the virus. The tobacco mosaic virus was crystallized in 1935, and in 1939 the first electron micrograph of a virus was recorded. The particulate nature of viruses was now an established fact. A further advance in animal virology was the use of embryonated eggs for culturing virus in 1931. In the same year, Shope identified influenza virus in swine; in 1933, influenza virus was isolated from human cases of the infection. The identification of the strain H1N1 in swine might be considered the first "emerging" disease in animals—that is, a virus crossing a species barrier and maintaining itself as an agent of disease in the new species. In an attempt to move away from large-animal experimentation, and to provide model systems for human diseases such as influenza, mice and rats became important tools for studying animal viruses. Thus we had the birth of laboratory animal medicine programs that have become the essential backbone of biomedical research.

The decade 1938–1948 saw major advances by Ellis, Delbruck and Luria in the use of bacteriophage to probe the mechanism of inheritance of phenotypic traits of these bacterial viruses. Advances in understanding the properties of viruses progressed much more rapidly with bacterial viruses, because the work could be done in artificial media, without any requirement for laborious and time-consuming propagation of viruses in either animals or plants. A key concept in virus replication, namely the latent period, was defined using one-step growth curve experiments with bacteriophage. This observation of the loss of infectivity for a period after the initiation of the infection directed research to define the mode of replication of viruses as totally distinct from that of all other replicating entities. Animal virus studies made a dramatic shift in emphasis with the development of reliable *in-vitro* animal cell cultures (1948–1955). As a result of intensive efforts to control poliovirus infections, single cell culture procedures were defined, cell culture media were standardized, a human cell line was developed, and growth of poliovirus in a non-neuronal cell demonstrated. These advances all permitted the development of a plaque assay for poliovirus 35 years after the concept was defined for bacteriophage. All the basic studies on animal viruses that were hindered by the necessity to work in animal systems were now possible, and the principles established for bacteriophage could be explored

for animal viruses. The cell culture era of animal virology had begun.

The advances in virology driven by human disease control efforts were directly applicable to animal virology. Bovine viral diarrhea virus was identified as a new disease-causing agent in cattle in 1946 and by the late 1950s was considered the most economically important disease of cattle in the United States. Cell culture procedures permitted isolation of the virus and the production of a vaccine by the early 1960s. Influenza virus was detected for the first time in wild birds in 1961, which led to the identification of water fowl and shore birds as the natural reservoir of influenza A viruses. An apparent cross-species incursion of a feline parvovirus variant produced the worldwide epizootic of canine parvovirus in the late 1970s. Again, standard *in-vitro* cell culture procedures identified the new agent and soon enabled the production of an effective vaccine. The entire arterivirus family (*Arteriviridae*) was identified in the cell culture era of virology—specifically, equine arteritis virus (1953), lactate dehydrogenase-elevating virus (1960), simian hemorrhagic fever virus (1964), and porcine reproductive and respiratory syndrome virus (1991). The discovery of human immunodeficiency virus (HIV) in 1983 attracted global attention, but the identification of simian immunodeficiency virus shortly thereafter may ultimately be of equal importance to the eventual control of human HIV infection. The primate system provided the animal models for studies of pathogenesis and vaccine development, and the existence of the simian virus in Old World primates provided the link to the origin of HIV as a cross-species (species jumper) infection.

The beginnings of the molecular era of virology reside in the late 1970s and early 1980s. Although not related to virology, the development of the polymerase chain reaction (PCR) in 1983 was to have an impact on virology as has no other technique to date. Cloning of nucleic acid sequences led to the first infectious molecular clone of a virus (poliovirus) in 1981. The impact of molecular techniques on virus detection and diagnostics was demonstrated with the identification of hepatitis C virus by molecular means without isolation (*in-vitro* culture of the virus). Viruses that could not be easily cultured *in vitro*—such as papillomaviruses, noroviruses, rotaviruses, and certain nidoviruses—could now be characterized and routinely detected by tests at the molecular level. A remarkably impressive feat spear-headed by Jeffrey Taubenberger was the molecular reconstruction of an infectious virus from RNA fragments representing the pandemic 1918 influenza A virus. Dreams of recreating extinct animals by molecular techniques may be farfetched, but the possibility exists for determining the early precursors of currently circulating viruses. Rapid and inexpensive nucleotide sequencing strategies are again redefining virology, and whole genomic sequencing is likely to replace less exact procedures for identifying and characterizing virus isolates. Metagenomic analyses of water and soil samples have identified myriads of new viruses, leaving some to estimate that viruses may contain more genetic information than all other species on earth combined.

In the early periods of virology, the discipline was dependent upon advances in the chemical and physical sciences. Defining the characteristics of the "filterable agents" was not possible by simply observing the impact of the agent on its host. However, as time went on, viruses became tools with which to probe the basic biochemical processes of cells, including gene transcription and translation. The bacterial viruses assisted in defining some of the basic principles of genetics through the study of mutations and the inheritance of phenotypic changes. As analytical chemical procedures developed, it was shown that viruses contained nucleic acids, and when Watson and Crick defined the structure of DNA, viruses became key players in defining the role of nucleic acids as the database for life. Progress was so rapid in the field of virology that, by the 1980s, some believed that the future value of viruses would simply be as tools for studying cellular processes. However, the unpredictable emergence of new viruses such as HIV, hepatitis C, Nipah and Hendra, and high-pathogenic H5N1 influenza, together with the expansion of individual viruses into previously free areas such as West Nile virus into North America and bluetongue virus into Europe, clearly confirm that much has yet to be learned about this class of infectious agents and the diseases that they cause.

Veterinary virology began as a discipline focusing on the effects of viral infections on animals of agricultural significance. Control of these infections relied on advances in understanding the disease process, in the characterization of the viruses, in the development of the fields of immunology and diagnostic technologies, and in the establishment of regulations controlling the movement of production animals. Initial experiences confirmed that eradication of some infectious diseases from defined areas could be achieved with a test and slaughter program, even in the absence of an effective vaccine. For example, the apparent recent global eradication of rinderpest was achieved through slaughter of infected animals, restriction of animal movement from enzootic areas to areas free of the infection, and vaccination of animals in enzootic areas. In this type of control program, the individual animal could be sacrificed for the good of the production unit. With the increase in the importance of companion animals in today's society, control programs based on depopulation of infected animals cannot be utilized simply because the individual animal is the important unit as in human medicine. Thus canine parvovirus infections cannot be controlled by killing the affected animals and restricting the movement of dogs, and effective vaccines must continue to be developed and utilized in a science-based immunization program. Diagnostic tests must be deployed that can rapidly detect infectious

agents in a time frame such that the test results can direct treatment. As we become more aware of the interaction between domestic animals and wildlife, we also must face the reality that there are viruses transmitted by insect vectors that do not respect national boundaries and for which the range may be expanding because of climatic changes. Enhanced surveillance programs, novel control strategies, and antiviral drugs will need to be developed continually in the future, particularly for those diseases in which vaccination is not cost-effective.

Viruses have traditionally been viewed in a rather negative context—disease-producing agents that must be controlled or eliminated. However, viruses have some beneficial properties that can be exploited for useful purposes. Specifically, viruses have been engineered to express proteins for production of non-viral proteins (baculovirus) or to express viral proteins for immunization purposes (e.g., poxvirus and adenovirus vectored vaccines). Lentiviruses have been modified for the purpose of inserting new genetic information into cells for research purposes and for possible use in gene therapy, as have a wide variety of other viruses, including adeno-associated viruses (parvoviruses). Bacteriophages are being considered in the context of controlling certain bacterial infections, and viruses have the hypothetical potential to be vectors that selectively target tumor cells for controlling cancers. In the broader context of the Earth's ecosystems, viruses are now viewed in a more positive sense, in that they may be a component of population control and perhaps a force in the evolution of species. Although restricting the population of agriculturally important animals is viewed as a negative from the human perspective, the ecosystem might benefit from the reduction of one species if its success is at the expense of others. We are happy to see an insect infestation curtailed by baculoviruses, but less pleased to see the loss of poultry by influenza virus, even though the two events may be ecologically equivalent. We are now fully comfortable with the concept of beneficial bacteria in the ecosystem of the human body. Do we need to start to consider that viruses that have evolved with the species may also have beneficial properties?

CHARACTERISTICS OF VIRUSES

Following the initial operational definition of a virus as a filterable agent, attempts were made to identify properties of viruses that made them distinct from other microorganisms. Even from the earliest times, it was evident that the filterable agents could not be cultivated on artificial media, and this particular characteristic has withstood the test of time, in that all viruses are obligate intracellular parasites. However, all obligate intracellular parasites are not viruses (Table 1.2). Members of certain bacterial genera also are unable to replicate outside a host cell (*Ehrlichia, Anaplasma, Legionella, Rickettsia*, are examples). These "degenerate" bacteria lack

TABLE 1.2 Properties of Unicellular Microorganisms and Viruses

Property	Bacteria	Rickettsiae	Mycoplasmas	Chlamydiae	Viruses
>300 nm diameter[a]	+	+	+	+	−
Growth on non-living medium	+	−	+	−	−
Binary fission	+	+	+	+	−
DNA and RNA[b]	+	+	+	+	−
Functional ribosomes	+	+	+	+	−
Metabolism	+	+	+	+	−

[a]*Some mycoplasmas and chlamydiae are less than 300 nm in diameter and mimiviruses are greater than 300 nm.*
[b]*Some viruses contain both types of nucleic acid but, although functional in some cases, are a minor component of the virion.*

key metabolic pathways, the products of which must be provided by the host cell. Viruses, by contrast, lack all metabolic capabilities necessary to reproduce, including energy production and the processes necessary for protein synthesis. Viruses do not possess standard cellular organelles such as mitochondria, chloroplasts, Golgi, and endoplasmic reticulum with associated ribosomes. However, cyanophages do encode proteins involved in photosynthesis that are viewed as increasing viral fitness by supplementing the host cell systems. Similarly, certain bacteriophages have genomes that encode enzymes involved in the nucleotide biosynthetic pathway. Outside the living cell, viruses are inert particles whereas, inside the cell, the virus utilizes the host cell processes to produce its proteins and nucleic acid for the next generation of virus. As will be noted later, the protein-coding capacity of viruses ranges from just a few proteins to nearly 1000. This range of complexity mirrors the diverse effects viral infections have on host cell metabolism, but the outcome of an infection is the same—the production of more progeny viruses.

A second inviolate property of viruses is that they do not reproduce by binary fission, a method of asexual reproduction in which a pre-existing cell splits into two identical daughter cells; in the absence of limiting substrate, the population of cells will double with each replication cycle, and at all points in the replication cycle there exists a structure that is identifiable as an intact cell. For viruses, the process of reproduction resembles an assembly line in which various parts of the virus come together from different parts of the host cell to form new virus particles. Shortly after the virus attaches to a host cell, it enters the cell and the intact virus particle ceases to exist. The viral genome then directs the production of new viral macromolecules, which results ultimately in the re-emergence of intact progeny virus particles. The period of time between the penetration of the virus particle into the host cell and the production of the first new virus particle is designated

as the *eclipse period*, and the duration of this period varies with each virus family. Disrupting cells during the eclipse period will not release significant numbers of infectious virus particles. Uninterrupted, a single infectious particle can replicate within a single susceptible cell to produce thousands of progeny virus particles.

As more sensitive analytical techniques became available and more viruses were identified, some of the criteria that defined a virus became less absolute. In general, viruses contain only one type of nucleic acid that carries the information for replicating the virus. However, is it now clear that some viruses do contain nucleic acid molecules other than the genomic DNA or RNA. For retroviruses, cellular transfer (t)RNAs are essential for the reverse transcriptase reaction, and studies have shown that 50–100 tRNA molecules are present in each mature virion. Similarly in herpesviruses, data show that host cell and viral transcripts localize to the tegument region of the mature virion. Early studies defined viruses by their tiny size; however, viruses now have been identified that are physically larger than some mycoplasma, rickettsia, and chlamydia. The newly discovered mimivirus group is an exception to existing rules: the virion is approximately 750 nm in diameter, with a DNA genome of 1.2 mbp. Because of the size of the virion, it would be retained by standard 300-nm filters traditionally used for separating bacteria from viruses. The genomic size is similar to that of the rickettsia and chlamydia, and more than 900 protein-encoding genes have been identified, at least 130 having been identified in mimivirus virions. Most surprising was the finding that the virus encodes genes involved in protein synthesis, such as aminoacyl-tRNA synthetases. The discovery of mimiviruses has revived the debate as to the origin of viruses, but sequence data indicate that this family of viruses is linked to the nucleocytoplasmic large DNA viruses, specifically viruses in the families *Poxviridae* and *Iridoviridae*.

Chemical Composition of the Virion

The chemical composition of virus particles varies markedly between those of individual virus families. For the simplest of viruses such as parvoviruses, the virion is composed of viral structural proteins and DNA; in the case of enteroviruses it comprises viral proteins and RNA. The situation becomes more complex with the enveloped viruses such as herpesviruses and pneumoviruses. These types of virus mature by budding through different cellular membranes that are modified by the insertion of viral proteins. For the most part, host-cell proteins are not a significant component of viruses, but minor amounts of cellular proteins can be identified in viral membranes and in the interior of the virus particle. Host-cell RNA such as ribosomal RNA can be found in virions, but there is no evidence for a functional role in virus replication. For enveloped viruses, glycoproteins are the major type of protein present on the exterior of the membrane. The existence/presence of a lipid envelope provides an operational method with which to separate viruses into two distinct classes—those that are inactivated by organic solvents (enveloped) and those that are resistant (non-enveloped).

Viral Nucleic Acids in the Virion

Viruses exhibit a remarkable variety of strategies for the expression of their genes and for the replication of their genome. If one considers the simplicity of RNA plant viroids (247–401 nt) at one extreme and the mimiviruses (1.2 mbp) at the other, one might conclude that viruses have perhaps exploited all possible means of nucleic acid replication for an entity at the subcellular level. The type of nucleic acid and the genomic structure of the nucleic acids are used to classify viruses. As viruses contain only one nucleic acid type with respect to transmitting genetic information, the virus world can simply be divided into RNA viruses and DNA viruses (Table 1.3). For RNA viruses, one major distinction is whether the virion RNA is of *positive sense* or polarity, directly capable of translation to protein, or of *negative sense* or polarity, which requires transcription of the genome to generate mRNA equivalents. Within the negative-strand group, there are single-strand whole-genome viruses (e.g., *Paramyxoviridae*) and segmented genome viruses (e.g., *Orthomyxoviridae*—six, seven, or eight segments; *Bunyaviridae*—three segments; *Arenaviridae*—two segments). The *Retroviridae* are considered diploid, in that the virion contains two whole-genomic positive-sense RNAs. Another unique configuration is the viruses with double-stranded RNA genomes. The *Birnaviridae* have two segments and the *Reoviridae* have 10, 11, or 12 segments, depending on the genus of virus. The size of animal RNA viral genomes ranges from less than 2 kb (*Deltavirus*) to more than 30 kb for the largest RNA viruses (*Coronaviridae*).

TABLE 1.3 Viral Properties that Distinguish and Define Virus Families

Family	Nature of the Genome	Presence of an Envelope	Morphology	Genome Configuration	Genome Size (kb or kbp)	Virion Size [diameter (nM)]
Poxviridae	dsDNA	+	pleomorphic	1 linear	130–375	250 × 200 × 200
Iridoviridae	dsDNA	+/−	isometric	1 linear	135–303	130–300
Asfarviridae	dsDNA	+	spherical	1 linear	170–190	173–215
Herpesviridae	dsDNA	+	isometric	1 linear	125–240	150
Adenoviridae	dsDNA	−	isometric	1 linear	26–45	80–100
Polyomaviridae	dsDNA	−	isometric	1 circular	5	40–45
Papillomaviridae	dsDNA	−	isometric	1 circular	7–8	55
Hepadnaviridae	dsDNA-RT	+	spherical	1 linear	3–4	42–50
Circoviridae	ssDNA	−	isometric	1 − or +/− circular	2	12–27
Parvoviridae	ssDNA	−	isometric	1 +/− linear	4–6	18–26
Retroviridae	ssRNA-RT	+	spherical	1 + (dimer)	7–13	80–100
Reoviridae	dsRNA	−	isometric	10–12 segments	19–32	60–80
Birnaviridae	dsRNA	−	isometric	2 segments	5–6	60
Paramyxoviridae	NssRNA	+	pleomorphic	1 − segment	13–18	~150
Rhabdoviridae	NssRNA	+	bullet-shaped	1 − segment	11–15	100–430 × 45–100
Filoviridae	NssRNA	+	filamentous	1 − segment	≈19	600–800 × 80 in diameter

(Continued)

TABLE 1.3 (Continued)

Family	Nature of the Genome	Presence of an Envelope	Morphology	Genome Configuration	Genome Size (kb or kbp)	Virion Size [diameter (nM)]
Bornaviridae	NssRNA	+	spherical	1 − segment	9	80–100
Orthomyxoviridae	NssRNA	+	pleomorphic	6–8 − segments	10–15	80–120
Bunyaviridae	NssRNA	+	spherical	3 − or +/− segments	11–19	80–120
Arenaviridae	NssRNA	+	spherical	2 +/− segments	11	50–300
Coronaviridae	ssRNA	+	spherical	1 + segment	38–31	120–160
Arteriviridae	ssRNA	+	spherical	1 + segment	13–16	45–60
Picornaviridae	ssRNA	−	isometric	1 + segment	7–9	≈30
Caliciviridae	ssRNA	−	isometric	1 + segment	7–8	27–40
Astroviridae	ssRNA	−	isometric	1 + segment	6–7	28–30
Togaviridae	ssRNA	+	spherical	1 + segment	10–12	≈70
Flaviviridae	ssRNA	+	spherical	1 + segment	10–12	40–60
Hepevirus (unassigned)	ssRNA	−	isometric	1 + segment	7	27–34
Anellovirus (unassigned)	ssDNA	−	isometric	1 − circular	3–4	30–32

dsDNA, double-stranded DNA; dsRNA, double-stranded RNA; kbp, kilobase pairs; NssRNA, negative single-stranded RNA; RT, reverse transcription; ssRNA, single-stranded RNA.

For the animal DNA viruses, the overall structure of the genomes is less complex, with either a single molecule of single-stranded (ss)DNA or a single molecule of double-stranded (ds)DNA. For the dsDNA viruses, the complexity ranges from the relatively simple circular super-coiled genome of the *Polyomaviridae* and *Papillomaviridae* (5–8 kbp) to the linear *Herpesvirinae* (125–235 kbp) with variable sequence rearrangements, which for the *Simplexvirus* can result in four isomeric forms. The ssDNA viral genomes are either linear (*Parvoviridae*) or circular (*Circoviridae* and *Anellovirus*), with sizes ranging from 2.8 to 5 kbp.

The size of the genome certainly reflects on the protein coding capacity of the virus, but in all cases there is not a simple calculation that reliably estimates this relationship. Parts of the viral genome are typically regulatory elements necessary for the translation of the proteins, replication of the genome, and transcription of viral genes (promoters, termination signals, polyadenylation sites, RNA splice sites, etc.). For synthesis of proteins, viruses have used a number of strategies to increase the relative coding capacity of the genome. For example, the *P* gene in Sendai virus (*Respirovirus*) directs the synthesis of at least seven viral proteins by several different mechanisms. One mechanism involves "RNA editing" whereby the RNA polymerase inserts G residues at specific sites in the growing mRNA molecule. This results in a series of proteins with the same amino terminus but with different ending points (different carboxyl termini). A different series of proteins are generated by using alternative start codons, which results in a series of proteins with different amino termini, but the same carboxyl terminus. For viruses such as the *Retroviridae*, RNA splicing is used to generate proteins that otherwise would not be produced using the linear coding capacity of the genome. Although the feature is not directly related to coding capacity, viruses also use the same protein for several functions. As an example, the NS3 protein of the member viruses of the family *Flaviviridae* is a multifunctional protein that has at its amino terminal region a serine protease activity and at its carboxyl terminal significant homology to supergroup 2 RNA helicases. One could easily envision that these two functions were on separate proteins that became fused to enhance functionality or to reduce the coding capacity of the genome.

Viral Proteins in the Virion

The genomes of animal viruses encode from as few as one protein to more than 100. Those that are present in virions (mature virus particles) are referred to as *structural* proteins whereas those involved in the assembly of the particle, replication of the genome, or modification of the host innate response to infection, are referred to as *non-structural* proteins. There is some ambiguity for enzymes that are essential for the initial stages of virus replication, such as the RNA polymerases for the negative-strand RNA viruses (*Paramyxoviridae, Rhabdoviridae*, etc.). As the first step in the replication cycle once the nucleocapsid enters the cytoplasm is transcription of the viral genome, the polymerase must be part of the mature virion. Whether the polymerase has a structural role in the mature particle in addition to its transcription activity remains unresolved. Numerous other viral proteins that occur within the virions of complex viruses (*Poxviridae, Herpesviridae, Asfarviridae*) have no apparent structural role.

Virion proteins fall into two general classes: modified proteins and unmodified proteins. The capsids of the non-enveloped viruses are composed of proteins with few modifications, as their direct amino acid interactions are essential for the assembly of the protein shells. Proteolytic cleavage of precursor proteins in the nascent capsid is not uncommon in the final steps of assembly of the mature capsid proteins. Glycoproteins are predominantly found in those viruses that contain a viral membrane. These structural proteins can be either a type I integral membrane protein (amino terminus exterior) (e.g., hemagglutinin [HA] of influenza virus) or type II (carboxyl terminus exterior) (e.g., neuraminidase (NA) of influenza virus). Glycosylation patterns may differ even amongst viruses that mature in the same cells, because *N*- and *O*-linked glycosylation sites on the virion proteins vary among the virus families. The glycoproteins involved in virion assembly have a cytoplasmic tail that communicates with viral proteins on the inner surface of the membrane to initiate the maturation process for production of the infectious virus particle. Structural proteins in the infectious virus particle have a number of key functions: (1) to protect the genomic nucleic acid and associated enzymes from inactivation; (2) to provide receptor-binding sites for initiation of infection; (3) to initiate or facilitate the penetration of the viral genome into the correct compartment of the cell for replication.

Viral Membrane Lipids

For viruses that mature by budding through a cellular membrane, a major constituent of the virion is phospholipid that forms the structural basis of the viral membrane. The maturation site for viruses can be the plasma membrane, nuclear membrane, Golgi, or the endoplasmic reticulum. For those viruses budding from the plasma membrane, cholesterol is a constituent of the viral membrane, whereas the envelopes of those viruses that bud from internal membranes lack cholesterol. The budding process is not random, in that specific viral glycoprotein sequences direct developing particles to the proper location within the inner membrane

surface. In polarized cells—cells with tight junctions, giving the cell a defined apical and basal surface—virus budding will be targeted to one surface over the other. For example, in Madin–Darby canine kidney (MDCK) cells, influenza virus will bud on the apical surface, whereas vesicular stomatitis virus buds from the basal surface. The transmembrane domain of viral glycoproteins targets specific regions of the cellular membrane for budding. For influenza virus, budding is associated with "lipid rafts," which are microdomains of the plasma membrane rich in sphingolipids and cholesterol.

VIRAL MORPHOLOGY

Early attempts to characterize viruses were hampered by the lack of appropriate technology. Filtration and sensitivity to chemical agents were two standard tests that were applied to new disease agents for nearly 40 years. Work with tobacco mosaic virus in the 1930s strongly suggested that the virus was composed of repeating protein subunits, and crystallization of the virus in 1935 supported this notion. However, it was not until 1939 that a virus was visualized using an electron microscope. Tobacco mosaic virus appeared as a rod-shaped particle, confirming the particulate nature of viruses. A major advance in determining virus morphology was the development of negative-stain electron microscopy in 1958. In this procedure, electron-dense stains were used to coat virus particles and produce a negative image of the virus with enhanced resolution (Figure 1.1). Figure 1.2 depicts the spectrum of morphological types represented by animal viruses. As indicated earlier, the size of virion ranges from 750 nm down to 20 nm. With this range, it is not surprising that there were inconsistencies noted in filtration studies.

Advances in determining virus morphology down to the atomic level came from studies initially using X-ray crystallography and then combining this technique with other structural techniques such as electron cryomicroscopy (cryo-EM). In this process, samples are snap frozen and examined at temperatures of liquid nitrogen or liquid helium (Figure 1.3). Cryo-EM offered the advantage that the samples are not damaged or distorted in the process of analyzing the structure, as occurs with negative-stain electron microscopy and X-ray crystallography. However, the individual images generated by this process are not as defined as those obtained with crystallography. Critical to these analyses were the developments in computer hardware and software that were able to capture, analyze, and construct the three-dimensional images from literally thousands of determinations. This "averaging" process can only work if the virus particles are uniformly the same size and shape. For many viruses, this uniformity is met by having the symmetry of a type of polyhedron known as an icosahedron. For intact virus particles showing icosahedral

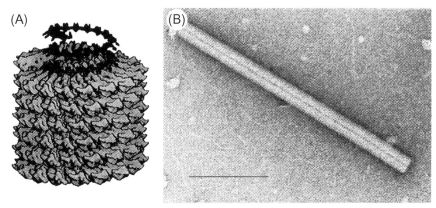

FIGURE 1.1   (A) Model of particle of Tobacco mosaic virus (TMV). Also shown is the RNA as it is believed to participate in the assembly process. (B) Negative-contrast electron micrograph of TMV particle stained with uranyl acetate. The bar represents 100 nm. *[From* Virus Taxonomy: Eighth Report of the International Committee on Taxonomy of Viruses *(C. M. Fauquet, M. A. Mayo, J. Maniloff, U. Desselberger, L. A. Ball, eds), p. 1009. Copyright © Elsevier (2005), with permission.]*

symmetry, the physical location of the individual peptides could be identified and the areas of the folded peptides that are on the surface of the virion were mapped. These areas could be linked to the specific epitopes recognized by monoclonal antibodies. In other studies, the binding site on the virion for the cellular receptor was mapped, which opened the possibility of developing antiviral drugs targeting these defined areas. X-ray crystallography can also be used to analyze subunits of a virus, such as was done for the HA protein of influenza virus (Figure 1.4). The impact of mutations in the HA peptide as they related to changes in the binding of antibodies or host-cell receptors could be determined with these advanced technologies.

Virion Structure

The *virion*—that is, the complete virus particle—of a simple virus consists of a single molecule of nucleic acid (DNA or RNA) surrounded by a morphologically distinct capsid composed of viral protein subunits (virus encoded polypeptides). The protein subunits can self-assemble into multimer units (structural units), which may contain one or several polypeptide chains. Structures without the nucleic acid can be detected and are referred to as empty capsids. The meaning of the term *nucleocapsid* can be somewhat ambiguous. In a strict sense, a capsid with its nucleic acid is a nucleocapsid, but for simple viruses such as poliovirus, this structure is also the virion. For flaviviruses, the nucleocapsid (capsid + RNA) is enclosed in a lipid envelope and the nucleocapsid does not represent the complete virion. For paramyxoviruses, the nucleocapsid refers to a structure composed of a single strand of RNA complexed to a viral protein that assembles in the form of an α helix. The nucleocapsid assembles into a complete virion by obtaining a lipid envelope from host cell membranes modified by the insertion of viral proteins.

Virion Symmetry

For reasons of evolutionary progression and genetic economy, virions are assembled from several copies of a few kinds of protein subunit. The repeated occurrence of similar protein–protein interfaces leads to assembly of the subunits into symmetrical nucleocapsids. This efficiency of design also depends on the principles of *self-assembly*, wherein structural units are brought into position through random thermal movement and are bonded in place through weak chemical bonds. Although it is possible to express viral proteins in bacteria such as *Escherichia coli* and have capsids self-assemble (simian virus 40 and hepatitis B, for example), it is now recognized that most viruses have some help in the virion assembly process. This help can come from the interaction of the viral proteins with the viral genome, with cellular membranes, or with cellular chaperone proteins. This "help" may be simply concentrating the viral proteins to enhance chances of interactions, providing an organization matrix, or inducing a conformational change needed to enhance binding. For large viruses (*Herpesvirinae* and *Adenoviridae*, for example) with icosahedral nucleocapsids, non-structural viral proteins referred to as scaffolding proteins take an active part in the assembly of the capsid, but are not present in the completed virion.

Viruses come in a variety of shapes and sizes that depend on the shape, size, and number of their protein subunits and the nature of the interfaces between these subunits (Figure 1.2). However, only two kinds of symmetry have been recognized in virus particles: icosahedral and helical. The symmetry found in isometric viruses is invariably that of an icosahedron; virions with icosahedron symmetry have 12 vertices (corners), 30 edges, and 20 faces, with each face an equilateral triangle. Icosahedra have two-, three-, and fivefold rotational symmetry, with the axes passing through their edges, faces, and vertices,

Families and Genera of Viruses Infecting Vertebrates

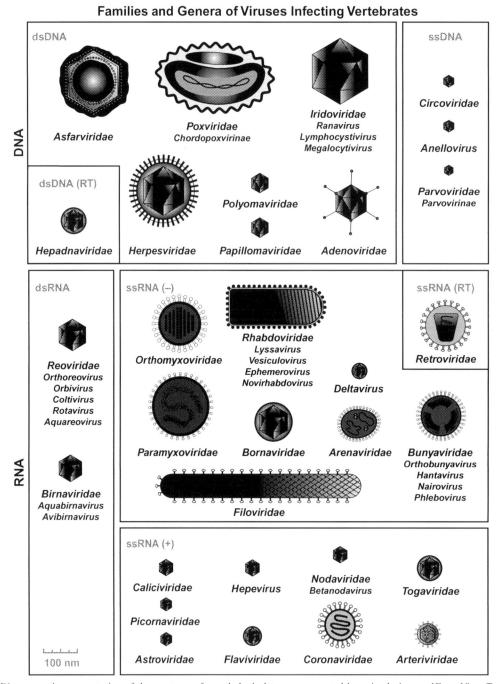

FIGURE 1.2   Diagrammatic representation of the spectrum of morphological types represented by animal viruses. *[From* Virus Taxonomy: Eighth Report of the International Committee on Taxonomy of Viruses *(C. M. Fauquet, M. A. Mayo, J. Maniloff, U. Desselberger, L. A. Ball, eds), p. 14. Copyright © Elsevier (2005), with permission.]*

respectively (Figure 1.5). The icosahedron is the optimum solution to the problem of constructing, from repeating subunits, a strong structure enclosing a maximum volume. Parvoviruses represent one of the simplest capsid designs, being composed of 60 copies of the same protein subunit— three subunits per face of the icosahedron. The protein is folded into a structure referred to as a "jelly-roll β-barrel"

that forms a block-like profile with an arm-like extension that provides the contact point with other subunits for stabilizing the protein–protein interactions. In the simplest arrangement, the size of the protein subunit determines the volume of the capsid. With a single capsid protein of 60 copies, only a small genome can be accommodated within the capsid (canine parvovirus = 5.3 kb ssDNA).

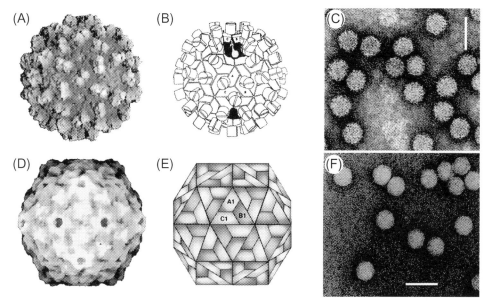

FIGURE 1.3 (A) Cryo-image reconstruction of recombinant Norwalk virus (NV)-like particles (rNV VLPs). (B) Cryo-image reconstruction of Primate calicivirus. A set of icosahedral five- and threefold axes is marked. (C) Central cross-section of rNV VLPs. (D) Electronic rendering of Norwalk virus. (E) Diagrammatic representation of a T = 3 icosahedral structure. (F) Negative-stain electron micrograph of bovine calicivirus particles. The bar represents 100 nm. *[From* Virus Taxonomy: Eighth Report of the International Committee on Taxonomy of Viruses *(C. M. Fauquet, M. A. Mayo, J. Maniloff, U. Desselberger, L. A. Ball, eds), p. 843. Copyright © Elsevier (2005), with permission.]*

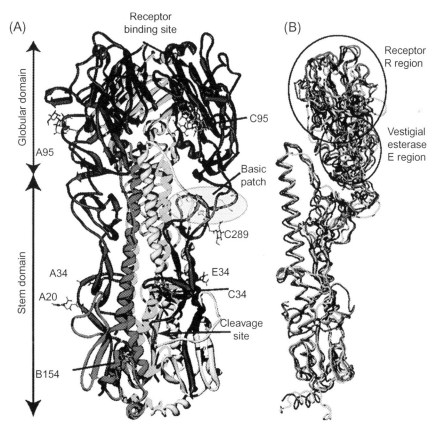

FIGURE 1.4 Crystal structure of the HA protein of influenza virus 1918 virus and comparison with other human, avian, and swine HAs. (A) Overview of the 18HA0 trimer, represented as a ribbon diagram. Each monomer is colored differently. (B) Structural comparison of the 18HA0 monomer (red) with human H3 (green), avian H5 (orange), and swine H9 (blue) HA0s. *[From J. Stevens, A. L. Corper, C. F. Basler, J. K. Taubenberger, P. Palese, I. A. Wilson.* Structure of the uncleaved human H1 hemagglutinin from the extinct 1918 influenza virus. *Science* **303***, 1866–1870 (2004), with permission.]*

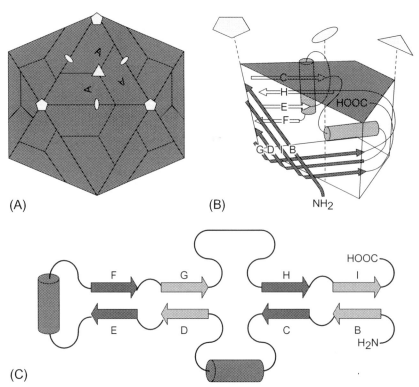

FIGURE 1.5 (A) An icosahedral capsid contains 60 identical copies of the protein subunit (blue) labeled A; these are related by fivefold (yellow pentagons at vertices), threefold (yellow triangles in faces), and twofold (yellow ellipses at edges) symmetry elements. For a given-sized subunit, this point group symmetry generates the largest possible assembly (60 subunits) in which every protein lies in an identical environment. (B) Schematic representation of the subunit building block found in many RNA and some DNA viral structures. Such subunits have complementary interfacial surfaces which, when they repeatedly interact, lead to the symmetry of the icosahedron. The tertiary structure of the subunit is an eight-stranded β-barrel with the topology of the jelly-roll. Subunit sizes generally range between 20 and 40 kDa, with variation among different viruses occurring at the N- and C-termini and in the size of insertions between strands of the β-sheet. These insertions generally do not occur at the narrow end of the wedge (B–C, H–I, D–E, and F–G turns). (C) The topology of viral β-barrel, showing the connections between strands of the sheets (represented by yellow or red arrows) and positions of the insertions between strands. The green cylinders represent helices that are usually conserved. The C–D, E–F, and G–H loops often contain large insertions. *[From* Encyclopedia of Virology *(B. W. J. Mahy, M. H. V. van Regenmortel, eds), vol 5, p. 394. Copyright © Academic Press/Elsevier (2008), with permission.]*

Viruses with larger genomes have solved the problem of limited capsid volume, but the basic structure of the capsid remains the icosahedron. The explanations for the ways viruses maintain the icosahedron symmetry with repeating structural units is beyond the scope of this text.

The nucleocapsid of several RNA viruses self-assembles as a cylindrical structure in which the protein structural units are arranged as a helix, hence the term *helical symmetry*. It is the shape and repeated occurrence of identical protein–protein interfaces of the structural units that lead to the symmetrical assembly of the helix. In helically symmetrical nucleocapsids, the genomic RNA forms a spiral within the core of the nucleocapsid. The RNA is the organizing element that brings the structural units into correct alignment. Many of the plant viruses with helical nucleocapsids are rod-shaped, flexible, or rigid without an envelope. However, with animal viruses, the helical nucleocapsid is wound into a secondary coil and enclosed within a lipoprotein envelope (e.g., *Rhabdoviridae*) (Figure 1.6).

VIRAL TAXONOMY

With the earliest recognition that infectious agents were associated with a given spectrum of clinical outcomes, it was natural for an agent to take on the name of the disease with which it was associated or the geographic location where it was found, as there was no other basis for assigning a name. Thus the agent that caused foot-and-mouth disease in cattle becomes "foot-and-mouth disease virus," or an agent that caused a febrile disease in the Rift Valley of Africa became "Rift Valley fever virus." It is not difficult at this time in history to see why this *ad hoc* method of naming infectious agents could lead to confusion and regulatory chaos. Different names may be given to the same virus that is both the agent causing a disease in a cow in England and that causing disease in a water buffalo in India. Hog cholera virus existed in North America whereas, in the rest of the world, it was classical swine fever virus, not to be confused with African swine fever virus. Within the same animal, one had infectious bovine rhinotracheitis

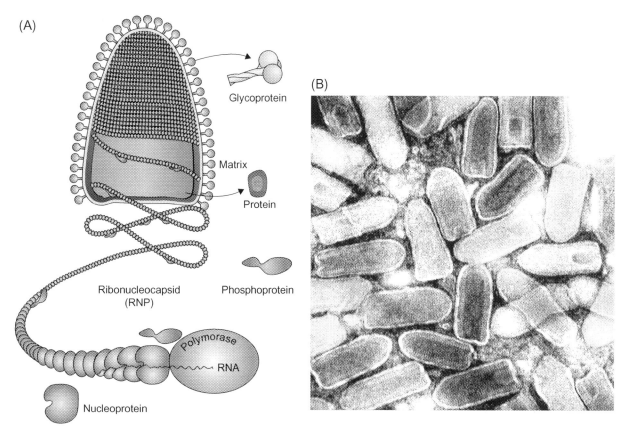

FIGURE 1.6 (A) Diagram illustrating a rhabdovirus virion and the nucleocapsid structure (courtesy of P. Le Merder). (B) Negative contrast electron micrograph of particles of an isolate of *Vesicular stomatitis Indiana virus* (courtesy of P. Perrin.). The bar represents 100 nm. *[From* Virus Taxonomy: Eighth Report of the International Committee on Taxonomy of Viruses *(C. M. Fauquet, M. A. Mayo, J. Maniloff, U. Desselberger, L. A. Ball, eds), p. 623. Copyright © Elsevier (2005), with permission.]*

(IBR) virus and infectious bovine pustular vulvovaginitis (IBPV) virus—both disease entities being caused by bovine herpesvirus 1. Even today, export documents ask for tests to certify animals free of IBR virus *and* IBPV virus. This disease-linked nomenclature could not be changed until such time as the tools became available to define the physical and chemical nature of viruses. With negative-stain electron microscopy as a readily available technology, the size and shape of viruses became a characteristic for defining them. This, along with the ability to define the type of nucleic acid in the virus particle, provided the beginnings of a more rational system of classifying and naming new viruses. Even with a defined shape and a type of nucleic acid, there were still ambiguities in the classification systems that were being developed. Viruses that were transmitted by insect vectors were loosely defined as "*arboviruses*"—arthropod-borne viruses. However, there were viruses that "looked like" arboviruses (togaviruses—viruses with a symmetrical lipid membrane) and had the same nucleic acid, but did not have an insect vector. These became "non-arthropod-borne" togaviruses. Similar ambiguities existed with the group of viruses collectively known as picornaviruses (small RNA viruses). The answer

to many of these issues came with the advances in the ability to determine the nucleotide sequences of these agents. Thus the "non-arbo" togaviruses became members of the genera *Rubivirus*, *Pestivirus*, and family *Arteriviridae*.

Even with advances in technologies to characterize individual viruses, there was the need to establish guidelines and procedures for developing a universally acceptable taxonomy for viruses. In 1966, the International Committee on Taxonomy of Viruses (ICTV) was established and charged with establishing, refining, and maintaining a universal virus taxonomy. Given the uncertain origins of viruses, establishing the initial framework for this classification system was not without controversy. Subcommittees and study groups meet periodically to assess new data submitted from the research community to refine the classification system and to place new viruses in their most logical position in the taxonomy scheme. It was not until the Seventh Report of the ICTV (2000) that the concept of virus species as the lowest group in the viral taxa was accepted. The advent of nucleotide sequence determination had a dramatic effect on all biological classification systems, and it has in many respects confirmed the major elements of the classification system. This textbook will use the information presented in the Eighth Report of the ICTV published in 2005. At that time, the ICTV had approved three orders, 73 families, 9 subfamilies, 287 genera, and more than 5000 viruses in 1950 approved species. As the process of classification and defining nomenclature is an ongoing one because of the discovery of new viruses and the generation of sequence data on older isolates, it is impossible for a textbook to be "current." For the most up-to-date information on classification and nomenclature, the reader is directed to the ICTV webpage (http://www.ictvonline.org/index.asp).

The hierarchy of recognized viral taxa is: (Order); Family; (Subfamily); Genus; Species. For example, human respiratory syncytial virus A2 would be found in this system as: *Mononegavirales* (order); *Paramyxoviridae* (family); *Pneumovirinae* (subfamily); *Pneumovirus* (genus); *Human respiratory syncytial virus* (species). To be a member of the taxa higher than species, a virus must have all properties defining the classification. In contrast, species are considered a *polythetic class*, in which members have several properties in common but all do not have to share a single defining property. For each genus, there has been designated a *type species*, which is a species that creates a link between the genus and the species. This designation is usually conferred on the species that necessitated the creation of the genus. The published virology literature contains obvious inconsistencies with regard to whether the name of a specific virus is written in italics: *Bovine viral diarrhea virus* versus bovine viral diarrhea virus, for example. In all cases dealing with taxonomy, the order, family, subfamily and genus names should be written in italics and capitalized. In discussing a virus in the context of taxonomy at the species level, the name is written in italics and the first word is capitalized: for example, *Canine distemper virus* is a species in the genus *Morbillivirus*. However, when a virus is written about in terms of tangible properties such as its ability to cause disease, growth in certain cell lines, or its physical characteristics, the name is neither written in italics nor capitalized unless the name contains a proper noun;

for example, one can grow canine distemper virus or West Nile virus in monkey cells. There are instances when the abstract (taxonomy) and the concrete aspects of a virus are not clear in the context of the sentence. In this textbook we will attempt to use the ICTV conventions when clearly appropriate, but as this text deals mainly with the tangible aspects of viruses, most virus names will not be in italics.

A basic question that has yet to be addressed is why we should bother with taxonomy at all. For some there seems to be a human need to place things into an ordered system. In characterizing an entity and defining a nomenclature, a basic understanding of the subject under study may be achieved. In a larger context, taxonomy provides a tool for comparing one virus with another or one virus family with another. It also enables one to assign biological properties to a new virus that is provisionally linked to a given family. For instance, if one has an electron micrographic image of a new virus that supports its identity as a coronavirus, then the discoverer can assume they have identified a single-stranded, positive-sense, non-segmented RNA virus. Further, one can extrapolate that coronaviruses are mainly associated with enteric disease, but can also cause respiratory disease in "atypical" hosts after "species jumping." As a group, coronaviruses are difficult to culture *in vitro*, and may require the presence of a protease to enhance growth in tissue culture. Conserved sequences—perhaps in the nucleocapsid—might provide a target for the development of a PCR test. Thus identification of the morphology of an unknown virus can be useful, as the general properties of specific virus families can assist in the interpretation of individual clinical cases. For example, confirming that an alphaherpesvirus was isolated from a particular case confers some basic knowledge about the virus without having explicitly to define the properties of the specific virus. Table 1.3 provided some of the basic properties of the animal virus families; Table 1.4 lists those discussed in the specific chapters. More detailed properties of the virus families that include significant pathogens of veterinary relevance will be found in specific chapters in Part II of this text.

TABLE 1.4 Universal Taxonomy System for Taxa Containing Veterinary and Zoonotic Pathogens[a]

Family	Subfamily	Genus	Type Species (Host if Not Vertebrate)
DNA Viruses			
Double-Stranded DNA Viruses			
Poxviridae	*Chordopoxvirinae*	*Orthopoxvirus*	*Vaccinia virus*
		Capripoxvirus	*Sheeppox virus*
		Leporipoxvirus	*Myxoma virus*
		Suipoxvirus	*Swinepox virus*
		Molluscipoxvirus	*Molluscum contagiosum virus*
		Avipoxvirus	*Fowlpox virus*
		Yatapoxvirus	*Yaba monkey tumor virus*
		Parapoxvirus	*Orf virus*
		Cervidpoxvirus[a]	*Deerpox virus W-848-83*

(Continued)

TABLE 1.4 (Continued)

Family	Subfamily	Genus	Type Species (Host if Not Vertebrate)
	Entomopoxvirinae	Entomopoxvirus genera	(Insect viruses, but probably also pathogens of fish)
Asfarviridae		Asfivirus	African swine fever virus
Iridoviridae		Ranavirus	Frog virus 3
		Lymphocystivirus	Lymphocystis disease virus 1
		Megalocytivirus	Infectious spleen and kidney necrosis virus
Alloherpesviridae		Ictalurivirus	Ictalurid herpesvirus 1
Herpesviridae	Alphaherpesvirinae	Simplexvirus	Human herpesvirus 1
		Varicellovirus	Human herpesvirus 3
		Mardivirus	Gallid herpesvirus 2
		Iltovirus	Gallid herpesvirus 1
	Betaherpesvirinae	Cytomegalovirus	Human herpesvirus 5
		Muromegalovirus	Murid herpesvirus 1
		Proboscivirus	Elephantid herpesvirus 1
		Roseolovirus	Human herpesvirus 6
	Gammaherpesvirinae	Lymphocryptovirus	Human herpesvirus 4
		Macavirus	Alcelaphine herpesvirus 1
		Percavirus	Equid herpesvirus 2
		Rhadinovirus	Saimiriine herpesvirus 2
Malacoherpesviridae		Osterovirus	Ostreid herpesvirus 1
Adenoviridae		Mastadenovirus	Human adenovirus C
		Aviadenovirus	Fowl adenovirus A
		Atadenovirus	Ovine adenovirus D
		Siadenovirus	Frog adenovirus
Polyomaviridae		Polyomavirus	Simian virus 40
Papillomaviridae		Alphapapillomavirus	Human papillomavirus 32
		Betapapillomavirus	Human papillomavirus 5
		Gammapapillomavirus	Human papillomavirus 4
		Deltapapillomavirus	European elk papillomavirus 1
		Epsilonpapillomavirus	Bovine papillomavirus 5
		Zetapapillomavirus	Equine papillomavirus 1
		Etapapillomavirus	Fringilla coelebs papillomavirus
		Thetapapillomavirus	Psittacus erithacus timneh papillomavirus
		Iotapapillomavirus	Mastomys natalensis papillomavirus
		Kappapapillomavirus	Cottontail rabbit papillomavirus
		Lambdapapillomavirus	Canine oral papillomavirus
		Mupapillomavirus	Human papillomavirus 1
		Nupapillomavirus	Human papillomavirus 41
		Xipapillomavirus	Bovine papillomavirus 3
		Omicronpapillomavirus	Phocoena spinipinnis papillomavirus
		Pipapillomavirus	Hamster oral papillomavirus
Single-Stranded DNA Viruses			
Parvoviridae	Parvovirinae	Parvovirus	Minute virus of mice
		Erythrovirus	B19 virus
		Dependovirus	Adeno-associated virus 2
		Amdovirus	Aleutian mink disease virus
		Bocavirus	Bovine parvovirus

(Continued)

TABLE 1.4 (Continued)

Family	Subfamily	Genus	Type Species (Host if Not Vertebrate)
Circoviridae		Circovirus	Porcine circovirus 1
		Gyrovirus	Chicken anemia virus

DNA and RNA Reverse-Transcribing Viruses

Family	Subfamily	Genus	Type Species (Host if Not Vertebrate)
Hepadnaviridae		Orthohepadnavirus	Hepatitis B virus
		Avihepadnavirus	Duck hepatitis B virus
Retroviridae	Orthoretrovirinae	Alpharetrovirus	Avian leukosis virus
		Betaretrovirus	Mouse mammary tumor virus
		Gammaretrovirus	Murine leukemia virus
		Deltaretrovirus	Bovine leukemia virus
		Epsilonretrovirus	Walleye dermal sarcoma virus
		Lentivirus	Human immunodeficiency virus 1
	Spumaretrovirinae	Spumavirus	Simian foamy virus

RNA viruses

Double-Stranded RNA Viruses

Family	Subfamily	Genus	Type Species (Host if Not Vertebrate)
Reoviridae		Orthoreovirus	Mammalian orthoreovirus
		Cardoreovirus	Eriocheir sinensis reovirus
		Orbivirus	Bluetongue virus 1
		Rotavirus	Rotavirus A
		Seadornavirus	Banna virus
		Coltivirus	Colorado tick fever virus
		Aquareovirus	Aquareovirus A
Birnaviridae		Avibirnavirus	Infectious bursal disease virus
		Aquabirnavirus	Infectious pancreatic necrosis virus

Single-Stranded Negative-Sense RNA Viruses

Family	Subfamily	Genus	Type Species (Host if Not Vertebrate)
Paramyxoviridae	Paramyxovirinae	Respirovirus	Sendai virus
		Morbillivirus	Measles virus
		Rubulavirus	Mumps virus
		Avulavirus	Newcastle disease virus
		Henipavirus	Hendra virus
	Pneumovirinae	Pneumovirus	Human respiratory syncytial virus
		Metapneumovirus	Avian pneumovirus
Rhabdoviridae		Vesiculovirus	Vesicular stomatitis Indiana virus
		Lyssavirus	Rabies virus
		Ephemerovirus	Bovine ephemeral fever virus
		Novirhabdovirus	Infectious hematopoietic necrosis virus
Filoviridae		Marburgvirus	Lake Victoria marburgvirus
		Ebolavirus	Zaire ebolavirus
Bornaviridae		Bornavirus	Borna disease virus
Orthomyxoviridae		Influenzavirus A	Influenza A virus
		Influenzavirus B	Influenza B virus
		Influenzavirus C	Influenza C virus
		Thogotovirus	Thogoto virus
		Isavirus	Infectious salmon anemia virus

(Continued)

TABLE 1.4 (Continued)

Family	Subfamily	Genus	Type Species (Host if Not Vertebrate)
Bunyaviridae		*Orthobunyavirus*	*Bunyamwera virus*
		Hantavirus	*Hantaan virus*
		Nairovirus	*Dugbe virus*
		Phlebovirus	*Rift Valley fever virus*
Arenaviridae		*Arenavirus*	*Lymphocytic choriomeningitis virus*
Single-Stranded Positive-Sense RNA Viruses			
Coronaviridae		*Coronavirus*	*Infectious bronchitis virus*
		Torovirus	*Equine torovirus*
Arteriviridae		*Arterivirus*	*Equine arteritis virus*
Roniviridae		*Okavirus*	*Gill-associated virus*
Picornaviridae		*Enterovirus*	*Human enterovirus C*
		Erbovirus	*Equine rhinitis B virus*
		Hepatovirus	*Hepatitis A virus*
		Cardiovirus	*Encephalomyocarditis virus*
		Aphthovirus	*Foot-and-mouth disease virus*
		Parechovirus	*Human parechovirus*
		Kobuvirus	*Aichi virus*
		Teschovirus	*Porcine teschovirus*
Caliciviridae		*Vesivirus*	*Vesicular exanthema of swine virus*
		Lagovirus	*Rabbit hemorrhagic disease virus*
		Norovirus	*Norwalk virus*
		Sapovirus	*Sapporo virus*
Astroviridae		*Mamastrovirus*	*Human astrovirus*
		Aviastrovirus	*Turkey astrovirus*
Togaviridae		*Alphavirus*	*Sindbis virus*
		Rubivirus	*Rubella virus*
Flaviviridae		*Flavivirus*	*Yellow fever virus*
		Pestivirus	*Bovine viral diarrhea virus 1*
		Hepacivirus	*Hepatitis C virus*
Unassigned or Subviral Agents			
Unassigned		*Hepevirus*	*Hepatitis E virus*
		Deltavirus	*Hepatitis delta virus*
		Anellovirus	*Torque teno virus*
Prions		Scrapie prion	

[a]*The terms used reflect the system of the International Committee on Taxonomy of Viruses as at November 2009.*

Virus Replication

Chapter Contents

In the previous chapter, viruses were defined as obligate intracellular parasites that are unable to direct any biosynthetic processes outside the host cell. It was further noted that the genetic complexity of viruses varies greatly between individual virus families, ranging from those viruses that encode just a few proteins to others that encode more than 900 proteins. Given this remarkable diversity, it is hardly surprising that the replication processes used by individual viruses would also be highly variable. However, all viruses must go through the same general steps for replication to occur—attach to a susceptible host cell, penetrate the cell, replicate its own genetic material and associated proteins, assemble new virus particles, and escape from the infected cell. This chapter will outline the general processes involved in each of these steps; however, more specific details are to be found in the chapters dealing with the individual virus families in Part II of this book.

GROWTH OF VIRUSES

Before the development of *in-vitro* cell culture techniques, all viruses had to be propagated in their natural host. For bacterial viruses, this was a relatively simple process that permitted an earlier development of laboratory-based research methods than was possible with plant or animal viruses. For animal viruses, samples from affected animals were collected and used to infect other animals, initially of the same species. When consistent results were obtained, attempts were usually made to determine whether other species might also be susceptible. These types of experiment were performed in an effort to determine the host range of any presumed viral agent. Although progress was made in defining the biological properties of viruses, this manner of propagation had obvious major drawbacks, especially with agents affecting large animals. A most serious issue was the infection status of the recipient animals. An undetected infectious agent in a sheep, for example, could alter the clinical signs observed after inoculation of that sheep with the test agent, and samples collected from this individual might now include several infectious agents, potentially confounding future experiments. In an attempt to avoid this type of contamination problem, groups of animals were raised under more defined conditions for use in research studies. As new infectious agents were discovered and tests developed for their detection, the research animals became more "clean" and the concept of "specific pathogen-free" (SPF) animals was born. It is noteworthy, however, that animals apparently "specific pathogen-free" could be infected with pathogens that were still undefined or undeclared. For example, pneumonia virus of mice (mouse pneumovirus) was discovered when "uninfected" control animals inoculated with lung extracts from other control animals died during experimental influenza virus infection studies. Many early viral and immunological studies were compromised by using rodents infected with mouse hepatitis virus, lactate dehydrogenase-elevating virus, or other agents unknown to the supplier of the research animals.

The search for suitable culture systems for viruses led to the discovery, in 1931, that vaccinia virus and herpes simplex virus could be grown on the chorioallantoic membrane of embryonated chicken eggs, as was also known for fowlpox virus, a naturally occurring pathogen of birds. The use of embryonated chicken eggs then became routine for propagation efforts, not only for avian viruses, but also for viruses infecting mammalian species. Viruses in most of the animal virus families can be grown in embryonated eggs, probably

Fenner's Veterinary Virology. DOI: 10.1016/B978-0-12-375158-4.00002-X because of the wide variety of cell and tissue types present in the developing embryo and its environment. In some cases, embryonated eggs entirely replaced research animals for the growth of virus stocks, and if the viral infection resulted in the death of the embryo, this system also provided a quantitative measure of the amounts of virus in individual stocks. Cell culture has largely replaced the egg system, which is labor-intensive and expensive, but the embryonated egg is still widely used for the isolation and growth of influenza viruses, in addition to many avian viruses.

The advent of *in-vitro* animal cell culture brought research studies in line with those involving bacterial viruses, thereby reducing the risks associated with adventitious viruses in animal inoculation systems and enhancing diagnostic testing. However, the problem of adventitious viruses was not entirely eliminated as, for example, early batches of the modified live poliovirus vaccine were contaminated with SV40 virus, a simian virus originating from the primary monkey kidney cultures used for vaccine production. Similarly, interpretation of the results of some early studies on newly described parainfluenza viruses is complicated because of viral contamination of the cell cultures used for virus isolation. In the veterinary world, contamination of ruminant cell cultures with bovine viral diarrhea virus has been an insidious and widespread problem. Some contaminated cell cultures and lines were probably derived from infected fetal bovine tissue, but—far more commonly—cells become infected through exposure to fetal bovine serum contaminated with bovine viral diarrhea virus. Fetal bovine serum became a standard supplement for cell culture medium in the early 1970s. The fact that many ruminant cell lines became infected from contaminated serum has compromised much research pertaining to ruminant virology and immunology, confounded diagnostic testing for bovine viral diarrhea virus, and caused substantial economic losses as a result of contaminated vaccines. The extent of the problem was not fully defined until the late 1980s when high-quality diagnostic reagents became available. As with experimental animals, problems with contaminating viral infections of cell cultures were only defined when the existence of the relevant infectious agent became known. Standard protocols for the use of serum in biological production systems now require irradiation of the serum to inactivate all viruses, known or unknown. With current technology allowing amplification of virtually all nucleic acid species in cells, coupled with rapid sequencing of these products, a complete profile of cell cultures for contaminating organisms is now feasible.

Various *in-vitro* cell culture systems have been utilized since artificial medium was developed to maintain cell viability outside the source species: organ cultures, explant cultures, primary cell cultures, and cell lines. Organ cultures maintain the three-dimensional structure of the tissue and are utilized for short-term experiments. Tracheal epithelial cells that remain attached to the cartilage matrix of the trachea during culture are an example of this type of system. The creation of primary cell cultures utilizes proteases such as trypsin or collagenase to produce individual cells of a given tissue such as fetal kidney or lung, and the individual cells are permitted to attach to a cell culture matrix and will divide for a limited number of cell divisions. The limited lifespan of these cells requires continual production of the cells from new tissue sources, which can lead to variation in quality between batches. In contrast, theoretically, cell lines have an unlimited capability of division, so that a more standard viral growth system can be developed. In the early period of cell culture, the development of these immortalized cells (transformation) was an empirical process with a low probability of success. More recently, procedures have been developed to immortalize virtually any cell type, so that the number of cell lines representing different species is increasing rapidly.

Recognition of Viral Growth in Culture

Recognition of the presence of a viral agent in a host system was dependent initially upon the recognition of signs not found in an unaffected (control) host, death being the most extreme outcome but easiest to determine. The same essentially applies to cells in culture—detection of viral growth is dependent upon the detection of a property of the inoculated cells that is not found in control cultures maintained under identical growth conditions. As with animals, the sign of a viral infection of a culture that is easiest to detect is death of the cells or a very significant change in cell morphology. This is usually referred to as a *cytopathic effect*, or "CPE," and is noted through microscopic examination of the test culture system (Figure 2.1). Careful observation of cultures showing cytopathic effect must be undertaken, as diagnostic samples may contain substances that are toxic for cultured cells, such as bacterial macromolecules. Other morphological changes may be manifest in virus-infected cell cultures; for example, a significant morphological change in cultured cells infected with avian reovirus is the formation of multinucleated cells or syncytia (Figure 2.1A). Many members of the family *Paramyxoviridae* can also cause this type of morphological change in cultured cells, but the extent of syncytium formation is cell-type-dependent. The type of cytopathology noted in culture can be characteristic for a given class of virus. For example, alphaherpesviruses produce a distinct cytopathic effect of rounded cells, with or without small syncytia, which spreads very rapidly through a susceptible cell culture (Figure 2.1B).

In the search for unknown viruses in cell cultures, early researchers took advantage of the property of some viruses to bind to red blood cells. For example, cells infected with bovine parainfluenza virus 3 will show the ability to adsorb chicken red blood cells to the plasma membrane. In the budding process of virus maturation (orthomyxoviruses, paramyxoviruses), viral proteins are inserted into the plasma membrane. If these proteins bind to receptors on the red blood cells, the infected cells show adherence of the cells on their surface (hemadsorption) (Figure 2.1D). This property

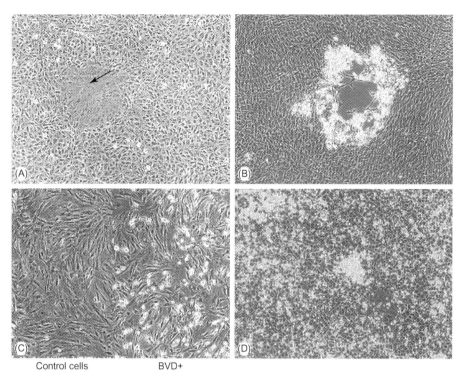

Control cells   BVD+

FIGURE 2.1 Cytopathic effects produced by different viruses. The cell monolayers are shown as they would normally be viewed by phase contrast microscopy, unfixed and unstained. (A) Avian reovirus in Vero cells. (B) Untyped herpesvirus in feline lung cell. (C) Bovine viral diarrhea virus in primary bovine kidney cells. (D) Parainfluenza virus 3 in Vero cells detected by hemadsorption of chicken red blood cells.

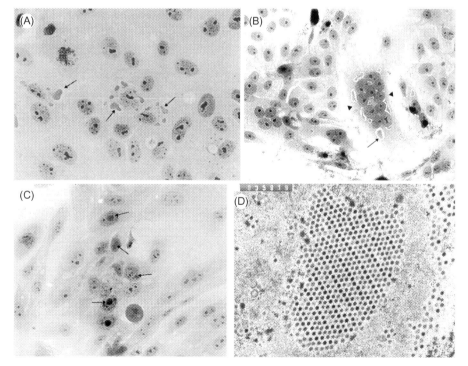

FIGURE 2.2 Typical inclusions and abnormal cell morphology in virus-infected cells. (A) Reovirus inclusions (arrows) in infected Vero cells. (B) Canine distemper virus inclusions (arrows) and syncytium (arrowheads) in infected Vero cells. (C) Bovine adenovirus 5 intranuclear inclusions (arrows) in primary bovine kidney cells. (D) Transmission electron micrograph of an untyped adenovirus nuclear inclusion in A459 cells.

of infected cells only occurs with viruses that bud from the plasma membrane, and may be specific for red blood cells of a given animal species. Viruses that induce hemadsorption also show the ability to hemagglutinate red blood cells in cell-free medium. The same viral proteins that permit hemadsorption are also responsible for the hemagglutination reaction. There are, however, viruses that can hemagglutinate red blood cells but not show hemadsorption of the infected cells—for example, adenoviruses and alphaviruses.

A characteristic morphological change in cells infected by certain viruses is the formation of inclusion bodies (Figure 2.2). These changes can be seen with a light microscope after fixation and treatment with cytological stains. As with hemadsorption, not all viruses will produce detectable inclusion bodies. The type of virus infecting a cell can be inferred by the location and shape of the inclusions: cells infected with herpesviruses, adenoviruses, and parvoviruses can have intranuclear inclusions, whereas cytoplasmic inclusions are characteristic of infections with poxviruses, orbiviruses, and paramyxoviruses (Figure 2.2B, 2.2C). The composition of the inclusions will vary with the virus type. The cytoplasmic Negri bodies identified in rabies-infected cells are composed of aggregates of nucleocapsids, whereas the intranuclear inclusions that occur in adenovirus-infected cells are crystalline arrays of mature virus particles (Figure 2.2D). Cytological stains are rarely used to identify cells infected with specific viruses, but are mainly used as a screening tests to assess the presence of any virus.

In the absence of a metagenomic screening test, detection of viruses that produce no cytopathology, do not induce hemadsorption or hemagglutinate, or produce no

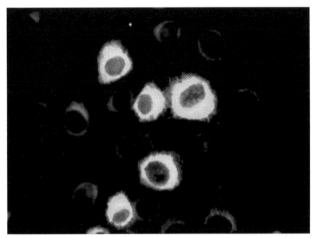

FIGURE 2.3 Indirect fluorescent antibody detection of non-cytopathic bovine viral diarrhea virus (BVDV) infected cells. Bovine cells exposed to BVDV for 72 hrs were fixed with cold acetone. Fixed cells were strained with BVDV monoclonal antibody 20.10.6 followed by a goat anti-mouse serum tagged with fluorescein isothiocyanate.

definable inclusions is carried out with virus-specific tests. This would be the case for screening bovine cells for the presence of non-cytopathic bovine viral diarrhea virus. The most commonly used tests in this type of situation are immunologically based assays such as fluorescent antibody tests or immunohistochemistry tests (Figure 2.3). The quality of the tests is dependent on the specificity of the antibodies used in the assay. With the development of monoclonal antibodies, this issue has been largely resolved. Other virus-specific tests depend on the detection of virus-specific nucleic acid in the infected cells. Hybridization tests have been replaced by assays based on polymerase chain reaction (PCR), because of their enhanced sensitivity and ease of test performance (see Chapter 5).

VIRUS REPLICATION

A fundamental characteristic that separates viruses from other replicating entities is the manner in which new virus particles are synthesized. Viruses do not use binary fission; virus particles are assembled *de novo* from the various structural components synthesized as somewhat independent but synchronized events. The earliest recognition of this unique replication pattern came from studies using bacteriophage. The outline of the experimental proof of concept was relatively simple: (1) add a chloroform-resistant phage to a culture of bacteria for several minutes; (2) rinse the bacteria to remove non-attached phage; (3) incubate the culture and remove samples at various periods of time; (4) treat sampled bacterial cultures with chloroform to stop growth; (5) quantify the amount of phage at each of the time periods. The result of this type of experiment is what we now refer to as a *one-step growth curve*, which can be achieved with any type of virus (Figure 2.4). The

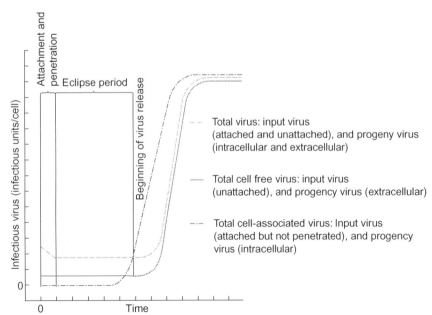

Total virus: input virus (attached and unattached), and progeny virus (intracellular and extracellular)

Total cell free virus: input virus (unattached), and progency virus (extracellular)

Total cell-associated virus: Input virus (attached but not penetrated), and progency virus (intracellular)

FIGURE 2.4 One-step growth curve of a non-enveloped virus. Attachment and penetration are followed by an eclipse period of 2–12 hours during which cell-associated infectivity cannot be detected. This is followed by a period of several hours during which virus maturation occurs. Virions of non-enveloped viruses are often released late and incompletely, when the cell lyses. The release of enveloped virions occurs concurrently with maturation by budding from the plasma membrane.

remarkable finding of this type of study was that infectious virus "disappeared" from the infected cultures for a variable period of time, depending on the virus–host-cell system. The period of time is referred to as the *eclipse period*, and represents the time needed for the various parts of the virus particle to be synthesized and assembled. Once assembly begins, there is an essentially exponential increase in infectious virus until the host cell is unable to maintain metabolic integrity. Depending on the type of virus, there may be sudden release of virus particles (lysis of the host cell, exemplified by T-even bacteriophage) or a more slow release (maturation of the virus particle at a cell membrane site, such as with influenza virus). A specific virus–host-cell system has its own inherent biological clock that cannot be significantly altered by a desire for faster test results, much to the frustration of the diagnostician, researcher, and clinician.

The one-step growth curve can be used to divide the virus replication cycle into its component parts for discussion of the general replication patterns. The basic components of the replication cycle are attachment, the eclipse period (penetration, uncoating, replication of component parts, maturation), and release of virus particles. Several of these patterns will be presented, but specific details of individual virus families are found in Part II of this book.

Attachment

The critical first step in the virus replication cycle is the binding of the virus particle to a host cell. This binding process may involve a series of interactions that define in part the host range of the virus and its tissue/organ specificity (tropism). Tissue and organ specificity largely defines the pathogenic potential of the virus and nature of the

disease it induces. Virus particles interact with cell-surface molecules referred to as attachment factors, entry factors, receptors, and co-receptors. Frequently, the term "viral receptor" is used to describe these cell-surface molecules, which is something of a misnomer, as cells certainly do not maintain receptors specifically for viruses—rather, viruses have evolved to use host cell-surface molecules critical for cellular processes. Although the exact series of events that occur on the cell surface may be complex, a general process can be envisioned. Initial contact of a virus particle with the cell surface may involve short-distance electrostatic interactions with charged molecules such as heparan sulfate proteoglycans. That charge is a key factor in this initial interaction is supported by the observation that positively charged compounds such as diethyl amino ethanol (DEAE) dextran can increase binding of virus to host cells. This initial contact may be one that simply helps to concentrate virus on the surface of the cell, permitting a more specific interaction with other receptor-like molecules. The affinity of binding for a given site may be low, but the large number of potential binding sites makes the interactions nearly irreversible. Attachment of a virus particle to the host cell is a temperature-independent process, but penetration is dependent upon the fluidity of the lipids in the plasma membrane which does have temperature constraints.

In recent years, the search for receptors/entry factors mediating virus attachment and entry has intensified such that numerous candidate receptors/entry factors have been identified. These include ligand-binding receptors (e.g. chemokine receptors), signaling molecules (e.g., CD4), cell adhesion/signaling receptors [e.g., intercellular cell adhesion molecule-1 (ICAM-1)], enzymes, integrins, and glycoconjugates with various carbohydrate linkages, sialic acid being a common terminal residue (Table 2.1). The number

TABLE 2.1 Examples of Cellular Macromolecules Used by Viruses as Receptors/Entry Factors

Virus	Family	Receptor
Human immunodeficiency virus	*Retroviridae*	CCR5, CCR3, CXCR4 (heparan sulfate proteoglycan)
Avian leukosis/sarcoma virus	*Retroviridae*	Tissue necrosis factor-related protein TVB
Murine leukemia virus E	*Retroviridae*	MCAT-1
Bovine leukemia virus	*Retroviridae*	BLV receptor 1
Poliovirus	*Picornaviridae*	PVR (CD155)—Ig family
Coxsackievirus B	*Picornaviridae*	CAR (coxsackie and adenovirus receptor)—Ig family
Human rhinovirus 14	*Picornaviridae*	ICAM-1 (intercellular cell adhesion molecule-1)—Ig family
Echovirus 1	*Picornaviridae*	$\alpha2\beta1$ integrin VLA-2

(Continued)

TABLE 2.1 (Continued)

Virus	Family	Receptor
Foot-and-mouth disease virus—wild-type virus	*Picornaviridae*	Various integrins
Foot-and-mouth disease virus—cell-culture-adapted	*Picornaviridae*	Heparan sulfate proteoglycan
Feline calicivirus	*Caliciviridae*	fJAM-A (feline junction adhesion molecule-A)
Adenovirus 2	*Adenoviridae*	CAR-Ig family
Adenoviruses	*Adenoviridae*	$\alpha v\beta 3$, $\alpha v\beta 5$ integrins
Herpes simplex virus 1	*Herpesviridae*	HveA (herpes virus entry mediator A), heparan sulfate proteoglycan, others
Human cytomegalovirus	*Herpesviridae*	Heparan sulfate proteoglycan
Epstein–Barr virus	*Herpesviridae*	CD21, complement receptor 2 (CR2)
Pseudorabies virus	*Herpesviridae*	CD155—Ig family
Feline parvovirus	*Parvoviridae*	TfR-1 (transferrin receptor-1)
Adenovirus-associated virus 5	*Parvoviridae*	$\alpha(2,3)$-linked sialic acid
Influenza A virus	*Orthomyxoviridae*	Sialic acid
Influenza C virus	*Orthomyxoviridae*	9-*O*-acetylsialic acid
Canine distemper virus	*Paramyxoviridae*	SLAM (signaling lymphocyte activation molecule)
Newcastle disease virus	*Paramyxoviridae*	Sialic acid
Bovine respiratory syncytial virus	*Paramyxoviridae*	Unknown
Hendra virus	*Paramyxoviridae*	Ephrin-B2
Rotavirus	*Reoviridae*	Various integrins
Reovirus	*Reoviridae*	JAMs (junction adhesion molecules)
Mouse hepatitis virus	*Coronaviridae*	CEA (carcinoembryonic antigen)—Ig family
Transmissible gastroenteritis virus	*Coronaviridae*	Aminopeptidase N
Lymphocytic choriomenigitis virus	*Arenaviridae*	α-Dystroglycan
Dengue virus	*Flaviviridae*	Heparan sulfate proteoglycan
Rabies virus	*Rhabdoviridiae*	Acetycholine, NCAM (neural adhesion molecule)

of specific molecules that play a part in the initial interactions of virus with host cells will certainly increase as new viruses are identified, and as existing viruses are better characterized. Different viruses may use the same receptor/entry factor, which simply reflects the fact that a similar host cell serves as the replication site of the viruses. The process of identification of receptors/entry factors is more complicated than initially imagined, as viruses within a given family may use different receptors. Furthermore, different strains of the same virus can utilize different receptors; for foot-and-mouth disease virus, the receptors in the bovine host are integrins, but cell-culture passaged virus can use heparan sulfate. This change in receptor specificity alters the pathogenicity of the virus, clearly indicating that receptor specificity is a key factor in the disease

process. For viruses with a wide host range, such as some of the alphaherpesviruses, it is speculated that these viruses can use several receptors, accounting for their ability to grow in cells from many hosts.

The story of virus–receptor interaction is further complicated by those viruses that require several entry factors to initiate an infection successfully. A prominent example of this phenomenon is human immunodeficiency virus (HIV). Initial cell interaction is through heparan sulfate, followed by binding to the CD4 receptor and a chemokine receptor such as CXCR4 or CCR5. For hepatitis C, at least four entry factors (CD81, SR-BI, CLDN1, and OCLN) must be expressed on the cell surface before the cell becomes fully susceptible to infection. It may well be that the highly restricted host range of some viruses is reflective of unique entry factor

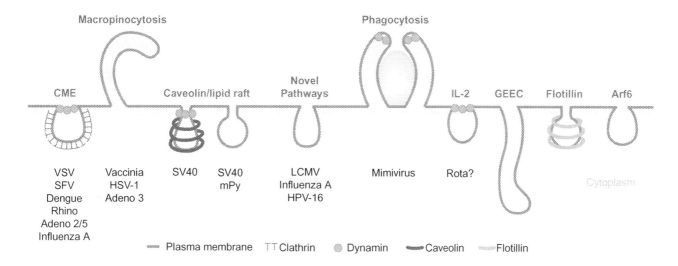

FIGURE 2.5 Endocytic mechanisms. Endocytosis in animal cells can occur via several different mechanisms. Several mechanisms are defined as pinocytic—that is, they involve the uptake of fluid, solutes, and small particles. These include clathrin-mediated, macropinocytosis, caveolar/raft-mediated mechanisms, in addition to several novel mechanisms. Some of these pathways involve dynamin-2, as indicated by the beads around the neck of the endocytic indentations. Large particles are taken up by phagocytosis, a process restricted to a few cell types. In addition, there are pathways such as IL-2, the so-called GEEC pathway, and the flotillin- and ADP-ribosylation factor 6 (Arf6)-dependent pathways that carry specific cellular cargo but are not yet used by viruses. Adeno 2/5, Adeno 3, adenoviruses 2/5 and 3; CME, clathrin-mediated endocytosis; HPV-16, human papillomavirus 16; HSV-1, herpes simplex virus 1; LCMV, lymphocytic choriomeningitis virus; mPy, mouse polyomavirus; SFV, Semliki Forest virus; SV40, simian virus 40; VSV, vesicular stomatitis virus. *[From J. Mercer. Virus entry by endocytosis. Annu. Rev. Biochem.* **79**, *6.1–6.31 (2010). Copyright © 2010 by Annual Reviews, with permission.]*

requirements found only on highly differentiated cells. A somewhat indirect entry factor system is exemplified by dengue virus. Virus particles bound to so-called non-neutralizing antibodies gain entry to macrophages by virtue of the Fc receptor binding to the immunoglobulin molecule. The antibody–virus complex is internalized, with infectious virus being released into the cytoplasm of the phagocytic cell. Foot-and-mouth disease virus and feline coronavirus can also use this antibody-dependent enhancement entry system *in vitro*, but its importance in the natural infection process is conjectural.

Penetration

The function of the receptors/entry factors is not simply to bind the virus particle, but also to assist or direct the process whereby the virus enters the cell. This assistance can occur through several different processes: (1) the interaction of the virus with its receptor can result in a conformational change in the virus particle or attachment protein that is necessary for entry; (2) the concentration and/or immobilization of the cell receptor can trigger a cellular response leading to internalization of the complexed receptors; (3) the bound receptor may induce the movement of the complex to an appropriate entry site or to a site permitting contact with a co-receptor. The individual cellular receptor utilized by a specific virus can determine the mode of entry of the virus into the host cell. All the signaling processes used by the host cell to internalize macromolecules and receptors are used in the virus entry process, as viruses rely on the normal cellular processes—specifically, activation of a myriad of protein kinases, GTPases, binding

proteins, second messengers, and structural element rearrangements. The specific pathways activated depend on the type of entry process. For virus particles, the internalization process can be divided into two general patterns: entry by way of membrane-bound vesicles or direct entry at the plasma membrane. Viruses that utilize the membrane vesicle route must still pass through a limiting membrane to gain access to the cytosol, so that the manner in which viruses move across the limiting membrane may be similar regardless of the site at which this event takes place.

The mechanism whereby viruses are internalized in membrane-bound vesicles is generally designated as endocytosis, a normal cellular process for internalizing macromolecules. The earliest example of this process involved the identification of virus particles in clathrin-coated "pits" in the plasma membrane (Figure 2.5). The cellular protein dynamin-2 induces the formation of a vesicle that enters the early endosomal system. The virus particle in the early endosome is subjected to a drop in pH that may induce structural changes in the particle. In the classic pathway, the vesicle is transformed into a late endosome with a corresponding lower pH. For some viruses, it is this lower pH that induces the structural changes. The late endosome will then fuse with lysosomal vesicles to initiate the degradation of the material internalized by this process. Virus particles that do not successfully escape the endosome are degraded and prevented from initiating the infection process. The one noted exception to this is reovirus that uses the lysosomal enzymes to activate the penetration process. The key factors in this entry process are the changes in pH which are necessary to induce structural changes in the virus particles that permit the breaching of the limiting membrane boundary. Compounds (balfilomycin A1, chloroquine, NH_4Cl) that can prevent the lowering of the pH in endosomes can significantly impair the infection process.

A second major vesicle internalization process involves the caveosome system. Caveolin-coated pits and lipid-raft-mediated pits containing cholesterol with associated virus particles are internalized and enter the caveosome system. Unlike the endosomal system, the caveosomes maintain a neutral pH within the vesicle, but there appears to be a pathway for caveosomes to enter the endosomal system, allowing pH activation of the virus particles. Another route for the caveosomes is to the endoplasmic reticulum, where viruses such as SV40 cross the limiting membrane boundary. As a general rule, the enveloped viruses do not use the caveosome system; this may be a function of particle size, as the vesicles formed by the endosomal system are larger and can accommodate the generally larger size of virions that possess lipid envelopes. The boundary between these systems may not be as clearly defined as was initially believed, and some viruses may use different systems depending on the cell type encountered. Earlier studies on virus particle entry mechanisms may be compromised by the possibility that these observations included predominantly non-infectious particles that were processed differently than infectious particles.

The true entry of the viral genetic material into the host cells occurs when the genome enters the cytosol. For the enveloped viruses, this process is conceptually simple, in that the viral envelope need only fuse with the cellular membrane, be it at the cell surface or within an endosomal vesicle. For many of the viruses in the family *Paramyxoviridae*, the fusion process occurs at the plasma membrane under neutral pH conditions. This group of viruses can induce a phenomenon referred to as "fusion from without" whereby, at high multiplicity of infection and in the absence of virus replication, the plasma membranes of adjacent cells fuse to form multinucleated cells known as syncytia. For many viruses, the fusion process is a pH-activated one, requiring the virus particles to be in the endosomal pathway. In all cases, regardless of the pH requirements, the surface glycoproteins of the virus particles must undergo changes in their tertiary or quaternary structures such that generally hydrophobic regions of the proteins can come into contact with the cellular membrane to produce a localized destabilization and induce fusion with the viral envelope. For many of the viruses (paramyxoviruses, orthomyxoviruses, flaviviruses, coronaviruses, and alphaviruses, for example), the surface glycoproteins must undergo a proteolytic processing step in order to permit these necessary conformational changes to occur. This finding was a major discovery in the early 1970s that allowed the routine propagation of influenza virus and parainfluenza viruses in cell culture.

The breaching of cellular membranes by non-enveloped virus particles is conceptually more difficult and potentially more confusing than the membrane fusion process. Several different mechanisms have been identified (Figure 2.6). For the picornaviruses, a "pore mechanism" has been proposed that operates under neutral or acid pH, depending on the specific virus. For poliovirus, the key event in penetration is the structural rearrangement of the virus particle induced by the binding of the cellular receptor. In the restructuring process, VP4 is released and the myristylated N-terminus of the VP-1 protein is inserted into the plasma membrane. The viral RNA then enters the cytoplasm through a pore in the membrane. In this model, the penetration and uncoating steps of the replication cycle occur simultaneously, with the viral capsid proteins remaining at the plasma membrane. For adenoviruses, a complex set of reactions occurs in the low pH of the endosomes, the result of which is the dissolution of the cellular membrane (lytic mechanism) such that a modified virus particle enters the cytoplasm along with the contents of the endosome. For polyomaviruses, the virus particle is transported to the endoplasmic reticulum by the caveosome system. In conjunction with cellular chaperone proteins, the virus particle is transported across the membrane (transfer mechanism) into the cytoplasm. In all cases, the virus particles are modified by rearrangements induced by receptor binding, pH, protease cleavages, or binding by cellular transport proteins.

The entry of the virus particle, nucleocapsid, or genomic nucleic acid into the cytoplasm in many cases is not the final step in the initiation of the replication process for the virus. In most cases, the nucleic acid is not in a form that would permit the synthesis of plus-strand RNA needed to direct the production of viral proteins, and the genome is not in a correct location for replication to occur. Again, cellular processes are involved in the transport of the viral units to the required locations. For most of the longer translocation needs, the microtubule transport system is used; actin filaments enable more localized movements. For the DNA viruses and RNA viruses such as influenza virus that utilize the nucleus for their replication site, nuclear localization signals exist on key viral proteins that interact with soluble cellular proteins of the nuclear import system. These proteins link the viral units to the nuclear pore complex, either permitting translocation of the viral unit into the nucleus (parvoviruses) or inducing the transport of the nucleic acid into the nucleus (adenoviruses, herpesviruses). The environment of the cytoplasm or the nucleus completes the uncoating process by inducing conformational changes in the nucleocapsid proteins by binding to "replication" sites, by allowing further proteolytic processing of proteins, or by destabilizing the viral protein–nucleic acid interactions. As an example, Semliki Forest virus capsid proteins, after release from the endosomes, bind to 60S ribosomal subunits that permit

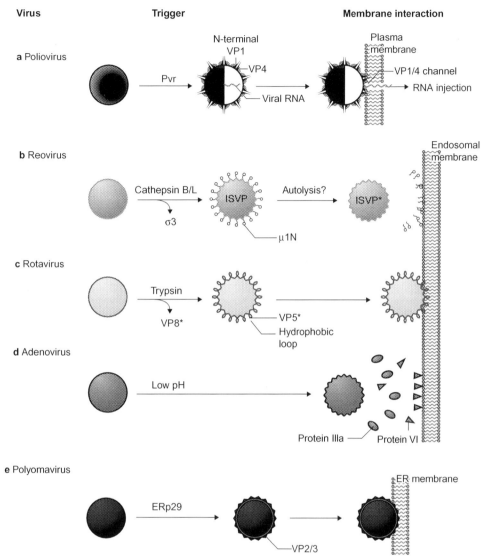

FIGURE 2.6   Different mechanisms that initiate the membrane penetration process. Interaction with a receptor (e.g., Pvr), proteases (e.g., cathepsin B/L or trypsin), or molecular chaperones (ERp29) or exposure to the low-pH environment triggers the structural rearrangements of non-enveloped viruses necessary for their membrane penetration. *[From B. Tsai. Penetration of nonenveloped viruses into the cytoplasm. Annu. Rev. Cell Dev. Biol. 23, 23–43 (2007), with permission.]*

the release of the viral RNA. For picornaviruses, the entry process produces a genomic RNA that is capable of interacting directly with ribosomes to initiate viral protein synthesis. Table 2.2 provides some general characteristics of the replication cycle of the families of viruses that are described in more detail in Part II of this book.

Viral Protein and Nucleic Acid Synthesis

Up to this point in the replication process, the virus has been somewhat passive in that, for the most part, no biosynthetic activity directed by the viral nucleic acid has occurred. The preliminary steps have put the viral genome in position to take active control of its replication cycle and to remodel the cell to assist in the production of mature virus particles.

The details of the next phases of the replication cycle are unique to each of the virus families, and those are outlined in each of the chapters on the specific virus families in Part II. A few selected examples of different replication strategies will be described in succeeding pages to emphasize specific aspects of their replication cycles.

Representative Examples of Virus Replication Strategies

Picornaviruses

For the picornaviruses, the entry process—whether at the plasma membrane or within an endosomal vesicle—results in an uncoated positive-sense single-stranded RNA genomic

TABLE 2.2 **Characteristics of Replication of Viruses of Different Families**

Family	Uptake Route	Site of Nucleic Acid Replication	Site of Maturation (Budding)
Poxviridae	Variable	Cytoplasm	Cytoplasm
Asfaviridae	Clathrin-mediated endocytosis	Cytoplasm	(Plasma membrane)
Iridoviridae	Variable	Nucleus/cytoplasm	Cytoplasm
Herpesviridae	Variable	Nucleus	(Nuclear membrane)
Adenoviridae	Clathrin-mediated endocytosis	Nucleus	Nucleus
Polyomaviridae	Caveolar endocytosis	Nucleus	Nucleus
Papillomaviridae	Clathrin/caveolar endocytosis	Nucleus	Nucleus
Parvoviridae	Clathrin-mediated endocytosis	Nucleus	Nucleus
Hepadnaviridae	Clathrin-mediated endocytosis	Nucleus/cytoplasm	(Endoplasmic reticulum)
Retroviridae	Plasma membrane fusion or clathrin-mediated endocytosis	Nucleus	(Plasma membrane)
Reoviridae	Clathrin-mediated endocytosis	Cytoplasm	Cytoplasm
Paramyxoviridae	Plasma membrane fusion	Cytoplasm	(Plasma membrane)
Rhabdoviridae	Plasma membrane fusion	Cytoplasm	(Plasma membrane)
Filoviridae	Plasma membrane fusion	Cytoplasm	(Plasma membrane)
Bornaviridae	Clathrin-mediated endocytosis	Nucleus	(Plasma membrane)
Orthomyxoviridae	Clathrin-mediated endocytosis	Nucleus	(Plasma membrane)
Bunyaviridae	Clathrin-mediated endocytosis	Cytoplasm	(Golgi membrane)
Arenaviridae	Clathrin-mediated endocytosis	Cytoplasm	(Plasma membrane)
Coronaviridae	Clathrin-mediated endocytosis/plasma membrane fusion	Cytoplasm	(Endoplasmic reticulum)
Arteriviridae	Clathrin-mediated endocytosis	Cytoplasm	(Endoplasmic reticulum)
Picornaviridae	Caveolar endocytosis/plasma membrane insertion	Cytoplasm	Cytoplasm
Caliciviridae	Caveolar endocytosis/plasma membrane insertion?	Cytoplasm	Cytoplasm
Astroviridae	Caveolar endocytosis/plasma membrane insertion?	Cytoplasm	Cytoplasm
Togaviridae	Clathrin-mediated endocytosis	Cytoplasm	(Plasma membrane)
Flaviviridae	Clathrin-mediated endocytosis	Cytoplasm	(Endoplasmic reticulum)

molecule free in the cytoplasm (Figure 2.7). In this environment, there are no cellular polymerases that are capable of replicating the genomic RNA. Accordingly, the first major event for the genomic RNA is to associate with the cellular protein translational system. Unlike most host-cell messenger RNAs (mRNAs), the picornavirus genomic RNA lacks a standard 5′ cap structure. However, these viruses have evolved to be able to initiate protein synthesis using an internal ribosome entry site (IRES). This alternative mechanism for binding ribosomes and translation factors provides the virus with the ability to restrict host-cell mRNA translation by directing the cleavage of translation initiation factors necessary for cap-dependent translation. This inhibition of cellular translation reduces competition for ribosomal complexes and

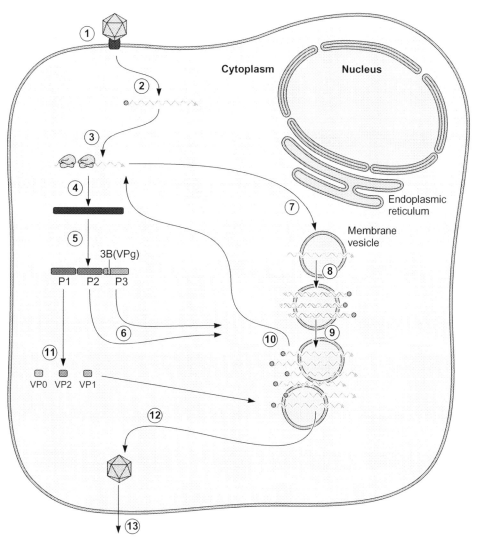

FIGURE 2.7 Single-cell reproductive cycle of a picornavirus, in this case poliovirus. The virion binds to a cellular receptor (1); release of the poliovirus genome occurs from within early endosomes located close (within 100 to 200 nm) to the plasma membrane (2). The VPg protein, depicted as a small orange circle at the 5′ end of the virion RNA, is removed, and the RNA associates with ribosomes (3). Translation is initiated at an internal site 741 nucleotides from the 5′ end of the viral mRNA, and a polyprotein precursor is synthesized (4). The polyprotein is cleaved during and after its synthesis to yield the individual viral proteins (5). Only the initial cleavages are shown here. The proteins that participate in viral RNA synthesis are transported to membrane vesicles (6). RNA synthesis occurs on the surfaces of these infected-cell-specific membrane vesicles. The (+) strand RNA is transported to these membrane vesicles (7), where it is copied into double-stranded RNAs (8). Newly synthesized (−) strands serve as templates for the synthesis of (+) strand genomic RNAs (9). Some of the newly synthesized (+) strand RNA molecules are translated after the removal of VPg (10). Structural proteins formed by partial cleavage of the PI precursor (11) associate with (+) strand RNA molecules that retain VPg to form progeny virions (12), which are released from the cell upon lysis (13). [*From* Principles of Virology, *S. J. Flint, L. W. Enquist, V. R. Racaniello, A. M. Skalka, 3rd ed., vol. 1, p. 519. Copyright © 2008 Wiley, with permission.*]

reduces the ability of the cells to produce an array of antiviral molecules that are made in response to the viral infection (see Chapter 4). The picornavirus proteins are synthesized from a single long open reading frame (ORF), with generation of specific proteins by a series of proteolytic cleavages that are mainly directed by virus-encoded proteases. It is one of these proteases that cleaves the cellular translation factor eIF4G.

A limited amount of viral protein can continue to be made from the input genome; however, the virus must begin to direct the synthesis of viral RNA if the infection is to be a

productive one. As cellular enzymes are incapable of doing this, a key viral protein is an RNA-dependent RNA polymerase—3D^pol for the picornaviruses. This protein, produced by a series of proteolytic cleavage reactions from precursor protein VP3, is found associated with remodeled smooth cellular membranes and this unit is referred to as the "RNA replication complex." Protein 3D^pol is a primer-dependent enzyme that also requires the presence of at least six other viral proteins for all aspects of RNA synthesis to be completed—synthesis of negative-stranded RNA as a template for the positive strand and more positive-stranded RNA to direct protein synthesis and for packaging into the virus particles. The mature virus particle of picornaviruses is composed of three or four proteins proteolytically processed by a virus-encoded protease from the precursor protein, VP1. The capsid proteins assemble into a 60-subunit particle with a single copy of the genomic RNA. The exact mechanism for the insertion of the RNA into the developing capsid remains unclear. The rate-limiting process for particle maturation appears to be the availability of the RNA molecule containing the VPg primer protein at the 5′ end. Picornaviruses do not have a specific mode of exit from the infected cell, as crystalline arrays of virus occur in the cytoplasm of infected cells awaiting dissolution of the cell structure.

The replication pattern of picornaviruses illustrates several common elements that are also found in other virus replication systems. Entry of the virus particle can occur at the plasma membrane or in membrane-bound vesicles. The first task of the positive-sense genomic RNA is to associate with ribosomes to produce new viral proteins that begin the process of replicating the viral RNA and taking control of the host-cell metabolic process. Viral proteins can be synthesized as larger precursor proteins that are cleaved by virus-specific proteases. They can induce the remodeling of cellular membrane structures to provide sites for viral RNA synthesis. Viral proteases perform several functions—generation of mature viral proteins and cleavage of various host-cell proteins that directly affect protein and RNA synthesis, in addition to inhibiting transcription of new proteins in response to the infection.

Rhabdoviruses

The rhabdoviruses present a different mode of replication (compared with picornaviruses) in that the input genomic RNA is of a negative sense—that is, it cannot serve as an mRNA for protein synthesis (Figure 2.8). The infection process is initiated by attachment of the virus particle to the plasma membrane and entry into an endosomal vesicle. The virion glycoproteins induce the fusion of the viral envelope with the endosomal membrane, with the release of the helical nucleocapsid into the cytoplasm. Unlike the picornaviruses, the virion RNA of rhabdoviruses is complexed throughout its length with N protein. Also unlike picornaviruses, the first event for the rhabdoviruses is to transcribe the virion RNA to make mRNA molecules. To do this, the nucleocapsid must contain an RNA transcriptase, because there are no cellular cytoplasmic enzymes that can fulfill this role. A series of capped, polyadenylated moncistronic RNAs are generated beginning at the 3′ end of the genomic RNA. This is achieved through a series of start and stop signals in the genomic RNA, and results in graded amounts of product from the 3′ to the 5′ end. As protein synthesis progresses, a complete plus strand (antigenome) of viral

RNA must be made to begin the process of producing more negative-sense virion RNA. The signal for this switch from discrete mRNA molecules to a complete genomic sequence appears to be the complexing of the RNA with N protein. Newly synthesized virion RNA can serve as template for more mRNA (secondary transcription) or can be incorporated into nucleocapsids for transport to a membrane maturation site.

Maturation of rhabdoviruses occurs through a series of coordinated movements of viral components. The virion glycoproteins are synthesized in association with the rough endoplasmic reticulum and transported to the surface of the cells through the exocytotic pathway. A key protein in the maturation process is the matrix (M) protein. This protein can bind to the nucleocapsid as well as to modified areas of the inner surface of the plasma membrane. These modified areas or "lipid rafts" have been identified as maturation sites for several of the virus families that contain membranes. It appears that the cytoplasmic tails of the surface glycoproteins are also critical for efficient budding of virus particles, but the exact signals that are necessary for the modified plasma membrane to produce the mature virion remain unknown. Unlike the picornaviruses, in the rhabdoviruses there are no mature virus particles in the infected cell. The maturation of the virus particles at the plasma membrane provides the mechanism for egress from the infected cell.

Like the picornaviruses, rhabdovirus activity is aimed towards specific inhibition of the host-cell innate antiviral defense systems described in Chapter 4. However, with a capped message system, modification of the translation process is not an option. In addition, viral proteases are not involved in the replication process, so direct degradation of host proteins is also not utilized. The paramyxoviruses and rhabdoviruses exert their inhibitory activity primarily on the interferon system—both the stimulation of interferon synthesis and the induction of an antiviral state by interferon. This appears to be achieved by competitive binding to internal pathogen recognition receptors (sensor-like elements such as MDA5 and RIG-I) that initiate the pathway for induction of interferon synthesis, or by preventing the transcription of interferon response genes (ISGs) by binding of viral proteins to the activators of transcription, resulting in their degradation. Inhibition of the induction of interferon is likely to be important during infection of animals, wherein interferon produced in one cell exerts its antiviral effect on its neighbors.

Retroviruses

The family *Retroviridae* provides several unique elements not found among viruses in the picorna- and rhabdovirus families (Figure 2.9). Penetration of the host cell is similar to that by the paramyxoviruses, in that most viruses appear

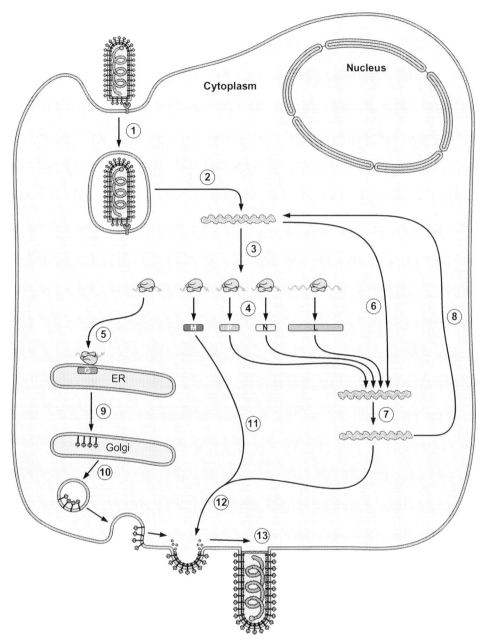

FIGURE 2.8   Single-cell reproductive cycle of a rhabdovirus. The virion binds to a cellular receptor and enters the cell via receptor-mediated endocytosis (1). The viral membrane fuses with the membrane of the endosome, releasing the helical viral nucleocapsid (2). This structure comprises (−) strand RNA coated with nucleocapsid protein molecules and a small number of L and P protein molecules, which catalyze viral RNA synthesis. The (−) strand RNA is copied into five subgenomic mRNAs by the L and P proteins (3). The N, P, M, and L mRNAs are translated by free cytoplasmic ribosomes (4), while G mRNA is translated by ribosomes bound to the endoplasmic reticulum (5). Newly synthesized N, P, and L proteins participate in viral RNA replication. This process begins with synthesis of a full-length (+) strand copy of genomic RNA, which is also in the form of a ribonucleoprotein containing the N, L, and P proteins (6). This RNA in turn serves as a template for the synthesis of progeny (−) strand RNA in the form of nucleocapsids (7). Some of these newly synthesized (−) strand RNA molecules enter the pathway for viral mRNA synthesis (8). Upon translation of G mRNA, the G protein enters the secretory pathway (9), in which it becomes glycosylated and travels to the plasma membrane (10). Progeny nucleocapsids and the M protein are transported to the plasma membrane (11 and 12), where association with regions containing the G protein initiates assembly and budding of progeny virions (13). *[From Principles of Virology, S. J. Flint, L. W. Enquist, V. R. Racaniello, A. M. Skalka, 3rd ed., vol. 1, p. 534. Copyright © Wiley (2008), with permission.]*

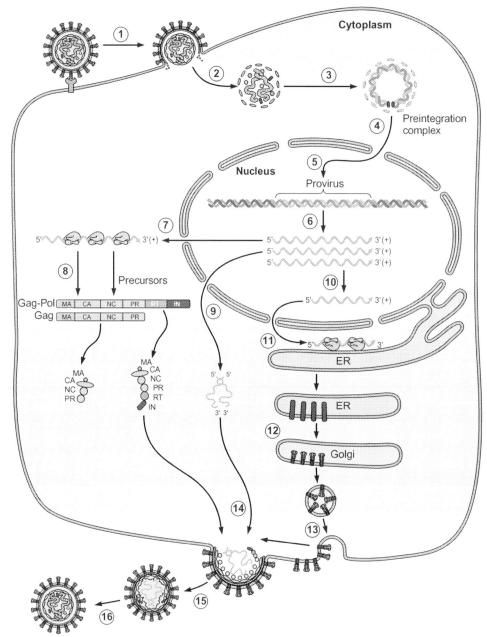

FIGURE 2.9   Single-cell reproductive cycle of a simple retrovirus. The virus attaches by binding of the viral envelope protein to specific receptors on the surface of the cell (1). The identities of receptors are known for several retroviruses. The viral core is deposited into the cytoplasm (2) following fusion of the virion and cell envelopes. Entry of some beta- and gammaretroviruses may involve endocytic pathways. The viral RNA genome is reverse transcribed by the virion reverse transcriptase (RT) (3) within a subviral particle. The product is a linear double-stranded viral DNA with ends that are shown juxtaposed in preparation for integration. Viral DNA and integrase (IN) protein gain access to the nucleus with the help of intracellular trafficking machinery or, in some cases, by exploiting nuclear disassembly during mitosis (4). Integrative recombination, catalyzed by IN, results in site-specific insertion of the viral DNA ends, which can take place at virtually any location in the host genome (5). Transcription of integrated viral DNA (the **provirus**) by host cell RNA polymerase II (6) produces full-length RNA transcripts, which are used for multiple purposes. Some full-length RNA molecules are exported from the nucleus and serve as mRNAs (7), which are translated by cytoplasmic ribosomes to form the viral Gag and Gag-Pol polyprotein precursors (8). Some full-length RNA molecules are destined to become encapsidated as progeny viral genomes (9). Other full-length RNA molecules are spliced within the nucleus (10) to form mRNA for the Env polyprotein precursor proteins. Env mRNA is translated by ribosomes bound to the endoplasmic reticulum (ER) (11). The Env proteins are transported through the Golgi apparatus (12), where they are glycosylated and cleaved by cellular enzymes to form the mature SU-TM complex. Mature envelope proteins are delivered to the surface of the infected cell (13). Virion components (viral RNA, Gag and Gag-Pol precursors, and SU-TM) assemble at budding sites (14) with the help of *cis*-acting signals encoded in each that exploit intracellular vesicular trafficking machinery. Type C retroviruses (e.g., alpharetroviruses and lentiviruses) assemble at the inner face of the plasma membrane, as illustrated. Other types (A, B, and D) assemble on internal cellular membranes. The nascent virions bud from the surface of the cell (15). Maturation (and infectivity) requires the action of the virus-encoded protease (PR), which is itself a component of the core precursor polyprotein. During or shortly after budding, PR cleaves at specific sites within the Gag and Gag-Pol precursors (16) to produce the mature virion proteins. This process causes a characteristic condensation of the virion cores. [*From* Principles of Virology, *S. J. Flint, L. W. Enquist, V. R. Racaniello, A. M. Skalka, 3rd ed., vol. 1, p. 531. Copyright © Wiley (2008), with permission.*]

to enter under neutral pH conditions at the plasma membrane. Specialized areas of the membrane may be selected through lateral movement of the virus–receptor complex. Structural rearrangements occur between the membrane proteins SU and TM during the entry process; the TM or transmembrane protein is believed to play the major role in membrane fusion. The nucleocapsid enters the cytoplasm and moves on cytoskeletal fibers to specified replication sites. The events in the uncoating process in the cytoplasm are poorly understood, but the genomic RNA becomes accessible to the RNA-dependent DNA polymerase found in the virion, as DNA synthesis is the first metabolic event in the retrovirus life cycle. Unlike picornaviruses that initially produce viral proteins, or rhabdoviruses that first produce mRNA, retroviruses use their unique polymerase to transcribe the plus-strand RNA into a double-stranded DNA copy. The virion RNA (two copies, making the virus essentially diploid) is capable of translation, but this is not the fate of the incoming genomic RNA.

A double-stranded linear DNA molecule is produced through a series of complex reactions, beginning with the priming of DNA using primer transfers RNAs (tRNAs) incorporated in the mature virion. The linear DNA molecule, still associated with a modified capsid structure, must be transported to the nucleus for integration into the host-cell genome. For many of the retroviruses, this transport and integration step is linked to cell division and the viral DNA is not available to integrate into host DNA until the nuclear membrane dissociates The exceptions to this rule are the lentiviruses and spumaviruses, which can integrate their DNA into non-dividing cells. The integration of the linear DNA into the host genome is directed by the viral integrase enzyme. It is from the integrated DNA that new viral RNA is synthesized. This process is carried out by the cellular transcription systems and the resulting RNA has all the properties of mRNA, such as a 5′ cap and a poly(A) tail at the 3′ end. A unique feature of the retroviruses is that viral messages may be spliced, thus joining two discontinuous pieces of RNA into a single virus-encoded message. This method of producing viral mRNA is not found with the picorna- or rhabdoviruses. The viral RNA molecules are transported to the cytoplasm as normal cellular mRNA, where they either associate with ribosomes for the synthesis of viral proteins or become incorporated into nucleocapsid structures.

As retroviruses are enveloped entities, the maturation process is similar but different from that of rhabdoviruses. The Env precursor protein is proteolytically processed during its synthesis in the endoplasmic reticulum and Golgi, and is transported to the cell surface as the TM and SU envelope proteins (C-type virions). A unique feature of the retroviruses is the manner in which the precursor proteins Gag and Gag-Pro-Pol participate in the maturation process. For many viruses, it is the mature proteins that are incorporated into the virion. For the retroviruses, the Gag protein enters the process as the precursor to matrix, capsid, and nucleocapsid proteins. A portion of the uncleaved precursor functions in a similar manner as the matrix protein of the paramyxoviruses and rhabdoviruses, providing a possible link with the cytoplasmic tail of the envelope protein and also binding to the membrane lipids. The presence of homologous viral glycoproteins is not essential for budding, as "bald" particles can be produced in addition to pseudotypes—virus particles with unrelated viral surface proteins. Another portion of Gag interacts with the virion RNA and may be responsible for the packaging of the RNA into the developing virion. As the Gag precursor associates with the inner surface of the plasma membrane, a budding site is established for the production of immature virus particles. Maturation for most retroviruses takes place once the virus particle is released from the plasma membrane. It is at this time that a viral protease cleaves the precursor proteins to produce the mature infectious particle. Inhibition of the protease produces non-infectious particles. As with picornaviruses, a virus-encoded protease has a key role in the replication process, but the stage in the replication process is very different for the retroviruses.

Adenoviruses

The adenoviruses are the last virus family to be described in this section, and for information on other families the reader is referred to Part II of this book. Adenoviruses are non-enveloped DNA viruses, approximately 90 nm in diameter with fibers projecting from the vertices of the icosahedron. The initial interaction with a host cell is through the fiber proteins and the coxsackievirus B and adenovirus receptor (CAR) receptor, which is the receptor for most human adenoviruses (Figure 2.10). This high-affinity binding brings the penton base protein into contact with cellular integrins, which are cell-surface receptors for extracellular matrix proteins. This binding initiates the endocytotic process involving clathrin-coated pits. Under the influence of the low pH of the endosome, the capsid structure of the virion undergoes modifications, with the loss of several virion proteins and the possible cleavage of others by the virion-associated protease. A "lytic" reaction releases the modified virion into the cytoplasm (Figure 2.6). After release from the endosome, the virions associate with the microtubule system for transport to the nucleus. At the nuclear membrane, the virion associates with the nuclear pore complex. Under the influence of the nuclear pore complex and histones, the viral DNA separates from the major virion proteins and is transported into the nucleus.

For large DNA viruses such as adenoviruses, viral gene expression can be divided into two major blocks, early and late, but these divisions have exceptions. Transcription of the viral DNA utilizes the host-cell transcription system, including the generation of spliced mRNAs. The early

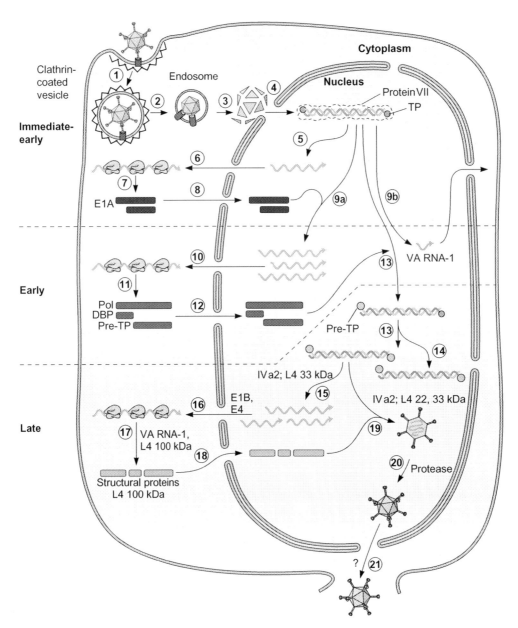

FIGURE 2.10   Single-cell reproductive cycle of human adenovirus type 2. The virus attaches to a permissive human cell via interaction between the fiber and (with most serotypes) the coxsackie-adenovirus receptor on the cell surface. The virus enters the cell via endocytosis (1 and 2), a step that depends on the interaction of a second virion protein, penton base, with a cellular integrin protein (red cylinder). Partial disassembly takes place prior to entry of particles into the cytoplasm (3). Following further uncoating, the viral genome associated with core protein VII is imported into the nucleus (4). The host cell RNA polymerase II system transcribes the immediate-early El A gene (5). Following alternative splicing and export of El A mRNAs to the cytoplasm (6), El A proteins are synthesized by the cellular translation machinery (7). These proteins are imported into the nucleus (8), where they regulate transcription of both cellular and viral genes. The larger El A protein stimulates transcription of the viral early genes by cellular RNA polymerase II (9a). Transcription of the VA genes by host cell RNA polymerase III also begins during the early phase of infection (9b). The early pre-mRNA species are processed, exported to the cytoplasm (10), and translated (11). These early proteins include the viral replication proteins, which are imported into the nucleus (12) and cooperate with a limited number of cellular proteins in viral DNA synthesis (13). Replicated viral DNA molecules can serve as templates for further rounds of replication (14) or for transcription of late genes (15). Some late promoters are activated simply by viral DNA replication, but maximally efficient transcription of the major late transcription unit (Fig. 1, ML) requires the late IVa2 and L4 proteins. Processed late mRNA species are selectively exported from the nucleus as a result of the action of the E1B 55-kDa and E4 Orf6 proteins (16). Their efficient translation in the cytoplasm (17) requires the major VA RNA. VA RNA-I, which counteracts a cellular defense mechanism, and the late L4 100-kDa protein. The latter protein also serves as a chaperone for assembly of trimeric hexons as they and the other structural proteins are imported into the nucleus (18). Within the nucleus, capsids are assembled from these proteins and the progeny viral genomes to form non-infectious immature virions (19). Assembly requires a packaging signal located near the end of the genome, as well as the IVa2 and L4 22/33-kDa proteins. Immature virions contain the precursors of the mature forms of several proteins. Mature infectious virions are formed (20) when these precursor proteins are cleaved by the viral L3 protease, which enters the virion core. Progeny virions are released (21), usually upon destruction of the host cell via mechanisms that are not well understood. *[From Principles of Virology, S. J. Flint, L. W. Enquist, V. R. Racaniello, A. M. Skalka, 3rd ed., vol. 1, p. 504. Copyright © Wiley (2008), with permission.]*

genes have at least three functions: (1) production of proteins needed for DNA replication; (2) establishment of systems for the inhibition of host-cell defenses; (3) stimulation of the cell to undergo cell division, which enhances virus replication. The first protein to be expressed is the large E1A protein, which has several effects on transcription units of other adenoviral proteins. With the onset of DNA synthesis, a large set of late genes are expressed, many from spliced mRNAs. The package of late genes includes the structural proteins of the mature virions. Structural proteins are synthesized in the cytoplasm and transported to the nucleus for assembly. Unlike the picornaviruses with a simple icosahedral structure, the adenovirus virion is a large and complex structure. Simple self-assembly models cannot account for this degree of complexity. Accordingly, viral proteins have been identified that act as chaperones for moving structural proteins to maturation sites and others that act as scaffolds for assembling the virion subunits. A virus-encoded protease that requires DNA as a co-factor to prevent premature proteolysis completes the maturation process by degrading scaffold proteins and cleaving precursor proteins. As with picornaviruses, adenovirus-infected cells show large crystalline arrays of virus particles but, in this instance, these are found as large intranuclear inclusion bodies.

The complexity of the adenovirus replication cycle and the long period (10–24 hours) to complete the cycle requires that the virus effectively inhibits the various antiviral responses available to the acutely infected cell. Adenoviruses effectively inhibit the cellular responses in many different ways. An early expressed protein of adenoviruses is the E1A protein, which can induce non-dividing cells to enter the S phase. This growth stimulation can be viewed by the cell as an abnormal event, with the induction of apoptosis (programmed cell death, see Chapter 4) that would not benefit the virus, so adenoviruses in turn produce several proteins (including E1B-19K) to block the induction of apoptosis. As with the picorna- and paramyxoviruses, adenoviruses also are capable of specifically suppressing both the production of interferon and the interferon response pathways. Part of this inhibition is mediated by small RNAs that inhibit the protein kinase (PKR) pathway that is important in interferon-mediated antiviral resistance (see Chapter 4). Viral RNAs can also interfere with the action of the interfering RNAs (RNAi) that the cell can use to inhibit the translation of viral mRNAs. Finally, adenoviruses can inhibit the synthesis of host-cell proteins by preventing the export of cellular mRNAs from the nucleus and by blocking translation of host-cell messages through modifications of the translation initiation factors. As with all viral infections, adenoviruses have evolved innovative strategies to circumvent the host-cell processes that limit virus replication and the production of new virus particles.

Assembly and Release

In the four examples just presented, two of the virus families were non-enveloped viruses and two were enveloped. All non-enveloped animal viruses have an icosahedral structure with varying degrees of complexity. The structural proteins of simple icosahedral viruses such as parvovirus and picornaviruses can associate spontaneously to form capsomers, which self-assemble to form capsids into which viral nucleic acid is packaged. Completion of the virion assembly often involves proteolytic cleavage of one or more species of capsid protein. Most non-enveloped viruses accumulate within the cytoplasm or nucleus and are released only when the cell eventually lyses. As indicated with adenovirus, the simple "self-assembly" model does not hold for the larger icosahedral viruses, as virus-encoded scaffolding proteins are needed to bring the capsids proteins into correct alignment to form a functional virus particle. Mutations in either the scaffolding proteins or the proteases that degrade these structures generate lethal mutations with respect to the production of infectious virus particles. These virus-encoded proteases can be targets for the development of antiviral agents.

All mammalian viruses with helical nucleocapsids, in addition to some with icosahedral nucleocapsids (e.g., herpesviruses, togaviruses, and retroviruses), mature by acquiring an envelope as they bud through cellular membranes. Enveloped viruses bud from the plasma membrane, from internal cytoplasmic membranes, or from the nuclear membrane. Viruses that acquire their envelope within the cell are then transported in exocytotic vesicles to the cell surface. Insertion of the viral glycoprotein(s) into the lipid bilayer of membranes occurs with lateral displacement of cellular proteins from that patch of membrane (Figure 2.8). Monomeric viral glycoprotein molecules associate into oligomers [homotrimers for the hemagglutination protein (HA) of influenza virus] to form the typical rod-shaped spike (peplomer) or club-shaped peplomer with a hydrophilic domain projecting from the external surface of the membrane, a hydrophobic transmembrane anchor domain, and a short hydrophilic cytoplasmic domain projecting slightly into the cytoplasm. In the case of icosahedral viruses (e.g., togaviruses), each protein molecule of the nucleocapsid binds directly to the cytoplasmic domain of the membrane glycoprotein oligomer, thus molding the envelope around the nucleocapsid. In the more usual case of viruses with helical nucleocapsids, it is the matrix protein that binds to the cytoplasmic domain of the glycoprotein spike (peplomer); in turn the nucleocapsid protein recognizes the matrix protein and this initiates budding of infectious virus particles. Release of each enveloped virion does not disrupt the integrity of the plasma membrane, hence thousands of virus particles may be shed over a period of several hours or days without significant cell damage.

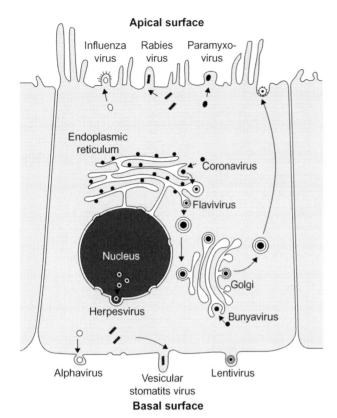

FIGURE 2.11 Sites of budding of various enveloped viruses. Viruses that bud from apical surfaces are in position to be shed in respiratory or genital secretions or intestinal contents. Viruses that bud from basal surfaces are in position for systemic spread via viremia or lymphatics. Some viruses, such as flaviviruses, bunyaviruses, and coronaviruses, take a more circuitous route in exiting the cell (see specific chapters in Part II). Viruses that do not bud usually are released only via cell lysis.

Epithelial cells display *polarity*—that is, they have an *apical* surface facing the outside world and a *basolateral* surface facing the interior of the body; the two are separated by lateral cell–cell tight junctions. These surfaces are chemically and physiologically distinct. Viruses that are shed to the exterior (e.g., influenza virus) tend to bud from the apical plasma membrane, whereas others (e.g., C-type retroviruses) bud through the basolateral membrane and are free to proceed to other sites in the body, sometimes entering the bloodstream and establishing systemic infection (Figure 2.11).

Flaviviruses, coronaviruses, arteriviruses, and bunyaviruses mature by budding through membranes of the Golgi complex or rough endoplasmic reticulum; vesicles containing the virus then migrate to the plasma membrane with which they fuse, thereby releasing the virions by the process of exocytosis (Figure 2.12). Uniquely, the envelope of the herpesviruses is acquired by budding through the inner lamella of the nuclear membrane; the enveloped virions then pass directly from the space between the two lamellae of the nuclear membrane to the exterior of the cell via the cisternae of the endoplasmic reticulum.

The budding process for some viruses may not be the final step in release of an infectious virus particle. As was noted for retroviruses, the Gag protein complex within the virus must be proteolytically processed to produce an infectious virus particle. For influenza virus, the virus must escape from the surface structures of the host cell. For this the virus needs to have an active neuraminidase enzyme to cleave the sialic acid residues from the macromolecules on the cell surface. Without the neuraminidase activity, the emerging virus particle becomes trapped at the cell surface.

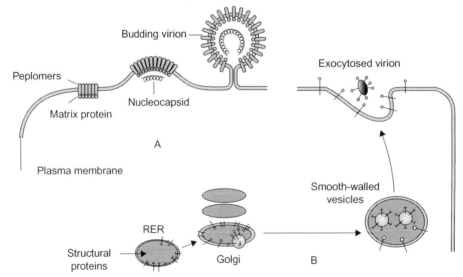

FIGURE 2.12 Maturation of enveloped viruses. (A) Viruses with a matrix protein (and some viruses without a matrix protein) bud through a patch of the plasma membrane in which glycoprotein spikes (peplomers) have accumulated over matrix protein molecules. (B) Most enveloped viruses that do not have a matrix protein bud into cytoplasmic vesicles [rough endoplasmic reticulum (RER) or Golgi], then pass through the cytoplasm in smooth vesicles and are released by exocytosis.

QUANTITATIVE ASSAYS OF VIRUSES

In dealing with virtually all aspects of viruses and viral diseases, there comes a time when it is necessary to determine how much virus exists in a given sample. The reproducibility of both *in-vitro* and *in-vivo* experiments depends upon using a consistent amount of virus to initiate an infection. In assessing clinical cases, it may be important to determine the quantity of virus in various tissues or fluids as a part of the determination of pathogenicity and to select the correct specimens for diagnostic testing. With the greater use of antivirals in treating viral infections, it is now commonplace to assess effectiveness by determining the viral load in clinical specimens. The answer to the question as to how much virus is present in an individual sample or specimen may not be simple, and is test dependent. There are basically two types of viral quantification tests—biological and physical. Tests performed on the same sample with different techniques will in some cases give vastly different answers, and it is essential to understand the reasons for these differences. Physical assays that do not depend on any biological activity of the virus particle include electron microscopic particle counts, hemagglutination, immunological assays such as antigen-capture enzyme-linked immunosorbent assay (ELISA) tests and, most recently, quantitative PCR assays. Biological assays that depend on a virus particle initiating a successful replication cycle include plaque assays and various endpoint titration methods.

The difference between the amount of virus detected using a physical assay such as particle counting by electron microscopy and a biological assay such as a plaque assay is often referred to as the particle to *plaque-forming unit* (pfu) ratio. In virtually all instances, the number of physical particles exceeds the number determined in a biological assay. For some viruses this ratio may be as high as 10,000:1, with ratios of 100:1 being common (Table 2.3). The reasons for the higher number of physical particles as compared with infectious particles are virus and assay dependent: (1) the assembly process for complete virus particles is inefficient, and morphologically complete particles are formed without the correct nucleic acid component; (2) the replication process is highly error prone (RNA viruses), and virus stocks contain particles with lethal mutations in the incorporated nucleic acid; (3) virus stocks are produced or maintained under suboptimum conditions such that infectious particles are inactivated; (4) tests for infectivity are performed in animals or cells that are not optimum for detecting infectious particles; (5) host-cell defenses prevent some infectious particles from successfully completing the replication process. The choice of host or host cell for the biological assays is a critical determinant for defining the amount of infectious virus in a sample. It is not unusual for assays in the natural host animal to provide the highest estimates of infectious units, as available cell cultures may be a poor substitute for the target cells in the animal (Table 2.3).

TABLE 2.3 Comparison of Quantitative Assay Efficiency

Method	Amount (per mL)
Direct electron microscope (EM) count	10^{10} EM particles
Quantal infectivity assay in eggs	10^9 egg ID_{50}
Quantal infectivity assay by plaque formation	10^8 pfu
Hemagglutination assay	10^3 HA units

ID_{50}, infectious dose 50; pfu, plaque-forming units; HA, hemagglutination.

Physical Assays

Direct Particle Counts by Electron Microscopy

The most direct method to determine the concentration of virus particles in a sample is to visually count the particles using an electron microscope. This process is not routinely carried out, because of the need for expensive equipment and highly trained technicians. For accuracy, the number of virus particles seen by electron microscopy must be compared with a known concentration of a standard particle such as latex beads that are added to the sample. This controls the sample volume variations that occur when preparing the samples on the solid matrix used for the procedure. Knowing the dilution of the virus preparation and the sample volume, one can calculate the concentration of virus particles. This procedure is most accurate for those viruses with unique geometric shapes such as picornaviruses, reoviruses, and adenoviruses. This process cannot assess biological activity of the preparation, but it can be used to assess whether the particles contain nucleic acid—empty capsids as opposed to complete particles.

Hemagglutination

As mentioned previously, some viruses can bind to red blood cells and produce an agglutination reaction: binding of virus to the red blood cells produces a lattice of cross-linked red blood cells. For this physical reactions to be visually detectable, the concentration of influenza virus particles must be in the range of 10^6/ml for a 0.5% chicken red blood cell suspension. A relative concentration of virus can be determined by serially diluting the sample and mixing the dilutions with red blood cells. The inverse of the greatest dilution that completely agglutinates the red blood cells is defined as the "HA titer" of the virus suspension (Figure 2.13). For influenza A viruses, this is a rapid way to assess the growth of the virus, keeping in mind the lower limits of detection. Also, this procedure does not require an intact or infectious virus particle to effect the agglutination reaction. Lipid micelles with the HA protein inserted are equally effective in agglutinating red blood cells.

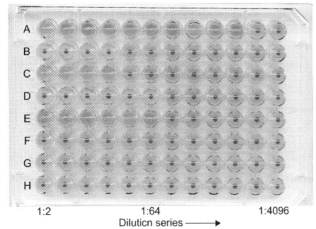

FIGURE 2.13 HA test for determining quantity of influenza virus in allantoic fluids. For determination of the quantity of influenza virus in allantoic fluid harvests from embryonated eggs using 96 well microtiter plates, the test material is serially diluted (twofold dilutions) in a buffered saline solution beginning in row 1. Following the dilution operation, an equal volume of 0.5% chicken or turkey red blood cells is added to all wells. End-point values are determined when the cell control wells show complete settling of the red blood cells ("button" formation). End-point titers are the reciprocal of the last dilution showing complete agglutination. Row A titer = 1024; Row B = <2; Row C = 16; Row D = <2; Row E = 64; Row F = <2; Row G = <2; Row H = red blood cell control.

Quantitative Polymerase Chain Reaction Assays

With the development of real-time PCR assays (see Chapter 5), it is now possible to determine the concentration of target nucleic acid in a test sample with proper controls and with special sample preparation. PCR can detect nucleic acid sequences in virtually any context, not just in a virus particle. The increased sensitivity of PCR over virus isolation in many instances is achieved by detecting non-virion nucleic acid in tissue samples. To use PCR correctly to quantify virus, it is necessary first to treat the suspension with nucleases to degrade all non-virion nucleic acid—virion nucleic acid being protected by the intact virus particle. With copy number controls in the assay system, the concentration of nucleic acid in the treated sample can be determined. This type of assay does not detect empty capsids (those that do not contain viral nucleic acid), and it does not relate to the infectivity of the preparation.

Biological Assays

Plaque Assays

Perhaps no other procedure in virology has contributed as much to the development of the field as the plaque assay. The test was originally developed by d'Herelle in 1915–1917, in his initial studies on bacteriophage. The assay is elegantly simple and is the most accurate of the quantitative biological assays. For the bacteriophage assay, serial

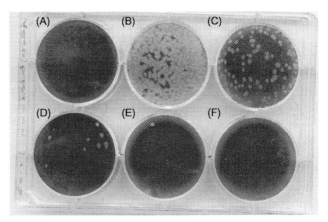

FIGURE 2.14 Plaque assay as means to determine concentration of infectious virus. Monolayer cultures of Vero cells were inoculated with serial 10-fold dilutions of vesicular stomatitis New Jersey virus. After a 1 hour period for adsorption, cultures were overlayered with 0.75% agarose in cell culture medium containing 5% fetal bovine serum. Cultures were incubated for 3 days at 37°C in a 5% CO_2-humidified atmosphere. The agarose overlay was removed and cultures fixed and stained with 0.75% crystal violet in 10% buffered formalin. A, control culture; B–F, serial 10-fold dilutions of virus: B, 10^{-3}; C, 10^{-4}; D, 10^{-5}; E, 10^{-6}; F, 10^{-7}.

10-fold dilutions of a virus sample are made in a bacterial culture medium. To these diluted samples are added a host bacterial suspension in a semi-solid culture medium (melted agar). This mixture is quickly poured onto a nutrient agar bacterial culture plate to distribute the bacterial suspension evenly. The agar hardens, preventing the movement of the initially seeded bacteria. With incubation, the host bacteria divide and produce a visible "lawn" of bacteria over the surface of the agar plate. In the control plates, there are no clear areas (plaques) in the bacterial lawn. If a high percentage of the bacterial cells are infected, the entire plate can be cleared, as all bacteria are killed by the phage. Serial dilution of the phage preparation facilitates the counting of discrete plaques so that, knowing the dilution, volume tested, and the plaque count, the concentration (titer) in the original sample can be determined. In 1953, the phage test was modified for use with the newly developed tissue culture system and animal viruses. Those viruses that produce a cytopathic effect in infected cells produced discrete "holes" in the monolayers that could be readily visualized when stained with vital dyes (Figure 2.14). More recently, immunohistochemical staining procedures have been used to develop plaque assays with non-cytopathic viruses.

In addition to its use to quantify the amount of virus in a sample, the plaque assay established a fundamental principle applicable to the vast majority of animal viruses, namely that a single virus particle was sufficient to establish a productive infection. This was proven by determining that the number of plaques in an assay increased in a linear fashion when plotted against the dilution factors—that is, the plaque number followed a one-hit kinetic curve. This is not the case

TABLE 2.4 Data for Calculating $TCID_{50}$ Endpoints

Virus Dilution	Mortality Ratio	Positive	Negative	Cumulative Positive	Cumulative Negative	Mortality Ratio	Percent Mortality
10^{-3}	8:8	8	0	23	0	23:23	100
10^{-4}	8:8	8	0	15	0	15:15	100
10^{-5}	6:8	6	2	7	2	7:9	78
10^{-6}	1:8	1	7	1	9	1:10	10
10^{-7}	0:8	0	8	0	17	0:17	0

For $TCID_{50}$ assays using microtiter plates, serial 10-fold dilutions of the virus sample are made in a cell culture medium. A sample volume (frequently 50 μl/ well) of each dilution is added to several wells (the example above is 8 wells/dilution) of the microtiter plate. A suspension of indicator cells is then added to all wells of the culture plate. Plates are then incubated for a period of time that permits clear development of cytopathology for cytopathic viruses or until such time that viral growth can be detected by immunocytochemistry. Each well is scored as positive (dead) or negative (survive) for viral growth. For calculation by Reed–Muench, a cumulative "mortality" is tabulated and the percent mortality calculated. To calculate the 50% endpoint, the following formula is followed:

$$\frac{(\% \text{ mortality at dilution next above } 50\%) - 50\%}{(\% \text{ mortality at dilution next above } 50\%) - (\% \text{ mortality at dilution next below})}$$

This gives the proportional distance between the dilutions spanning the 50% endpoint. For the data in Table 2.4, this gives:

$$\frac{78 - 50}{78 - 10} = \frac{28}{68} = 0.41$$

Adding this proportional factor to the dilution next above 50% (10^{-5}) yields a dilution of $10^{-5.4}$ to give one $TCID_{50}/50\,\mu l$ (test volume). The reciprocal of this value, adjusting for the sample volume, gives the titer of the virus stock as: 5×10^6 $TCID_{50}/ml$.

for many plant viruses, in which segmented genomes are incorporated into separate virus particles. Plaque assays were also instrumental in early studies of viral genetics, as plaque variants either occurring naturally or induced chemically could be selected (biologically cloned) and studied to determine the impact of the mutation on viral growth properties.

Endpoint Titration Assays

Before the development of the plaque assay for animal viruses, and for those viruses that do not produce plaques, the quantification of virus stocks was achieved by inoculating either test animals or embryonated eggs. As with plaque assays, serial dilutions of the sample or specimen were used to infect test animals or eggs. A successful infection could be scored directly—death of the animal or egg—or indirectly by showing an immune response to the virus in the infected host. At low dilutions, all animals would become infected whereas, at high dilutions, none of the animals would show infection. At some intermediate dilution only some of the animals or eggs would show infection. Two methods were devised (Reed–Muench or Spearman–Karber) to calculate the dilution of the virus that would infect 50% of the test animals, and the titer of the stock virus was expressed as an infectious dose 50 (ID_{50}) (Table 2.4). If the animals died, one had a lethal dose 50 (LD_{50}); for eggs one had an egg infectious dose 50 (EID_{50}); for cell-culture determinations one has a tissue culture

infectious dose 50 ($TCID_{50}$). Although not as accurate as plaque assays and not as amenable to statistical analysis, the $TCID_{50}$ endpoint system is easier to set up and automate than the plaque assay.

SPECIAL CASE OF DEFECTIVE INTERFERING MUTANTS

As noted previously, not all physical virus particles can initiate a productive infection. A special class of defective particles—*defective interfering particles*—has been demonstrated *in vitro* in most families of viruses. These mutants cannot replicate by themselves, but need the presence of the parental wild-type virus; at the same time they can interfere with and usually decrease the yield of the parental virus. All defective interfering particles of RNA viruses that have been characterized are deletion mutants. In influenza viruses and reoviruses, which have segmented genomes, defective virions lack one or more of the larger segments and contain instead smaller segments consisting of an incomplete portion of the encoded gene(s). In the case of viruses with a non-segmented genome, defective interfering particles contain RNA that is shortened: as much as two-thirds of the genome may have been deleted in the defective interfering particles of vesicular stomatitis viruses. Morphologically, defective interfering particles usually resemble the parental virions; however, with vesicular stomatitis viruses, their normally bullet-shaped virions are shorter than wild-type virions. In the jargon used to describe these particles, normal vesicular stomatitis virions are called *B particles* and the defective interfering particles are called truncated or *T particles.*

In cell culture, the concentration of defective interfering particles increases greatly with serial passage at a high multiplicity of infection—that is, infection of a cell with a high number of virus particles. This increase in defective interfering particles is the result of several possible mechanisms: (1) their shortened genomes require less time to be replicated; (2) they are less often diverted to serve as templates for transcription of mRNA; (3) they have enhanced affinity for the viral replicase, giving them a competitive advantage over their full-length counterparts. These features also explain why defective interfering particles interfere with the replication of infectious virions with full-length RNA genomes, with progressively greater efficiency on serial passage. Production of defective interfering particles can be cell-line-dependent, in that some cell types produce more of these unique particles than others with the same virus growth conditions. It is possible that the generation of these particles is part of the host-cell defense system resulting in the production of fewer infectious particles.

The generation of other defective DNA virus genomes can occur by any of a great variety of modes of DNA rearrangement, thus defective interfering particles may contain reiterated copies of the genomic origins of replication, sometimes interspersed with DNA of host-cell origin.

Our knowledge of defective interfering particles derives mostly from studies of viral infections of cultured cells, and evidence for their role in the pathogenesis of *in-vivo* infections is very limited. In experimental animal studies, inoculation with defective interfering particles and infectious virus can show some decrease in virulence, but whether this can occur naturally is unknown. One well defined instance of a defective particle being linked to disease expression occurs in cattle persistently infected with bovine viral diarrhea virus, in which the defective particle generates expression of the NS3 protein that is linked to the development of mucosal disease. In this unique situation where the animal is persistently infected with a wild-type virus, many cells can harbor both the defective genome and the complete viral genome. The non-defective virus facilitates expression of the NS3 protein sequence encoded by the defective genome. Expression of the viral NS3 protein induces cell death (cytopathology) *in-vitro*, and expression of NS3 is characteristic of all viruses that produce the mucosal disease syndrome in cattle. Defective interfering mutants may be involved in a variety of chronic animal diseases, but because their defective and variable nature makes them difficult to detect in animals, their role in disease is still obscure.

Chapter 3

Pathogenesis of Viral Infections and Diseases

Chapter Contents

Viral infection is not synonymous with disease, as many viral infections are subclinical (i.e., asymptomatic, inapparent), whereas others result in disease of varying severity that is typically accompanied by characteristic clinical signs in the affected host (Figure 3.1). Amongst many other potentially contributing factors, the outcome of the virus—host encounter is essentially the product of the virulence of the infecting virus on the one hand and the susceptibility of the host on the other. The term *virulence* is used as a quantitative or relative measure of the pathogenicity of the infecting virus—that is, a virus is said to be either pathogenic or non-pathogenic, but its virulence is stated in relative terms ("virus A is more virulent than virus B" or "virus strain A is more virulent in animal species Y than species Z"). The terms *pathogenicity* and *virulence* refer to the capacity of a virus to cause disease in its host, and are unrelated to the infectivity or transmissibility (contagiousness) of the virus.

For viruses to cause disease they must first infect their host, spread to (and within) and damage target tissues. To ensure their perpetuation, viruses must then be transmitted to other susceptible individuals—that is, they must be shed with secretions or excretions into the environment, be taken up by another host or a vector, or be passed congenitally from mother to offspring. Viruses have developed a remarkable variety of strategies to ensure their own survival. Similarly, individual viruses cause their associated diseases through a considerable variety of distinct pathogenic mechanisms.

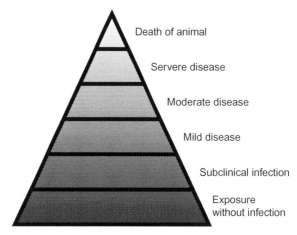

FIGURE 3.1 The iceberg concept of viral infection and diseases.

INTERPLAY OF VIRAL VIRULENCE AND HOST RESISTANCE, OR SUSCEPTIBILITY FACTORS IN EXPRESSION OF VIRAL DISEASES

Viruses differ greatly in their virulence, but even in a population infected by a particular virus strain there are usually striking differences in the outcome of infection of individual animals. Similarly, there is much variation amongst viruses

Fenner's Veterinary Virology. DOI: 10.1016/B978-0-12-375158-4.00003-1

of the same species and the determinants of viral virulence are often multigenic, meaning that several viral genes contribute to the virulence of individual viruses. Similarly, the determinants of host resistance/susceptibility are usually multifactorial, and include not only a variety of host factors but environmental ones as well.

The advent and application of molecular technologies has facilitated mapping of virulence determinants in the genome of many viruses (e.g., by whole-genomic sequencing of virus strains, and manipulation of molecular clones), as well as the location of resistance/susceptibility determinants in the genome of experimental animals. Virus strain differences may be quantitative, involving the rate and yield of virus replication, lethal dose, infectious dose, the number of cells infected in a given organ, or they may be qualitative, involving organ or tissue tropism, extent of host-cell damage, mode and efficacy of spread in the body, and character of the disease they induce.

Assessment of Viral Virulence

There is wide variation in the virulence of viruses, ranging from those that almost always cause inapparent infections, to those that usually cause disease, to those that usually cause death. Meaningful comparison of the virulence of viruses requires that factors such as the infecting dose of the virus and the age, sex, and condition of the host animals and their immune status be equal; however, these conditions are never met in nature, where heterogeneous, outbred animal populations are the rule and the dynamics of exposure and viral infection are incredibly varied. Hence, subjective and vague terminology may be used to describe the virulence of particular viruses in domestic and wild animals. Precise measures of virulence are usually derived only from assays in inbred animals such as mice. Of course, such assays are only feasible for those viruses that grow in mice, and care must always be exercised in extrapolating data from mice to the host species of interest.

The virulence of a particular strain of virus administered in a particular dose, by a particular route, to a particular age and strain of laboratory animal may be assessed by determining its ability to cause disease, death, specific clinical signs, or lesions. The dose of the virus required to cause death in 50% of animals [lethal dose 50 (LD_{50})] has been a commonly used measure of virulence, but is now passing out of favor in the research arena for ethical reasons. For example, in the susceptible BALB/c strain of mouse, the LD_{50} of a virulent strain of ectromelia virus is 5 virions, as compared with 5000 for a moderately attenuated strain and about 1 million for a highly attenuated strain. Viral virulence can also be measured in experimental animals by determining the ratio of the dose of a particular strain of virus that causes infection in 50% of individuals [infectious dose 50 (ID_{50})] to the dose that kills

50% of individuals (the $ID_{50}:LD_{50}$ ratio). Thus, the ID_{50} of a virulent strain of ectromelia virus in BALB/c mice is 2 virions and the LD_{50} about 5 virions, whereas for resistant C57BL strain mice the ID_{50} is the same but the LD_{50} is 1 million virions. The severity of an infection, therefore, depends on the interplay between the virulence of the virus and the resistance of the host. Viral virulence also can be estimated through assessment of the severity, location, and distribution of gross, histologic, and ultrastructural lesions in affected animals.

Determinants of Viral Virulence

The advent of molecular biology has facilitated determination of the genetic basis of virulence of many viruses, along with other important aspects of their replication. Specifically, the role of potential determinants of virulence identified by genetic sequence comparison of viruses of defined virulence can be confirmed unequivocally by manipulation of molecular clones of the virus in question. This "reverse genetics" strategy utilizing molecular (infectious) clones was first widely employed using complementary DNA (cDNA) copies of the entire genome of simple positive-strand RNA viruses such as alphaviruses and picornaviruses, as RNA transcribed from full-length cDNA copies (clones) of these viruses is itself infectious after transfection into cells. The virion RNA of negative-sense RNA viruses such as rhabdoviruses is not infectious, but infectious virus can be recovered from cDNA clones if the necessary proteins are also produced in cells transfected with full-length RNA transcripts. Even the considerable logistical challenges posed by RNA viruses with segmented genomes (such as influenza viruses, bunyaviruses, arenaviruses, and reoviruses) have been overcome, and molecular clones of these viruses are now used for reverse genetic manipulation. It is also now possible to specifically manipulate the genomes of even the very large DNA viruses as artificial chromosomes. Of necessity, most experimental work has been carried out in inbred laboratory animals, although molecular clones of a substantial number of pathogenic animal viruses have now been evaluated in their respective natural animal hosts. It is apparent from these reverse genetic studies that several viral genes can contribute to the virulence of individual viruses, as described under each virus family in Part II of this book.

Viruses exhibit host and tissue specificity (tropism), usually more than is appreciated clinically. Mechanistically, the organ or tissue tropism of the virus is an expression of all the steps required for successful infection, from the interaction of virus attachment molecules and their cellular receptors to virus assembly and release (see Chapter 2). Organ and tissue tropisms also involve all stages in the course of infection in the whole host animal, from the site of entry, to the major target organs responsible for the clinical signs, to the site involved in virus release and shedding.

Caution should be exercised in attributing characteristics of viral epidemics or epizootics solely to the virulence of the causative virus, as there typically is considerable variation in the response of individual infected animals, both within and between animal species. For example, during the epizootic of West Nile virus infection that began in North America in 1999, approximately 10% of infected horses developed neurological disease (encephalomyelitis) and, of these, approximately 30–35% died. Neuroinvasive disease was even less common in humans infected with this same strain of West Nile virus, whereas infected corvids (crows and their relatives) almost uniformly developed disseminated, rapidly fatal infections.

Determinants of Host Resistance/ Susceptibility

As just described for West Nile virus, genetic differences in host resistance/susceptibility to viral infections are most obvious when different animal species are compared. Viral infections tend to be less pathogenic in their natural host species than in exotic or introduced species. For instance, myxoma virus produces a small benign fibroma in its natural host, which are wild rabbits of the Americas (*Sylvilagus* spp.), but an almost invariably fatal generalized infection in the European rabbit, *Oryctolagus cuniculus*. Likewise, zoonotic (transmitted from animal to human) infections caused by arenaviruses, filoviruses, and many arboviruses are severe in humans but mild or asymptomatic in their reservoir animal hosts.

The innate and adaptive immune responses to particular viral infections differ greatly from one individual to another (see Chapter 4). Studies with inbred strains of mice have confirmed that susceptibility to specific viruses may be associated with particular major histocompatibility antigen haplotypes, presumably because of their central role in directing the nature of the adaptive immune response generated to the infecting virus. Similarly, studies with genetically modified mice have unequivocally confirmed the critical role of innate immune responses, especially those associated with the interferon system, in conferring antiviral resistance and protection.

Expression of critical receptors on target cells is a fundamental determinant of host resistance/susceptibility to a particular virus. The more conserved or ubiquitous the receptor, the wider the host range of the virus that exploits it; for example, rabies virus, which uses sialylated gangliosides in addition to the acetylcholine receptor, has a very wide host range, but infection is restricted narrowly to a few host cell types, including myocytes, neurons, and salivary gland epithelium. Changes in viral attachment proteins can lead to the emergence of variant viruses with different tropism and disease potential. For example, porcine respiratory coronavirus arose from transmissible gastroenteritis virus, which is strictly an enteric pathogen, through a substantial deletion in the gene encoding the viral spike protein that mediates virus attachment. This change affected the tropism of the virus as well as its transmissibility.

Physiologic Factors Affecting Host Resistance/ Susceptibility

In addition to innate and adaptive immune responses, a considerable variety of physiologic factors affect host resistance/susceptibility to individual viral diseases, including age, nutritional status, levels of certain hormones, and cell differentiation.

Viral infections tend to be most serious at both ends of life—in the very young and the very old. Rapid physiologic changes occur during the immediate postpartum period and resistance to the most severe manifestations of many intestinal and respiratory infections builds quickly in the neonate. Maturation of the immune system is responsible for much of this enhanced, age-related resistance, but physiologic changes also contribute. Malnutrition can also potentially impair immune responsiveness in adults, but it often difficult to distinguish adverse nutritional effects from other factors found in animals living in very adverse environments.

Certain infections, particularly herpesvirus infections, can be reactivated during pregnancy, leading to abortion or perinatal infection of the progeny of infected dams. The fetus itself is uniquely susceptible to a number of different viral infections.

Cellular differentiation and the stage of the cell cycle may affect susceptibility to infection with specific viruses. For example, parvoviruses replicate only in cells that are in the late S phase of the cell cycle, so the rapidly dividing cells of bone marrow, intestinal epithelium, and the developing fetus are vulnerable. The rapidly dividing, often migratory cell populations that occur during embryogenesis in the developing fetus are exquisitely susceptible to infection and injury by a number of viruses, notably several highly teratogenic viruses that infect the developing central nervous system.

Almost all viral infections are accompanied by fever. In classic studies of myxoma virus infection in rabbits, it was shown that increasing body temperature increased protection against disease, whereas decreasing temperature increased the severity of infection. Blocking the development of fever with drugs (e.g., salicylates) increased mortality. Similar results have been obtained with ectromelia and coxsackievirus infections in mice. In contrast, fever does not accompany viral infection in certain poikilotherms (e.g., fish), in which this response is probably of no or lesser selective advantage.

The immunosuppressive effects of increased concentrations of corticosteroids, whether endogenous or exogenous in origin, can reactivate latent viral infections or exacerbate active mild or subclinical viral infections, such as those caused by herpesviruses. This mechanism probably contributes to the increased incidence of severe viral infections that occurs in settings in which animals are transported or brought into crowded environments, such as animal shelters and feedlots. Products of host inflammatory and innate immune responses also probably contribute to the transient immunosuppression and other general signs that can accompany viral infections.

MECHANISMS OF VIRAL INFECTION AND VIRUS DISSEMINATION

At the level of the cell, infection by viruses (see Chapters 1 and 2) is quite different from that caused by bacteria and other microorganisms, whereas at the level of the whole animal and animal populations there are more similarities than differences. Like microorganisms, viruses must gain entry into their host's body before they can exert their pathogenic effects; entry of virus into the host can occur through any of a variety of potential routes, depending on the properties of the individual virus (Figure 3.2; Table 3.1).

Routes of Virus Entry

Viruses are obligate intracellular parasites that are transmitted as inert particles. To infect its host, a virus must first attach to and infect cells at one of the body surfaces, unless these potential barriers are bypassed by parenteral inoculation via a wound, needle, or the bite of an arthropod or vertebrate. Cedric Mims represented the animal body as a set of surfaces, each covered by a sheet of epithelial cells separating host tissues from the outside world (Figure 3.2). The skin that covers the animal body externally has a relatively impermeable outer layer of keratin, whereas the mucosal epithelial lining of the respiratory tract and much of the gastrointestinal and urogenital tracts lacks this protective layer. Similarly, in and around the eyes, the protective keratinized layer of skin is replaced by the non-keratinized epithelial lining of the conjunctiva and cornea. Each of these sites is the target for invasion by specific viruses. In animals without significant areas of keratinized epithelium (e.g., fish), the skin and gills serve as an extensive mucosal surface that is the initial site of infection with many viruses.

Entry via the Respiratory Tract

The mucosal surfaces of the respiratory tract are lined by epithelial cells that can potentially support the replication of viruses, so defenses are necessary to minimize the risk of infection. The respiratory tract from the nasal passages to the

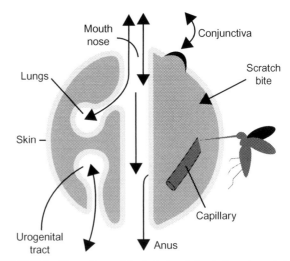

FIGURE 3.2 The surfaces of the body in relation to the entry and shedding of viruses. *(Courtesy of C. A. Mims.)*

TABLE 3.1 Obligatory Steps in Viral Infection

Step in Infection Process	Requirement for Virus Survival and Progression of Infection
Entry into host and primary virus replication	Evade host's natural protective and cleansing mechanisms
Local or general spread in the host, cell and tissue tropism, and secondary virus replication	Evade immediate host defenses and natural barriers to spread; at the cellular level the virus takes over necessary host-cell functions for its own replication processes
Evasion of host inflammatory and immune defenses	Evade host inflammatory, phagocytic, and immune defenses long enough to complete the virus transmission cycle
Shedding from host	Exit host body at site and at concentration needed to ensure infection of the next host
Cause damage to host	Not necessary, but this is the reason we are interested in the virus and its pathogenetic processes

distal airways in the lungs is protected by the "mucociliary blanket," which consists of a layer of mucus produced by goblet cells that is kept in continuous flow by the coordinated beating of cilia on the luminal surface of the epithelial cells that line the nasal mucosa and airways. The airspaces (alveoli) are protected by resident alveolar macrophages. The distance to which inhaled particles penetrate into the respiratory tract is inversely related to their size, so that larger particles (greater than 10 μm in diameter) are trapped on the mucociliary blanket lining the nasal cavity and airways and small particles (less than 5μm in diameter) can be inhaled directly into the airspaces, where they are ingested by alveolar macrophages. Most inhaled virions are trapped in mucus and then carried by ciliary action from the nasal cavity and airways to the pharynx, and then swallowed or coughed out.

The respiratory system is also protected by the innate and adaptive immune mechanisms that operate at all mucosal surfaces (see Chapter 4), including specialized lymphoid aggregates [e.g., nasal associated lymphoid tissue (NALT) and tonsils- and bronchus-associated lymphoid tissue (BALT)] that occur throughout the respiratory tree. Despite its protective mechanisms, however, the respiratory tract is perhaps the most common portal of virus entry into the body. Viruses can infect the host via the respiratory tract by first attaching to specific receptors on epithelial cells within the mucosa, thus avoiding clearance by either the mucociliary blanket or phagocytic cells. After invasion, some viruses remain localized to the respiratory system, or spread from cell to cell to invade other tissues, whereas many others become widely disseminated via lymphatics and/or the bloodstream.

Entry via the Gastrointestinal Tract

A substantial number of viruses (enteric viruses) are spread to susceptible hosts by ingestion of virus-contaminated food or drink. The mucosal lining of the oral cavity and esophagus (and forestomachs of ruminants) is relatively refractory to viral infection, with the notable exception of that overlying the tonsils, thus enteric viral infections typically begin within the mucosal epithelium of the stomach and/or intestines. The gastrointestinal tract is protected by several different defenses, including acidity of the stomach, the layer of mucus that tenaciously covers the mucosa of the stomach and intestines, the antimicrobial activity of digestive enzymes as well as that of bile and pancreatic secretions, and innate and adaptive immune mechanisms, especially the activity of defensins and secretory antibodies such as immunoglobulin (Ig) A, the latter produced by B lymphocytes in the gastrointestinal mucosa and mucosal associated lymphoid tissues. Despite these protective mechanisms, enteric infection is characteristic of certain viruses that first infect the epithelial cells lining the gastrointestinal mucosa or the specialized M cells that overlie intestinal lymphoid aggregates (Peyer's patches).

In general, viruses that cause purely enteric infection, such as rotaviruses and enteroviruses, are acid and bile resistant. However, there are acid- and bile-labile viruses that cause important enteric infections; for example, coronaviruses such as transmissible gastroenteritis virus are protected during passage through the stomach of young animals by the buffering action of suckled milk. Not only do some enteric viruses resist inactivation by proteolytic enzymes in the stomach and intestine, their infectivity is actually increased by such exposure. Thus cleavage of an outer capsid protein by intestinal proteases enhances the infectivity of rotaviruses and some coronaviruses. Rotaviruses, coronaviruses, toroviruses, and astroviruses are all major causes of viral diarrhea in animals, whereas the great majority of enteric infections caused by enteroviruses and adenoviruses are asymptomatic. Parvoviruses, morbilliviruses, and many other viruses can also cause gastrointestinal infection and diarrhea, but only after reaching cells of the gastrointestinal tract in the course of generalized (systemic) infection after viremic spread.

Entry via the Skin

The skin is the largest organ of the body, and its dense outer layer of keratin provides a mechanical barrier to the entry of viruses. The low pH and presence of fatty acids in skin provide further protection, as do various other components of innate and adaptive immunity, including the presence of migratory dendritic cells (Langerhans cells) within the epidermis itself. Breaches in skin integrity such as insect or animal bites, cuts, punctures, or abrasions predispose to viral infection, which can either remain confined to the skin, such as the papillomaviruses, or disseminate widely. Deeper trauma can introduce viruses into the dermis and subcutis, where there is a rich supply of blood vessels, lymphatics, and nerves that can individually serve as routes of virus dissemination. Generalized infection of the skin, such as occurs in lumpy skin disease, sheeppox, and others, is the result, not of localized cutaneous infection but of systemic viral spread via viremia.

One of the most efficient ways by which viruses are introduced through the skin is via the bite of arthropods, such as mosquitoes, ticks, *Culicoides* spp. (hematophagous midges), or sandflies. Insects, especially flies, may act as simple mechanical vectors ("flying needles"); for example, equine infectious anemia virus is spread among horses, rabbit hemorrhagic disease virus and myxoma virus are spread among rabbits, and fowlpox virus among chickens in this way. However, most viruses that are spread by arthropods replicate in their vector. Viruses that are both transmitted by and replicate in arthropod vectors are called *arboviruses*.

Infection can also be acquired through the bite of an animal, as in rabies, and introduction of a virus by skin penetration may be iatrogenic—that is, the result of veterinary or husbandry procedures. For example, equine infectious anemia virus has been transmitted via contaminated needles, twitches, ropes, and harnesses, and orf virus and papillomaviruses can be transmitted via ear tagging, tattooing, or virus-contaminated inanimate objects (*fomites*).

Entry via Other Routes

Several important pathogens (e.g., several herpesviruses and papillomaviruses) are spread through the genital tract.

Small tears or abrasions in the penile mucosa and the epithelial lining of the vagina may occur during sexual activity and facilitate transmission of venereal virus. The conjunctiva, although much less resistant to viral invasion than the skin, is constantly cleansed by the flow of secretion (tears) and mechanical wiping by the eyelids; some adenoviruses and enteroviruses gain entry at this site, and a substantial number of viruses can be experimentally transmitted by this route.

Host Specificity and Tissue Tropism

The capacity of a virus to infect cells selectively in particular organs is referred to as tropism (either cell or organ tropism), which is dependent on both viral and host factors. At the cellular level, there must be an interaction between viral attachment proteins and matching cellular receptors. Although such interactions are usually studied in cultured cells, the situation is considerably more complex *in vivo*. Not only do some viruses require several cellular receptors/co-receptors (see Chapter 2), some viruses utilize different receptors on different cells; for example, the cell attachment glycoprotein of human immunodeficiency virus can bind several receptors (including CD4, CXCR4 and CCR5), which allows it to infect both T lymphocytes and macrophages. Expression of receptors can be dynamic; for example, it has been shown experimentally that animals treated with neuraminidase have substantial protection against intranasal infection with influenza virus that lasts until the neuraminidase-sensitive receptors have regenerated. Receptors for a particular virus are usually restricted to certain cell types in certain organs, and only these cells can be infected. In large part, this accounts for both the tissue and organ tropism of a given virus and the pathogenesis of the disease caused by the virus.

The presence of critical receptors is not the only factor that determines whether the cell may become infected—intracellular factors that exert their effect subsequent to virus attachment, such as viral enhancers, may also be required for productive infection. Viral enhancers are gene activators that increase the efficiency of transcription of viral or cellular genes; specifically, they are short, often tandem-repeated sequences of nucleotides that may contain motifs representing DNA-binding sites for various cellular or viral site-specific DNA-binding proteins (transcription factors). Viral enhancers augment binding of DNA-dependent RNA polymerase to promoters, thereby accelerating transcription. Because many of the transcription factors affecting individual enhancer sequences in viruses are restricted to particular cells, tissues, or host species, they can determine the tropism of viruses and can act as specific virulence factors. The genomic DNA of papillomavirus contains such enhancers, which are active only in keratinocytes and, indeed, only in the subset of these cells in which papillomavirus replication occurs. Enhancer sequences have also been defined in the genomes of retroviruses and several herpesviruses, amongst others, where they also appear to influence tropism by regulating the expression of viral genes in specific cell types.

Mechanisms of Viral Spread and Infection of Target Organs

Virus replication may be restricted to the body surface through which the virus entered—for example, the skin, respiratory tract, gastrointestinal tract, genital tract, or conjunctiva. Alternatively, the invading virus may breach the epithelial barrier and be spread through the blood (hematogenous spread), lymphatics, or nerves to cause a generalized infection, or infection in a specific site such as the central nervous system (brain and spinal cord).

In pioneering experiments in 1949, Frank Fenner used ectromelia virus (the agent of mousepox) as a model system that first revealed the sequence of events leading to systemic infection and disease. Groups of mice were inoculated in the footpad of a hind limb, and at daily intervals their organs were titrated to determine the amount of virus present. Fenner showed that, during the incubation period, infection spread through the mouse body in a stepwise fashion (Figure 3.3). The virus first replicated locally in tissues of the footpad and then in the draining lymph nodes. Virus produced in these sites then gained entry into the bloodstream, causing a primary viremia, which brought the virus to its initial target organs (organ tropism), especially the spleen, lymph nodes, and the liver. This stage of infection was accompanied by the development of focal necrosis, first in the skin and draining lymph nodes in the inoculated hind limb and then in the spleen and liver. Within days there was extensive necrosis in both the spleen and liver, and rapid death. However, this was not the entire pathogenetic sequence because, to complete the viral life cycle, shedding and infection of the next host had to be explained. Fenner found that the virus produced in the target organs—that is, the spleen and liver—caused a secondary viremia that disseminated virus to the skin and mucosal surfaces. Infection in the skin caused a macular and papular rash from which large amounts of virus were shed, leading to contact exposure of other mice. Fenner's studies with ectromelia virus stimulated similar studies that have defined the pathogenesis of many other viral infections.

Local Spread on Epithelial Surfaces

Viruses first replicate in epithelial cells at the site of entry and produce a localized infection, often with associated virus shedding directly into the environment from these sites. The spread of infection along epithelial surfaces

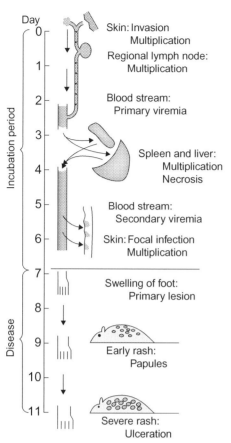

Day

0 — Skin: Invasion
Multiplication

1 — Regional lymph node:
Multiplication

2 — Blood stream:
Primary viremia

3 —

4 — Spleen and liver:
Multiplication
Necrosis

5 — Blood stream:
Secondary viremia

6 — Skin: Focal infection
Multiplication

7 — Swelling of foot:
Primary lesion

8 —

9 — Early rash:
Papules

10 —

11 — Severe rash:
Ulceration

Incubation period

Disease

FIGURE 3.3 Frank Fenner's classic study of the pathogenesis of ectromelia (mousepox) viral infection. This was the first study ever done using serial (daily) titration of the viral content of organs and tissues, and the model for many studies that have since advanced knowledge of the pathogenesis of systemic viral infections. *[From F. Fenner. Mousepox (infectious ectromelia of mice): a review. J. Immunol. 63, 341–373 (1949), with permission.]*

occurs by the sequential infection of neighboring cells, which, depending on the individual virus, may or may not precede spread into the adjacent subepithelial tissues and beyond.

In the skin, papillomaviruses and poxviruses such as orf virus remain confined to the epidermis, where they induce localized proliferative lesions, whereas other poxviruses such as lumpy skin disease virus, spread widely after cutaneous infection. Viruses that enter the body via the respiratory or intestinal tracts can quickly cause extensive infection of the mucosal epithelium, thus diseases associated with these infections progress rapidly after a short incubation period. In mammals, there is little or no productive invasion of subepithelial tissues of the respiratory tract after most influenza and parainfluenza virus infections, or in the intestinal tract following most rotavirus and coronavirus infections. Although these viruses apparently enter lymphatics and thus have the potential to spread, they usually do not do so, because appropriate

viral receptors or other permissive cellular factors such as cleavage-activating proteases or transcription enhancers are restricted to epithelial cells, or because of other physiological constraints.

Restriction of viral infection to an epithelial surface should never be equated with any lack of virulence or disease severity. Although localized, injury to the intestinal mucosa caused by rotaviruses and coronaviruses can result in severe and, especially in neonates, even fatal diarrhea. Similarly, influenza virus infection can cause extensive injury in the lungs, leading to acute respiratory distress syndrome and possibly death.

Subepithelial Invasion and Lymphatic Spread

A variety of factors probably contribute to the ability of some viruses to breach the epithelial barrier and to invade the subepithelial tissues, including (1) targeted migration of virus within phagocytic leukocytes, specifically dendritic cells and macrophages, and (2) directional shedding of viruses from the infected epithelium (see Chapter 2). Dendritic cells are abundant in the skin and at all mucosal surfaces, where they constitute a critical first line of immune defense, both innate and adaptive (see Chapter 4). Migratory dendritic cells (such as Langerhans cells in the skin) "traffic" from epithelial surfaces to the adjacent (draining), regional lymph node, and infection of these cells may be responsible for the initial spread of alphaviruses, bluetongue and other orbiviruses, and feline and simian human immunodeficiency viruses, amongst many others. Directional release of virus into the lumen of the respiratory or intestinal tracts facilitates local spread to the surface of contiguous epithelial cells and immediate shedding into the environment, whereas shedding from the basolateral cell surface of epithelial cells potentially facilitates invasion of subepithelial tissues and subsequent virus dissemination via lymphatics, blood vessels, or nerves.

Many viruses that are widely disseminated in the body following infection at epithelial surfaces are first carried to the adjacent (local) lymph nodes through the afferent lymphatic drainage (Figure 3.4). Within the draining lymph node, virions may be inactivated and processed by macrophages and dendritic cells so that their component antigens are presented to adjacent lymphocytes to stimulate adaptive immune responses (see Chapter 4). Some viruses, however, replicate efficiently in macrophages (e.g., many retroviruses, orbiviruses, canine distemper virus and other morbilliviruses, arteriviruses such as porcine reproductive and respiratory syndrome virus, and some herpesviruses), and/or in dendritic cells and lymphocytes. From the regional lymph node, virus can spread to the bloodstream in efferent lymph, and then quickly be disseminated throughout the body, either within cells or as cell-free virions. Blood-filtering organs, including the lung, liver, and

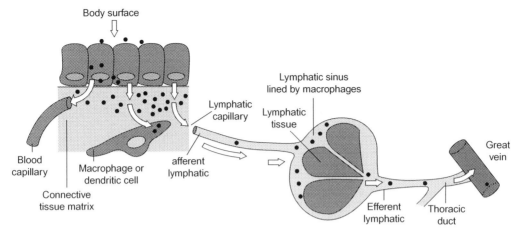

FIGURE 3.4 Subepithelial invasion and lymphatic spread of infection. *(Adapted from the work of C. A. Mims.)*

spleen, are often target organs (tropism) of viruses that cause disseminated infections.

Normally, there is a local inflammatory response at the site of viral invasion, the severity of which reflects the extent of tissue damage. Inflammation leads to characteristic alterations in the flow and permeability of local blood vessels, as well as leukocyte trafficking and activity; some viruses take advantage of these events to infect cells that participate in this inflammatory response, which in turn can facilitate spread of these viruses either locally or systemically. Local inflammation may be especially important to the pathogenesis of arthropod-transmitted viruses because of the marked reaction at the site of virus inoculation induced by the bite of the arthropod vector.

Spread via the Bloodstream: Viremia

The blood is the most effective vehicle for rapid spread of virus through the body. Initial entry of virus into the blood after infection is designated primary viremia, which, although usually inapparent clinically, leads to the seeding of distant organs—as exemplified in Fenner's pioneering studies of ectromelia virus infection. Virus replication in major target organs leads to the sustained production of much higher concentrations of virus, producing a secondary viremia (Figure 3.5) and infection in yet other parts of the body that ultimately results in the clinical manifestations of the associated disease.

In the blood, virions may circulate free in the plasma or may be contained in, or adsorbed to, leukocytes, platelets, or erythrocytes. Parvoviruses, enteroviruses, togaviruses, and flaviviruses typically circulate free in the plasma. Viruses carried in leukocytes, generally lymphocytes or monocytes, are often not cleared as readily or in the same way as viruses that circulate in the plasma. Specifically, cell-associated viruses may be protected from antibodies and other plasma components, and they can be carried as

"passengers" when leukocytes that harbor the virus emigrate into tissues. Individual viruses exhibit tropism to different leukocyte populations; thus monocyte-associated viremia is characteristic of canine distemper, whereas lymphocyte-associated viremia is a feature of Marek's disease and bovine leukosis. Erythrocyte-associated viremia is characteristic of infections caused by African swine fever virus and bluetongue virus. The association of bluetongue virus with erythrocytes facilitates both prolonged viremia by delaying immune clearance, and infection of the hematophagous (blood feeding) *Culicoides* midges that serve as biological vectors of the virus. A substantial number of viruses, including equine infectious anemia virus, bovine viral diarrhea virus, and bluetongue virus, associate with platelets during viremia—an interaction that might facilitate infection of endothelial cells. Neutrophils, like platelets, have a very short lifespan; neutrophils also possess powerful antimicrobial mechanisms and they are rarely infected, although they may contain phagocytosed virions.

Virions circulating in the blood are removed continuously by macrophages, thus viremia can typically be maintained only if there is a continuing introduction of virus into the blood from infected tissues or if clearance by tissue macrophages is impaired. Although circulating leukocytes can themselves constitute a site for virus replication, viremia is usually maintained by infection of the parenchymal cells of target organs such as the liver, spleen, lymph nodes, and bone marrow. In some infections, such as African horse sickness virus and equine arteritis virus infections of horses, viremia is largely maintained by the infection of endothelial cells and/or macrophages and dendritic cells. Striated and smooth muscle may also be an important site of replication of some certain viruses.

There is a general correlation between the magnitude of viremia generated by blood-borne viruses and their capacity to invade target tissues, thus the failure of some attenuated vaccine viruses to generate a significant viremia may

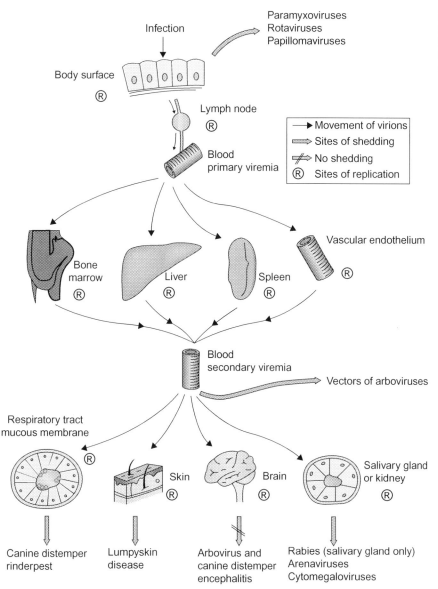

FIGURE 3.5 The role of viremia in the spread of viruses through the body, indicating sites of replication and important routes of shedding of various viruses. *(Adapted from the work of C. A. Mims and D. O. White.)*

account for their lack of tissue invasiveness. Certain neurotropic viruses are virulent after intracerebral inoculation, but avirulent when given peripherally, because they do not attain viremia titers sufficient to facilitate invasion of the nervous system. The capacity to produce viremia and the capacity to invade tissues from the bloodstream are thus two different properties of a virus. For example, some strains of Semliki Forest virus (and certain other alphaviruses) have lost the capacity to invade the central nervous system while retaining the capacity to generate a viremia equivalent in duration and magnitude to that produced by neuroinvasive strains.

Viruses that circulate in blood, especially those that circulate free in plasma, encounter, amongst many others, two cell types that exert especially important roles in determining the subsequent pathogenesis of infection: macrophages and vascular endothelial cells.

Virus Interactions with Macrophages

Macrophages are bone marrow-derived mononuclear phagocytic cells that are present in all compartments of the body, including those that occur "free" in plasma (monocytes) or the pulmonary airspaces (alveolar macrophages), and those that are present in all tissues, including the subepithelial connective tissues beneath mucosal surfaces, fixed tissue macrophages such as osteoclasts (bone), microglia (central nervous system), and those that line the sinusoids of the lymph nodes and liver, spleen, bone marrow, etc. Together with dendritic cells, macrophages have a critical role in antigen processing and presentation to other immune cells that is central to the initiation of adaptive immune responses (see Chapter 4). They also initiate innate immune responses because of their ability to detect the presence of pathogen-associated molecular patterns

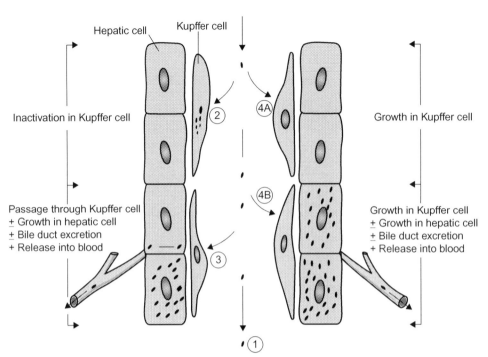

FIGURE 3.6   Types of interaction between viruses and macrophages, exemplified by Kupffer cells, the macrophages that line the sinusoids in the liver. (1) Macrophages may fail to phagocytose virions; e.g., in Venezuelan equine encephalitis virus infection this is an important factor favoring prolonged high viremia. (2) Virions may be phagocytosed and destroyed: because the macrophage system is so efficient, viremia can be maintained only if virions enter the blood as fast as they are removed. (3) Virions may be phagocytosed and then transferred passively to adjacent cells (hepatocytes in the liver); e.g., in Rift Valley fever virus infection, the virus replicates in hepatocytes and causes severe hepatitis—the virus produced in the liver sustains the high viremia. (4) Virions may be phagocytosed by macrophages and then may replicate in them: (4A) with some viruses, such as lactate dehydrogenase elevating virus in mice, only macrophages are infected and progeny from that infection are the source of the extremely high viremia; (4B) more commonly, as in infectious canine hepatitis, the virus replicates in both macrophages and hepatocytes, producing severe hepatitis. *(Adapted from the work of C. A. Mims and D. O. White.)*

(PAMPs) through specific receptors—for example, Toll-like receptors. Macrophages are heterogeneous in their functional activity, which can vary markedly depending on their location and state of activation; even in a given tissue or site there are subpopulations of macrophages that differ in phagocytic activity and in susceptibility to viral infection. The various kinds of interactions that can occur between macrophages and virions may be described in relation to Kupffer cells, the macrophages that line the sinusoids of the liver, as shown in Figure 3.6. Not shown in this model is tissue invasion via carriage of virus inside monocytes/macrophages that emigrate through the walls of small blood vessels—sometimes referred to as the "Trojan Horse" mechanism of invasion, which is especially important in the pathogenesis of lentivirus infections.

Differences in virus–macrophage interactions may account for differences in the virulence of individual strains of the same virus, and differences in host resistance. Although macrophages are inherently efficient phagocytes, this capacity is even further enhanced after their activation by certain microbial products and cytokines such as interferon-γ. Macrophages also have Fc receptors and C3 receptors that further augment their ability to ingest opsonized

virions, specifically those virions that are coated with antibody or complement molecules. Viruses in many families are capable of replicating in macrophages, thus opsonization of virions by antibody can actually facilitate antibody-mediated enhancement of infection, which may be a major pathogenetic factor in human dengue and several retrovirus infections.

Viral infection can itself lead to transcriptional activation of macrophages and dendritic cells, with production of inflammatory and vasoactive mediators such as tissue necrosis factor that contribute to the pathogenesis of viral diseases, particularly hemorrhagic viral fevers such as Ebola and bluetongue.

Virus Interactions with Vascular Endothelial Cells

The vascular endothelium with its basement membrane and tight cell junctions constitutes the blood–tissue interface and a barrier for particles such as virions. Parenchymal invasion by circulating virions depends on crossing this barrier, often in capillaries and venules, where blood flow is slowest and the vascular wall is thinnest. Virions may move passively between or through endothelial cells and

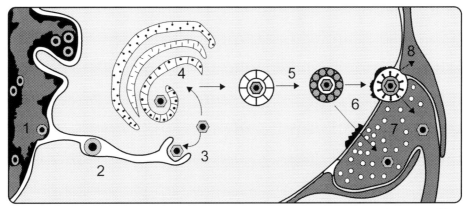

FIGURE 3.7 Events leading to the passage of pseudorabies virus across the junction between nerve cells on its centripetal intra-axonal transit to the brain. (1) Virions replicate in the nucleus of a peripheral nerve cell, acquiring an envelope as they bud from the inner lamella of the nuclear envelope. (2) Virions traverse the endoplasmic reticulum. (3) Virions are subsequently released into the cytoplasm after a fusion event between the virion envelope and endoplasmic reticulum membrane. (4) Virions acquire another envelope at the Golgi apparatus. (5) Virions are transported across the cytoplasm in vacuoles. (6) Virions enter the next neuron by fusion of the viral envelope and plasma membrane at a synaptic terminus. (7) Virions, now without their envelope, are carried centrally by retrograde axoplasmic flow, reaching the cell body and nucleus of the neuron, where further replication occurs. The process continues, eventually bringing the virus to the brain, where necrotizing encephalitis follows. (8) Some virions invade and replicate in the Schwann cells of the myelin sheaths surrounding neurons, thereby amplifying the amount of virus available to invade neurons. *[From J. P. Card, L. Rinaman, R. B. Lynn, B. H. Lee, R. P. Meade, R. R. Miselis, and L. W. Enquit. Pseudorabies virus infection of the rat central nervous system: ultrastructural characterization of virus replication, transport and pathogenesis. J. Neurosci. **13**, 2515–2539 (1993), with permission.]*

the basement membrane of small vessels, be carried within infected leukocytes (Trojan horse mechanism), or infect endothelial cells and "grow" their way through this barrier, with infection of the luminal aspect of the cell and release from the basal aspect. This subject has been studied most intensively in relation to viral invasion of the central nervous system, but it also applies to secondary invasion of many tissues during generalized infections.

Infection of endothelial cells is also important to the pathogenesis of viral diseases characterized by vascular injury that results in widespread hemorrhage and/or edema, the so-called hemorrhagic viral fevers. Virus-induced endothelial injury leads to coagulation and vascular thrombosis and, if widespread, disseminated intravascular coagulation (DIC). However, it is likely that inflammatory and vasoactive mediators produced by virus-infected macrophages and dendritic cells, such as tissue necrosis factor, also contribute to the pathogenesis of vascular injury in hemorrhagic viral fevers.

Spread via Nerves

Although infection of the central nervous system can occur after hematogenous spread, invasion via the peripheral nerves is also an important route of infection—for example, in rabies, Borna disease, and several alphaherpesvirus infections (e.g., B virus encephalitis, pseudorabies, and bovine herpesvirus 5 encephalitis). Herpesvirus capsids travel to the central nervous system in axon cytoplasm and, while doing so, also sequentially infect the Schwann cells of the nerve sheath. Rabies virus and Borna disease virus also travel to

the central nervous system in axon cytoplasm, but usually do not infect the nerve sheath. Sensory, motor, and autonomic nerves may be involved in the neural spread of these viruses. As these viruses move centripetally, they must cross cell–cell junctions. Rabies virus and pseudorabies virus are also known to cross at synaptic junctions (Figure 3.7).

In addition to passing centripetally from the body surface to the sensory ganglia and from there to the brain, herpesviruses can move through axons centrifugally from ganglia to the skin or mucous membranes. This is the same phenomenon that occurs after reactivation of latent herpesvirus infections and in the production of recrudescent epithelial lesions.

Rabies virus, Borna disease virus, respiratory mouse hepatitis virus, some togaviruses, and certain other viruses are able to use olfactory nerve endings in the nares as sites of entry. They gain entry in the special sensory endings of the olfactory neuroepithelial cells, cause local infection and progeny virus (or subviral entities containing the viral genome) then travel in axoplasm of olfactory nerves directly to the olfactory bulb of the brain.

Mechanisms of Virus Shedding

Shedding of infectious virions is crucial to the maintenance of infection in populations (see Chapter 6). For viruses that replicate only at epithelial surfaces, exit of infectious virions usually occurs from the same organ system involved in virus entry (e.g., the respiratory or gastrointestinal system; Figure 3.2). In generalized viral infections, shedding can occur from a variety of sites (Figure 3.5), and some viruses are shed from several sites. The amount of virus shed in an excretion or secretion is important in relation to transmission. Very low concentrations may be irrelevant unless very large volumes of infected material are involved; however, some viruses occur in such high concentrations that a minute quantity of virus-laden secretion or excretion can readily lead to transmission to the next animal host. Enteric viruses are in general more resistant to inactivation by environmental conditions than respiratory viruses; especially when suspended in water, such viruses can persist for some time.

Viruses such as influenza and the pneumoviruses that typically cause localized infection and injury of the respiratory tract are shed in mucus and are expelled from the respiratory tract during coughing or sneezing. Viruses are also shed from the respiratory tract in several systemic infections. Enteric viruses such as rotaviruses are shed in the feces, and the more voluminous the fluid output the greater is the environmental contamination they cause. A few viruses are shed into the oral cavity from infected salivary glands (e.g., rabies virus and cytomegaloviruses) or from the lungs or nasal mucosa during infection of the respiratory system. Salivary spread depends on activities such as licking, nuzzling, grooming, or biting. Virus shedding in saliva may continue during convalescence or recurrently thereafter, especially with herpesviruses.

The skin is an important source of virus in diseases in which transmission is by direct contact or via small abrasions: papillomaviruses and some poxviruses and herpesviruses employ this mode of transmission. Although skin lesions are produced in several generalized diseases, in only a few is virus actually shed from the skin lesions. However, in vesicular diseases such as foot-and-mouth disease, vesicular stomatitis, and swine vesicular disease, the causative viruses are produced in great quantities in vesicles within the mucosa and skin of affected animals; virus is shed from these lesions after the vesicles rupture. Localization of virus in the feather follicles is important in the shedding of Marek's disease virus by infected chickens.

Urine, like feces, tends to contaminate food sources and the environment. A number of viruses (e.g., infectious canine hepatitis virus, foot-and-mouth disease viruses, and arenaviruses) replicate in tubular epithelial cells in the kidney and are shed in urine. Viruria is prolonged and common in equine rhinitis A virus infection and life-long in arenavirus infections of reservoir host rodents; it constitutes the principal mode of contamination of the environment by these viruses.

Several viruses that cause important diseases of animals are shed in the semen and are transmitted during coitus; for example, equine arteritis virus can be shed for months or years in the semen of apparently healthy carrier stallions, long after virus has been cleared from other tissues. Similarly, viruses that replicate in the mammary gland are excreted in milk, which may serve as a route of transmission—for example, caprine arthritis–encephalitis virus, mouse mammary tumor virus, and some of the tick-borne flaviviruses. In salmonid fish, the fluid surrounding eggs oviposited during spawning may contain high concentrations of viruses such as infectious hemopoietic necrosis virus, which is an important mode of virus transmission in both hatchery and wild fish populations.

Although not "shedding" in the usual sense of the word, blood and tissues from slaughtered animals must be considered important sources of viral contagion. Virus-laden blood is also the basis for transmission when it contaminates needles and other equipment used by veterinarians and others treating or handling sick animals. Similarly, the use of virus-contaminated fetal bovine serum can result in similar contamination of biological products.

Virus Infection Without Shedding

Many sites of virus replication might be considered "dead ends" from the perspective of natural spread; however, replication at these sites can indirectly facilitate virus transmission as, for instance, carnivores and omnivores may be infected by consuming virus-laden meat or tissues. Similarly, classical swine fever (hog cholera), African swine fever, and vesicular exanthema of swine viruses have been previously translocated to different regions and countries through feeding garbage containing contaminated pork scraps. The epizootic of bovine spongiform encephalopathy (mad cow disease) in the United Kingdom was spread widely amongst cattle by the feeding of contaminated meat and bone meal containing bovine offal that included nervous tissue.

Many retroviruses are not shed at all, but instead are transmitted directly in the germ plasm or by infection of the avian egg or developing mammalian embryo. Despite the lack of horizontal transmission, these vertically transmitted viruses accomplish the same ends as those shed into the environment—that is, transmission to new hosts and perpetuation in nature.

MECHANISMS OF VIRAL INJURY AND DISEASE

The outcome of a viral infection is dependent on the ability of the infecting virus to infect, colonize and then cause tissue- or organ-specific injury in the host, in addition to its ability to avoid clearance by the host's innate and adaptive immune responses (see Chapter 4). After successful infection, viruses can cause disease in their hosts either by direct injury to target cells or by inducing immune or inflammatory responses that themselves mediate tissue injury and cause disease.

Virus–Cell Interactions

An appreciation of the potential adverse outcomes of infection in the individual cell is key to understanding the impact of viral infection in complex tissues and organs—and, indeed, the whole host animal. As described in the preceding section, cellular tropism of viruses is determined by the presence of appropriate cellular receptors and, frequently, cell-type specific transcription factors (enhancers). Viruses typically encode genes that modulate host-cell functions for their own benefit and, of course, the host has elaborate innate defenses to restrict viral functions. Thus the viral and cellular factors that influence the outcome of infection are often in delicate balance and easily shifted one way or the other.

Virus infection can cause a wide variety of potentially deleterious changes in the many different kinds of cells that occur in the animal host. The disruption of cellular functions, the induction of cell death or transformation, or the activation of an inappropriate immune response are all potentially manifested as disease by the infected host (Figure 3.8). Although virus-induced changes at the cellular, subcellular, and molecular levels are most commonly studied in cultured cells, additional insight has been gained through the use of explant and organ cultures, transplantation of infected cells and tissues back into experimental animals, and the extensive recent use of genetically modified laboratory animals in conjunction with molecular clones of individual viruses.

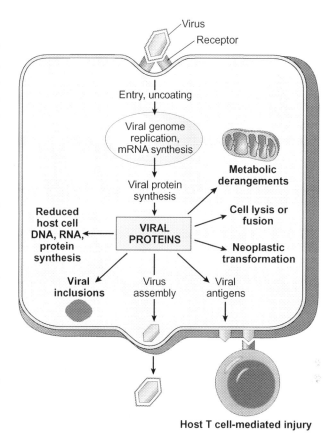

FIGURE 3.8 Potential mechanisms by which viruses cause injury to cells. [*From* Robbins & Cotran Pathologic Basis of Disease, *V. Kumar, A. K. Abbas, N. Fausto, J. Aster, 8th ed., p. 343. Copyright © Saunders/ Elsevier (2010), with permission.*]

Types of Virus–Cell Interaction

Viral infections may be cytocidal (cytolytic, cytopathic) or non-cytocidal, and productive or non-productive (abortive)—that is, not all infections lead to cell death or the production and release of new virions. However, critical changes can occur in virus-infected cells regardless of whether the infection is productive or not. Certain kinds of cells are permissive—that is, they support complete replication of a particular virus—whereas others are non-permissive—that is, virus replication may be blocked at any point from virus attachment through to the final stages of virion assembly and release, and this outcome can be determined by either cellular factors, such as the presence of specific proteolytic enzymes or cellular transcription enhancers, or viral factors, such as the deletion in defective interfering particles of key genes required for virus replication.

Some of the most important of all non-productive virus–cell interactions are those associated with persistent infections or latent viral infections, which will be described in a subsequent section. The term *persistent infection* simply describes an infection that lasts a long time, considerably beyond the interval when infection normally would be expected to be cleared. The term *latent infection* describes a specific type of persistent infection that "exists but is not

exhibited"—that is, an infection in which infectious virions are not formed. In either case, the virus or its genome is maintained indefinitely in the cell, either by the integration of the viral nucleic acid into the host-cell DNA or by carriage of the viral nucleic acid in the form of an episome, and the infected cell survives and may divide repeatedly; in some instances persistently infected cells never release virions, whereas in others the infection may become productive when induced by an appropriate stimulus, such as the periodic reactivation and virus shedding associated with many latent herpesvirus infections. Persistent or latent infections with oncogenic viruses may also lead to cell transformation, as described later in this chapter. The various types of interaction that can occur between virus and cell are summarized in Table 3.2 and in Figure 3.8.

Cytocidal Changes in Virus-Infected Cells

Cytopathic viruses kill the cells in which they replicate, by preventing synthesis of host macromolecules (as described below), by producing degradative enzymes or toxic products, or by inducing apoptosis (see Chapter 4). After inoculation of a cytopathic virus into a monolayer of cultured cells, the first

TABLE 3.2 Types of Virus–Cell Interaction

Type of Infection	Effects on Cell	Production of Infectious Virions	Examples
Cytocidal	Morphologic changes in cells (cytopathic effects); inhibition of protein, RNA, and DNA synthesis; cell death	Yes	Alphaherpesviruses, enteroviruses, reoviruses
Persistent, productive	No cytopathic effect; little metabolic disturbance; cells continue to divide; may be loss of the special functions of some differentiated cells	Yes	Pestiviruses, arenaviruses, rabies virus, most retroviruses
Persistent, non-productive	Usually nil	No, but virus may be induced[a]	Canine distemper virus in brain
Transformation	Alteration in cell morphology; cells can be passaged indefinitely; may produce tumors when transplanted to experimental animals	No, oncogenic DNA viruses	Polyomavirus, adenoviruses
		Yes, oncogenic retroviruses	Murine, avian leukosis and sarcoma viruses

[a]By co-cultivation, irradiation, or chemical mutagens.

round of virus replication yields progeny virions that spread through the medium to infect both adjacent and distant cells; all cells in the culture may eventually become infected. The resulting cell damage is known as a cytopathic effect (CPE). Cytopathic effects can usually be observed by low-power light microscopy of unstained cell cultures (Figure 3.9). The nature of the cytopathic effect is often characteristic of the particular virus involved, and is therefore an important preliminary clue in the identification of clinical isolates in the diagnostic laboratory (see Chapters 2 and 5).

So many pathophysiologic changes occur in cells infected with cytopathic viruses that the death of the cell usually cannot be attributed to any particular event; rather, cell death may be the final result of the cumulative action of many insults. Nevertheless, a variety of specific mechanisms have been identified that might in the future be potentially targeted for therapeutic intervention. General mechanisms of virus-induced cell injury and death (Figure 3.8) include:

Inhibition of Host-Cell Nucleic Acid Synthesis is an inevitable consequence of viral inhibition of host-cell protein synthesis and its effect on the cellular machinery of DNA replication. Some viruses, especially the large DNA viruses, use specific mechanisms to promote their own synthetic processes through production of virus-encoded regulatory proteins.

Inhibition of Host-Cell RNA Transcription occurs during replication of viruses in several different families, including poxviruses, rhabdoviruses, reoviruses, paramyxoviruses, and picornaviruses. In some instances, this inhibition may be the indirect consequence of viral effects on host-cell protein synthesis that decrease the availability of transcription factors required for RNA polymerase activity. Certain viruses encode specific transcription factors to regulate the expression of their own genes, and these factors sometimes modulate the expression of cellular genes as well. For example, herpesviruses encode proteins that bind directly to specific viral DNA sequences, thereby regulating the transcription of viral genes.

Inhibition of Processing of Host-Cell Messenger RNAs occurs during replication of vesicular stomatitis viruses, influenza viruses, and herpesviruses, through interference with the splicing of cellular primary mRNA transcripts that are needed to form mature mRNAs. In some instances, spliceosomes are formed, but subsequent catalytic steps are inhibited. For example, a protein synthesized in herpesvirus-infected cells suppresses RNA splicing and leads to reduced amounts of cellular mRNAs and the accumulation of primary mRNA transcripts.

Inhibition of Host-Cell Protein Synthesis while viral protein synthesis continues is a characteristic of many viral infections. This shutdown is particularly rapid and profound in picornavirus infections, but it is also pronounced in togavirus, influenzavirus, rhabdovirus, poxvirus, and herpesvirus infections. With some other viruses, the shutdown occurs late in the course of infection and is more gradual, whereas with non-cytocidal viruses, such as pestiviruses, arenaviruses, and retroviruses, there is no dramatic inhibition of host-cell protein synthesis, and no cell death. The mechanisms underlying the shutdown of host-cell protein synthesis are varied, including those just described in

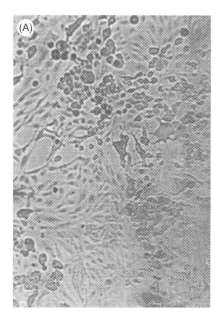 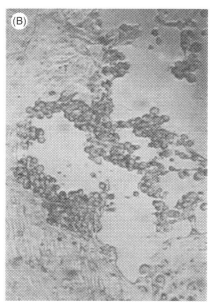

FIGURE 3.9 Cytopathic effects produced by different viruses. The cell monolayers are shown as they would normally be viewed in the laboratory, unfixed and unstained. (A) Typical cytopathology of an enterovirus: rapid rounding of cells, progressing to complete cell lysis. (B) Typical cytopathology of a herpesvirus: focal areas of swollen rounded cells. Magnification: ×60. (*Courtesy of I. Jack.*)

addition to the production of viral enzymes that degrade cellular mRNAs, the production of factors that bind to ribosomes and inhibit cellular mRNA translation, and the alteration of the intracellular ionic environment favoring the translation of viral mRNAs over cellular mRNAs. Most importantly, some viral mRNAs simply outcompete cellular mRNAs for cellular translation machinery by mass action—the large excess of viral mRNA outcompetes cellular mRNA for host ribosomes. Viral proteins may also inhibit the processing and transport of cellular proteins from the endoplasmic reticulum, and this inhibition may lead to their degradation. This effect is seen in lentivirus and adenovirus infections.

Cytopathic Effects of "Toxic" Viral Proteins reflect the accumulation of large amounts of various viral components in the cell late in infection. It was previously believed that cytopathic effect was simply a consequence of the intrinsic toxicity of these proteins, but most cell damage probably represents the supervening of virus replication events on cellular events. Hence, the list of "toxic proteins" has been shortened, but some remain. For example, the toxicity of adenovirus penton and fiber proteins appears to be direct and independent of adenovirus replication.

Interference with Cellular Membrane Function can affect the participation of cellular membranes in many phases of virus replication, from virus attachment and entry, to the formation of replication complexes, to virion assembly. Viruses may alter plasma membrane permeability, affect ion exchange and membrane potential, or induce the synthesis of new intracellular membranes or the rearrangement of previously existing ones. For example, a generalized increase in membrane permeability occurs early

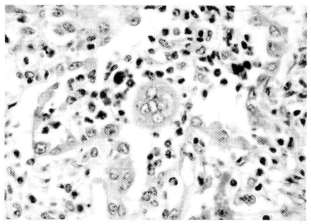

FIGURE 3.10 Syncytial cell with an intracytoplasmic inclusion in the lung of a calf infected with bovine respiratory syncytial virus. (*Courtesy of M. Anderson, University of California, Davis.*)

during picornavirus, alphavirus, reovirus, rhabdovirus, and adenovirus infections.

Enveloped viruses specifically direct the insertion of their surface glycoproteins, including fusion proteins, into host-cell membranes as part of their budding process, often leading to membrane fusion and syncytium formation. Syncytia are a conspicuous feature of infection of cell monolayers by lentiviruses, coronaviruses, paramyxoviruses, respiroviruses, morbilliviruses, pneumoviruses, henipaviruses and some herpesviruses, which result from the fusion of an infected cell with neighboring infected or uninfected cells (Figure 3.10). Such multinucleate syncytia (*syn.* multinucleated giant cells) may also occur in the tissues of animals infected with these viruses; for example, in horses infected with Hendra virus and cattle infected with respiratory syncytial virus. Syncytia may represent an important mechanism of spread of viruses in tissues: fusion bridges may allow subviral entities, such as viral nucleo-capsids and nucleic acids, to spread while avoiding host defenses. Cell membrane fusion is mediated by viral fusion proteins or fusion domains on other viral surface proteins. For example, the fusion activity of influenza viruses is carried on the hemagglutinin spikes, whereas the fusion activity of paramyxoviruses such as parainfluenza virus 3 is carried on separate spikes composed of fusion (F) protein. At high multiplicity of infection, paramyxoviruses may cause a rapid fusion of cultured cells without any requirement for virus replication; this phenomenon occurs simply as a result of the action of fusion protein activity of input virions as they interact with plasma membranes.

Cells in monolayer cultures infected with influenza viruses, paramyxoviruses, and togaviruses, all of which bud from the plasma membrane, acquire the ability to adsorb erythrocytes. This phenomenon, known as hemadsorption (Figure 3.11), is the result of incorporation of viral spike glycoprotein into the plasma membrane of infected cells, which then serves as a receptor for ligands on the surface of erythrocytes. The same glycoprotein spikes are responsible for hemagglutination *in vitro*—that is, the agglutination of erythrocytes. Although hemadsorption and hemagglutination are not known to play a part in the pathogenesis of viral diseases, both phenomena are used in laboratory diagnostics (see Chapter 5).

Viral proteins (antigens) inserted into the host-cell plasma membrane may also constitute targets for specific humoral and cellular immune responses that cause the lysis of the cell. This may happen before significant progeny virus is produced, thus slowing or arresting the progress of infection and hastening recovery (see Chapter 4). Alternatively, in some instances the immune response may cause immune-mediated tissue injury and disease. Viral antigens may also be incorporated in the membrane of cells transformed by viruses, and play an important role in immune-mediated resolution, or regression—of viral papillomas, for example.

Changes in cell shape are characteristic of many viral infections of cultured cells. Such changes are caused by damage to the cytoskeleton, which is made up of several filament systems, including microfilaments (e.g., actin), intermediate filaments (e.g., vimentin), and microtubules (e.g., tubulin). The cytoskeleton is responsible for the structural integrity of the cell, for the transport of organelles through the cell, and for certain cell motility activities. Particular viruses may damage specific filament systems: for example, canine distemper virus, vesicular stomatitis viruses, vaccinia virus, and herpesviruses cause a depolymerization of actin-containing microfilaments, and enteroviruses induce extensive damage to microtubules. Such damage contributes to the drastic cytopathic changes that precede cell lysis in many infections. The elements of the cytoskeleton are also employed by many viruses in the course of

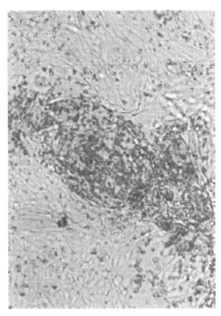

FIGURE 3.11 Hemadsorption: erythrocytes adsorb to infected cells that have incorporated hemagglutinin into the plasma membrane. The cell monolayers are shown as they would normally be viewed in the laboratory, unfixed and unstained. Magnification: ×60. *(Courtesy of I. Jack.)*

their replication: in virus entry, in the formation of replication complexes and assembly sites, and in virion release.

Non-Cytocidal Changes in Virus-Infected Cells

Non-cytocidal viruses usually do not kill the cells in which they replicate. On the contrary, they often cause persistent infection during which infected cells produce and release virions but overall cellular metabolism is little affected. In many instances, infected cells even continue to grow and divide. This type of interaction can occur in cells infected with several kinds of RNA viruses, notably pestiviruses, arenaviruses, retroviruses, and some paramyxoviruses. Nevertheless, with few exceptions (e.g., some retroviruses), there are slowly progressive changes that ultimately lead to cell death. In the host animal, cell replacement occurs so rapidly in most organs and tissues that the slow fallout of cells as a result of persistent infection may have no effect on overall function, whereas terminally differentiated cells such as neurons, once destroyed, are not replaced, and persistently infected differentiated cells may lose their capacity to carry out specialized functions.

Viruses such as the pestiviruses, arenaviruses, Bornavirus, and retroviruses that do not shut down host-cell protein, RNA, or DNA synthesis and that do not rapidly kill their host cells, can produce important pathophysiologic changes in their hosts by affecting crucial functions that are associated neither with the integrity of cells nor their basic housekeeping functions. Damage to the specialized functions of differentiated cells may still affect complex regulatory, homeostatic, and metabolic functions, including those of the central nervous system, endocrine glands, and immune system.

Ultrastructural Changes in Virus-Infected Cells

Electron microscopy is useful for evaluation of changes in virus-infected cells. Early changes in cell structure often are dominated by proliferation of various cell membranes: for example, herpesviruses cause increased synthesis, even reduplication, of nuclear membranes; flaviviruses cause proliferation of the endoplasmic reticulum; picornaviruses and caliciviruses cause a distinctive proliferation of vesicles in the cytoplasm; and many retroviruses cause peculiar fusions of cytoplasmic membranes. Other ultrastructural changes that are prominent in many viral infections include disruption of cytoskeletal elements, mitochondrial damage, and changes in the density of the cytosol. Late in the course of infection, many cytolytic viruses cause nuclear, organelle, and cytoplasmic rarefaction and/or condensation, with terminal loss of host-cell membrane integrity. In many instances the inevitability of cell death is obvious, but in others host-cell functional loss is subtle and cannot be attributed to particular ultrastructural changes. In non-cytolytic infections, most functional losses cannot be attributed to damage that is morphologically evident. Specific examples reflecting the range of host-cell changes occurring in virus-infected cells are included in many of the chapters in Part II of this book.

In addition to changes directly attributable to virus replication, most virus-infected cells also show non-specific changes, very much like those induced by physical or chemical insults. The most common early and potentially reversible change is cloudy swelling, a change associated with increasing permeability of the cellular membranes leading to swelling of the nucleus, distention of the endoplasmic reticulum and mitochondria, and rarefaction of the cytoplasm. Later in the course of many viral infections the nucleus becomes condensed and shrunken, and cytoplasmic density increases. Cell destruction can be the consequence of further loss of osmotic integrity and leakage of lysosomal enzymes into the cytoplasm. This progression is consistent with the so-called common terminal pathway to cell death.

Virus-Mediated Tissue and Organ Injury

The severity of a viral disease is not necessarily correlated with the degree of cytopathology produced by the causative virus in cells in culture. Many viruses that are cytocidal in cultured cells do not produce clinical signs *in vivo* (e.g., many enteroviruses), whereas some that are non-cytocidal *in vitro* cause lethal disease in animals (e.g., retroviruses and rabies virus). Further, depending on the organ affected, cell and tissue damage can occur without producing clinical signs of disease—for example, a large number of hepatocytes (liver cells) may be destroyed in Rift Valley fever in sheep without significant clinical signs. When damage to cells does impair the function of an organ or tissue, this may be relatively insignificant in a tissue such as skeletal muscle, but potentially devastating in organs such as the heart or the brain. Likewise, virus-induced inflammation and edema are especially serious consequences in organs such as the lungs and central nervous system.

Mechanisms of Viral Infection and Injury of Target Tissues and Organs

The mechanisms by which individual viruses cause injury to their specific target organs are described in detail under individual virus families in Part II of this book, thus the objective of this section is to provide a brief overview of potential pathogenic mechanisms that viruses can use to cause injury in their target tissues.

Viral Infection of the Respiratory Tract

Viral infections of the respiratory tract are extremely common, especially in animals housed in crowded settings. Individual viruses exhibit tropism for different levels of the respiratory tract, from the nasal passages to the pulmonary airspaces (terminal airways and alveoli), but there is considerable overlap. Tropism of respiratory viruses is probably a reflection of the distribution of appropriate receptors and intracellular transcriptional enhancers, as well as physical barriers, physiological factors, and immune parameters. For example, bovine rhinoviruses replicate in the nasal passages because their replication is optimized at lower temperatures, whereas bovine respiratory syncytial virus preferentially infects epithelial cells lining the terminal airways; thus rhinoviruses may cause mild rhinitis, whereas respiratory syncytial virus is the cause of bronchiolitis and bronchointerstitial pneumonia. Some viruses cause injury to the type I or type II pneumocytes lining the alveoli, either directly or indirectly; if extensive, injury to type I pneumocytes leads to acute respiratory distress syndrome, whereas injury to type II pneumocytes delays repair and healing in the affected lung.

Influenza viruses replicate in both the nasal passages and airways of infected mammals, but influenza virus infection is typically confined to the lung because of the requirement for hemagglutinin cleavage by tissue-specific proteases. However, highly virulent influenza viruses such as the current Eurasian–African H5N1 virus can spread beyond the lungs to cause severe generalized (systemic) infection and disease. The ability of this virus to escape the lung may be related to its tropism to type I pneumocytes that line alveoli, and its ability to cause systemic disease may reflect that its hemagglutinin can be cleaved by ubiquitous proteases that are present in many tissues. Similarly in birds, high-pathogenicity avian influenza viruses have several basic amino acids at the hemagglutinin cleavage site, which expands the range of cells capable of producing infectious virus because cleavage can be affected intracellularly by ubiquitous endopeptidase furins located in the trans-Golgi network. In contrast, the hemagglutinin protein of low pathogenicity avian influenza viruses is cleaved extracellularly by tissue-restricted proteases that are confined to the respiratory and gastrointestinal tracts (see Chapter 21).

Regardless of the level of the respiratory tree that is initially infected, viral infection typically leads to local cessation of cilial activity, focal loss of integrity of the lining mucus layer, and multifocal destruction of small numbers of epithelial cells (Figure 3.12). Initial injury is followed by progressive infection of epithelial cells within the mucosa, and inflammation of increasing severity, with exudation of fluid and influx of inflammatory cells. Fibrin-rich inflammatory exudate and necrotic cellular debris (degenerate neutrophils and sloughed epithelium) then accumulate in the lumen of the affected airways or passages, with subsequent obstruction and, in severe cases, increasing hypoxia and respiratory distress. The mucosa is quickly regenerated in animals that survive, and adaptive immune responses clear the infecting virus and prevent reinfection for variable periods of time (depending on the particular virus).

In addition to their direct adverse consequences, viral infections of the respiratory tract often predispose animals to secondary infections with bacteria, even those bacteria that constitute the normal flora in the nose and throat. This predisposition can result from interference with normal mucociliary clearance as a consequence of viral injury to the mucosa, or suppression of innate immune responses. For example, cellular expression of Toll-like receptors is depressed in the lung after influenza virus infection, and thus convalescent animals may be less able to quickly recognize and neutralize invading bacteria. This potential synergy between respiratory viruses and bacteria is compounded by overcrowding of animals as occurs during shipping and in feedlots and shelters.

Viral Infection of the Gastrointestinal Tract

Infection of the gastrointestinal tract can be acquired either by ingestion of an enteric virus (e.g., rotaviruses, coronaviruses, astroviruses, toroviruses) of which infection is confined to the gastrointestinal tract or as a consequence of generalized hematogenous spread of a systemic viral infection such as with certain parvoviruses (e.g., feline panleukopenia, canine parvovirus), pestiviruses (e.g., bovine viral diarrhea virus), and morbilliviruses (e.g., canine distemper, rinderpest). Enteric virus infections usually result in rapid onset of gastrointestinal disease after a short incubation period, whereas systemic infections have a longer incubation period and are typically accompanied by clinical signs that are not confined to dysfunction of the gastrointestinal tract.

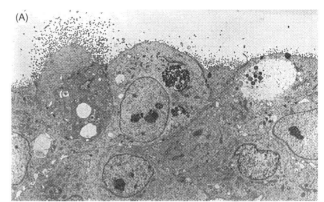
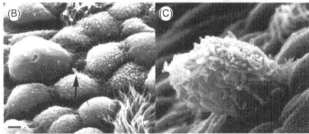

FIGURE 3.12 (A) Avian influenza virus infection in the respiratory tract of a chicken. The normal side-by-side position of columnar epithelial cells has been replaced by cuboidal cells without cilia, several of which exhibit massive virus budding from their apical surface. Thin-section electron microscopy. Magnification: ×10,000. (B, C) Scanning electron micrographs showing desquamating cells in an influenza-virus-infected mouse trachea and the adherence of *Pseudomonas aeruginosa*. Bar: 2 μm. (B) Normal mouse trachea showing a single bacterium (arrow) on a serous cell. (C) Microcoliny of *P. aeruginosa* adhering to a residual epithelial cell on an otherwise denuded surface. [*B, C: Courtesy of P. A. Small, Jr.*]

Virus-induced diarrhea is a result of infection of the epithelial cells (enterocytes) lining the gastrointestinal mucosa. Rotaviruses, astroviruses, coronaviruses, and toroviruses characteristically infect the more mature enterocytes that line the intestinal villi, whereas parvoviruses and pestiviruses infect and destroy the immature and dividing enterocytes present in the intestinal crypts. Regardless of their site of predilection, these infections all destroy enterocytes in the gastrointestinal mucosa and so reduce its absorptive surface, leading to malabsorption diarrhea with attendant loss of both fluid and electrolytes. The pathogenesis of enteric virus infections can be even more complex than simple virus-mediated destruction of enterocytes; for example, rotaviruses produce a protein (nsp4) that itself causes secretion of fluid into the bowel (intestinal hypersecretion), even in the absence of substantial virus-mediated damage. In suckling neonates, undigested lactose from ingested milk passes through the small bowel to the large bowel, where it exerts an osmotic effect that further exacerbates fluid loss. Animals with severe diarrhea can rapidly develop pronounced dehydration, hemoconcentration, acidosis that inhibits critical enzymes and metabolic pathways, hypoglycemia, and systemic electrolyte disturbances (typically, decreased sodium and increased potassium), and diarrhea can be quickly fatal in very young or otherwise compromised animals.

Enteric virus infections generally begin in the stomach or proximal small intestine, and they then spread caudally as a "wave" that sequentially affects the jejunum, ileum, and large bowel. As the infection progresses through the bowel, absorptive cells destroyed by the infecting virus are quickly replaced by immature enterocytes from the intestinal crypts. The presence of increased numbers of these immature entero-cytes contributes to malabsorption and intestinal hypersecre-tion (fluid and electrolyte loss). Similarly, adaptive immune responses lead to mucosal IgA and systemic IgG production in animals that survive, conferring resistance to reinfection. Enteric virus infections in neonates are frequently associated with infections by other enteric pathogens, including bacte-ria (e.g., enterotoxigenic or enteropathogenic *Escherichia coli*) and protozoa such as *Cryptosporidium* spp., probably because of the common factors (crowding, poor sanitation) that predispose to these infections.

Viral Infection of the Skin

In addition to being a site of initial infection, the skin may be invaded secondarily via the blood stream. Thus skin lesions that accompany viral infections can be either local-ized, such as papillomas, or disseminated. In animals, ery-thema (reddening) of the skin as a consequence of systemic viral infections is most obvious on exposed, hairless, non-pigmented areas such as the snout, ears, paws, scrotum, and udder. In addition to papillomas (warts), virus-induced lesions that commonly affect the skin of virus-infected ani-mals are variously described as macules, papules, vesicles, and pustules. Viruses of particular families tend to produce characteristic cutaneous lesions, frequently in association with similar lesions in the oral and nasal mucosa, the teats and genitalia, and at the junction of the hooves and skin of ungulates. Vesicles are especially important cutaneous lesions, because they are characteristic of foot-and-mouth disease and other viral diseases that can mimic it, although vesicles clearly can occur in diseases that are not caused by viruses. Vesicles are essentially discrete "blisters" that result from accumulation of edema fluid within the affected epidermis, or separation of the epidermis from the underly-ing dermis (or mucosal epithelium from the submucosa). Vesicles rupture quickly to leave focal ulcers.

Papules are either localized (e.g., orf) or disseminated (e.g., lumpy skin disease) epithelial proliferations that are characteristic of poxvirus infections. These proliferative and raised lesions frequently become extensively encrusted with inflammatory exudate.

Virus infections that result in widespread endothelial injury in blood vessels throughout the body, including those of the subcutaneous tissues, can produce subcutane-ous edema and erythema or hemorrhages in the skin and elsewhere (including the oral cavity and internal organs).

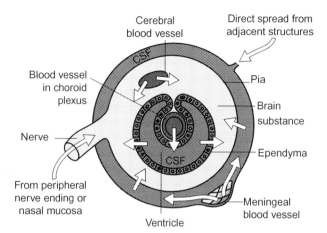

FIGURE 3.13 Routes of viral invasion of the central nervous system. CSF, cerebrospinal fluid. [*From* Medical Microbiology, *C. A. Mims, J. H. Playfair, I. M. Roitt, D. Wakelin, R. Williams. Mosby, St. Louis, MO (1993), with permission.*]

Viral Infection of the Central Nervous System

The central nervous system (brain and spinal cord) is exquisitely susceptible to serious, often fatal injury by cer-tain viral infections. Viruses can spread from distal sites to the brain via nerves (as previously described), or via the blood. To spread from the blood, viruses first must over-come the obstacle of the blood–brain barrier formed by the endothelial lining and mesenchymal wall of blood vessels within the brain and spinal cord. It remains somewhat enig-matic as to how most viruses cross this barrier to assess the parenchyma of the central nervous system, whether by passage in virus-infected leukocytes or by active or passive transport through the vascular wall (Figure 3.13).

Once present within the central nervous system, a number of viruses can quickly spread to cause progressive infection of neurons and/or glial cells (astrocytes, micro-glia, and oligodendrocytes). Lytic infections of neurons, whether caused by togaviruses, flaviviruses, herpesviruses, or other viruses, leads to encephalitis or encephalomyeli-tis characterized by neuronal necrosis, phagocytosis of neurons (neuronophagia), and perivascular infiltrations of inflammatory cells (perivascular cuffing). In contrast, virulent rabies virus infection of neurons is non-cytocidal and evokes little inflammatory reaction, but it is uniformly lethal for most mammalian species.

Other characteristic pathologic changes are produced by various viruses, and by prions that cause slowly progressive diseases of the central nervous system. In bovine spongi-form encephalopathy in cattle and scrapie in sheep, for example, there is slowly progressive neuronal degeneration and vacuolization. In contrast, infection of glial cells in dogs with canine distemper leads to progressive demyelination.

In most cases, central nervous system infection seems to be a dead end in the natural history of viruses—shedding and transmission of most neurotropic viruses do not depend on pathogenetic events in the nervous system. There are important exceptions, however. Rabies virus infection causes behavioral changes in the host that favor transmission of the virus to other hosts. The alphaherpesviruses depend on the delivery of virus from cranial and spinal sensory ganglia to epithelial sites. Epithelial shedding, which follows virus emergence from ganglia during recrudescence, is important because it offers the opportunity for transmission long after primary lesions have resolved. The prion agent of bovine spongiform encephalopathy is iatrogenically spread by the inclusion of ruminant central nervous system tissue in meat and bone meal fed to cattle. All in all, it seems anomalous that neurotropism should be the outstanding characteristic of so many of the most notorious pathogens of animals and zoonotic pathogens of humans, and yet be the pathogenetic characteristic least related to virus perpetuation in nature, emphasizing perhaps that the irreparable damage that is of such grave consequence to the host is of such little consequence to the virus.

Viral Infection of the Hemopoietic System and Immune Effects

The hemopoietic system includes: (1) the myeloid tissues, specifically the bone marrow and cells derived from it—erythrocytes, platelets, monocytes, and granulocytes, and (2) the lymphoid tissues, which include the thymus, lymph nodes, spleen, mucosal-associated lymphoid tissues and, in birds, the cloacal bursa. As cells that populate the myeloid and lymphoid systems, including lymphocytes, dendritic cells, and cells of the mononuclear phagocytic system (monocytes and macrophages) are all derived from bone marrow (or equivalent hemopoietic tissue) precursors, it is convenient to group them together under the heading of the hemopoietic system and to dispense with obsolete terminology such as "lymphoreticular" or "reticuloendothelial" systems. Importantly, lymphocytes and mononuclear phagocytes (blood monocytes, tissue macrophages, dendritic cells) are responsible for adaptive immunity (see Chapter 4), thus viral infections of these cells can have profound effects on immunity.

Infection and damage to mononuclear phagocytes can protect an invading virus from phagocytic removal, and suppress or inhibit both the innate and adaptive immune response to it. Some of the most destructive and lethal viruses known exhibit this tropism: filoviruses, arenaviruses, hantaviruses, orbiviruses such as African horse sickness and bluetongue viruses, certain bunyaviruses such as Rift Valley fever virus, alphaviruses such as Venezuelan equine encephalitis virus, and flaviviruses such as yellow fever virus. After initial invasion, infection with these viruses begins with their uptake by dendritic cells and/or

macrophages in lymphoid tissues (lymph nodes, thymus, bone marrow, Peyer's patches, and the white pulp of the spleen). Viral infection can then spread in these tissues, frequently leading to cytolysis of adjacent lymphocytes and immune dysfunction.

Viral infections can result in either specific acquired immunodeficiency or generalized immunosuppression. A relevant example of this phenomenon is provided by infection of the cloacal bursa (bursa of Fabricius) in chickens (the site of B cell differentiation in birds) with infectious bursal disease virus, which leads to atrophy of the bursa and a severe deficiency of B lymphocytes, equivalent to bursectomy. The result is an inability of severely affected birds to develop antibody-mediated immune responses to other infectious agents, which in turn leads to an increase in susceptibility to bacterial infections such as those caused by *Salmonella* spp. and *E. coli*, and other viruses. Since the discovery of acquired immunodeficiency syndrome (AIDS) in humans and its etiologic agent, human immunodeficiency virus (HIV), similar viruses have been discovered in monkeys (simian immunodeficiency viruses), cattle (bovine immunodeficiency virus), and cats (feline immunodeficiency virus). In susceptible animals, these viruses individually can infect and destroy specific but different cells of the immune system, thereby causing immunosuppression of different types and severity.

Many other viruses (e.g., classical swine fever virus, bovine viral diarrhea virus, canine distemper virus, feline and canine parvoviruses) that cause systemic infections, especially those that infect mononuclear phagocytes and/or lymphocytes, may temporarily but globally suppress adaptive immune responses, both humoral and cell-mediated. Affected animals are predisposed to diseases caused by other infectious agents during the period of virus-induced immunosuppression, a phenomenon that can also occur following vaccination with certain live-attenuated vaccines. The immune response to unrelated antigens may be reduced or abrogated in animals undergoing such infections.

Virus-induced immunosuppression may in turn lead to enhanced virus replication, such as the reactivation of latent herpesvirus, adenovirus, or polyomavirus infections. Similarly, immunosuppression associated with administration of cytotoxic drugs or irradiation for chemotherapy or organ transplantation can predispose to recrudescence of herpesviruses and, potentially, others.

Viral Infection of the Fetus

Most viral infections of the dam have no harmful effect on the fetus, although severe infections of the dam can sometimes lead to fetal death and expulsion (abortion) in the absence of fetal infection. However, some viruses can cross

TABLE 3.3 Viral Infections of the Fetus or Embryo

Animal	Family/Genus	Virus	Syndrome
Cattle	Herpesviridae/Varicellovirus	Infectious bovine rhinotracheitis virus	Fetal death, abortion
	Retroviridae/Deltaretrovirus	Bovine leukemia virus	Inapparent infection, leukemia
	Reoviridae/Orbivirus	Bluetongue virus	Fetal death, abortion, congenital defects
	Bunyaviridae/Bunyavirus	Akabane virus	Fetal death, abortion, stillbirth, congenital defects
	Flaviviridae/Pestivirus	Bovine viral diarrhea virus	Fetal death, abortion, congenital defects, inapparent infection with life-long carrier status and shedding
Horses	Herpesviridae/Varicellovirus	Equine herpesvirus 1	Fetal death, abortion, neonatal disease
	Arteriviridae/Arterivirus	Equine arteritis virus	Fetal death, abortion
Swine	Herpesviridae/Varicellovirus	Pseudorabies virus	Fetal death, abortion
	Parvoviridae/Parvovirus	Swine parvovirus	Fetal death, abortion, mummification, stillbirth, infertility
	Flaviviridae/Flavivirus	Japanese encephalitis virus	Fetal death, abortion
	Flaviviridae/Pestivirus	Classical swine fever (hog cholera) virus	Fetal death, abortion, congenital defects, inapparent infection with life-long carrier status and shedding
Sheep	Reoviridae/Orbivirus	Bluetongue virus	Fetal death, abortion, congenital defects
	Bunyaviridae/Phlebovirus	Rift Valley fever virus	Fetal death, abortion
	Bunyaviridae/Nairovirus	Nairobi sheep disease virus	Fetal death, abortion
	Flaviridae/Pestivirus	Border disease virus	Congenital defects
Dogs	Herpesviridae/Varicellovirus	Canine herpesvirus	Perinatal death
Cats	Parvoviridae/Parvovirus	Feline panleukopenia virus	Cerebellar hypoplasia
	Retroviridae/Gammaretrovirus	Feline leukemia virus	Inapparent infection, leukemia, fetal death
Mice	Parvoviridae/Parvovirus	Rat virus	Fetal death
	Arenaviridae/Arenavirus	Lymphocytic choriomeningitis virus	Inapparent infection, with life-long carrier status and shedding
Chicken	Picornaviridae/Enterovirus	Avian encephalomyelitis virus	Congenital defects, fetal death
	Retroviridae/Alpharetrovirus	Avian leukosis/sarcoma viruses	Inapparent infection, leukemia, other diseases

the placenta to infect the fetus (Table 3.3). Such infections occur most commonly in young dams (such as first-calf heifers) that are exposed during pregnancy to pathogenic viruses to which they have no immunity, as a consequence of lack of either appropriate vaccination or natural infection. The outcome of fetal viral infection is dependent upon the properties (virulence and tropism) of the infecting virus, as well as the gestational age of the fetus at infection. Severe cytolytic infections of the fetus, especially in early gestation, are likely to cause fetal death and resorption or abortion, which also is dependent on the species of animal affected—abortion is especially common in those species in which pregnancy is sustained by fetal production of progesterone (such as sheep), whereas pregnancy is less

likely to be terminated prematurely in multiparous species in which pregnancy is maintained by maternally derived progesterone (such as swine).

Teratogenic viruses are those that can cause developmental defects after *in-utero* infection. The outcome of infections of pregnant animals with teratogenic viruses is influenced to a great extent by gestational age. Thus, viral infections that occur during critical stages of organogenesis in the developing fetus can have devastating consequences from virus-mediated infection and destruction of progenitor cells before they can populate organs such as the brain. For example, Akabane virus, Cache Valley virus, bovine viral diarrhea virus, and bluetongue virus can all cause teratogenic brain defects in congenitally infected ruminants.

Although immune competence generally is developed by mid-gestation, viral infections before this time can lead to a weak and ineffectual immune response that leads to persistent postnatal infection, such as persistent bovine viral diarrhea virus infection in cattle and congenital lymphocytic choriomeningitis virus infection in mice.

Viral Infection of Other Organs

Almost any organ may be infected with one or another kind of virus via the blood stream, but most viruses have well-defined organ and tissue tropisms that reflect the factors described earlier (presence of receptors, intracellular and other physiological or physical co-factors, etc.). The clinical importance of infection of various organs and tissues depends, in part, on their role in the physiologic well-being of the animal. In addition to the organs and tissues already described (respiratory tract, gastrointestinal tract, skin, brain and spinal cord, hemopoietic tissues), viral infections of the heart and liver can also have especially devastating consequences. The liver is the target of relatively few viral infections of animals, in marked contrast to the numerous hepatitis viruses (hepatitis A, B, and C viruses in particular) and other viruses (e.g., yellow fever virus) that are important causes of severe liver disease in humans. In animals, Rift Valley fever virus, mouse hepatitis virus, and infectious canine hepatitis virus characteristically affect the liver, as do several abortigenic herpesviruses after fetal infections (e.g., infectious bovine rhinotracheitis virus, equine herpesvirus 1, pseudorabies virus). Virus-mediated cardiac injury is relatively uncommon in animals, but is characteristic of bluetongue and some other endotheliotrophic viral infections, and alphavirus infections of Atlantic salmon and rainbow trout.

Non-specific Pathophysiological Changes in Viral Diseases

Some of the adverse consequences of viral infections cannot be attributed to direct cell destruction by the virus, to immunopathology, or to the effects of increased concentrations of endogenous adrenal glucocorticoids in response to the stress of the infection. Viral diseases are accompanied frequently by a number of vague general clinical signs, such as fever, malaise, anorexia, and lassitude. Cytokines (interleukin-1 in particular) produced in the course of innate immune responses to infection may be responsible for some of these signs, which collectively can significantly reduce the animal's performance and impede recovery. Less characterized are the potential neuropsychiatric effects of persistent viral infection of particular neuronal tracts, such as that caused by Borna disease virus. Borna disease virus infection is not lytic in neurons, but induces bizarre changes in the behavior of rats, cats, and horses.

Viruses that cause widespread vascular injury can result in disseminated hemorrhages and/or edema as a result of increased vascular permeability. Vascular injury in these so-called hemorrhagic viral fevers, which include Dengue hemorrhagic fever, yellow fever, Ebola, and different hantavirus infections in humans, and bluetongue in ruminants, can result either from viral infection of endothelial cells or the systemic release from other infected cells of vasoactive and inflammatory mediators such as tissue necrosis factor. Widespread endothelial injury leads to coagulation and thrombosis that may precipitate disseminated intravascular coagulation, which is the common pathway that leads to death of animals and humans infected with a variety of viruses that directly or indirectly cause vascular injury.

Virus-induced Immunopathology

Viruses typically cause direct damage to the host cells they infect cells by subverting their metabolic machinery. Inflammatory responses that accompany most viral infections also can potentially contribute to disease pathogenesis, as described earlier. However, in certain instances, it is the host's immune response triggered by viral infection that mediates tissue injury and disease, particularly in those viruses that cause persistent, non-cytocidal infections. Thus the immune response can exert a two-edged role in the pathogenesis of viral diseases. Infiltration of virus-infected tissues by lymphocytes and macrophages, release of cytokines and other mediators, and the resultant inflammation are all typical of viral infections. These responses are critical to the initial control of infection, as well as to eventual virus clearance and induction of protective immunity (see Chapter 4). However, there is a delicate balance between the protective and destructive effects of host antiviral immune responses, and between the ability of the virus to replicate and spread in the face of the host's protective response. Indeed, there are viral infections in which such manifestations of the immune response are the cardinal factors in the onset and progression of the associated disease.

Immune-mediated tissue injury caused by individual viruses involves any one or more of the four types (I–IV) of immunopathologic (hypersensitivity) reactions. The distinction between these various mechanisms is increasingly less defined, but this classification system is useful for mechanistic understanding. Most viruses that cause diseases with a defined immune-mediated component involve type IV hypersensitivity reactions, and a few involve type III reactions. Type I reactions are anaphylactic-type reactions mediated by antigen-specific IgE and mast-cell-derived mediators such as histamine and heparin, and the activation of serotonin and plasma kinins; with the exception of its potential role in inflammation, this mechanism is probably unimportant in the pathogenesis of most viral infections. Similarly, type II hypersensitivity reactions that involve antibody-mediated lysis of cells, either directly through complement activation or via cells that bind to the Fc portion of bound antibodies, are of uncertain significance in the pathogenesis of viral diseases in animals.

Type III hypersensitivity reactions are caused by complexes of antigen and antibody (immune complexes) that initiate inflammation and tissue damage. Immune complexes circulate in blood in the course of most viral infections. The fate of the immune complexes depends on the ratio of antibody to antigen. In infections in which there is a large excess of antibody as compared with circulating virus, or even if there are equivalent amounts of antibody and virus, the virus is typically cleared by tissue macrophages. However, in some persistent infections, viral proteins (antigens) and/or virions are released continuously into the blood but the antibody response is weak and antibodies are of low avidity. In these instances, immune complexes are deposited in small blood vessels that function as filters, especially those of the renal glomeruli. Immune complexes continue to be deposited in glomeruli over periods of weeks, months, or even years, leading to their accumulation and subsequent immune-complex mediated glomerulonephritis.

Lymphocytic choriomeningitis virus infection in mice infected *in utero* or as neonates provides a classic example of immune complex disease associated with a persistent viral infection. Viral antigens are constantly present in the blood and, although there is specific immune dysfunction ("tolerance"), small amounts of non-neutralizing antibody are formed as mice age, leading to the formation of immune complexes that are deposited progressively within the walls of the glomerular capillaries. Depending on the strain of mouse, the end result may be glomerulonephritis leading to death from renal failure. Circulating immune complexes may also be deposited in the walls of the small blood vessels in the skin, joints, and choroid plexus, where they also cause tissue injury. A similar disease pathogenesis can occur in other persistent viral infections of animals, such as Aleutian mink disease (parvovirus infection), feline leukemia, and equine infectious anemia.

Unlike the other hypersensitivity reactions, type IV reactions, also called delayed hypersensitivity reactions, are mediated by T lymphocytes and macrophages. Cytotoxic T lymphocytes are critical components of the adaptive immune response that leads to clearance of virus-infected cells. Specifically, cytotoxic T lymphocytes recognize viral antigens expressed along with major histocompatibility (MHC) class I molecules on the surface of infected cells, which they then bind and lyse (see Chapter 4). This mechanism, however, can lead to ongoing destruction of host cells during certain viral infections, including those persistent infections caused by non-cytocidal viruses. Examples include neurological diseases induced by Borna disease virus. The respiratory tract is especially vulnerable to this type of immune-mediated disease, including infection with influenza

and parainfluenza viruses. For example, Sendai virus is a non-cytolytic respiratory pathogen in rodents. Disease is minimal following Sendai virus infection of T-cell-deficient animals, whereas disease is severe in immunocompetent animals. T cells induce severe necrotizing bronchiolitis and interstitial pneumonia, with destruction of type II pneumocytes, rendering the alveoli incapable of repair.

Experimental lymphocytic choriomeningitis virus infection of adult mice has been extensively studied as a type IV immune-mediated disease accompanying a non-cytolytic viral infection (Figure 3.14). After intracerebral inoculation, the virus replicates harmlessly in the meninges, ependyma, and choroid plexus epithelium until about the seventh day, when (CD)8+ class I MHC-restricted cytotoxic T cells invade the central nervous tissues to lyse the infected cells, which in turn results in extensive inflammation producing meningitis, cerebral edema, neurological

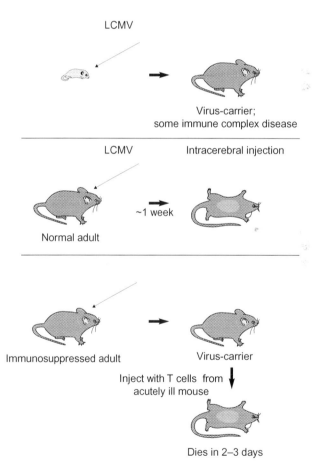

FIGURE 3.14   Injection of lymphocytic choriomeningitis virus (LCMV) into a newborn mouse produces a persistent infection with only minor pathological changes (top). Intracerebral injection of a normal adult mouse produces a fulminating disease that quickly kills the animal (middle). However, a T-deficient mouse (e.g. neonatally thymectomized or treated with anti-thymocyte serum) tolerates an intracerebral injection of LCMV (bottom). This carrier state can be broken by an injection of T cells (but not serum) from a mouse acutely ill with LCM. (*Adapted from Introduction to Immunology. J. W. Kimball, p. 462. Copyright 1983 MacMillan Publishing, with permission.*)

signs such as convulsions, and death. Likewise, intraperitoneal inoculation of virus results in immune-mediated hepatitis and severe lymphoid depletion in the spleen. The death of infected mice can be prevented by chemical immunosuppression, by X-irradiation, or by prior treatment with antilymphocyte serum.

Viruses and Autoimmune Disease

It repeatedly has been proposed, with little definitive evidence, that subtle (subclinical or asymptomatic) viral infections are responsible for autoimmune diseases in animals and humans. Proposed mechanisms for this largely hypothetical phenomenon focus on either unregulated or misdirected immune responses precipitated by a viral infection, or the presence of shared or equivalent antigens on infectious agents and host cells (molecular mimicry). Molecular mimicry clearly is responsible for immune-mediated diseases initiated by microbial infection, as classically illustrated by rheumatic heart disease in humans that is initiated by group A *Streptococcus* infection. In viruses, individual epitopes have been identified in several viruses that are also present in animal tissue, such as muscle or nervous tissue (e.g., myelin basic protein). These antibodies to these epitopes potentially might contribute to immune-mediated tissue during the course of viral infection, but their pathogenic role, if any, in initiating and potentiating autoimmune disease remains uncertain.

Persistent Infection and Chronic Damage to Tissues and Organs

Persistent infections of one type or another are produced by a wide range of viruses, and are common in veterinary medicine. Apart from enteric and respiratory viruses that cause transient infections that remain localized to their respective target organs, most other categories of viral infections include examples of chronic infection. Foot-and-mouth disease, for example, usually is an acute, self-limiting infection, but a carrier state of uncertain epidemiological relevance occurs in which virus persists in the oropharynx of low numbers of convalescent animals. In other instances, such as those associated with immunodeficiency viral infections, persistent viral infections lead to chronic diseases, even when the acute manifestations of infection have been trivial or subclinical. Finally, persistent infections can lead to continuing tissue injury, often with an immune-mediated basis.

Persistent viral infections are important for several reasons. For example, they may be reactivated and cause recrudescent episodes of disease in the individual host, or they may lead to immunopathologic disease or to neoplasia. Persistent infection may allow survival of a particular virus in individual animals and herds, even after vaccination. Similarly, persistent infections may be of epidemiologic importance—the source of contagion in long-distance virus transport and in reintroduction after elimination of virus

from a given herd, flock, region, or country. For convenience, persistent viral infections may be subdivided into several categories:

Persistent infections, *per se*, in which infectious virus is demonstrable continuously, whether or not there is ongoing disease. Disease may develop late, often with an immunopathologic or neoplastic basis. In other instances, disease is not manifest in persistently infected animals; for example, in the deer mouse (*Peromyscus maniculatus*), the reservoir rodent host of Sin Nombre virus, and the etiologic agent of hantavirus pulmonary syndrome in humans, virus is shed in urine, saliva, and feces probably for the life of the animal, even in the face of neutralizing antibody.

A striking proportion of persistent infections involve the central nervous system. The brain is somewhat sequestered from systemic immune activity by the blood–brain barrier and, further, neurons express very little MHC antigen on their surface, thereby conferring some protection against destruction by cytotoxic T lymphocytes.

Latent infections, in which infectious virus is not demonstrable except when reactivation occurs. For example, in infectious pustular vulvovaginitis, the sexually transmitted disease caused in cattle by bovine herpesvirus 1, virus usually cannot be isolated from the latently infected carrier cow except when there are recrudescent lesions. Viral latency may be maintained by restricted expression of genes that have the capacity to kill the cell. During latency, herpesviruses express only a few genes that are necessary in the maintenance of latency, notably so-called latency-associated transcripts. During reactivation, which is often stimulated by immunosuppression and/or by the action of a cytokine or hormone, the whole viral genome is transcribed again. This strategy protects the virus during its latent state from all host immune actions that would normally result in virus clearance.

Slow infections, in which quantities of infectious virus gradually increase during a very long preclinical phase that eventually leads to a slowly progressive disease (e.g., ovine progressive pneumonia).

Acute infections with late clinical manifestations, in which continuing replication of the causative virus is not involved in the progression of the disease. For example, in the cerebellar atrophy syndrome that occurs in young cats as a result of fetal infection with feline panleukopenia virus, virus cannot be isolated at the time neurologic damage is diagnosed. In fact, because of this, the cerebellar syndrome was for many years considered to be an inherited malformation.

It may be noted that these categories are defined primarily in terms of the extent and continuity of virus replication during the long period of persistence. The presence or absence of shedding and disease are secondary issues as far as this categorization is concerned. Further, some persistent infections possess features of more than one of these categories. For example, all retrovirus infections are persistent and most exhibit features of latency, but the

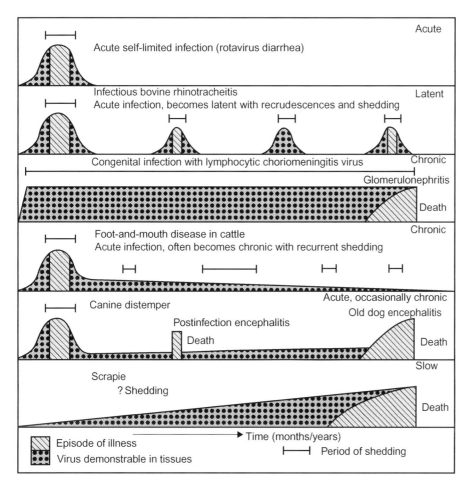

FIGURE 3.15 The shedding of virus and the occurrence of clinical signs in acute self-limited infections and various kinds of persistent infection, as exemplified by the diseases indicated. The time scale is notional and the duration of various events approximate.

diseases they cause may be delayed following infection or only manifest as slowly progressive diseases. The variety of patterns of persistent viral infections is shown diagrammatically in Figure 3.15.

Individual viruses employ a remarkable variety of strategies for successful evasion of host immune and inflammatory responses *in vivo*. These mechanisms include non-cytocidal infections without expression of immunogenic proteins, replication in cells of the immune system or subversion of host innate and adaptive immunity (see Chapter 4), and infection of non-permissive, resting, or undifferentiated cells. Some viruses have evolved strategies for evading neutralization by the antibody they elicit. Ebola virus, for example, uses an "immune decoy" to evade neutralizing antibody—specifically, a secreted viral protein that binds circulating antibody. The surface glycoproteins of filoviruses, arenaviruses, bunyaviruses (e.g., Rift Valley fever virus) and some arteriviruses (e.g., porcine reproductive and respiratory syndrome virus and lactate dehydrogenase-elevating virus) are heavily glycosylated, which may serve to mask the neutralizing epitopes contained in these proteins. Antigenic drift is especially characteristic of persistent RNA viral infection, particularly persistent RNA

virus infections such as those associated with lentiviruses (e.g., equine infectious anemia virus). During persistent infection, sequential antigenic variants are produced, with each successive variant sufficiently different to evade the immune response raised against the preceding variant. In equine infectious anemia, clinical signs occur in periodic cycles, with each cycle being initiated by the emergence of a new viral variant. In addition to providing a mechanism for escape from immune elimination, each new variant may be more virulent than its predecessor, and this may directly affect the severity and progression of the disease.

The integration of retroviral proviral DNA into the genome of the host germ-line cells assures indefinite maintenance from one generation to the next; such proviral DNA can also lead to induction of tumors (oncogenesis).

VIRUS-INDUCED NEOPLASIA

The revolution in molecular cell biology has provided remarkable insights into the mechanisms of regulation of cell growth and differentiation, and these insights have, in turn, advanced understanding of the mechanisms underpinning failures of regulatory processes that are expressed as neoplasia. The genetic changes that are ultimately responsible for neoplasia may be caused by chemical or physical agents or viruses, but all involve certain common cellular pathways. Interestingly, while there are a substantial number of both RNA and DNA viruses that are oncogenic in animals, only a relatively few viruses have been definitively linked to human cancer.

The discoveries of the viral etiology of avian leukemia by Ellerman and Bang and of avian sarcoma by Rous, in 1908 and 1911 respectively, were long regarded as curiosities unlikely to be of any fundamental significance. However, study of these avian viruses and related retroviruses of mice has increased our overall understanding of neoplasia greatly, and since the 1950s there has been a steady stream of discoveries clearly incriminating other viruses in a variety of benign and malignant neoplasms of numerous species of mammals, birds, amphibians, reptiles, and fish. Many avian retroviruses are major pathogens of poultry, and other retroviruses produce neoplasms in domestic animals. Similarly, several different DNA viruses have been determined to be responsible for cancers in humans and animals.

Any discussion of virus-induced neoplasia requires that a few commonly used terms are defined: a neoplasm is a new growth (*syn.* tumor); neoplasia is the process that leads to the formation of neoplasms (*syn.* carcinogenesis); oncology is the study of neoplasia and neoplasms; a benign neoplasm is a growth produced by abnormal cell proliferation that remains localized and does not invade adjacent tissue; in contrast, a malignant neoplasm (*syn.* cancer) is locally invasive and may also be spread to other parts of the body (metastasis). Carcinomas are cancers of epithelial cell origin, whereas sarcomas are cancers that arise from cells of mesenchymal origin. Solid neoplasms of lymphocytes are designated lymphosarcoma or malignant lymphoma (*syn.* lymphoma), whereas leukemias are cancers of hemopoietic origin characterized by circulation of cancerous cells.

Neoplasms arise as a consequence of the dysregulated growth of cells derived from a single, genetically altered progenitor cell. Thus, although neoplasms are often composed of several cell types, they are considered to originate from a monoclonal outgrowth of a single cell. It recently has been proposed that neoplasms arise from cells with properties and function similar to those of the stem cells that are present in normal tissue. Specifically, many normal tissues contain a small population of resident, long-lived stem cells that are tissue progenitors; these cells can divide to produce either terminally differentiated, relatively short-lived cells with limited replicative ability, or additional long-lived stem cells. As cancers are immortal and have unlimited ability to replicate, it is assumed that they, too, must contain stem cells that arise either from normal tissue stem cells or from differentiated cells that assume stem cell-like properties.

The Cellular Basis of Neoplasia

Neoplasia is the result of non-lethal genetic injury, as may be acquired by chemical or physical damage, or from viral infections. Some cancers, however, arise randomly through the accumulation of spontaneous genetic mutations. A neoplasm results from the clonal expansion of a single cell that has suffered genetic damage, typically in one of four types of normal regulatory genes: (1) proto-oncogenes, which are cellular genes that regulate growth and differentiation; (2) tumor suppressor genes that inhibit growth, typically by regulating the cell cycle; (3) genes that regulate apoptosis (programmed cell death; see Chapter 4); (4) genes that mediate DNA repair. Carcinogenesis involves a multi-step progression resulting from the cumulative effects of multiple mutations.

Once developed, neoplasms are: (1) self-sufficient, in that they have the capacity to proliferate without external stimuli; for example, as the result of unregulated oncogene activation; (2) insensitive to normal regulatory signal that would limit their growth, such as transforming growth factor-β and the cyclin-dependent kinases that normally regulate orderly progression of cells through the various phases of the cell cycle; (3) resistant to apoptosis because of either the activation of anti-apoptotic molecules or the inhibition of mediators of apoptosis such as p53; (4) limitless potential for replication. Cancers also may have the ability to invade and spread to distant tissues (metastasis), and neoplasms typically promote the proliferation of new blood vessels that support their growth.

Neoplasia, regardless of cause, is the result of unregulated cellular proliferation. In the normal sequence of events during cellular proliferation, a growth factor binds to its specific cellular receptor, leading to signal transduction that ultimately results in nuclear transcription, which in turn leads to the cell entering and progressing through the cell cycle until it divides. Proto-oncogenes are normal cellular genes that encode proteins that function in normal cellular growth and differentiation; they include (1) growth factors; (2) growth factor receptors; (3) intracellular signal transducers; (4) nuclear transcription factors; (5) cell-cycle control proteins. Oncogenes are derived by mutation of their normal cellular proto-oncogene counterparts, and the expression of oncogenes results in production of onco-proteins that mediate autonomous (unregulated) growth of neoplastic cells.

The development of cancer (malignant neoplasia) is a protracted, multi-step process that reflects the accumulation of multiple mutations. A potentially neoplastic clone of cells must bypass apoptosis (programmed death), circumvent the need for growth signals from other cells, escape from immunologic surveillance, organize its own blood supply, and possibly metastasize. Thus, tumors other than those induced by rapidly transforming retroviruses like Rous sarcoma virus generally do not arise as the result of a single event, but by a series of steps leading to progressively greater loss of regulation of cell division.

Oncogenic DNA and RNA viruses have been identified in both animals and humans, including retroviruses, papillomaviruses, herpesviruses, and several other DNA viruses. Cells transformed by non-defective retroviruses also express the full range of viral proteins, and new virions bud from their membranes. In contrast, transformation by DNA viruses usually occurs in cells undergoing non-productive infection in which viral DNA is integrated into the cellular DNA of the transformed cells or, in the case of papillomaviruses and herpesviruses, in which the viral DNA remains episomal. Certain virus-specific antigens are demonstrable in transformed cells. Some tumor-associated antigens are expressed on the plasma membrane where, *in vivo*, they constitute potential targets for immunologic attack.

Oncogenic RNA Viruses

Retrovirus Pathogenesis

Retroviruses are a significant cause of neoplasia in many species of animals, including cattle, cats, non-human primates, mice, and chickens, among others. Their pathogenesis is linked to their propensity to integrate randomly within the genome of host cells, thereby being infectious mutagens. The consequences of such integration are largely innocuous and clinically silent, and only seldom result in oncogenesis. As described in Chapter 14, retroviruses can be biologically divided into *exogenous* (horizontally transmissible) agents, or *endogenous*, in which case they are integrated within the host genome. Retroviruses can be either replication-competent or replication-defective.

Rarely, a replication-competent retrovirus will integrate into the genome of host germ cells. A complete DNA copy of the viral genome (known as the *provirus*) may thereafter be transmitted in the germ line DNA from parent to progeny (i.e., via ova or sperm) and, over the course of evolution, may be perpetuated in every individual of an animal species. Such retroviruses are said to be *endogenous*. As long as endogenous retroviruses remain replication-competent, they may also be horizontally transmissible like their exogenous relatives. Over the course of time, multiple endogenous retroviruses become integrated throughout the genome, either through new exposures, or more commonly when provirus genomes are replicated during cell division, they can then be integrated elsewhere in the genome as *retrotransposons*. As millennia pass, many of these "retroelements" become replication-defective but their DNA continues to have the potential to reintegrate as retrotransposons, and their partial genes may continue to encode proteins. These reintegration events, when involving functioning host genes, may result in spontaneous mutations

within the germ line of the species. This process is known as *insertional mutagenesis*. It is not necessarily in the best interest of the host to carry potentially deleterious viral mutagens within its genome, so the host evolves to lack somatic cell receptors for its endogenous viruses, or the host may mutate, truncate, methylate, or even evict proviral sequences over time. In essence, endogenous retroviruses and their hosts are in a constant state of co-evolution. Some anciently acquired endogenous retroviruses have actually become vital to host physiology. During pregnancy of mammals (except monotremes), endogenous retro-elements are expressed to high levels during embryo implantation and placental development, inducing immunosuppressive and cell fusion (syncytium formation) effects that are vital to mammalian placental and fetal development. Syncytin-1 is one such gene product that is an endogenous retro-element *env*-derived fusigenic glycoprotein that is critical in syncytial trophoblast formation. It is a highly conserved and essential gene among placental animals.

Endogenous proviruses, like other host genes, are expressed differentially in different tissues, at different ages, and under the control of various stimuli, including hormones and immune states. When a dividing cell is co-expressing two or more proviruses, proviral genomes may recombine to form new retroviral variants with novel ability to infect somatic cells through alternate receptors. This has been illustrated in lymphoma-prone inbred mouse strains, with each mouse strain having different constellations of proviral integrations that recombine to become replication-competent infectious viruses that can target vulnerable tissues through novel receptor–ligand interactions. Although this has been extensively studied, the consequences of proviral recombination and induction of neoplasia by viral recombinants is largely an artificial phenomenon that is unique to the inbred mouse.

Retrovirus-Induced Neoplasia

Oncogenic retroviruses are classified as *chronic transforming* or *acute transforming* retroviruses. These two major types of transforming retroviruses induce neoplasia in significantly different ways.

Chronic Transforming Retroviruses

Chronic transforming retroviruses induce neoplasia through random integrations into the genome of somatic cells. They exert their effect as "*cis*-activating" retroviruses that transform cells by becoming integrated in the host-cell DNA close to a cell growth regulating gene, and thus usurping normal cellular regulation of this gene. These cell growth regulating host genes are termed "oncogenes," or cellular oncogenes (c-*onc*). Despite the terminology implying that they are oncogenic, c-*onc* genes are host genes that encode important cell signaling products that regulate normal cell proliferation and quiescence. The presence of an integrated provirus, with its strong promoter and enhancer elements, upstream from a c-*onc* gene may amplify the expression of the c-*onc* gene greatly. This is the likely mechanism whereby the weakly oncogenic endogenous avian leukosis viruses produce neoplasia. When avian leukosis viruses cause malignant neoplasia, the viral genome has generally been integrated at a particular location, immediately upstream from a host c-*onc* gene. Integrated avian leukosis provirus increases the synthesis of the normal c-*myc* oncogene product 30- to 100-fold. Experimentally, only the viral long-terminal repeats (LTR) need be integrated to cause this effect; furthermore, by this mechanism c-*myc* may also be expressed in cells in which it is not normally expressed or is normally expressed at much lower levels.

Not all chronic transforming retroviruses require insertional mutagenesis in regions of c-*onc* genes to be oncogenic. Both exogenous and endogenous mouse mammary tumor viruses carry an extra viral gene sequence that encodes a super-antigen (*Sag*) that stimulates proliferation of lymphocytes. Expression of *Sag* stimulates massive B cell proliferation and mouse mammary tumor virus replication in the dividing B cells, with subsequent homing of virus-expressing lymphocytes to mammary tissue. Both lymphomas and mammary tumors may ensue, but oncogenesis does not require alteration of host oncogenes. The exogenous ovine retroviruses that cause nasal carcinomas and pulmonary adenocarcinomas (Jaagsiekte) infect epithelial target cells, and transformation is related to expression of the viral *env* gene. Bovine leukemia virus is an exogenous retrovirus that causes chronic leukosis and B cell lymphoma. The virus encodes *tax*, *rex*, *R3*, and *G4* genes in the 3′ end of its viral genome. The *tax* gene functions as a transactivator of host genes. Bovine leukemia virus is closely related to human T lymphotrophic virus 1 (HTLV-1), which has a similar viral genome. In contrast to *cis*-activating retroviruses, these viruses are examples of "trans-activating" retroviruses.

Acute Transforming Retroviruses

Acute transforming retroviruses are directly oncogenic by carrying an additional viral oncogene, v-*onc*, and are classified as "transducing" retroviruses. The retroviral v-*onc* originates from a host c-*onc* gene, and the transforming activity of the v-*onc* is accentuated by mutation. Given the high error rate of reverse transcription, v-*onc* gene homologs of c-*onc* genes will always carry mutations and the strongly promoted production of the viral oncoprotein will readily exceed that of the normal cellular oncoprotein. The result can be uncontrolled cell growth. Because c-*onc* genes are the precursors of v-*onc* genes, c-*onc* genes are also called "proto-oncogenes." Wherever acute transforming retroviruses

integrate in the host genome, it is the v-*onc* that is directly responsible for the rapid malignant change that occurs in cells infected with these viruses. Over 60 different v-*onc* genes have been identified, and retroviruses have been instrumental in identifying their cellular homologues.

The v-*onc* is usually incorporated into the viral RNA in place of part of one or more normal viral genes. Because such viruses have lost some of their viral genetic sequences, they are usually incapable of replication, and are therefore termed "defective" retroviruses. Defective retroviruses circumvent their defective replicative ability by utilizing non-defective "helper" retroviruses for formation of infectious virions. An exception is Rous sarcoma virus, in that its genome contains a viral oncogene (v-*src*) in addition to its full complement of functioning viral genes (*gag*, *pol*, and *env*); thus Rous sarcoma virus is both replication-competent and an acute transforming virus. Rous sarcoma virus is one of the most rapidly acting carcinogens known, transforming cultured cells in a day or so and causing neoplasia and death in chickens in as little as 2 weeks after infection.

Although retrovirus v-*onc* genes often preclude virus replication, v-*onc* genes have been acquired over time by retroviruses, most likely because they cause cellular proliferation. As most retroviruses replicate during cell division, this favors virus growth and perpetuation in nature. Defective retroviruses carrying a v-*onc* gene are always found in the company of a replication-competent helper virus that supplies missing functions, such as an environmentally stable envelope. The advantage to both viruses is presumably that when they are together they can infect more cells and produce more progeny of both viruses.

The various v-*onc* genes and the proteins they encode are assigned to major classes: growth factors (such as v-*sis*); growth factor receptors and hormone receptors (such as v-*erbB*); intracellular signal transducers (such as v-*ras*); and nuclear transcription factors (such as v-*jun*). The oncoprotein products of the various retroviral v-*onc* genes act in many different ways to affect cell growth, division, differentiation, and homeostasis:

- v-*onc* genes usually contain only that part of their corresponding c-*onc* gene that is transcribed into messenger RNA—in most instances they lack the introns that are so characteristic of eukaryotic genes
- v-*onc* genes are separated from the cellular context that normally controls gene expression, including the normal promoters and other sequences that regulate c-*onc* gene expression
- v-*onc* genes are under the control of the viral LTRs, which not only are strong promoters but also are influenced by cellular regulatory factors. For some retrovirus v-*onc* genes, such as *myc* and *mos*, the presence of viral LTRs is all that is needed for tumor induction

- v-*onc* genes may undergo mutations (deletions and rearrangements) that alter the structure of their protein products; such changes can interfere with normal protein–protein interactions, leading to escape from normal regulation

- v-*onc* genes may be joined to other viral genes in such a way that their functions are modified. For example, in Abelson murine leukemia virus the v-*abl* gene is expressed as a fusion protein with a gag protein; this arrangement directs the fusion protein to the plasma membrane where the Abl protein functions. In feline leukemia virus, the v-*onc* gene *fms* is also expressed as a fusion protein with a gag protein, thus allowing the insertion of the Fms oncoprotein in the plasma membrane.

Many acute transforming retroviruses induce solid tumors in addition to hemopoietic tumors. These viruses are termed "sarcoma" viruses. In addition to many avian leukosis virus-derived sarcoma viruses that have incorporated various v-*onc* genes, several acute transforming defective sarcoma viruses have been isolated from sarcomas of cats naturally infected with exogenous feline leukemia virus, a woolly monkey infected with a simian retrovirus, and several sarcoma viruses have been isolated from laboratory rodents infected with both exogenous and endogenous retroviruses. Acute transforming defective retroviruses are significant as oncogens in individual animals, but are not naturally transmissible agents.

Oncogenic DNA Viruses

Although retroviruses are the most important oncogenic viruses in animals, certain DNA viruses are also significant, including papillomaviruses, polyomaviruses, herpesviruses, and potentially others (Table 3.4). DNA tumor viruses

TABLE 3.4 Viruses that can Induce Tumors in Domestic or Laboratory Animals or Humans

Family / Genus	Virus	Kind of Tumor
DNA Viruses		
Poxviridae[a] / *Leporipoxvirus*	Rabbit fibroma virus and squirrel fibroma virus	Fibromas and myxomas in rabbits and squirrels (hyperplasia rather than neoplasia)
Poxviridae[a] / *Yatapoxvirus*	Yaba monkey tumor virus	Histiocytoma in monkeys
Herpesviridae / Alphaherpesvirinae / Mardivirus	Marek's disease virus	T cell lymphoma in fowl
Herpesviridae / Gammaherpesvirinae / Rhadinovirus	Ateline herpesvirus 2 and saimirine herpesvirus 2	Nil in natural hosts, lymphomas and leukemia in certain other monkeys
Herpesviridae / Gammaherpesvirinae / Lymphocryptovirus	Epstein–Barr virus	Burkitt's lymphoma, nasopharyngeal carcinoma, and B cell lymphomas in humans and monkeys
	Baboon herpesvirus	Lymphoma in baboons
Herpesviridae / Gammaherpesvirinae / Rhadinovirus	Cottontail rabbit herpesvirus	Lymphoma in rabbits
Alloherpesviridae / ranid herpesvirus	Lucké frog herpesvirus	Renal adenocarcinoma in frogs and tadpoles
Adenoviridae / Mastadenovirus	Many adenoviruses	Tumors in newborn rodents, no tumors in natural hosts
Papillomaviridae / multiple genera	Cottontail rabbit papillomavirus	Papillomas, skin cancers in rabbits
	Bovine papillomavirus 4	Papillomas, carcinoma of intestine, bladder
	Bovine papillomavirus 7	Papillomas, carcinoma of eye
	Human papillomaviruses 5, 8	Squamous cell carcinoma
	Human papillomaviruses 16, 18	Genital carcinomas
Polyomaviridae / Polyomavirus	Murine polyomavirus and simian virus 40	Tumors in newborn rodents

(Continued)

TABLE 3.4 (Continued)

Family / Genus	Virus	Kind of Tumor
Reverse Transcribing Viruses		
Hepadnaviridae/Orthohepadnavirus	Human, woodchuck hepatitis viruses	Hepatocellular carcinomas in humans and woodchucks
Hepadnaviridae/Avihepadnavirus	Duck hepatitis virus	Hepatocellular carcinomas in ducks
Retroviridae/Alpharetrovirus	Avian leukosis viruses	Leukosis (lymphoma, leukemia), osteopetrosis, nephroblastoma in fowl
	Rous sarcoma virus	Sarcoma in fowl
	Avian myeloblastosis virus	Myeloblastosis in fowl
Retroviridae/Betaretrovirus	Mouse mammary tumor virus	Mammary carcinoma in mice
	Mason–Pfizer monkey virus	Sarcoma and immunodeficiency disease in monkeys
	Ovine pulmonary adenocarcinoma virus (Jaagsiekte virus)	Pulmonary adenocarcinoma in sheep
Retroviridae/Gammaretrovirus	Feline leukemia virus	Leukemia in cats
	Feline sarcoma virus	Sarcoma in cats
	Murine leukemia and sarcoma viruses	Leukemia, lymphoma, and sarcoma in mice
	Avian reticuloendotheliosis virus	Reticuloendotheliosis in fowl
Retroviridae/Deltaretrovirus	Bovine leukemia virus	Leukemia (B cell lymphoma) in cattle
	HTLV 1 and 2 viruses and simian HTLV viruses	Adult T cell leukemia and hairy cell leukemia in humans, leukemia in monkeys
RNA Viruses		
Flaviviridae/Hepacivirus	Hepatitis C virus	Hepatocellular carcinoma in humans

[a]Not true oncogenic viruses. They differ from all other viruses listed in that poxviruses replicate in cytoplasm and do not affect the cellular genome.

interact with cells in one of two ways: (1) productive infection, in which the virus completes its replication cycle, resulting in cell lysis, or (2) non-productive infection, in which the virus transforms the cell without completing its replication cycle. During such non-productive infection, the viral genome or a truncated version of it is integrated into the cellular DNA; alternatively, the complete genome persists as an autonomously replicating plasmid (episome). The genome continues to express early gene functions. The molecular basis of oncogenesis by DNA viruses is best understood for polyomaviruses, papillomaviruses, and adenoviruses, all of which contain genes that behave as oncogenes, including tumor suppressor genes. These oncogenes appear to act by mechanisms similar to those described for retrovirus oncogenes: they act primarily in the nucleus, where they alter patterns of gene expression and regulation of cell growth. In every case the relevant genes encode early proteins having a dual role in virus replication and cell transformation. With a few possible exceptions, the oncogenes of DNA viruses have no homologue or direct ancestors (c-onc genes) among cellular genes of the host.

The protein products of DNA virus oncogenes are multifunctional, with particular functions that mimic functions of normal cellular proteins related to particular domains of the folded protein molecule. They interact with host-cell proteins at the plasma membrane or within the cytoplasm or nucleus.

Oncogenic Polyomaviruses and Adenoviruses

During the 1960s and 1970s, two members of the family *Polyomaviridae*, murine polyomavirus and simian virus 40 (SV40), as well as certain human adenoviruses (types 12, 18, and 31) were shown to induce malignant neoplasms following their inoculation into baby hamsters and other rodents. With the exception of murine polyomavirus, none of these viruses induces cancer under natural conditions in its natural host, rather they transform cultured cells of certain other species and provide experimental models for analysis of the molecular events in cell transformation.

Polyomavirus- or adenovirus-transformed cells do not produce virus. Viral DNA is integrated at several sites in the chromosomes of the cell. Most of the integrated viral genomes are complete in the case of the polyomaviruses, but defective in the case of the adenoviruses. Only certain early viral genes are transcribed, albeit at an unusually high rate. By analogy with retrovirus genes, they are now called oncogenes. Their products, demonstrable by immunofluorescence, used to be known as *tumor (T) antigens*. A great deal is now known about the role of these proteins in transformation. Virus can be rescued from polyomavirus-transformed cells—that is, virus can be induced to replicate, by irradiation, treatment with certain mutagenic chemicals, or co-cultivation with certain types of permissive cells. This cannot be done with adenovirus-transformed cells, as the integrated adenovirus DNA contains substantial deletions.

It should be stressed that the integration of viral DNA does not necessarily lead to transformation. Many or most episodes of integration of polyomavirus or adenovirus DNA have no recognized biological consequence. Transformation by these viruses in experimental systems is a rare event, requiring that the viral transforming genes be integrated in the location and orientation needed for their expression. Even then, many transformed cells revert (abortive transformation). Furthermore, cells displaying the characteristics of transformation do not necessarily produce neoplasms.

Oncogenic Papillomaviruses

Papillomaviruses produce papillomas (warts) on the skin and mucous membranes of most animal species (see Chapter 11). These benign neoplasms are hyperplastic epithelial outgrowths that generally regress spontaneously. Occasionally, however, they may progress to malignancy, which in part is a property of specific virus strains. Virus-induced papillomas occur in many species, and papillomaviruses are also the cause of sarcoids in horses, some human oropharyngeal carcinomas, and cervical carcinoma in women, and are associated with some squamous cell carcinomas in cats and dogs.

In benign warts, the papillomavirus DNA is episomal, meaning it is not integrated into the host-cell DNA and persists as an autonomously replicating episome, whereas in papillomavirus-induced cancers the viral DNA is integrated into that of the host. Thus, integration probably is necessary for malignant transformation, as the pattern of integration is clonal within cancers: each cancer cell carries at least one, and often many incomplete copies of the viral genome. The site of virus integration is random, and there is no consistent association with cellular proto-oncogenes. For some papillomaviruses, integration disrupts one of the early genes, *E2*, which is a viral repressor. Other viral genes may also be deleted, but the viral oncogenes (e.g., *E6* and *E7*) remain intact, are expressed efficiently, and cause the malignant transformation. The proteins expressed by the viral oncogenes interact with cellular growth regulating proteins produced by proto-oncogenes and tumor suppressors such as p53 to block apoptosis and promote cellular proliferation. Another relevant example is bovine papillomavirus type 1 E5 oncoprotein, which alters the activity of cell membrane proteins involved in regulating cellular proliferation—for example, platelet derived growth factor receptor.

Oncogenic Hepadnaviruses

Mammalian, but not avian, hepadnaviruses are associated strongly with naturally occurring hepatocellular carcinomas in their natural hosts. Woodchucks that are chronically infected with woodchuck hepatitis virus almost inevitably develop hepatocellular carcinoma, even in the absence of other carcinogenic factors. Oncogenesis induced by mammalian hepadnaviruses is a multifactorial process, and there are differences in the cellular mechanisms responsible for carcinogenesis associated with different viruses. Whereas ground squirrel and woodchuck hepatitis viruses activate cellular oncogenes, the mode of action of human hepatitis B virus is uncertain, as it apparently has no consistent site of integration or oncogene association. The hepatocellular regeneration accompanying cirrhosis of the liver also promotes the development of neoplasia in hepatitis virus-infected humans, but there is no cirrhosis in the animal models. The likelihood of hepadnavirus-associated carcinoma is greatest in animals (and humans) infected at birth.

Oncogenic Herpesviruses

Oncogenic Alphaherpesviruses

Marek's disease virus of chickens transforms T lymphocytes, causing them to proliferate to produce a generalized polyclonal T lymphocyte neoplasm. The disease is preventable by vaccination with live-attenuated virus vaccines that lack the retrovirus v-*onc* genes that are present in Marek's disease virus.

Oncogenic Gammaherpesviruses

Herpesviruses of the subfamily *Gammaherpesvirinae* are lymphotropic and the etiologic agents of lymphomas and carcinomas in hosts ranging from amphibians to primates, including humans. Epstein–Barr virus (human herpesvirus 4) in otherwise healthy young human adults causes infectious mononucleosis (glandular fever), in which there is B lymphocyte proliferation that resolves. The mechanism by which the virus goes on to produce malignancy in some individuals has been best studied in Burkitt's lymphoma, a malignant B cell lymphoma that occurs in children in East Africa and less frequently in children in other parts of the world. The Epstein–Barr viral genomic DNA is present in multiple copies of episomal DNA in each cell of most African Burkitt's lymphomas. Lymphoma cells express viral nuclear antigen, but do not produce virus. These cells also contain a characteristic 8 : 14 chromosomal translocation. Burkitt's lymphoma may develop as a consequence of c-*myc* deregulation resulting from this translocation, which in turn causes an arrest of normal cellular maturation and differentiation processes. Some Burkitt's lymphomas also have mutations in the cellular tumor suppressor gene, *p53*.

The subfamily *Gammaherpesvirinae* includes several other viruses that cause lymphomas in heterologous primate hosts (e.g., herpesvirus siamiri), human herpesvirus 8, associated with Kaposi sarcoma mostly in humans with AIDS, and bovine malignant catarrhal fever virus, an acute fatal lymphoproliferative disease of cattle and certain wild ruminants (see Chapter 9). These viruses are lymphotropic and contain numerous unspliced genes that appear to have been captured from the host during virus replication, over considerable evolutionary time. These captured genes typically encode proteins that (1) regulate cell growth, (2) are immunosuppressive, or (3) are enzymes involved in nucleic acid metabolism—they include genes encoding cytokine or cytokine receptor homologues, regulatory proteins such as cyclins that control the cell cycle, and proteins such as bcl2 that can block apoptosis. The function of these various virus-encoded proteins is consistent with the lymphotropic and transforming properties of these viruses. Thus these herpesviruses seem to have evolved/acquired different strategies to overcome cell cycle arrest, apoptosis, and activation of cellular immunity, all to favor virus replication and survival, all also causing lymphocyte proliferation and transformation.

Certain members of the family *Alloherpesviridae* are associated with neoplasia in their respective hosts, including renal adenocarcinomas of frogs and epithelial tumors of salmonid fish.

Oncogenic Poxviruses

Although some poxviruses are regularly associated with the development of benign tumor-like lesions (see Chapter 7), there is no evidence that these ever become malignant, nor is there evidence that poxvirus DNA is ever integrated into cellular DNA. A very early viral protein produced in poxvirus-infected cells displays homology with epidermal growth factor and is probably responsible for the epithelial hyperplasia characteristic of many poxvirus infections. For some poxviruses (e.g., fowlpox, orf, and rabbit fibroma viruses), epithelial hyperplasia is a dominant clinical manifestation and may be a consequence of a more potent form of the poxvirus epidermal growth factor homologue.

Antiviral Immunity and Prophylaxis

As obligate intracellular parasites, viruses have co-evolved with their respective hosts, and eukaryotic host organisms have developed diverse and sophisticated defenses to protect themselves against viral infections and their associated diseases. In turn, viruses have also developed a remarkable variety of strategies to avoid or subvert these host defenses. Antiviral immunity in higher animals is complex, and reflects a combination of innate and acquired (adaptive) immune response mechanisms, although there is considerable interplay between these two broad categories. Cytokines, dendritic cells, natural antibodies and certain T lymphocytes ($\gamma\delta$ T cells) provide especially important bridging linkage between innate and adaptive immune responses. Antiviral immunity in animals is mediated by both cellular and humoral factors, and the nature of the immune response generated by different individuals infected with the same virus can be different, depending on the individual's genetic constitution, environmental influences, and other factors that can determine the course and pathogenesis of the infection.

Innate immune defenses (also referred to as native or natural immunity) are constantly present to protect multicellular organisms against viral infections, and previous exposure to a particular virus is not required to activate these mechanisms. In contrast, adaptive immunity develops only after exposure to a virus, and is specific to that particular virus and, sometimes, its close relatives. Adaptive immunity involves cellular and antibody (humoral) effector mechanisms, mediated respectively by T and B lymphocytes. In further contrast to innate immunity, adaptive immune responses exhibit memory, such that the response may be

quickly reactivated after re-exposure to the same virus. With many systemic viral infections, immunological memory after natural infection confers long-term, often life-long, protection against the associated disease.

The development of efficacious vaccines has substantially reduced the deleterious impact of viral diseases of humans and animals. The goal of vaccination is to stimulate the adaptive immune responses that protect animals after reinfection with specific viruses. An increasing variety of vaccine types are now commercially available for use in animals, especially companion and production animal species, including livestock, poultry and fish; these include inactivated (*syn.* "killed"), live-attenuated (*syn.* modified-live), and various types of recombinant and genetically engineered vaccines. Vaccines are used extensively in regulatory programs for the control of individual viral diseases of livestock, often in combination with specific management procedures. Other strategies for antiviral treatment and prophylaxis include drugs that interfere with viral infection and/or replication, as well as molecules that stimulate or mimic protective host responses.

HOST IMMUNITY TO VIRAL INFECTIONS

Innate Immunity

Innate immune defenses exhibit neither antigen specificity nor memory, but they provide a critical line of first defense against viral infections because they are constantly present and are operational immediately after viral infection. Innate immunity

Fenner's Veterinary Virology. DOI: 10.1016/B978-0-12-375158-4.00004-3

is often considered separate from acquired immune responses, but they are inextricably linked, and innate responses modulate subsequent acquired responses in many ways. Several distinct activities mediate innate immune defense, including: (1) epithelial barriers; (2) antimicrobial serum proteins such as complement; (3) natural antibodies produced by B1 lymphocytes; (4) the activities of phagocytic cells such as neutrophils, macrophages, and dendritic cells; (5) natural killer (NK) cells that can lyse virus-infected cells; (6) various cell types present at sites of virus invasion that possess receptors that generically recognize and quickly respond to invading viruses by transcriptional activation that results in production of a wide variety of protective molecules, the interferon (IFN) system being an especially critical and central component of antiviral resistance; (7) apoptosis, a process of programmed cell death that can eliminate virus-infected cells; (8) small RNA molecules that interfere with virus replication (RNAi).

Viruses that are transmitted horizontally between individuals must first breach the barriers at their portal of entry before they can cause infection in their respective hosts. For example, the epithelial lining of the skin and respiratory, gastrointestinal, and urogenital tracts provides a mechanical barrier against infection at these common sites of virus entry. Secretions and other activities at mucosal surfaces provide further non-specific protection against viral infection. For example, surfactant and the mucociliary apparatus confer non-specific antimicrobial protection to the respiratory tract. Similarly, antimicrobial protection in the gastrointestinal tract is mediated by, amongst others, the mucous barrier, regional pH extremes, sterilizing action of secretions (e.g., from the liver (bile) and pancreas), and specific antimicrobial peptides such as defensins that are present within the mucosa and its secretions.

A variety of plasma proteins exert antimicrobial activity, including the various complement proteins, C-reactive protein, mannose-binding protein, and broadly reactive natural antibodies. These proteins can exert either a direct antimicrobial effect, or they can promote the uptake of microorganisms into phagocytic cells by coating their surface to facilitate receptor binding (opsonization).

Phagocytic cells—macrophages and neutrophils—provide a critical antimicrobial function, as they are attracted to sites of inflammation, where they efficiently ingest and digest foreign materials, including microorganisms. These cells possess the intracellular machinery to destroy ingested microbes, particularly bacteria, through the actions of hydrolytic lysosomal enzymes as well as the production of activated oxygen and nitrogen metabolites within phagocytic vacuoles. Various soluble mediators can both attract these cells to sites of inflammation, and activate them to enhance their antimicrobial activity.

Dendritic cells are key players in both adaptive and innate immunity to viral infections (and will be discussed in detail in the section below on Adaptive Immunity). In addition to being highly efficient antigen-presenting cells, dendritic cells

are an especially important source of type I IFN and various other cytokines that inhibit viral infection and replication. Interdigitating dendritic cells are abundant at portals of virus entry (such as the respiratory, urogenital, and gastrointestinal tracts, and skin), and they are endowed with pattern recognition receptors that allow them quickly to initiate protective innate immune responses to invading viruses.

Natural Killer Cells

Natural killer cells are specialized lymphocytes that are capable of rapid killing of virus-infected cells; thus they provide early and non-specific resistance against viral infections. Specifically, natural killer cells recognize host cells that express altered levels of major histocompatibility complex (MHC) class I molecules and/or heat shock (or similar) proteins. The function of natural killer cells is stringently regulated by the balance of activating and inhibitory signals expressed on the surface of target cells. Virus-infected cells typically express reduced levels of inhibitory class I MHC molecules and increased levels of ligands specific for activating receptors on natural killer cells. In summary, natural killer cells are not antigen specific; rather, their activation requires differential engagement of cell-surface receptors in combination with stimulation by proinflammatory cytokines (Figure 4.1).

Natural killer cells mediate death of virus-infected cells via apoptosis; this cytocidal activity is central to the control of viral infections, because it can eliminate infected cells before they release progeny virions. Natural killer cells also possess surface receptors for the Fc portion of immunoglobulin molecules, which allows them to bind and lyse antibody-coated target cells through the process of antibody-dependent cell-mediated cytotoxicity. Lastly, natural killer cells synthesize and release a variety of cytokines, including type II IFN and several interleukins that stimulate their own proliferation and cytolytic activity.

Cellular Pattern Recognition Receptors

Cells at portals of virus entry possess surface receptors (*pattern recognition receptors* (PRR)) that recognize specific *pathogen-associated molecular patterns* (PAMPs), which are macromolecules present in microbes but not on host cells. These pattern recognition receptors are expressed on and in a variety of different cells, including macrophages, dendritic cells, neutrophils, natural killer cells, endothelial cells, and mucosal epithelial cells. The binding of microbial macromolecules (PAMPs) to these receptors immediately triggers innate immune responses that protect the host against microbial invasion. Activation of these responses does not require prior exposure of the host to the specific virus.

The *toll-like receptors* (TLRs; the name reflects the similarity of these proteins to the *Drosophila* protein Toll) are important examples of pattern recognition receptors. They are located both on the cell surface and in endosomal vesicles, which allows these receptors to detect the presence of microbial

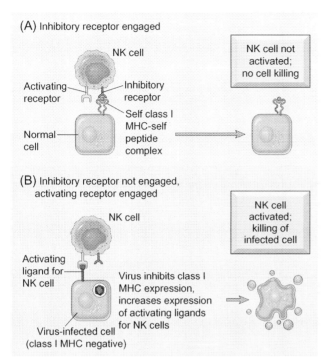

(A) Inhibitory receptor engaged

NK cell

Activating receptor

Inhibitory receptor

Self class I MHC-self peptide complex

Normal cell

NK cell not activated; no cell killing

(B) Inhibitory receptor not engaged, activating receptor engaged

NK cell

Activating ligand for NK cell

Virus inhibits class I MHC expression, increases expression of activating ligands for NK cells

Virus-infected cell (class I MHC negative)

NK cell activated; killing of infected cell

FIGURE 4.1   Activating and inhibitory receptors of natural killer (NK) cells. A. Healthy cells express self class I MHC molecules, which are recognized by inhibitory receptors, thus ensuring that NK cells do not attack normal cells. Note that healthy cells may express ligands for activating receptors (not shown) or may not express such ligands (as shown), but they do not activate NK cells because they engage the inhibitory receptors. B. In virus-infected cells, class I MHC expression is reduced so that the inhibitory receptors are not engaged, and ligands for activating receptors are expressed. The result is that NK cells are activated and the infected cells are killed. [*From* Robbins & Cotran Pathologic Basis of Disease, *V. Kumar, A. K. Abbas, N. Fausto, J. Aster, 8th ed., p. 188. Copyright © Saunders/Elsevier (2010), with permission.*]

"triggers" (PAMPs) in the extracellular environment, in addition to those internalized into the cell following phagocytosis or receptor-mediated endocytosis. There are at least 10 mammalian TLRs, and different TLRs recognize different PAMPs. TLR3 is especially important for antiviral immunity, because its ligand is double-stranded RNA (dsRNA), which is produced in virus-infected cells. All TLRs have an extracellular portion that includes leucine- and cysteine-rich domains, and a conserved cytoplasmic portion that interacts with cellular signaling proteins. Other pathogen recognition/detection systems are also operational within the cell cytoplasm, and activation of the TLRs and/or any of the other sensors results in activation of common signaling pathways that involve cellular transcriptional factors, notably nuclear factor κB (NF-κB) that causes, depending on cell type: (1) expression of IFNs and inflammatory cytokines such as tissue necrosis factor and interleukins-1 and -12 (IL-1, IL-12); (2) activation of phagocytic cells and endothelial cells with increased production of inflammatory mediators and cell-surface expression of adhesion molecules; (3) production in phagocytic cells of microbicidal products such as

nitric oxide. Collectively, these cellular responses that are triggered by activation of pattern recognition receptors are potent stimulators of inflammation and inhibitors of viral infection and replication.

Cytokines

Cytokines are messengers of the immune system that are responsible for the induction and regulation of both innate and adaptive immune responses. Specifically, cytokines are soluble mediators that facilitate communication between key cell populations, including the various subpopulations of lymphocytes, macrophages, dendritic cells, endothelial cells, and neutrophils. By way of general properties, cytokines are typically inducible glycoproteins that are transiently synthesized after appropriate stimulation of the cell that produces them. Individual cytokines usually are produced by more than one cell type and perform several, frequently divergent activities. There is much overlap (redundancy) in the activity of different cytokines; thus their interactions and activities are highly complex. Cytokines bind to specific receptors on the surface of target cells, with subsequent transcriptional activation of that cell. These activities can manifest as:

- autocrine effects on the same cell type that produces them
- paracrine effects on adjacent cells of different types
- endocrine effects, which are systemic effects on many cell types

Key cytokines involved in innate immune responses include the type I IFNs, tissue necrosis factor (TNF), IL-6, and the chemokines. *Chemokines* are a family of small proteins that are chemotactic for leukocytes, including, among many others, IL-8. Other cytokines such as IL-12 and type II IFN are critical to both innate and adaptive immune responses. The IFNs are especially critical to antiviral immunity and are discussed in detail in the following section.

Interferons

In 1957, Isaacs and Lindenmann reported that cells of the chorioallantoic membrane of embryonated hen's eggs infected with influenza virus release into the medium a non-viral protein—"interferon" (IFN)—that protects uninfected cells against the same or unrelated viruses. It has since been determined that there are several types and subtypes of interferon (IFN), and that these proteins are key elements of antiviral resistance and are central to both innate and adaptive immune responses to viral infections.

There are three distinct types of IFN, designated as types I, II, and III, that each utilize different cellular receptors (Figure 4.2).

- *Type I interferon (type I IFN).* Type I IFNs include IFN-α, of which there are several types depending on species, and a single type of IFN-β; many cell types can

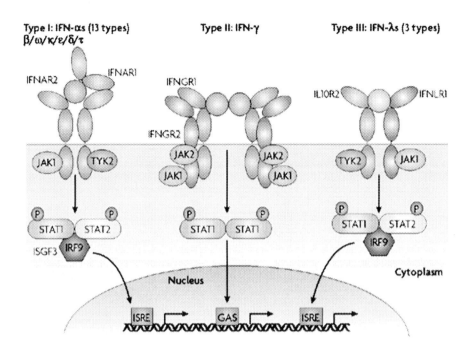

Nature Reviews | Drug Discovery

FIGURE 4.2   Receptor activation or ligand–receptor complex assembled by type I, type II, or type III interferons (IFNs). Type I IFNs (α, β, δ, ϵ, κ, and ω in pigs; τ in ruminants) interact with IFN (-α, -β, and -ω) receptor 1 (IFNAR1) and IFNAR2; type II IFN-γ interacts with IFN-γ receptor 1 (IFNGR1) and IFNGR2; type III IFN-λs interact with IFN-λ receptor 1 (IFNRL1; also known as IL28RA) and IL-10 receptor 2 (IL10R2; also known as IL10RB). Type II IFN-γ is an antiparallel homodimer exhibiting a twofold axis of symmetry. It binds two IFNGR1 receptor chains, assembling a complex that is stabilized by two IFNGR2 chains. These receptors are associated with two kinases from the JAK family: Janus (JAK)1 and tyrosine (TYK)2 for types I and III IFNs; JAK1 and JAK2 for type II IFN. All IFN receptor chains belong to the class 2 helical cytokine receptor family, which is defined by the structure of the extracellular domains of their members: approximately 200 amino acids structured in two subdomains of 100 amino acids (fibronectin type III modules), themselves structured by seven β-strands arranged in a β-sandwich. The 200 amino acid domains usually contain the ligand binding site. IFNAR2, IFNLR1, IL10R2, IFNGR1, and IFNGR2 are classical representatives of this family, whereas IFNAR1 is atypical, as its extracellular domain is duplicated. GAS, IFN-γ-activated site; IRF9, IFN regulatory factor 9; ISGF3, IFN-stimulated gene factor 3 (refers to the STAT1–STAT2–IRF9 complex); ISRE, IFN-stimulated response element; P, phosphate, STAT1/2, signal transducers and activators of transcription 1/2. *[From E. C. Borden, G. C. Sen, G. Uze, R. H. Silverman, R. M. Ransohoff, G. R. Foster, G. R. Stark. Interferons at age 50: past, current and future impact on biomedicine. Nat. Rev. Drug Discov.* **6***, 975–990 (2007), with permission.]*

produce these type I IFNs. Additional type I IFNs with specific functions include IFN-δ, -ϵ, -κ, -o, and -τ. Type I IFNs bind the IFN-α receptor (IFNAR), a heterodimer of IFNARs 1 and 2, to activate a signaling cascade of enzymes including the tyrosine (TYK) and Janus (JAK) kinases, signal transducers and activators of transcription (STATs), and IFN regulatory factor 9 (IRF9). Activation of this signaling cascade ultimately results in induction of the IFN response genes [IFN-stimulated response elements (ISRE)] in the treated cell (Figure 4.2). The importance of type I IFN to innate resistance is graphically confirmed by the fact that IFN receptor (IFNAR)-deficient mice are highly susceptible to lethal infections with viruses, but not with intracellular pathogens such as the bacteria *Listeria monocytogenes*. Similarly, humans with deficits in signaling pathways triggered by IFN (STAT, TYK, IFNAR) often die of viral diseases.

- *Type II interferon (type II IFN).* There is a single form of type II IFN designated IFN-γ, which is a product of T cells and NK cells. Activated T cells are especially important sources of IFN-γ production, which is central to the expression of the cell-mediated immune aspects of adaptive immunity. Type II IFN binds the IFN-γ receptor (IFNGR), which is a tetramer composed of two heterodimers of IFNGRs 1 and 2, to activate a cell signaling pathway (involving JAK and STAT) to induce the cellular IFN-γ-activated site (GAS). This transcriptional activation induced by IFN-γ generates broad antimicrobial immunity in the treated cell, especially macrophages. IFN-γ is particularly important in conferring immunity to intracellular microorganisms other than viruses.

- *Type III interferon (type III IFN).* Type III IFN represented by IFN-λ was only recently described and appears to represent an ancestral type I IFN, perhaps one with regulatory function.

In addition to their important antiviral activities, particularly those of type I IFN, the IFNs also stimulate

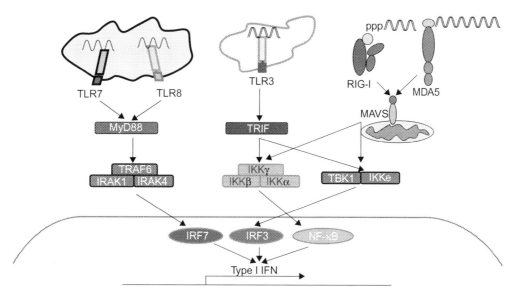

FIGURE 4.3 Endosomal and cytoplasmic pathways for virus recognition and IFN production. In dendritic cells, TLR7 and TLR8 located in endosomal compartments recognize viral ssRNA through direct infection, autophagocytic uptake of viral material from cytoplasm, or phagocytic uptake of other infected cells or vial particles. Both TLR7 and TLR8 signal through the adapter MyD88, which through interaction with the IRAK4–IRAK1–TRAF6 complex leads to phosphorylation and activation of IRF7 and subsequent IFN transcription. TLR3 located in endosomes of DCs, macrophages, epithelial cells, and fibroblasts is activated by encountering dsRNA. Following its activation, TLR3 signals through its adapter, TRIF, which leads to activation of non-canonical IKK kinases (TBK1/IKKε) and subsequent phosphorylation and nuclear translocation of IRF3. Nuclear factor κB (NFκB) is also activated by TRIF-mediated signaling through canonical IKK kinases (IKKα, β, and γ). Cytoplasmically located RIG-1 and MDA5 are expressed in most cells and recognize 5′ppp-containing dsRNA or long dsRNA, respectively. Both of these cytoplasmic sensors upon activation interact and signal through the mitochondrially located adapter, MAVS. This signaling pathway, analogous to that of TLR3, leads to activation of the canonical and non-canonical IKK kinases and the following nuclear translocation of NFκB and IRF3. Concurrent activation of IRF3 and NFκB in turn allows for transcription of IFN genes and its synthesis and export. DC, dendritic cells; IKK, IκB kinases; IRAK, interleukin receptor-associated kinase; IRF, IFN regulatory factor; MDA5, melanoma differentiation-associated gene 5; MVAS, mitochondrial antiviral signaling protein; RIG, retinoic-acid-inducible gene; TBK, TRAF family member-associated NFκB activator binding kinase; TLR, Toll-like receptor; TRAF, tumor necrosis factor receptor-associated factor; TRIF, TIR-domain-containing adapter-inducing IFN-β. *[From A. Baum, A. Garcia-Sastre. Amino Acids* **38***, 1283–1299 (2010), with permission.]*

adaptive immune responses, including enhanced cytotoxic T-lymphocyte-mediated cell lysis through increased expression of class I MHC on virus-infected cells. Similarly, IFN-γ promotes expression of class II MHC on macrophages, activates macrophages and NK cells, and modulates immunoglobulin synthesis by B lymphocytes. Type II IFN also exerts systemic effects including pyrexia and myalgia.

Induction of IFN Production

Induction of type I IFN involves activation via cellular pattern recognition receptors, which are non-specific sensors of viral infections that detect unique viral signatures (PAMPs), leading to transcription of numerous genes encoding proteins that are involved in innate and adaptive immune responses, including type I IFN. Importantly, these responses may be triggered by several redundant pathways, both cytoplasmic and extracytoplasmic (Figure 4.3). The TLRs are largely responsible for pathogen detection in extracytoplasmic compartments, and subsequent induction of production of type I IFN. The TLRs detect PAMPs and signal via cytoplasmic Toll/IL-1 receptor (TIR) domains to transcriptionally activate critical genes, including those encoding the type 1 IFNs. Different TLRs detect different PAMPs; thus TLR7

and TLR8 detect single-stranded RNA (ssRNA) and are important in type I IFN production in influenza and human immunodeficiency viral infections, TLR9 detects viral DNA, as in herpesvirus infection, and TLR3 detects dsRNA, which characteristically is produced during viral infections but is not present in normal cells. These receptors are predominantly located in the endosome, where they can readily detect viruses internalized after endocytosis, including viruses or their nucleic acid released from adjacent apoptotic or lysed cells. Induction of type I IFN transcription following activation of the extracytoplasmic path is dependent on the specific TLR that is activated; thus TLR3 utilizes a specific adapter designated TRIF (TIR-domain-containing adapter-inducing IFN-β) that mediates activation of: (1) NFκB, (2) IRF3, and (3) activating protein 1 (AP1), leading to upregulation of IFN-β gene transcription. In contrast, activation of TLRs 7, 8, and 9 is mediated by the myeloid differentiation primary response protein 88 (MyD88) adapter molecule associated with the TIR domain, which results in activation of IRF7, NFκB, and AP1, which results in transcriptional activation of both the IFN-α and IFN-β genes (Figure 4.3). Especially high levels of expression of this latter pathway occur in dendritic cells, presumably because of their critical central role in both innate and adaptive immune responses.

Cytoplasmic pathways for pathogen sensing and type I IFN induction also can occur via TLR-independent signaling involving cytoplasmic RNA helicase proteins such as retinoic acid inducible gene (RIG-1) and melanoma differentiation-associated gene 5 (MDA5) (Figure 4.3). The cytoplasmic pathway includes mitochondrial antiviral signaling protein (MAVS; also referred to as IPS-1) and leads to activation of NFκB, AP-1, and IRF3, with resultant transcriptional activation of innate response genes including type 1 IFN. There are also TLR- and RIG-1-independent signaling pathways that provide further redundancy in the detection of microorganism triggers (PAMPs), which is so critical to a prompt antiviral response and, ultimately, to host survival.

Action of Type I IFN

Type I IFN produced and released from virus-infected cells (as described in the preceding section) exerts its effects on adjacent cells via receptor (IFNAR) binding and signaling that leads to induction of the IFN response element, with transcriptional activation of more than 300 IFN-stimulated genes (ISGs). Most of these ISGs encode cellular pattern recognition

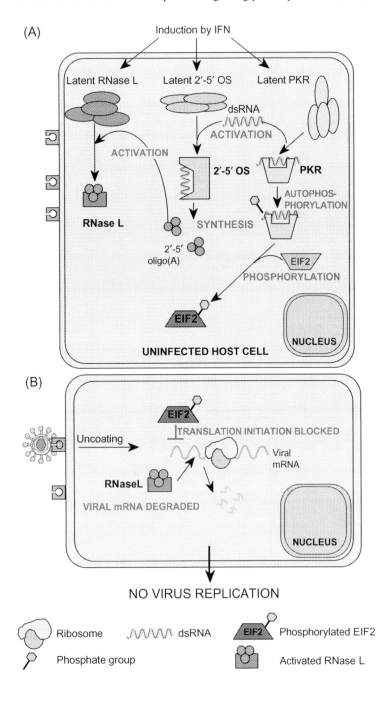

FIGURE 4.4 The antiviral state. (A) Development of the antiviral state begins with the action of interferon on an uninfected cell. The result of the signal transduction cascade shown in Figure 4.2 is the induction of expression of up to 300 genes, of which three are shown here: RNase L, the 2′-5′ oligo(A) synthetase (2′-5′ OS), and the double-stranded DNA (dsRNA)-dependent protein kinase (PKR). These proteins are latent until they are activated by viral infection. PKR and 2′-5′ OS are activated by dsRNA that is produced during viral infection. Once activated, PKR autophosphorylates, and then phosphorylates eukaryotic initiation factor 2 (EIF2). The activated synthetase makes trimeric oligonucleotides, which in turn activate RNase L. (B) Phosphorylated EIF2 and activated RNase L are characteristic of the "antiviral state," in which a eukaryotic cell is refractory to infection by a wide variety of viruses. Phosphorylated EIF2 cannot serve to initiate translation of mRNA by ribosomes, and activated RNase L degrades mRNAs, both viral and cellular, so protein synthesis stops. Without protein synthesis, no virus replication can take place, but the inhibition of protein synthesis is transient and the cell may recover. [*From* Viruses and Human Disease, *J. H. Strauss, E. G. Strauss, 2nd ed., p. 401. Copyright © Academic Press/Elsevier (2007), with permission.*]

receptors or proteins that regulate either signaling pathways or transcription factors that amplify IFN production, whereas others promote an antiviral state via cytoskeletal remodeling, apoptosis, post-transcriptional events (mRNA editing, splicing, degradation), or post-translational modification (Figure 4.4). Those proteins proven to be critical to the induction of the IFN-induced antiviral state include:

- ISG15, which is a ubiquitin homolog that is not constitutively expressed in cells. Addition of ubiquitin to cellular proteins is key to regulation of the innate immune response, and ISG15 apparently can exert a similar function with more than 150 target proteins in IFN-stimulated cells. Activities of ISG15 can regulate all aspects of the IFN pathway, including induction, signaling, and action.

- MxGTPase is a hydrolyzing enzyme that, like ISG15, is not constitutively expressed. The enzyme is located in the smooth endoplasmic reticulum, where it affects vesicle formation, specifically targeting the viral nucleocapsid in virus-infected cells to prevent virus maturation.

- The protein kinase (PKR) pathway is constitutively expressed at only a very low level, but is quickly upregulated by IFNAR signaling. In the presence of dsRNA, protein kinase phosphorylates elongation (translation) initiation factor eIF-2α and prevents recycling of cyclic nucleotides (GDP), which in turn halts protein synthesis. This IFN-induced pathway is especially important for inhibiting replication of reoviruses, adenoviruses, vaccinia and influenza viruses, amongst many others.

- The 2′-5′ oligoadenylate synthetase (OAS) pathway, like the PKR pathway, is constitutively expressed only at low level. After IFNAR stimulation and in the presence of dsRNA, this enzyme produces oligoadenylates with a distinctive 2′-5′ linkage, as contrasted with the normal 3′-5′ lineage. These 2′-5′ oligoadenylates in turn activate cellular RNase that degrades RNA, which cleaves viral messenger and genomic RNA. Picornaviruses are especially susceptible to inhibition by this pathway, as is West Nile virus.

- Many other pathways have been identified in IFN-treated cell cultures, but their individual significance remains to be unequivocally proven in knockout mice.

In summarized, type I IFN is produced after viral infection of many different types of cells, and the IFN released from these cells then induces an antiviral state in adjacent cells (autocrine or paracrine effect). The multiple antiviral pathways that are activated in IFN-treated cells are stringently regulated by requirement for the presence of co-factors such as dsRNA, meaning that these pathways can only be activated when the IFN-treated cell is subsequently infected with a virus. This stringent regulation is necessary because some of these antiviral defense mechanisms also compromise normal cellular functions.

Apoptosis

It was long thought that viruses killed cells by direct means such as usurping their cellular machinery or disrupting membrane integrity, ultimately leading to necrosis of the virus-infected cell. However, it is now clear that apoptosis is an important and common event during many viral infections. *Apoptosis* is the process of programmed cell death, which is essentially a mechanism of cell suicide that the host activates as a last resort to eliminate viral factories before progeny virus production is complete. There are two distinct cellular pathways that trigger apoptosis (Figure 4.5), both of which culminate in the activation of host-cell caspase enzymes that mediate death of the cell (the so-called executioner phase). Once activated, caspases are responsible for degradation of the cell's own DNA and proteins. Cell membrane alterations in the doomed cell promote its recognition and removal by phagocytic cells. The two initiation pathways are:

1. *The Intrinsic (Mitochondrial) Pathway.* The mitochondrial pathway is activated as a result of increased permeability of mitochondrial membranes subsequent to cell injury, such as that associated with a viral infection. Severe injury alters the delicate balance between anti-apoptotic (e.g., Bcl-2) and pro-apoptotic (e.g., Bax) molecules in mitochondrial membranes and the cytosol, resulting in progressive leakage of mitochondrial proteins (such as cytochrome *c*) into the cytosol where these proteins activate cellular caspases.

2. *The Extrinsic (Death Receptor) Pathway.* The extrinsic pathway is activated by engagement of specific cell-membrane receptors, which are members of the TNF receptor family (TNF, Fas, and others). Thus binding of the cytokine TNF to its cellular receptor can trigger apoptosis. Similarly, cytotoxic T lymphocytes that recognize virus-infected cells in an antigen-specific manner can bind the Fas receptor, activate the death domain, and trigger the executioner caspase pathway that then eliminates the cell before it becomes a functional virus factory.

In addition to death-receptor-mediated cytolysis, cytotoxic T lymphocytes and natural killer cells can initiate apoptosis of virus-infected target cell, utilizing preformed mediators such as perforin and granzyme that directly activate caspases in the target cell.

Gene Silencing (Interfering RNA)

Cells utilize small, interfering, RNA molecules (RNAi) to silence genes as a means of regulating normal developmental and physiological processes, and potentially to interfere with virus replication. The RNAi are produced from longer segments of either ssRNA or dsRNA, after their cleavage by an endoribonuclease (DICER). Production of RNAi initiates formation of the RNA-silencing complex that includes an endonuclease (argonaute) that degrades those

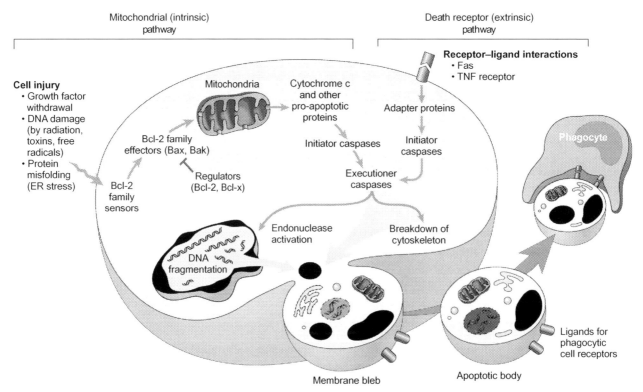

FIGURE 4.5   Mechanisms of apoptosis. The two pathways of apoptosis differ in their induction and regulation, and both culminate in the activation of "executioner" caspases. [*From* Robbins & Cotran Pathologic Basis of Disease, *V. Kumar, A. K. Abbas, N. Fausto, J. Aster, 8th ed., p. 28. Copyright © Saunders/Elsevier (2010), with permission.*]

mRNAs with a sequence that is complementary to that of the RNAi (Figure 4.6). Cells can utilize this mechanism to disrupt virus replication through the production of RNAi that are complementary to specific viral genes; however, RNAi also may be produced during viral infections that specifically inhibit protective cellular antiviral pathways.

Adaptive Immunity

Adaptive immunity includes humoral and cellular components. Humoral immunity is mediated principally by antibodies released from B lymphocytes, whereas cellular immunity is mediated by T lymphocytes (Figure 4.7). In addition, dendritic cells, macrophages, NK cells, and cytokines are all critical to adaptive immune responses. Adaptive immunity is antigen specific, so that these responses take time (several days at least) to develop, and this type of immunity is mediated by lymphocytes that possess surface receptors that are specific to each pathogen. Adaptive immunity stimulates long-term memory after infection, meaning that protective immune responses can quickly be reactivated on re-exposure of the organism to the same pathogen.

Cytokines were described above in the section on innate immunity, but they are also critical to adaptive immune responses, emphasizing how innate and acquired immune responses are inter-related. Those cytokines that are

especially important to adaptive immunity are principally produced by CD4$^+$ T cells after antigenic stimulation, and they promote the proliferation, differentiation, and activation of lymphocytes. Important cytokines of adaptive immunity include interleukins IL-2, IL-4, IL-5, and IL-17 and IFN-γ (type II IFN).

B lymphocytes produce antibodies that are responsible for, amongst other activities, neutralization and clearance of cell-free viruses. Antibodies also mediate long-term protection against reinfection by many viruses. B lymphocytes express surface receptors that are specific to particular antigens: after exposure to antigen such as a viral infection, B cells develop into plasma cells that secrete antibodies with the same antigen specificity as that of the surface receptors of the B cells from which they were derived. Receptor diversity is generated by rearrangement of the genes encoding portions of individual immunoglobulin molecules. The acquired B cell response to infection involves immunoglobulin class switching and progressive specificity, known as *affinity maturation.*

A subclass of B lymphocytes, designated B1 cells, secrete broadly reactive immunoglobulin, known as natural antibody, without specific antigen stimulation. Thus natural antibodies provide linkage between the innate and acquired humoral responses and provide a first line of humoral defense.

T lymphocytes also possess antigen-specific surface receptors. Like B-cell antigen recognition, diversity and

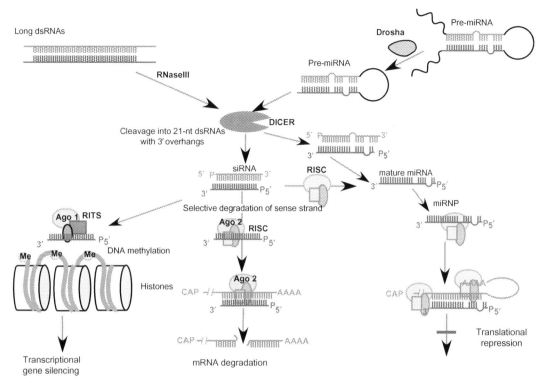

FIGURE 4.6 Mechanisms of RNA interference. Long double-stranded RNAs (dsRNAs) are cleaved by RNaseIII and subsequently processed by DICER into short interfering RNAs (siRNAs), which are short dsRNAs of 21–22 nts with 2-nt overhangs on the 3′ termini. siRNAs then enter the *R*NA-*i*nduced *s*ilencing *c*omplex (RISC), where the sense strand is selectively degraded. miRNAs are encoded as incompletely self-complementary hairpins in viral and cellular genomes. They are cleaved by Drosha in the nucleus and the pre-micro RNA (pre-miRNA) is exported to the cytoplasm by Exportin 5. There they are also processed by DICER. siRNAs silence genes by binding in the context of RISC to mRNAs that are exactly complementary, and causing mRNA degradation. miRNAs often contain some mismatches and generally exert their effects by inhibiting translation. siRNAs can also enter *R*NA*i*nduced *t*ranscriptional *s*ilencing complexes (RITS), which recruit an enzyme to methylate DNA in chromatin, turning it into inactive heterochromatin. Both RITS and RISC contain argonaute proteins (Agos). miRNP, micro ribonucleoprotein. [*From* Viruses and Human Disease, *J. H. Strauss, E. G. Strauss, 2nd ed., p. 403. Copyright © Academic Press/Elsevier (2007), with permission.*]

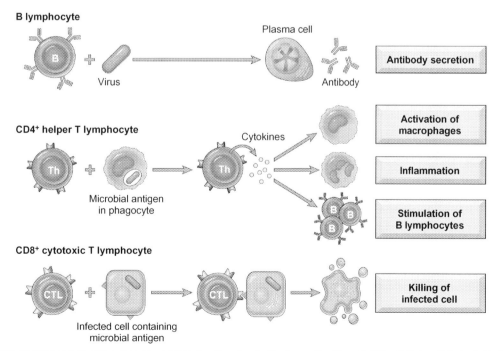

FIGURE 4.7 The principal classes of lymphocytes and their functions in adaptive immunity. [*From* Robbins & Cotran Pathologic Basis of Disease, *V. Kumar, A. K. Abbas, N. Fausto, J. Aster, 8th ed., p. 185. Copyright © Saunders/Elsevier (2010), with permission.*]

receptor specificity is generated by somatic rearrangement of the genes that encode the T cell receptor. There are two major classes of T cells: those with receptors that consist of a heterodimer of α and β chains (so-called α/β T cells), and those with a receptor composed of a heterodimer of γ and δ chains (γ/δ T cells). The α/β T cells recognize small peptides expressed on the surface of cells in association with MHC antigens, which confers exquisite specificity to the cellular immune mechanisms mediated by these cells. In contrast, although γ/δ T cells also recognize small peptides expressed on the cell surface, they do so without the requirement for MHC restriction. This lack of MHC restriction, coupled with the fact that γ/δ T cells are especially abundant at mucosal surfaces that serve as portals of virus entry (like the mucosal lining of the gastrointestinal tract), suggests that these cells serve as sentinels to remove virus-infected cells. Thus γ/δ T cells probably constitute a critical "bridge" between innate and adaptive antiviral immunity.

Cellular immunity (cell-mediated immunity) is mediated by effector lymphocytes and macrophages that specifically eliminate virus-infected cells. The lymphocytes that mediate cell lysis are *cytotoxic T lymphocytes* (CTLs) that typically express (CD8) on their cell surface (CD8$^+$ CTLs), and which lyse cells that express viral antigen in the context of appropriate class I MHC molecules. Portions of immunogenic viral proteins produced in the cytosol of the infected cell are transported to the endoplasmic reticulum, where they associate with class I MHC molecules. This complex is directed to the cell surface, where the viral peptides can be recognized by antigen-specific cytotoxic T lymphocytes that then lyse the virus-infected cell by inducing apoptosis.

Dendritic cells are also key players in adaptive and innate immunity; they derive their names from their abundant fine cytoplasmic processes ("dendrites"). There are two major types of dendritic cells:

- *Interdigitating dendritic cells* are critical antigen-presenting cells that are located at portals of virus entry, such as the skin and within/beneath the mucosal epithelial surfaces lining the gastrointestinal, respiratory, and urogenital tracts. They are also present within the interstitium of virtually all tissues. These dendritic cells express surface pattern-recognition receptors that can quickly and generically respond to the presence of viral triggers (PAMPs) by the production and release of antiviral cytokines such as IFN. In addition, these cells migrate to the T cell regions of lymphoid tissues, where they can present antigen to T cells and, because they express high levels of stimulatory molecules such as MHC antigens, they are potent inducers of T cell activation.
- *Follicular dendritic cells* occur within germinal centers of lymphoid tissues such as lymph node and spleen. These cells efficiently capture (phagocytose) circulating antigens, which they then present to B lymphocytes that

express the relevant surface receptor specificity, leading to B cell activation and development of humoral (antibody-mediated) immunity.

Macrophages are important bone-marrow-derived cells that are responsible for microbial phagocytosis and killing. They can be activated by cytokines into effector cells that mediate cellular immunity through their enhanced antimicrobial capacity. Macrophage activation is mediated by IFN-γ that is released by antigen-specific T cells, and by NK cells.

Major histocompatibility complex (MHC) antigens expressed on the surface of relevant cells are central to adaptive immunity. Major histocompatibility antigens are polymorphic proteins the major function of which is to display portions of immunogenic proteins to antigen-specific T lymphocytes (Figure 4.8). Class I MHC antigens are expressed on the surface of all nucleated cells, and class I MHC molecules on the surface of virus-infected cells typically display

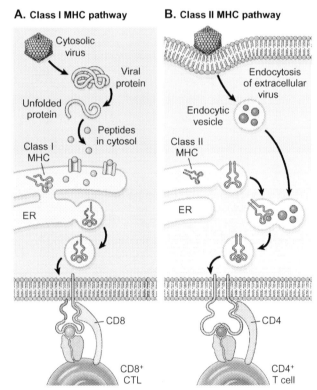

A. Class I MHC pathway

B. Class II MHC pathway

FIGURE 4.8 Antigen processing and display by major histocompatibility complex (MHC) molecules. A. In the class I MHC pathway, peptides are produced from proteins in the cytosol and transported to the endoplasmic reticulum (ER), where they bind to class I MHC molecules. The peptide MHC complexes are transported to the cell surface and displayed for recognition by CD8$^+$ T cells. B. In the class II MHC pathway, proteins are ingested into vesicles and degraded into peptides, which bind to class II MHC molecules being transported in the same vesicles. The class II-peptide complexes are expressed on the cell surface and recognized by CD4$^+$ T cells. [*From Robbins & Cotran Pathologic Basis of Disease, V. Kumar, A. K. Abbas, N. Fausto, J. Aster, 8th ed., p. 192. Copyright © Saunders/Elsevier (2010), with permission.*]

immunogenic proteins from the infecting virus that are recognized by antigen-specific cytotoxic T lymphocytes. Specifically, viral proteins produced in the cytoplasm of infected cells are degraded within proteasomes, and fragments of these proteins are then transported to the endoplasmic reticulum where they bind to newly synthesized class I MHC molecules. Association of $\beta2$ microglobulin with the class I MHC and viral peptide complex forms a stable heterotrimer that is transported to the cell surface, where the viral antigen can be recognized by antigen-specific cytotoxic T lymphocytes. This T-cell-mediated killing is restricted to target cells that express the same class I MHC haplotype. Class II MHC antigen, in contrast, is expressed principally on antigen-presenting cells, namely B lymphocytes, macrophages, and dendritic cells. Class II MHC molecules display viral proteins at the cell surface that are recognized by antigen-specific $CD4^+$ T lymphocytes—that is, those with surface receptors that specifically recognize and bind to the displayed peptide. In this scenario, viral proteins are degraded into peptides within endocytic vesicles and these peptides then associate with class II MHC molecules that are synthesized within these same vesicles. The complex of class II MHC molecule and viral peptide is then transported to the cell surface for display and recognition by antigen-specific $CD4^+$ T lymphocytes.

Passive Immunity

Specific antibody alone is highly effective in preventing many viral infections. For example, artificial passive immunization (injection of antibodies) temporarily protects animals against infection with the viruses that cause canine distemper, feline panleukopenia, and porcine reproductive and respiratory syndrome, amongst many others. Furthermore, natural passive immunization—that is, the transfer of maternal antibody from dam to fetus or newborn—protects the newborn for the first few months of life against most of the infections that the dam has experienced.

Natural passive immunity is important for two major reasons: (1) it is essential for the protection of young animals, during the first weeks or months of life, from the myriad of microorganisms and viruses that are present in the environment into which animals are born; (2) maternally derived antibody interferes with active immunization of the newborn and must therefore be taken into account when designing vaccination schedules.

Maternal antibodies may be transmitted in the egg yolk in birds, across the placenta in primates and rodents, or via colostrum and/or milk in ungulates and other mammals. Different species of mammals differ strikingly in the predominant route of transfer of maternal antibodies, depending on the structure of the placenta of the species. In those species such as primates in which the maternal and fetal circulations are in relatively close apposition, antibody of the immunoglobulin (Ig) G (but not IgM) class is able to cross the placenta, and maternal immunity is transmitted mainly by this route. Some species with more complex placentation, such as mice, acquire maternal antibody through yolk-sac immunoglobulin receptors. In contrast, the complex placenta of most domestic animals serves as a barrier to maternal immunoglobulins; in these species, maternal immunity is transmitted to the newborn via colostrum and, to a much lesser extent, via milk. Different species differ in regard to the particular class or subclass of immunoglobulin that is transferred preferentially to the newborn in colostrum, but in most domestic animals it is mainly IgG. In cattle and sheep there is a selective transfer of IgG1 from the serum across the alveolar epithelium of the mammary gland during the last few weeks of pregnancy. Antibodies of the IgG1 class are important in protection against enteric infections as long as suckling continues.

The very substantial amounts of IgG present in colostrum are ingested and translocated in large intracytoplasmic vesicles by specialized cells present in the upper part of the small intestine to reach the circulation of the newborn. Small amounts of other antibodies (IgM, IgA) present in colostrum or milk may, in some species, also be translocated across the gut, but disappear quickly from the circulation of the young animal. The period after birth during which antibody, ingested as colostrum, is translocated is sharply defined and very brief (about 48 hours) in most domestic animals, but can be very prolonged in rodents; mice continue to acquire maternal IgG for up to 3 weeks.

In birds there is a selective transfer of IgG from the maternal circulation, so that IgG is concentrated in the egg yolk. IgG enters the vitelline circulation, and hence that of the chick, from day 12 of incubation. Some IgG is also transferred to the amniotic fluid and is swallowed by the chick. Close to the time of hatching, the yolk sac with the remaining maternal immunoglobulin is completely taken into the abdominal cavity and absorbed by the chick.

Maternal antibody in the blood stream of the newborn mammal or newly hatched chick is destroyed quite rapidly, with first-order kinetics. The half-life, which is somewhat longer than in adult animals, ranges from about 21 days in the cow and horse, to 8–9 days in the dog and cat, to only 2 days in the mouse. Of course, the newborn animal will be protected against infection with any particular virus only if the dam's IgG contains specific antibodies, and protection may last much longer than one IgG half-life if the initial titer against that virus is high.

Although the concentrations of IgA transferred via colostrum to the gut of the newborn animal are considerably lower than those of IgG, antibodies of this isotype are important in protecting the neonate against enteric viruses against which the dam has developed immunity. Moreover, there is evidence that even after intestinal translocation ceases, immunoglobulins present in ordinary milk—principally IgA but also IgG and IgM—may continue to provide some protective immunity against gut infections. Often the newborn encounters viruses while still partially protected. Under these circumstances the virus replicates, but only to a limited extent, stimulating an immune response without causing significant disease, and the infected newborn thus acquires active immunity while partially protected by maternal immunity.

Failure of Maternal Antibody Transfer

The failure or partial failure of maternal antibody transfer is the most common immunodeficiency disease of livestock, and predisposes affected animals to infectious diseases, particularly enteric and respiratory diseases. Maternal immunization to ensure passive protection of newborn animals has become an important strategy in veterinary medical practice, in conjunction with sound management practices that ensure newborn animals quickly receive adequate amounts of colostrum.

VIRAL MECHANISMS OF AVOIDANCE AND ESCAPE

In the ongoing war and détente between virus and host, viruses have developed remarkably sophisticated mechanisms to avoid the various host protective responses. In addition to the many different strategies utilized by viruses to facilitate persistent infection [including growth in immune cells and/or in immunologically privileged sites, latency, integration, antigenic drift (see Chapter 3)], individual viruses have developed diverse and complex mechanisms of avoiding protective host innate and adaptive immune responses. Examples of these mechanisms include the following:

- Shutdown of host macromolecular synthesis
- Avoidance of CTL-mediated killing of virus-infected cells
- Prevention of NK-cell-mediated lysis of virus-infected cells
- Interference with apoptosis
- Counter defenses against cytokines
- Evasion of the antiviral state
- Virus-specific gene-silencing pathways

Shutdown of Host Macromolecule Synthesis

Many viruses, soon after infection, inhibit normal transcription and/or translation of cellular proteins, and rapidly subvert the machinery of the infected cell for production of progeny virions. This rapid shutdown of the host cell quickly impairs the innate immune response to the infecting virus, including the production of critical proteins such as class I MHC antigen and antiviral cytokines such as type I IFN. The result is that, without effective innate immune responses, the infecting virus can quickly replicate and disseminate before the host can develop an adaptive immune response. This strategy is widely used by RNA viruses, many of which have very rapid replication cycles.

Avoidance of CTL-Mediated Killing of Virus-Infected Cells

Cytotoxic T lymphocyte (CTL)-mediated killing of virus-infected cells requires the presentation of viral antigens on the surface of the infected cell in the context of the appropriate class I MHC molecule; thus viruses have developed different strategies to suppress the normal expression of class I MHC proteins so as to inhibit CTL-mediated lysis. These strategies include: (1) suppression of cellular production of class I MHC molecules by shutdown of host protein synthesis; (2) production of virus-encoded proteins that disrupt normal production of class I MHC proteins, or their transport from the endoplasmic reticulum to the Golgi apparatus or to the cell surface; (3) production of virus-encoded proteins that disrupt the function or viability of class I MHC molecules; (4) production of virus-encoded homologs of class I MHC molecules that can bind $\beta 2$ microglobulin and viral peptides, but are otherwise dysfunctional in terms of mediating CTL activity.

Prevention of NK-Cell-Mediated Lysis of Virus-Infected Cells

In contrast to CTL-mediated lysis, which requires the presence of appropriate concentrations of class I MHC antigen on the surface of virus-infected cells, NK-cell-mediated cytolysis is promoted by reduced levels of class I MHC antigen on the cell surface. Also important to NK cell activity is the balance of inhibitory molecules (such as class I MHC antigen) and stimulatory molecules (such as heat-shock proteins) on the cell surface; thus some viruses selectively inhibit cellular production and expression of molecules that provide stimulatory signals for NK cell activity. Other viruses inhibit host-cell production of both stimulatory and inhibitory molecules, such that the infected cell is somewhat protected against both CTL- and NK-cell-mediated lysis.

Interference with Apoptosis

In addition to apoptosis induced by NK-cell or CTL-mediated cell lysis (as described in the preceding sections), viral infection alone can initiate apoptosis via either the extrinsic (death receptor) or intrinsic (mitochondrial) pathways (see pages 82/83). Apoptosis is especially deleterious to the relatively slow-growing DNA viruses, including poxviruses, herpesviruses, and adenoviruses, because apoptosis can result in death of cells infected with these viruses before maximal levels of virus replication have been completed. Thus these DNA viruses, in particular, have developed a remarkable variety of strategies to optimize their replication by inhibiting the various pathways that normally lead to apoptosis. The need for these viruses to prevent apoptosis to promote their own survival is reflected by the fact that individual viruses may use a combination of strategies, including: (1) inhibition of the activity of executioner caspases that mediate cellular injury—notably by the serpins, which are protease inhibitors produced by poxviruses that bind to and block the proteolytic activity of caspases; (2) inhibition of the expression, activation, and signaling of death receptors, such as by production of viral receptor homologs that bind TNF so that it cannot initiate the extrinsic pathway, or molecules that specifically block the signaling cascade initiated by death receptor activation; (3) production of virus-encoded homologs of anti-apoptotic proteins such as Bcl-2; (4) production of proteins that sequester p53, which is a pro-apoptotic molecule that accumulates in cells infected with certain viruses; (5) other as yet poorly defined mechanisms of inhibition of apoptosis, apparently used by a myriad of viral proteins.

Counter Defenses against Cytokines

Cytokines are central to both innate and adaptive immune responses of animals to viral infections, thus viruses also have developed effective strategies to combat the activities of these important mediators of antiviral immunity. Certain viruses have acquired and modified cellular genes, creating viral genes that encode proteins that are homologs of cytokines or their receptors. Virus-encoded cytokine homologs can be functional (so-called virokines) and mimic the biological effect of the authentic molecule, or they can be non-functional and simply bind and block the specific cytokine receptor to neutralize that activity. Similarly, virus-encoded receptor homolog proteins typically bind to and neutralize the relevant cytokine. Other virus-encoded proteins interfere with dsRNA-activated pattern recognition receptor signaling pathways (such as TLR3 or RIG-1) that trigger production of type I IFN and other antiviral cytokines, or with the signaling pathways activated by the binding of IFN to its receptor (IFNAR). Collectively, these virus-encoded proteins can modulate the activities of a wide variety of critical cytokines such as IL-1, IL-6, IL-8, types I and II IFN, and TNF to the replicative benefit of the virus, by either inhibiting or promoting specific cytokine-mediated functions.

Evasion of the Antiviral State

Predictably, viruses also have evolved elaborate strategies to circumvent the activity of important IFN-induced antiviral effector mechanisms such as the protein kinase (PKR) and $2'$-$5'$ oligoadenylate synthetase (OAS) pathways. These include the production of virus-encoded proteins or RNA molecules (RNAi) that bind but do not activate critical enzymes (or genes encoding them) involved in these pathways, the production of non-functional enzyme homologs, and the stimulation of pathways that downregulate activity and function of these protective antiviral pathways. Other virus-encoded proteins sequester dsRNA, which is a critical co-factor for both PKR and OAS. Viruses in many different families of both DNA and RNA viruses have incorporated strategies for evading the host antiviral pathways, and additional examples undoubtedly will be identified in the future.

Virus-Specific Gene Silencing Pathways

Viruses have also developed counter defenses to cellular antiviral RNA interference pathways, either by the production of virus-encoded proteins or small interfering mRNA (siRNA) molecules that inhibit key steps of the cellular pathway depicted in Figure 4.4. Other viruses themselves produce RNAi molecules to silence key cellular genes involved in antiviral immunity.

VACCINES AND VACCINATION AGAINST VIRAL DISEASES

Vaccination is the most effective way of preventing viral diseases. Although deliberate exposure to virulent viruses such as smallpox (*syn.* variolation) was long recognized as an effective, albeit dangerous, method of prophylaxis, the concept of vaccination is considered to have been widely introduced by Edward Jenner in 1798 to protect humans against smallpox. Nearly a century later, the concept was shown by Louis Pasteur to have wider applications and, most notably, could be used to prevent rabies. With the advent of cell culture techniques in the 1950s, a second era of vaccination was introduced and many live-attenuated virus and inactivated-virus vaccines were developed. More recently, the field of vaccinology has witnessed the introduction of a number of novel "new generation" vaccines produced through various forms of recombinant DNA and related technologies. While live-attenuated and inactivated virus vaccines of the second era are still the "work horses" of veterinary practice, new generation vaccines are now complementing and, increasingly, replacing them.

There are some important differences between vaccination practices in humans and animals. Economic constraints are generally of less importance in human medicine than in veterinary medicine. There is also greater agreement about the safety and efficacy of vaccines in use in human medicine than there is with animal vaccines, and better mechanisms for reporting potential adverse consequences associated with the use of specific products. At the international level, the World Health Organization (WHO) exerts persuasive leadership for human vaccine usage, and maintains a number of programs that have no equivalents for animal vaccine usage by its sister agencies, the Food and Agriculture Organization and the Office International des Epizooties (OIE; *syn.* the World Organization for Animal Health). Furthermore, within countries, greater latitude is allowed in the manufacture and use of vaccines for veterinary diseases than is allowed by national regulatory authorities for human vaccines.

Before the recent advent of the new generation vaccines based on recombinant DNA technology, there were just two major strategies for the production of virus vaccines: one employing live-attenuated (*syn.* modified-live) virus strains and the other employing chemically inactivated (*syn.* killed) virus preparations. Live-attenuated virus vaccines replicate in the vaccine recipient and, in so doing, amplify the amount of antigen presented to the host's immune system. There are important benefits in this approach, because the replication of vaccine virus mimics infection to the extent that the host immune response is more similar to that occurring after natural infection than is the case with inactivated or some subunit vaccines. When inactivated virus vaccines are produced, the chemical or physical treatment used to eliminate infectivity may be damaging enough to diminish the immunogenicity of the vaccine virus, especially the induction of virus-specific cell-mediated immune responses. As a result, inactivated vaccines often induce an immune response that is shorter in duration, narrower in antigenic spectrum, weaker in cell-mediated and mucosal immune responses, and possibly less effective in inducing sterilizing immunity. Nonetheless, very serviceable and safe inactivated vaccines are available and widely used.

The majority of vaccines in large-scale production for use in animals continue to include either live-attenuated or inactivated virus; however, new generation vaccines developed through recombinant DNA technologies offer significant improvements and potential advantages in terms of both their safety and their efficacy. A remarkable variety of such vaccines have recently been developed, an increasing number of which are now in commercial production.

Live-Attenuated Virus Vaccines

Live-attenuated virus vaccines, when they have been proven to be safe, have historically been the best of all vaccines. Several of them have been dramatically successful in reducing the incidence of important diseases of animals and humans. Most attenuated virus vaccines are injected intradermally, subcutaneously, or intramuscularly, but some are delivered orally, and a few by aerosol or to poultry in their drinking water. For these vaccines to be successful, the vaccine virus must replicate in the recipient, thereby eliciting a lasting immune response while causing little or no disease. In effect, a live-attenuated virus vaccine mimics a subclinical infection. The individual virus strain incorporated in a live-attenuated virus vaccine may be derived from any one of several sources.

Vaccines Produced from Naturally Occurring Attenuated Viruses

The original vaccine (*vacca* = cow), introduced by Jenner in 1798 for the control of human smallpox, utilized cowpox virus, a natural pathogen of the cow. This virus produced only a mild infection and lesions in humans, but, because it is antigenically related to smallpox virus, it conferred protection against the human disease. The same principle has been applied to other diseases—for example, the protection of chickens against Marek's disease using a vaccine derived from a related herpesvirus of turkeys, and the protection of piglets against porcine rotavirus infection using a vaccine derived from a bovine rotavirus. Similarly, rabbits can be effectively protected against the pox viral disease, myxomatosis, with the naturally avirulent Shope rabbit fibroma virus.

Vaccines Produced by Attenuation of Viruses by Serial Passage in Cultured Cells

Most of the live-attenuated virus vaccines in common use today were derived empirically by serial passage of virulent "field" virus (*syn.* "wild-type" virus) in cultured cells. The cells may be of homologous or, more commonly, heterologous host origin. Typically, adaptation of virus to more vigorous growth in cultured cells is accompanied by progressive loss of virulence for the natural host. Loss of virulence may be demonstrated initially in a convenient laboratory model such as a mouse, before being confirmed by clinical trials in the species of interest. Because of the practical requirement that the vaccine must not be so attenuated that it fails to replicate satisfactorily in its natural host, it is sometimes necessary to compromise by using a virus strain that replicates sufficiently well that it may induce mild clinical signs in a few of the recipient (vaccinated) animals.

During repeated passage in cultured cells, viruses typically accumulate nucleotide substitutions in their genome, which in turn lead to attenuation. With the recent advent of high-throughput, whole-genome sequencing, the genetic basis of virulence and attenuation has been established with many viruses, which allows better prediction of vaccine efficacy and safety. Furthermore, it is increasingly clear that several genes can contribute to virulence and tropism of individual viruses, and do so in different ways. For example, in contrast to the severe, systemic infections associated with some wild-type or "field" viruses, live-attenuated vaccine strains of these same viruses administered by the respiratory route may replicate, for instance, only in the upper respiratory tract, or undergo only limited replication in the intestinal epithelium after oral administration.

Despite the outstanding success of empirically derived attenuated virus vaccines, there is a strong perceived need to replace what some veterinarians and veterinary scientists consider to be "genetic routlette" with rationally designed, specifically engineered vaccines. In these engineered live-attenuated vaccines, the mutations associated with attenuation of the parental virus are defined and predictable, as is the potential for reversion to virulence.

Vaccines Produced by Attenuation of Viruses by Serial Passage in Heterologous Hosts

Serial passage in a heterologous host was a historically important means of empirically attenuating viruses for use as vaccines. For example, rinderpest and classical swine fever (hog cholera) viruses were each adapted to grow in rabbits and, after serial passage, became sufficiently attenuated to be used as vaccines. Other viruses were passaged in embryonated hens' eggs in similar fashion, although some such passaged viruses acquired novel and very undesirable properties. For example, live-attenuated bluetongue virus vaccines propagated in embryonated eggs can cross the placenta of ruminants vaccinated during pregnancy, with resultant fetal infection and developmental defects or loss. Similarly, embryonated-egg-propagated African horse sickness virus caused devastating consequences in humans infected after aerosol exposure to this vaccine virus.

Vaccines Produced by Attenuation of Viruses by Selection of Cold-Adapted Mutants and Reassortants

The observation that temperature-sensitive mutants (viruses that are unable to replicate satisfactorily at temperatures much higher than normal body temperature) generally display reduced virulence suggested that they might make satisfactory live-attenuated vaccines, although some viruses with temperature-sensitive mutations have displayed a disturbing tendency to revert toward virulence during replication in vaccinated animals. Attention accordingly moved to cold-adapted mutants, derived by adaptation of virus to grow at suboptimal temperatures. The rationale is that such mutant viruses would be safer vaccines for intranasal administration, in that they would replicate well at the lower temperature of the nasal cavity (about 33°C in most mammalian species), but not at the temperature of the more vulnerable lower respiratory tract and pulmonary airspaces. Cold-adapted influenza vaccines that contain mutations in most viral genes do not revert to virulence, and influenza vaccines based on such mutations are now licensed for human use; vaccines against equine influenza have been developed utilizing the same principle.

Non-Replicating Virus Vaccines

Vaccines Produced from Inactivated Whole Virions

Inactivated (*syn.* killed) virus vaccines are usually made from virulent virus; chemical or physical agents are used to destroy infectivity while maintaining immunogenicity. When prepared properly, such vaccines are remarkably safe, but they need to contain relatively large amounts of antigen

to elicit an antibody response commensurate with that induced by a much smaller dose of live-attenuated virus vaccine. Normally, the primary vaccination course comprises two or three injections, and further ("booster") doses may be required at regular intervals thereafter to maintain immunity. Killed vaccines usually must be formulated with chemical adjuvants to enhance the immune response, but these also can result in more adverse reactions to vaccination.

The most commonly used inactivating agents are formaldehyde, β-propiolactone, and ethylenimine. One of the advantages of β-propiolactone, which is used in the manufacture of rabies vaccines, and ethylenimine, which is used in the manufacture of foot-and-mouth disease vaccines, is that they are completely hydrolyzed, within hours, to nontoxic products. Because virions in the center of aggregates may be shielded from inactivation, it is important that aggregates be broken up before inactivation. In the past, failure to do this occasionally resulted in vaccine-associated disease outbreaks—for example, several foot-and-mouth disease outbreaks have been traced to this problem.

Vaccines Produced from Purified Native Viral Proteins

Lipid solvents such as sodium deoxycholate are used in the case of enveloped viruses, to solubilize the virion and release the components, including the glycoprotein spikes of the viral envelope. Differential centrifugation is used to semi-purify these glycoproteins, which are then formulated for use as so-called split vaccines. Examples include vaccines against herpesviruses, influenza viruses, and coronaviruses.

Vaccines Produced by Recombinant DNA and Related Technologies

The relatively recent advent of molecular biology and its many associated technologies has facilitated the development of new vaccine strategies, each with inherent potential advantages and, in some instances, disadvantages as compared with those of the traditional vaccines. Such novel technologies have been used in the creation of new vaccines that already are in use and, given their substantial inherent potential advantages, it is anticipated that the availability and types of such products will only increase in the future.

Vaccines Produced by Attenuation of Viruses by Gene Deletion or Site-Directed Mutagenesis

The problem of the reversion to virulence of live-attenuated virus vaccines (i.e., a mutation by which the vaccine virus regains virulence) may be largely avoided by deliberate insertion of several attenuating mutations into key viral genes, or by completely deleting non-essential genes that contribute to virulence. Gene deletion is especially feasible with the large DNA viruses that carry a significant number of genes that are not essential for replication, at least for replication in cultured cells. "Genetic surgery" is used to construct deletion mutants that are stable over many passages. Several herpesvirus vaccines have been constructed using this strategy; including a thymidine kinase (*TK*) deletion pseudorabies vaccine for swine that also includes a deletion of one of the glycoprotein genes (*gE*). The deleted glycoprotein may be used as capture antigen in an enzyme-linked immunosorbent assay, so that vaccinated, uninfected pigs, which would test negative, can be distinguished from naturally infected pigs [the differentiation/discrimination of infected from vaccinated animals (DIVA) strategy], enabling eradication programs to be conducted in parallel with continued vaccination. A gE-deleted marker vaccine also is available for infectious bovine rhinotracheitis virus (bovine herpesvirus-1).

Site-directed mutagenesis facilitates the introduction of defined nucleotide substitutions into viral genes at will. As the particular genes that are influential in virulence and immunogenicity of individual viruses are increasingly defined, it is anticipated that existing empirically derived live-attenuated virus vaccines will be replaced by those engineered for attenuation through "customized" alteration of critical genes. The production of live-attenuated virus vaccines from molecular clones facilitates both the deliberate introduction of defined attenuating nucleotide substitutions into the vaccine virus, and consistent production of vaccine virus from a genetically defined "seed" virus. This strategy also potentially enables the use of differential serological tests to distinguish vaccinated and naturally infected animals (DIVA).

Subunit Vaccines Produced by Expression of Viral Proteins in Eukaryotic (Yeast, Mammalian, Insect), Bacterial, or Plant Cells

Eukaryotic expression vectors offer the potential for large-scale production of individual viral proteins that can be purified readily and formulated into vaccines. Once the critical viral protein conferring protection has been identified, its gene [or, in the case of an RNA virus, a complementary DNA (cDNA) copy of the gene] may be cloned into one of a wide choice of expression plasmids and expressed in any of several cell systems. Mammalian cells offer the advantage over cells from lower eukaryotes in that they are more likely to possess the machinery for correct post-translational processing and authentic maturation of complex viral proteins.

Useful eukaryotic expression systems include plant and yeast cells (*Saccharomyces cerevisiae*), insect cells (*Spodoptera frugiperda*), and various mammalian cells. Yeast offers the advantage that there is extensive experience with scale-up for industrial production; the first vaccine produced by expression of a cloned gene, human hepatitis B vaccine, was produced in yeast. Insect cells offer the advantage

of simple technology derived from the silk industry: moth cell cultures (or caterpillars!) may be made to express very large amounts of viral proteins through infection with recombinant baculoviruses carrying the gene(s) of the virus of interest. The promoter for the gene encoding the baculovirus polyhedrin protein is so strong that the product of a viral gene of interest inserted within the baculovirus polyhedrin gene may comprise up to half of all the protein the infected cells make. For example, immunization of pigs with the capsid protein of porcine circovirus 2 expressed in insect cells from a recombinant baculovirus vector confers protective immunity against porcine-circovirus-associated diseases such as multisystemic wasting disease. Similarly, baculovirus-expressed E2 protein alone provides an effective recombinant subunit vaccine against classical swine fever virus.

Expression of protective viral antigens in plant cells can theoretically provide a very cost-effective and efficient method of vaccinating production animals. For example, plant cell lines have been developed that express the hemagglutinin and neuraminidase proteins of Newcastle disease virus for protective immunization of birds.

Vaccines Produced by Expression of Viral Proteins that Self-Assemble into Virus-like Particles

The expression of genes encoding the capsid proteins of viruses within certain families of non-enveloped icosahedral viruses leads to the self-assembly of the individual capsid proteins into virus-like particles (VLPs) that can be used as a vaccine. This strategy has been developed for various picornaviruses, caliciviruses, rotaviruses, and orbiviruses, and an effective VLP-vaccine has been developed recently against human genital papillomaviruses. The advantage of recombinant virus-like particles over traditional inactivated vaccines is that they are devoid of viral nucleic acid, and therefore completely safe. They may also be equated to an inactivated whole-virus vaccine, but without the potentially damaging loss of immunogenicity that can accompany chemical inactivation. However, the potential limitations of the strategy include production costs and low yields, stability of the VLP after production, and less effective immunity as compared with some existing vaccines.

Vaccines Utilizing Viruses as Vectors for Expression of Other (Heterologous) Viral Antigens

Recombinant DNA techniques allow foreign genes to be introduced into specific regions of the genome of either RNA or DNA viruses, and the product of the foreign gene is then carried into and expressed in the target cell. Specifically, the gene(s) encoding key protective antigens (those against which protective responses are generated in the host) of the virus causing a disease of interest are inserted into the genome of an avirulent virus (the recombinant vector). This modified avirulent virus is then administered either as a live-attenuated virus vector or as a non-replicating ("suicide") expression vector. Infected cells within the immunized host express the foreign protein, to which the animal will in turn mount an adaptive immune response (humoral and/or cellular). The approach is safe, because only one or two genes of the disease-causing virus typically are inserted into the expression vector, and because well-characterized viruses (such as existing live-attenuated vaccine viruses) can be used as the expression vector. Furthermore, animals vaccinated with such recombinant vaccines can be distinguished readily from infected animals (or those vaccinated with live-attenuated virus vaccines) using serological tests that detect antibodies to viral proteins that are not included in the vaccine construct (the so-called DIVA strategy).

DNA Viruses as Vectors

Individual genes encoding antigens from a variety of viruses have been incorporated into the genome of DNA viruses, especially vaccinia and several other poxviruses, adenoviruses, herpesviruses, and adeno-associated viruses (which are parvoviruses).

Vaccination of animals with a significant number of different recombinant poxvirus-vectored vaccine constructs has effectively generated antibody and/or cell-mediated immune responses that confer strong protective immunity in the recipient animals against challenge infection with virulent strains of the heterologous viruses from which the genes were derived. For example, recombinant vaccinia virus vectored rabies vaccines incorporated into baits administered orally protect both foxes and raccoons against this zoonotic disease; this vaccine contains only the gene encoding the surface glycoprotein (G) of rabies virus. Similarly, the avian poxviruses have been increasingly used as expression vectors of heterologous genes in recombinant vaccine constructs. Fowlpox virus is a logical choice as a vector for avian vaccines but, perhaps surprisingly, fowlpox virus has also been shown to be a very useful expression vector in mammals: even though this virus, and the closely related canarypox virus, do not complete their replication cycle in mammalian cells, the inserted genes are expressed and induce strong cellular and humoral immune responses in inoculated animals. Because the large genome of poxviruses can accommodate at least a dozen foreign genes and still be packaged satisfactorily within the virion, it is theoretically possible to construct, as a vector, a single recombinant virus capable of protecting against several different viral diseases.

Recombinant poxvirus vectored vaccines that have been widely used to immunize mammals include vaccinia–rabies constructs used for the vaccination of foxes in Europe and raccoons and coyotes in the United States, and canarypox virus vectored vaccines to prevent influenza and West Nile disease in horses, distemper in dogs, ferrets and certain zoo animals/wildlife species, and feline leukemia and rabies in cats. Amongst many others, experimental recombinant canarypox virus vectored vaccines also have been successfully developed to prevent

African horse sickness, bluetongue, Japanese encephalitis, and Nipah, and extensive trials have been carried out in humans with an experimental human immunodeficiency virus (HIV)–recombinant canarypox virus vaccine. Raccoonpox, capripox, and other poxviruses have also been successfully developed as recombinant expression vectors for potential use as vaccines in mammals. Rabbits can be effectively immunized against both myxomatosis (pox virus) and rabbit hemorrhagic disease (calicivirus) with a recombinant live-attenuated myxoma virus that expresses the *VP60* gene of rabbit hemorrhagic disease virus. This combined vaccination strategy has the considerable advantage that rabbit hemorrhagic disease virus cannot be grown in cell culture, so that vaccination against rabbit hemorrhagic disease alone currently requires inactivation of virus collected from livers of virus-infected rabbits.

A number of DNA virus vectored vaccines have also been developed for use in poultry, including recombinant herpesvirus of turkey vectored vaccines against Newcastle disease virus, infectious laryngotracheitis virus, and infectious bursal disease virus; these vaccines include only genes encoding the protective antigens of the heterologous viruses, but they generate protective immunity in chickens against both Marek's disease and the other respective disease (Newcastle disease, infectious laryngotracheitis, infectious bursal disease). Fowlpox virus vectored vaccines against Newcastle disease and H5 influenza viruses have also been developed, and the latter has been widely used in Mexico and Central America.

Chimeric DNA viruses also have been developed as vaccines in which the genes of a virulent virus are inserted into the genetic backbone of a related avirulent virus. For example, a chimeric circovirus vaccine used in swine includes a genetic backbone of porcine circovirus 1, which is avirulent (non-pathogenic) in swine, with the gene encoding the immunogenic capsid protein of pathogenic porcine circovirus 2. Antibodies to the capsid protein of porcine circovirus 2 confer immunity in vaccinated pigs. Like porcine circovirus 1, the chimeric virus replicates to high titer in cell culture, which makes vaccine production more efficient and cost effective.

It is anticipated that commercially available veterinary vaccines increasingly will utilize DNA viruses as expression vectors in the future, because of their inherent advantages in terms of safety and efficacy, and the ability in control programs to distinguish vaccinated animals from those exposed to infectious virus (DIVA).

RNA Viruses as Vectors

As with DNA virus vectored vaccines, RNA viruses, especially virus strains of proven safety, can be used as "genetic backbones" for insertion of critical immunogenic genes from other (heterologous) viruses. Chimeric RNA viruses utilize the replicative machinery of one virus for expression of the protective antigens of the heterologous virus. For example, chimeric vaccines have been developed in which the genes encoding the envelope proteins of the traditional live-attenuated vaccine strain of yellow fever virus are replaced with corresponding genes of other flaviviruses such as Japanese encephalitis virus, West Nile virus, or dengue virus, or even with genes encoding critical immunogenic proteins of distinct viruses such as influenza. A chimeric vaccine based on yellow fever virus that includes the premembrane (preM) and envelope (E) proteins of West Nile virus was used for protective immunization of horses.

Positive-sense RNA viruses are especially convenient for use as molecular clones for the insertion of foreign genes because the genomic RNA of these viruses is itself infectious. Nevertheless, infectious clones also have been developed for negative-sense RNA viruses by including the replicase proteins at transfection. In poultry, a recombinant Newcastle disease virus vaccine that expresses the *H5* gene of influenza virus has been developed and widely used in China for protective immunization of birds against both Newcastle disease and H5 avian influenza. Additional negative-sense RNA viruses such as rhabdoviruses are also being evaluated as potential gene vectors, along with positive-sense RNA viruses such as Nidoviruses (coronaviruses, arteriviruses).

Recombinant replicon particles offer a similar but slightly different strategy that has been developed with certain RNA viruses, including flaviviruses and alphaviruses such as Venezuelan equine encephalitis, Semliki Forest, and Sindbis viruses. Recombinant alphavirus replicon particles are created exclusively from the structural proteins of the donor alphavirus, but the genomic RNA contained in these particles is chimeric, in that the genes encoding the structural proteins of the replicon alphavirus are replaced by those from the heterologous virus. As an example, replicon particles derived from the vaccine strain of Venezuelan equine encephalitis virus that co-express the GP5 and M envelope proteins of equine arteritis virus induce virus-neutralizing antibody and protective immunity in immunized horses; neither infectious Venezuelan equine encephalitis virus nor equine arteritis virus is produced in immunized horses, as the replicon genome includes only the non-structural proteins of Venezuelan equine encephalitis virus and the structural protein genes of equine arteritis virus.

For influenza viruses and other viruses with segmented genomes, the principle of chimeric viruses was well established before the advent of recombinant DNA technology. Reassortant viruses were produced by homologous reassortment (segment swapping) by co-cultivation of an existing vaccine strain virus with the new isolate. Viruses with the desirable growth properties of the vaccine virus but with the immunogenic properties of the recent isolate were selected, cloned, and used as vaccine. For example, inactivated chimeric H5N3 influenza virus has been developed as a vaccine for use in poultry.

Vaccines Utilizing Viral DNA ("DNA Vaccines")

The discovery, in the early 1990s, that viral DNA itself can be used for protective immunization offered a potentially revolutionary new approach to vaccination. Specifically, a plasmid construct that included the *β-galactosidase* gene expressed the enzyme for up to 60 days after it was inoculated into mouse skeletal muscle. From this early observation, there has been an explosion of interest in the development of DNA vaccines and this methodology has been utilized experimentally for a wide range of potential applications. The first commercially available DNA vaccine was developed to protect salmon against infectious hemopoietic necrosis virus, and a DNA-based vaccine to prevent West Nile disease in horses is now available. However, commercial utilization of this strategy in veterinary vaccines has otherwise been slow.

With hindsight, the discovery that DNA itself could confer protective immunity was perhaps not that surprising. In 1960, it was shown that cutaneous inoculation of DNA from Shope papillomavirus induced papillomas at the site of inoculation in rabbit skin. Subsequently, it was shown for many viruses that genomic viral DNA, RNA, or cDNA of viral RNA, could complete the full replicative cycle following transfection into cells. The strategy of DNA vaccines is to construct recombinant plasmids that contain genes encoding key viral antigens. The DNA insert in the plasmid, on injection, transfects cells and the expressed protein elicits an immune response that in turn simulates a response to the respective viral infection. DNA vaccines usually consist of an *E. coli* plasmid with a strong promoter with broad cell specificity, such as the human cytomegalovirus immediate early promoter. The plasmid is amplified, commonly in *E. coli*, purified, and then simply injected into the host. Intramuscular immunization is most effective. Significant improvement in response to vaccination has been achieved by coating the plasmid DNA onto microparticles—commonly gold particles 1–3 μm in diameter—and injecting them by "bombardment," using a helium-gas-driven gun-like apparatus (the "gene gun").

Theoretical advantages of DNA vaccines include purity, physiochemical stability, simplicity, a relatively low cost of production, distribution, and delivery, potential for inclusion of several antigens in a single plasmid, and expression of antigens in their native form (thereby facilitating processing and presentation to the immune system). Repeated injection may be given without interference, and DNA immunization can induce immunity in the presence of maternal antibodies. However, DNA vaccination is yet to be widely used, because the practical application of the technology is considerably more challenging in humans and animals than it is in laboratory animals. Unsubstantiated concerns have also been raised regarding the fate and potential side-effects of the foreign, genetically engineered DNA and, for animals that will enter the human food chain, the costs of proving safety are likely to be significant.

Other Potential Vaccine Strategies

Vaccines Utilizing Bacteria as Vectors for Expression of Viral Antigens

Viral proteins (or immunogenic regions thereof) can be expressed on the surface of engineered bacteria that infect the host directly. The general approach is to insert the DNA encoding a protective viral antigen into a region of the genome of a bacterium, or one of its plasmids, which encodes a prominent surface protein. Provided that the added viral protein does not seriously interfere with the transport, stability, or function of the bacterial protein, the bacterium can multiply and present the viral epitope to the immune system of the host. Enteric bacteria that multiply naturally in the gut are the ideal expression vectors for presenting protective epitopes of virulent enteric viruses to the gut-associated lymphoid tissue, and attenuated strains of *E. coli*, *Salmonella* spp., and *Mycobacterium* spp. are being evaluated for immunization against enteric pathogens, including viruses, and/or for the preferential stimulation of mucosal immunity.

Synthetic Peptide Vaccines

With the increased ability to locate and define critical epitopes on viral proteins, it is also possible to synthesize peptides chemically that correspond to these antigenic determinants. Appropriately designed synthetic peptides can elicit neutralizing antibodies against many viruses, including foot-and-mouth disease virus and rabies virus, but in general this approach has been disappointing, probably because of the conformational nature of many critical epitopes included in the authentic protein. Specifically, conformational epitopes are not composed of linear arrays of contiguous amino acids, but rather are assembled from amino acids that, while separated in the primary sequence, are brought into close apposition by the folding of the polypeptide chain(s). An effective antigenic stimulus requires that the three-dimensional shape that an epitope has in the native protein molecule or virus particle be maintained in a vaccine. Because short synthetic peptides lack any tertiary or quaternary conformation, most antibodies raised against them are incapable of binding to virions, hence neutralizing antibody titers may be orders of magnitude lower than those induced by inactivated whole-virus vaccines or purified intact proteins. In contrast, the epitopes recognized by T lymphocytes are short linear peptides (bound to MHC protein). Some of these T cell epitopes are conserved between strains of virus and therefore elicit a cross-reactive T cell response.

Vaccines Utilizing Anti-Idiotypic Antibodies

The antigen-binding site of the antibody produced by each B cell contains a unique amino acid sequence known as its idiotype or idiotypic determinant. Because anti-idiotypic antibody is capable of binding to the same idiotype as binds the combining epitope on the original antigen, the anti-idiotypic antibody mimics the conformation of that epitope. Thus the anti-idiotypic antibody raised against a neutralizing monoclonal antibody to a particular virus can conceivably be used as a vaccine. It remains uncertain whether this points the way to a practical vaccine strategy, but there are situations, probably in human rather than veterinary medicine, in which such vaccines, if efficacious, would have advantages over orthodox vaccines, primarily because of their safety.

Methods for Enhancing Immunogenicity of Virus Vaccines

The immunogenicity of inactivated vaccines, especially that of purified protein vaccines and synthetic peptides, usually needs to be enhanced; this may be achieved by mixing the antigen with an adjuvant, incorporation of the antigen in liposomes, or incorporation of the antigen in an immunostimulating complex. Similar approaches are also used to enhance the immunogenicity of recombinant vaccines, and the immunogenicity of these vaccines can be potentially even further enhanced through incorporation of immunopotentiating agents into or along with the expression vector. There is a considerable research effort currently focused on strategies for more efficient and effective antigen delivery for vaccination.

Adjuvants are formulations that, when mixed with vaccines, potentiate the immune response, humoral and/or cellular, so that a lesser quantity of antigen and/or fewer doses will suffice. Adjuvants differ greatly in their chemistry and in their modes of action, but they typically can prolong the process of antigen degradation and release and/or enhance the immunogenicity of the vaccine by recruiting and activating key immune cells (macrophages, lymphocytes, and dendritic cells) at the site of antigen deposition. Alum and mineral oils have been used extensively in veterinary vaccines, but many others have been developed or are currently under investigation, some of which remain proprietary. Among many examples, synthetic biodegradable polymers such as polyphospazene can serve as potent adjuvants, especially when used with microfabricated needles for intradermal inoculation of antigen. Immunomodulatory approaches to enhance the immunogenicity of vaccines also continue to be investigated—specifically, molecules that can enhance critical innate and adaptive immune responses or inhibit suppressors thereof.

Liposomes consist of artificial lipid membrane spheres into which viral proteins can be incorporated. When purified viral envelope proteins are used, the resulting "virosomes" (or "immunosomes") somewhat resemble the original envelope of the virion. This not only enables a reconstitution of viral envelope-like structures lacking nucleic acid and other viral components, but also allows the incorporation of non-pyrogenic lipids with adjuvant activity. When viral envelope glycoproteins or synthetic peptides are mixed with cholesterol plus a glycoside known as Quil A, spherical cage-like structures 40 nm in diameter are formed. Several veterinary vaccines include this "immunostimulating complex adjuvant (ISCOM)" technology.

The recognition of the innate immune system as defined by pattern recognition receptor (PRR) mediated stimulation of transcription of cytokines and regulatory proteins established the link between innate and adaptive immunity. Attempts to enhance the adaptive immune response by utilizing the innate immune system have taken several different approaches. TLR-9 recognizes DNA molecules with methylation patterns not routinely found in eukaryotic cells. Cytosine guanine oligonucleotides (CpG ODNs) have been developed to activate the TLR-9 pathway in conjunction with various antigens and DNA vaccines. Although enhanced immune responses have been noted in mouse models, positive responses may be linked to a given species and to the sequence and size of the CpG ODN. CpG ODNs did not accelerate an immune response to a foot-and-mouth-disease virus vaccine, but positive responses were noted in chickens immunized with a killed influenza virus vaccine and CpG ODNs. Enhanced production of cytokines induced by the innate immune response can be achieved by expressing the cytokines in a viral expression vector along with the antigen of interest. Alternatively, a DNA vaccine expressing a viral antigen can be given along with a DNA molecule coding for a given cytokine. Numerous studies have shown enhanced immune responses when cytokines are used to augment the response naturally induced by an immunization process.

Given the recent development and increasing commercial production of new vaccine types and adjuvants, be they natural or artificial, it anticipated that vaccine formulations and their methods of delivery will change quickly in the coming years.

Factors Affecting Vaccine Efficacy and Safety

In much of the world, vaccines are made under a broad set of guidelines, termed *Good Manufacturing Practices.* Correctly prepared and tested, all vaccines should be safe in immunocompetent animals. As a minimum standard, licensing authorities insist on rigorous safety tests for residual infectious virus in inactivated virus vaccines. There are other safety problems that are inherent to live-attenuated virus vaccines and, potentially, new generation recombinant virus vaccines.

The objective of vaccination is to protect against disease and, ideally, to prevent infection and virus transmission within the population at risk. If infection with wild-type virus occurs as immunity wanes after vaccination, the infection is likely to be subclinical, but it will boost immunity. For enzootic viruses, this is a frequent occurrence in farm animals, cats and dogs in shelters, and birds in crowded pens.

The efficacy of live-attenuated virus vaccines delivered by either the mouth or nose is critically dependent on subsequent replication of the inoculated virus in the intestinal or respiratory tract, respectively. Interference can occur between the vaccine virus and enteric or respiratory viruses, incidentally infecting the animal at the time of vaccination. In the past, interference occurred also between different attenuated viruses contained in certain vaccine formulations; for example, it has been proposed by some that canine parvovirus infection may be immunosuppressive to such an extent that it interferes with the response of dogs to vaccination against canine distemper.

IgA is the most important class of immunoglobulin relevant to the prevention of infection of mucosal surfaces, such as those of the intestinal, respiratory, genitourinary, and ocular epithelia. One of the inherent advantages of orally administered live-attenuated virus vaccines is that they often induce prolonged synthesis of local IgA antibody, which confers relatively transient immunity to those respiratory and enteric viruses the pathogenic effects of which are manifested mainly at the site of entry. In contrast, IgG mediates long-term, often life-long, immunity to reinfection against most viruses that reach their target organ(s) via systemic (viremic) spread. Thus the principal objective of vaccination is to mimic natural infection—that is, to elicit a high titer of neutralizing antibodies of the appropriate class, IgG and/or IgA, directed against the relevant epitopes on the virion in the hope of preventing infection.

Special difficulties also attend vaccination against viruses known to establish persistent infections, such as herpesviruses and retroviruses: a vaccine must be remarkably effective if it is to prevent, not only the primary disease, but also the establishment of life-long latency. Live-attenuated virus vaccines are generally more effective in eliciting cell-mediated immunity than inactivated ones; however, they also carry some risk of themselves establishing persistent infections in the immunized host.

Adverse Effects from Live-Attenuated Virus Vaccines

Underattenuation

Some live-attenuated virus vaccines may cause clinical signs in some vaccinated animals—in effect, a mild case of the disease. For example, some early canine parvovirus vaccines that had undergone relatively few cell culture passages produced an unacceptably high incidence of disease. However, attempts to attenuate virulence further by additional passages in cultured cells may lead to a decline in the ability of the virus to replicate in the vaccinated animal, with a corresponding loss of immunogenicity.

Such side-effects are typically minimal with current animal virus vaccines, and do not constitute a significant disincentive to vaccination. However, it is important that live-attenuated virus vaccines are used only in the species for which they were produced; for example, canine distemper vaccines cause fatalities in some members of the family *Mustelidae*, such as the black footed ferret, so that recombinant or inactivated whole-virus vaccines must be used.

Genetic Instability

Some vaccine virus strains may revert toward virulence during replication in the recipient or in contact animals to which the vaccine virus has spread. Ideally, live-attenuated vaccine viruses are incapable of such spread, but in those that do there may be an accumulation of back mutations that gradually can result in restoration of virulence. The principal example of this phenomenon is the very rare reversion to virulence of Sabin poliovirus type 3 oral vaccine in humans, which eventually led to its replacement by the safer, although not necessarily more efficacious, non-replicating vaccine. Temperature-sensitive mutants of bovine viral diarrhea virus have also proven to be genetically unstable.

Heat Lability

Live-attenuated virus vaccines are vulnerable to inactivation by high ambient temperatures, a particular problem in the tropics, where maintenance of the "cold chain" from manufacturer to the point of administration to animals in remote, hot, rural areas can be challenging. To some extent the problem has been alleviated by the addition of stabilizing agents to the vaccines, selection of vaccine strains that are inherently more heat stable, and by packaging them in freeze-dried form for reconstitution immediately before administration. Simple portable refrigerators for use in vehicles and temporary field laboratories are invaluable.

Presence of Contaminating Viruses

Because vaccine viruses are grown in animals or in cells derived from them, there is always a possibility that a vaccine will be contaminated with another virus from that animal or from the medium used for culturing its cells. An early example, which led to restrictions on international trade in vaccines and sera that are still in effect, was the introduction into the United States in 1908 of foot-and-mouth disease virus as a contaminant of smallpox vaccine produced in calves. Similarly, the use of embryonated eggs to produce vaccines for use in chickens may pose problems (e.g., the contamination of Marek's disease vaccine with reticuloendotheliosis virus). Another important source of viral contaminants is fetal bovine serum, used universally in cell cultures; all batches must be screened for contamination with bovine viral diarrhea virus in particular.

Likewise, porcine parvovirus is a common contaminant of crude preparations of trypsin prepared from pig pancreases, which is used commonly in the preparation of animal cell cultures. The risk of contaminating viruses is greatest with live-attenuated virus vaccines, but may also occur with inactivated whole-virus vaccines, as some viruses are more resistant to inactivation than others; the prion agents are notoriously resistant to traditional methods of sterilization, for example.

Adverse Effects in Pregnant Animals

Attenuated virus vaccines are not generally recommended for use in pregnant animals, because they may be abortigenic or teratogenic. For example, live-attenuated infectious bovine rhinotracheitis vaccines can be abortigenic, and the live-attenuated feline panleukopenia, classical swine fever, bovine viral diarrhea, Rift Valley fever, and bluetongue vaccines are all teratogenic if they cross the placenta to infect the fetus at critical stages of gestation. These adverse effects are usually the result of primary immunization of a non-immune pregnant animal at a susceptible stage of gestation, so that it may be preferable to immunize pregnant animals with inactivated vaccines, or to immunize the dam with a live-attenuated vaccine before mating. Contaminating viruses in vaccines sometimes go unnoticed until used in pregnant animals; for example, the discovery that bluetongue virus contamination of canine vaccines caused abortion and death in pregnant bitches was most unexpected.

Adverse Effects from Non-Replicating Vaccines

Some inactivated whole-virus vaccines have been found to potentiate disease. The earliest observations were made with inactivated vaccines for measles and human respiratory syncytial virus, in which immunized individuals developed more severe disease than did those that remained unvaccinated before infection. Similar events have occurred in veterinary medicine, including the enhanced occurrence of feline infectious peritonitis in cats immunized with a recombinant vaccinia virus that expressed the feline coronavirus E2 protein before challenge infection. Despite the production of neutralizing antibodies after immunization, the kittens were not protected and died quickly of feline infectious peritonitis after challenge. There are numerous instances of disease induced by incomplete inactivation of non-replicating vaccines, and others wherein contaminating viruses survived the inactivation process.

Vaccination Frequency and Inoculation Site Reactions

Beyond the schedule of primary vaccination, there is little agreement and much current debate as to how often animals need to be revaccinated. For most vaccines, there is comparatively little definitive information available on the duration of immunity. For example, it is well recognized that immunity after vaccination with live-attenuated canine distemper vaccine is of long duration, perhaps lifelong. However, the duration of immunity to other viruses or components in a combined vaccine may not be of such long duration. In companion-animal practice, the cost of vaccination, relative to other costs, is small when clients visit their veterinarian, so it has been argued that, if revaccination does no harm, it may be considered a justified component of the routine annual "check-up" in which a wide spectrum of healthcare needs may be addressed. In many countries, annual revaccination has become a cornerstone of broad-based companion-animal preventive healthcare programs, although the rationale for this approach is conjectural at best.

This concept of annual vaccination was further disturbed in the mid-1990s by reports of highly aggressive subcutaneous fibrosarcomas in cats at sites of vaccination (often behind the shoulder). All the factors responsible for these vaccine-associated cancers remain to be thoroughly proven; however, a contaminating virus within the vaccines themselves is not responsible, and the prevailing suspicion is that irritation induced by the vaccine constituents is responsible. Regardless, this phenomenon rekindled the debate of frequency of revaccination in companion animals, leading to new recommendations on the preferred vaccination site, vaccination interval (extended from 1 to 3 years for some vaccines), and systems for reporting adverse responses.

Vaccination Policy and Schedules

The available range of vaccines, often in multivalent formulations and with somewhat different recommendations from each manufacturer regarding vaccination schedules, means that the practicing veterinarian needs to educate her/himself constantly about vaccine choice and usage. Multivalent vaccine formulations confer major practical advantages by reducing the number of visits the owner must make to the veterinarian. Also, multivalent vaccines allow more extensive use of vaccines against agents of secondary importance. Unlike the situation in human medicine, however, where there is general agreement on vaccine formulations and schedules for vaccination against all the common viral diseases of childhood, there is no such consensus in veterinary medicine. Furthermore, unlike the situation in human medicine in which there are few vaccine manufacturers, there are many veterinary vaccine manufacturers, each promoting their own products. The reader is referred to the specific resources on vaccination schedules specific for each animal species provided at the end of this section, but some general considerations for vaccination are described here.

Optimal Age for Vaccination

The risk of most viral diseases is greatest in young animals. Most vaccines are therefore given during the first 6 months of life. Maternal antibody, whether transferred transplacentally in primates or, as in domestic animals and birds, in the colostrum or via the yolk sac, inhibits the immune response of the newborn or newly hatched to vaccines. Optimally, vaccination should be delayed until the titer of maternal antibody in the young animal has declined to near zero. However, any delay in vaccine administration may leave the animal defenseless during the resulting "window of susceptibility." This is potentially life threatening in crowded, highly contaminated environments or where there is intense activity of arthropod vectors. There are a number of approaches to handling this problem in different animal species, but none is fully satisfactory. The problem is complicated further because young animals do not necessarily respond to vaccines in the same way as older animals do. In horses, for example, antibody responses to inactivated influenza vaccines are poor until recipients become yearlings.

Because the titer of passively acquired antibody in the circulation of newborn animals after receiving colostrum is proportional to that in the dam's blood, and because the rate of its subsequent clearance in different animal species is known, it is possible to estimate, for any given maternal antibody titer, the age at which no measurable antibody remains in the offspring. This can be plotted as a nomograph, from which the optimal age of vaccination against any particular disease can be read. The method is seldom used, but might be considered for exceptionally valuable animals in a "high-risk" environment.

In practice, relatively few vaccine failures are encountered if one simply follows the instructions from the vaccine manufacturers, who have used averaged data on maternal antibody levels and rate of IgG decay in that animal species to estimate an optimal age for vaccination. It is recommended commonly, even in the case of live-attenuated virus vaccines, that a number of doses of vaccine be administered, say at monthly intervals, to cover the window of susceptibility in animals with particularly high maternal antibody titers. This precaution is even more relevant to multivalent vaccine formulations, because of the differences in levels of maternal antibody against each virus.

Dam Vaccination

The aim of vaccination is generally thought of as the protection of the vaccinee. This is usually so, but in the case of certain vaccines [e.g., those for equine herpes (abortion) virus-1, rotavirus infection in cattle, parvovirus infection in swine, infectious bursal disease of chickens] the objective is to protect the vaccinee's offspring either *in utero* (e.g., equine abortion) or as a neonate/hatchling. This is achieved by vaccination of the dam. For neonates/hatchlings, the level of maternal antibody transferred in the colostrum and milk or in the egg ensures that the offspring have a protective level of antibody during the critical early days. Because many attenuated virus vaccines are abortigenic or teratogenic, inactivated vaccines are recommended for dam vaccination.

Available and Recommended Vaccines

The types of vaccines available for each viral disease (or the lack of any satisfactory vaccine) are discussed in each chapter of Part II of this book. There is clearly enormous geographic variation in the requirements for individual vaccines, particularly for highly regulated diseases such as foot-and-mouth disease. There are also different requirements appropriate to various types of livestock husbandry (e.g., for dairy cattle, beef cows, and their calves on range, or cattle in feedlots and in poultry for breeders, commercial egg layers, and broilers). Similarly, vaccination schedules for dogs, cats, horses, pet birds, and other species such as rabbits should reflect science-based criteria in addition to individual risk. Thus the reader is referred to specialty organizations that publish guidelines for the vaccination of, for example: horses [the American Association of Equine Practitioners (http://www.aaep.org/vaccination_guidelines.htm)], cats [the American Association of Feline Practitioners (http://www.catvets.com/professionals/guidelines/publications/?Id=176)], and dogs [the American Animal Hospital Association (http://secure.aahanet.org/eweb/dynamicpage.aspx?site=resource&webcode=CanineVaccineGuidelines)]. Relatively few vaccines are widely available for use in pet birds, but those that are include vaccines for polyoma virus, Pacheco's disease virus, canarypox and, in enzootic areas, West Nile virus.

For some species, including production animals, protection against viral infections and diseases is by exclusion. Laboratory rodents, for example, are maintained in various types of microbial barrier environments. Rarely, laboratory mice at high risk for ectromelia virus infection during outbreaks in highly valuable mouse populations may be individually vaccinated with the IHD-T strain of vaccinia virus.

Commercially raised rabbits, as well as pet rabbits, are often vaccinated against myxoma virus and rabbit hemorrhagic disease virus, where these agents are highly prevalent, such as in Europe. These rabbit diseases also illustrate the political context of veterinary vaccination: vaccines may not be available in some countries, such as the United States, because vaccination may obscure surveillance for natural outbreaks of disease.

Vaccination of Poultry and Fish

In the United States alone, the annual production of poultry birds exceeds $22 billion. All commercially produced birds are vaccinated against several different viral diseases, although there is variation in the types of vaccines used in different countries. The strategy for vaccination of poultry against viral diseases is no different than that for mammals, but the cost of each vaccine dose is tiny; much of this economy of scale is linked to low-cost delivery systems (aerosol and drinking water). Further economies have been achieved by the introduction of *in-ovo* immunization of 18-day-old embryonated eggs; an instrument (called an Inovoject), capable of immunizing 40,000 eggs per hour, is used. The most frequently used vaccines are against Marek's disease; formerly inoculated individually into 1-day-old chicks, these are now delivered in this way. By 2009, more than 95% of meat chickens (broilers) in the United States were vaccinated by this method.

Vaccination is used to prevent infectious hemopoietic necrosis and infectious pancreatic necrosis in fish. Vaccines to these diseases include DNA and subunit protein vaccines that are administered either by injection or orally. The objective of vaccination in fish is the same as in mammals; indeed, the phylogenetic origins of the vertebrate immune system can be traced to the first jawed vertebrates, including bony fish (teleosts). Antiviral immunity, although less understood in fish as compared with mammals or birds, involves both innate and acquired response mechanisms. Specifically, cellular and humoral innate responses involve equivalent cell types, signaling molecules, and soluble factors as are found in mammals. These include phagocytes equipped with pattern recognition receptors (PRRs) such as TLRs that lead to pro-inflammatory responses and interferon induction; induction of type 1-like interferons is essential for antiviral innate immune responses in fish, and their production is stimulated by dsRNA and signaling pathway in a manner analogous to that in mammals. Increasing evidence demonstrates that the innate immune response induces an antiviral state in addition to priming adaptive immunity. Similarly, adaptive responses involving T and B lymphocytes and specific immunoglobulin production are critical for antiviral immunity in fish. The structure of the T cell receptor complex ($\alpha\beta$ $\gamma\delta$) has remained virtually constant throughout the evolution of jawed vertebrates, including teleosts, whereas the organization and usage of the B cell receptors in fish varies from that of other vertebrates, as fish possess two distinct B-cell lineages (sIgM$^+$ or sIgτ/ζ^+)—both of which are important for antiviral immunity and affinity maturation of immunoglobulins—and a less pronounced memory response is typical of the adaptive response in fish as compared with mammals or birds. As fish are poikilotherms, the magnitude of the immune response in most fish is profoundly influenced by water temperature, which may play a causal role in seasonal viral disease patterns in both captive and wild fish populations.

OTHER STRATEGIES FOR ANTIVIRAL PROPHYLAXIS AND TREATMENT

Passive Immunization

It is possible to confer short-term protection against specific viral disease by the subcutaneous administration of an appropriate antibody, such as immune serum, immunoglobulin, or a monoclonal antibody. Homologous immunoglobulin is preferred, because heterologous protein may provoke a hypersensitivity response, as well as being more rapidly cleared by the recipient. Pooled normal immunoglobulin contains sufficiently high concentrations of antibody against all the common viruses that cause systemic disease in the respective species. Higher titers occur in convalescent serum from donor animals that have recovered from infection or have been hyperimmunized by repeated vaccinations; such hyperimmune globulin is the preferred product if available commercially.

A more common practice is to vaccinate (preferably using an inactivated virus vaccine) the pregnant dam or female bird approximately 3 weeks before anticipated parturition or egg laying. This provides the offspring with passive (maternal) immunity via antibodies present in the egg (in birds) or in colostrum and milk (in many wild and domestic mammals). This is particularly important for diseases in which the major impact occurs during the first few weeks of life, when active immunization of the newborn cannot be accomplished early enough. Furthermore, this strategy avoids the use of live-attenuated vaccines that may themselves be pathogenic to neonates.

Chemotherapy of Viral Diseases

If this had been a book about bacterial diseases of domestic animals, there would have been a large section on antimicrobial chemotherapy. However, the antibiotics that have been so effective against bacterial diseases have few counterparts in our armamentarium against viral diseases. The reason is that viruses are intimately dependent on the metabolic pathways of their host cell for their replication, hence most agents that interfere with virus replication are toxic to the cell. In recent years, however, and spurred in large part by investigation of devastating human viral diseases such as acquired immunodeficiency syndrome, influenza, and B-hepatitis, increased knowledge of the biochemistry of virus replication has led to a more rational approach in the search for antiviral chemotherapeutic agents, and a number of such compounds have now become a standard part of the armamentarium against particular human viruses. Antiviral chemotherapeutic agents are not in common use in veterinary practice, partly because of their very high cost, but some of the antiviral drugs used in human medicine have already also been utilized in veterinary

medicine. Accordingly, it is appropriate to outline briefly some potential developments in this field.

Several steps in the virus replication cycle represent potential targets for selective antiviral drug attack. Theoretically, all virus-encoded enzymes are vulnerable, as are all processes (enzymatic or non-enzymatic) that are more essential to the replication of the virus than to the survival of the cell. Table 4.1 sets out the most vulnerable steps and provides examples of antiviral drugs that display activity, indicating some that have already been licensed for use in humans.

A logical approach to the development of new antiviral drugs is to isolate or synthesize substances that might be predicted to serve as inhibitors of a known virus-encoded enzyme such as a transcriptase, replicase, or protease. Analogs of this prototype drug are then synthesized with a view to enhancing activity and/or selectivity. A further refinement of this approach is well illustrated by the nucleoside analog, acycloguanosine (aciclovir)—an inhibitor of herpesvirus DNA polymerase. Aciclovir is in fact an inactive prodrug that requires another herpesvirus-coded enzyme, thymidine kinase, to phosphorylate it to its active form. Because this viral enzyme occurs only in infected cells, aciclovir is non-toxic for uninfected cells, but very effective in herpesvirus-infected cells. Aciclovir and related analogs (e.g., valacyclovir, ganciclovir) are now available for treatment of herpesvirus infections in humans, and they have also been used on a limited scale in veterinary medicine, such as for treatment of feline herpesvirus 1 induced corneal ulcers and equine herpesvirus-1 induced

TABLE 4.1 Possible Targets for Antiviral Chemotherapy in Veterinary Medicine

Target	Prototype Drug
Attachment of virion to cell receptor	Receptor analogs
Uncoating	Rimantadine[a]
Primary transcription from viral genome	Transcriptase inhibitors
Reverse transcription	Zidovudine—AZT[a]
Regulation of transcription	Lentivirus tat inhibitors
Processing of RNA transcripts	Ribavirin[a]
Translation of viral RNA into protein	Interferons[a]
Post-translational cleavage of proteins	Protease inhibitors
Replication of viral DNA genome	Acycloguanosine (Acyclovir[a])
Replication of viral RNA genome	Replicase inhibitors

[a]Licensed for human use.

encephalomyelitis. They have also been used in humans exposed to the zoonotic herpes virus of macaques, herpes simiae (B virus) that may have catastrophic consequences in infected humans.

Drugs also have been developed to treat influenza virus infections in people and, potentially, animals. For example, oseltamivir phosphate (Tamiflu) is a prodrug that, after its metabolism in the liver, releases an activate metabolite that inhibits neuraminidase, the virus-encoded enzyme that releases budding virions from the surface of infected cells and cleaves the virus receptor so that released virions do not bind to already infected cells. Inhibition of neuraminidase, therefore, slows virus spread, giving the immune system the opportunity to "catch up" and mediate virus clearance.

Ribavirin is also a prodrug that is metabolized to purine RNA metabolites that interfere with the RNA metabolism that is required for virus replication. This drug has been used in the treatment of human respiratory syncytial virus and hepatitis C virus infections.

X-ray crystallography has opened a major new approach in the search for antiviral drugs. Now that the three-dimensional structure of many viruses is known, it has been possible to characterize receptor-binding sites on capsid proteins at the atomic level of resolution. Complexes of viral proteins with bound cellular receptors can be crystallized and examined directly. For example, for some rhinoviruses, receptor-binding sites on virions are in "canyons"—that is, clefts in the capsid surface. Drugs have been found that fit into these clefts, thereby preventing virus attachment to the host cell. Further information is provided by mapping the position of the particular amino acid residues that form these clefts, thereby allowing the design of drugs that better fit and better interfere with the viral infection process. This approach also lends itself to the development of drugs that block virus penetration of the host cell or uncoating of virus once inside the cell. If any of these strategies are successful in human medicine, adaptation to veterinary usage may follow.

VIRUSES AS VECTORS FOR GENE THERAPY

In addition to their central role as pathogens, viruses also have contributed much to the current understanding of both cellular and molecular biology. Individual viruses, or components thereof, have been exploited as molecular tools, and viruses also offer a novel and useful system for the expression of heterologous genes. Specifically, with the advent of cloning and genetic manipulation, foreign genes can readily be inserted into the genome of many viruses so that they can be used as expression vectors. These viral gene vectors include those that deliver the gene of interest without replicating in the host ("suicide" vectors) and those that do replicate in the host, with or without integration into the genome.

The use of both DNA and RNA viruses as recombinant vaccine vectors was described earlier in this chapter, but this same strategy also can potentially be exploited for therapeutic use. Viral-vector gene therapy strategies offer a novel and especially attractive approach to the correction of specific genetic disorders, particularly those with a defined missing or dysfunctional gene. Correction of such disorders requires the long-term expression of the specific protein that is absent or dysfunctional; thus viruses with the capability of safely and stably inserting the target gene into the genome of the affected individual are a logical choice as vectors for this purpose. To this end, a variety of viruses have been evaluated as potential gene vectors, including retroviruses because of their inherent ability to integrate into the host genome, poxviruses, adenoviruses, adeno-associated viruses (which are parvoviruses), herpesviruses, and various positive- and negative-sense RNA viruses.

Adeno-associated viruses have received much recent attention as potential vectors for gene therapy. They are small DNA viruses (family *Parvoviridae*, genus *Dependovirus*) that can infect both dividing and non-dividing cells, and they can insert their genome into that of the host cell. Furthermore, integration of the viral genome of adeno-associated viruses occurs at specific sites within the host genome, as opposed to that of retroviruses, insertion of which is typically random and potentially mutagenic. Adeno-associated viruses are considered to be avirulent (non-pathogenic), and the capacity for integration is readily abolished by genetic manipulation. Recombinant adeno-associated viruses that express appropriate proteins have been evaluated for the correction of a variety of human genetic disorders, including hemophilia and muscular dystrophy.

The strategy of targeted gene delivery is also potentially applicable for therapeutic intervention by the delivery of molecules with the capacity to modulate disease processes, especially chronic diseases with an immune-mediated pathogenesis that might be susceptible to regional expression of immunomodulatory molecules.

Another potential application of targeted gene delivery using recombinant viruses is to control the reproduction of wildlife and feral species, including those species considered to be pests, by targeted delivery of immunogenic proteins critical for reproductive activity.

Chapter 5

Laboratory Diagnosis of Viral Infections

Chapter Contents

Tests to support or establish a specific diagnosis of a viral infection are of five general types: (1) those that demonstrate the presence of infectious virus; (2) those that detect viral antigens; (3) those that detect viral nucleic acids; (4) those that demonstrate the presence of an agent-specific antibody response; (5) those that directly visualize ("see") the virus. Most available routine tests are agent dependent—that is, they are designed to detect a specific virus and will give a negative test result even if other viruses are present in the sample. For this reason, agent-independent tests such as virus isolation and electron microscopy are still used to identify the unexpected or unknown agent in a clinical sample. Traditional methods such as virus isolation are still widely used; however, many are too slow to have any direct influence on clinical management of an index case. A major thrust of the developments in diagnostic sciences continues to be toward rapid methods that provide a definitive answer in less than 24 hours or, optimally, even during the course of the initial examination of the animal. A second major area of interest and focused effort is the development of multiplexed tests that can screen simultaneously for several pathogens from a single sample. The best of these methods fulfill five prerequisites: speed, simplicity, diagnostic sensitivity, diagnostic specificity, and low cost. For some economically important viruses: (1) standardized diagnostic tests and reagents of good quality are available commercially; (2) assays have been miniaturized to conserve reagents and decrease costs; (3) instruments have been developed to automate tests, again often decreasing costs; (4) computerized analyses aid in making the interpretation of results as objective as possible in addition to facilitating reporting, record keeping, and billing.

Although less impressive in veterinary medicine in comparison with human medicine (for reasons of economic return on investment and range of tests required across each species), there has been recent expansion in the number of commercially available rapid diagnostic kits. These tests detect viral antigens, allowing a diagnosis from a single specimen taken directly from the animal during the acute phase of the illness, or they test for the presence of virus-specific antibody. Solid-phase enzyme immunoassays (EIAs) or enzyme-linked immunosorbent assays (ELISAs), in particular, have revolutionized diagnostic virology for both antigen and antibody detection, and are now methods of choice in many situations. For laboratory-based diagnosis, polymerase chain reaction (PCR) technology is now widely used to detect viral nucleic acids in clinical specimens, offering a very rapid alternative to other methods of virus detection. Quantitative PCR assays, in particular, facilitate the very rapid, sensitive, and specific identification of many known pathogenic viruses, and automation of these assays allows the processing of large numbers of samples in short periods of time (high sample-throughput). Another major advantage of quantitative PCR assays is that they provide an objective estimate of viral load in a clinical sample. Research efforts in PCR continue, to move testing from the laboratory to the field, particularly for high-consequence agents with which rapidity of diagnosis is critically important.

The provision, by a single laboratory, of a comprehensive service for the diagnosis of viral infections of domesticated animals is a formidable undertaking. Viruses in more than 130 different genera and belonging to 35 families cause infections of veterinary significance. Add to these numbers the rapidly expanding array of viruses that occur in wildlife and fish, and it is not surprising that no single laboratory can have the necessary specific reagents available or the skills and experience for the detection and identification of all viruses of all animal species. For this reason, veterinary diagnostic laboratories tend to specialize [e.g., in diseases of food animals, companion animals, poultry, fish, or laboratory species, or in diseases caused by exotic viruses (foreign animal diseases)]. Contacting the laboratory to determine its specific capabilities should be a first step in submitting specimens for testing. Table 5.1 provides a general guide to diagnostic tests currently used in veterinary medicine. These will be defined in more detail later in this chapter.

RATIONALE FOR SPECIFIC DIAGNOSIS

Why bother to establish a definitive laboratory diagnosis of a viral infection? In earlier times when laboratory diagnostic testing was in its infancy, diagnosis of diseases related to viral infections was achieved mainly on the basis of clinical history and signs, and/or gross pathology and histopathology; laboratory test results were viewed as confirmatory data. This is no longer the case, for several reasons: (1) the recent development of rapid test formats for specific and sensitive identification of individual viral infections; (2) many clinical cases occur as disease complexes that cannot be diagnosed on the basis of clinical signs or pathology alone—for example, the canine and bovine respiratory disease complexes; (3) diagnostic medicine, especially that pertaining to companion animals, increasingly demands reliable and specific antemortem diagnoses; (4) legal/regulatory actions for diseases of production animals and zoonoses can require identification of the specific agents involved, avian influenza being a relevant contemporary example. Other areas in which laboratory testing data is essential are considered below.

At the Individual Animal or Individual Herd Level

Diseases in which the management of the animal or its prognosis is influenced by the diagnosis. Respiratory diseases (e.g., in a broiler facility, acute respiratory disease in a boarding kennel, shipping fever in a cattle feedlot), diarrheal diseases of neonates, and some mucocutaneous

diseases may be caused by a variety of different infectious agents, including viruses. Rapid and accurate identification of the causative agent can be the basis for establishing a management plan (biosecurity, vaccination, antimicrobial treatment) that prevents additional losses in the stable, kennel, flock, or herd.

Certification of freedom from specific infections. For diseases in which there is life-long infection—such as bovine and feline leukemia virus infection, persistent bovine viral diarrhea virus infection, equine infectious anemia, and certain herpesvirus infections—a negative test certificate or history of appropriate vaccination is often required as a condition of sale, for exhibition at a state fair or show, or for competitions and/or international movement.

Artificial insemination, embryo transfer, and blood transfusion. Males used for semen collection and females used in embryo transfer programs, especially in cattle, and blood donors of all species are usually screened for a range of viruses to minimize the risk of viral transmission to recipient animals.

Zoonoses. Viruses such as rabies, Rift Valley fever, Hendra, influenza, eastern, western, and Venezuelan equine encephalitis are all zoonotic, and are of sufficient public health significance as to require relevant veterinary diagnostic laboratories to establish the capability for accurate detection of these agents. Early warning of a potential influenza virus epidemic through diagnosis of infection and/or disease in an individual poultry flock or in affected swine allows the implementation of control programs to eradicate the infection and/or restrict movement of exposed animals. As an example, laboratory identification of rabies virus in a dog, skunk, or bat that has bitten a child provides the basis for treatment decisions.

At the State, Country, and International Level

Epidemiologic and economic awareness. Provision of a sound veterinary service in any state or country depends on knowledge of prevailing diseases, hence epidemiologic studies to determine the prevalence and distribution of particular viral infections are frequently undertaken. Such programs are also directed against specific zoonotic, food-borne, water-borne, rodent-borne, and arthropod-borne viruses. Internationally, the presence of specific livestock diseases in a country or region requires notification to the Office Internationale des Epizooties (the OIE, *syn.* the World Organization for Animal Health), which records the occurrence of these notifiable diseases in the approximately 175 member countries of the organization.

Test and removal programs. For infections caused by viruses such as equine infectious anemia virus, Marek's disease virus, bovine herpesvirus 1, pseudorabies virus, and bovine viral diarrhea virus, it is possible to reduce substantially the incidence of disease or eliminate the causative

TABLE 5.1 Principles and Objectives of Diagnostic Methods

Principle	Method	Specimens/Findings	Characteristics
Visual Information Leading to a Presumptive Diagnosis			
	Review of the disease history, clinical examination, chemistry, hematology, etc.	Subject animal and its body fluids/Abnormal values	Essence of differential and rule out diagnoses; presumptive diagnosis determines the specimens and methods for further testing
	Pathology, histopathology, ultrastructural pathology	Animals, organs, tissues, cells/Characteristic lesions, inclusion bodies	Although slow and expensive, still important in veterinary diagnostics
	Detection of viruses by electron microscopy	Tissues, cells, secretions, excretions, vesicular contents/Particles of uniform, characteristic morphology	Rapid; sensitive enough with many diseases, especially diarrheas; expensive; technically demanding, expertise unavailable in many settings
Detection and Identification of Viral Antigens			
	Enzyme immunoassay methods (e.g., antigen-capture enzyme immunoassay)	Tissues, cells, secretions, excretions/Reaction of viral antigen with antibody of known specificity	Rapid, sensitive and specific. Most common methods in use today
	Immunochromatography, immunogold-binding assays (the equivalent of the home pregnancy test)	Blood, secretions, excretions/Viral antigen identified by reaction with antibody of known specificity	Rapid, sensitive, specific, suitable for testing of individual specimens in the clinical setting
	Immunofluorescence	Tissues and cells/Viral antigen identified in situ by reaction with antibody of known specificity	Rapid, sensitive and specific. Localization of antigen in specific cells adds to confidence in diagnosis; technically demanding
	Immunohistochemistry (immunoperoxidase staining)	Tissues and cells/Viral antigen identified in situ by reaction with antibody of known specificity	Slow, but sensitive and specific. Localization of antigen in specific cells adds to confidence in diagnosis; technical expertise involved is more like an extension of histopathology
	Immunoelectron microscopy	Tissues, cells, secretions, excretions/Character and aggregation of virus by specific antibody of known specificity	Extension of diagnostic electron microscopy. Rapid, sensitive and specific. Expensive and technically demanding; expertise unavailable in many settings
Direct Detection and Identification of Viral Nucleic Acids			
	Hybridization methods, including in-situ hybridization, Southern blot hybridization and dot-blot filter hybridization methods	Extracts from tissues, cells, secretions, excretions/Viral nucleic acid identified by reaction with specific DNA probe	Dot-blot methods are rapid, simple to carry out, very sensitive, and with suitable reagents very specific. Largely being replaced with polymerase chain reaction (PCR) procedures
	PCR, reverse transcriptase-PCR, real-time PCR, and amplification by isothermal amplification	Extracts from tissues, cells, secretions, excretions/Viral nucleic acid specifically amplified using primer sets and then identified by various methods such as fragment size analysis, labeled DNA probes, probe hydrolysis, and partial sequencing	Some methods can be subject to contamination, causing false-positive results. Nevertheless, because of incredible sensitivity and specificity, becoming used very widely in circumstances where the "state of the art" is required. Automation and new methods for identifying amplified products are leading to quicker, more reliable, and less expensive tests
	Viral genomic sequencing and partial sequencing	Extracts from tissues, cells, secretions, excretions/Viral nucleic acid specifically amplified, usually via PCR and then subjected to automated sequencing, usually of only 100–300 bases in selected genomic regions	When combined with automated genome amplification methods and computer-based analyses of results, this becomes the new "gold standard" in identifying a virus

(Continued)

TABLE 5.1 (Continued)

Principle	Method	Specimens/Findings	Characteristics
	Oligonucleotide fingerprinting and restriction endonuclease mapping	Extracts from tissues, cells, secretions, excretions/Viral nucleic acid amplified, usually via PCR or growing the virus in cell culture, then restriction enzyme digestion and gel electrophoresis to determine characteristic banding patterns ("viral bar-coding")	Very slow, expensive, difficult to automate, and complex to analyze. Methods largely being replaced with PCR and sequencing
Virus Isolation and Identification			
	Virus isolation in cultured cells	Tissues, cells, secretions, excretions/Specimens inoculated into suitable cell cultures and presence of virus detected by various methods, usually immunological methods	Relatively slow, expensive, and technically demanding. However, this is the only method that provides a virus isolate for further testing (e.g., strain typing) and is therefore widely used in reference centers
	Virus isolation in animals	Tissues, cells, secretions, excretions/Specimens inoculated into animals, usually newborn or 3-week-old mice, usually by the intracerebral or intraperitoneal routes, with sickness or death as indication of viral growth. Identification of virus by various methods, usually immunological methods	Even slower, more expensive, and technically demanding than virus isolation in cell culture. However, for viruses that do not grow well in cell culture, this is the only method that provides a virus isolate for further testing (e.g., strain typing) and is therefore still used in reference centers in special circumstances
Detection and Quantitation of Antiviral Antibodies (Serologic Diagnosis)			
	Enzyme immunoassay (EIA)—enzyme-linked immunosorbent assay (ELISA)	Serum/Specimens tested for presence of specific antibodies indicating recent or past infection	Rapid, sensitive, and specific; the pillar of retrospective diagnosis for many clinical and epidemiological purposes. In many cases, paired sera are needed to confirm infection or recent vaccination
	IgM class-specific antibody EIA–ELISA	Serum/Specimens tested for presence of specific IgM antibodies indicating recent infection	Rapid, sensitive, and specific; becoming the pillar of serologic diagnosis of recent infection in human medicine, with limited development in veterinary medicine. In many cases a single serum suffices
	Serum (virus) neutralization assay	Serum/Specimens tested for presence of specific antibodies indicating recent or past infection	Cell culture-based method; slow, expensive, and technically demanding. However, this is the "gold standard" of serology, as neutralizing antibodies correlate best with immune protection
	Immunoblotting (Western blotting)	Serum/Specimens tested for presence of specific antibodies indicating recent or past infection	Slow, expensive, and technically demanding, mostly used as confirmatory test
	Indirect immunofluorescence assay	Serum/Specimens tested for presence of specific antibodies indicating recent or past infection	Rapid, sensitive, but subject to uncontrollable, non-specific reactions
	Hemagglutination-inhibition assay	Serum/Specimens tested for presence of specific antibodies indicating recent or past infection	Rapid, sensitive, and specific; widely used for retrospective diagnosis for epidemiological and regulatory purposes. Still a pillar in avian virus diagnostics and for many mammalian virus diseases
	Immunodiffusion	Serum/Specimens tested for presence of specific antibodies indicating recent or past infection	Rapid, but can lack sensitivity and subject to specificity problems. There are very good tests available for some diseases

virus from herds or flocks by test and removal programs. The elimination of pseudorabies virus from commercial swine facilities in the United States is an example of where differential laboratory tests [the so-called differentiation/discrimination of infected from vaccinated animals (DIVA) test, which discriminates between naturally infected and vaccinated animals] were essential to the eradication effort.

Surveillance programs in support of enzootic disease research and control activities. Surveillance of viral infections based on laboratory diagnostics is central to all epidemiologic research, whether to determine the significance of a particular virus in a new setting, to unravel the natural history and ecology of a virus in a particular host animal population, to establish priorities and means of control, or to monitor and evaluate control programs.

Surveillance programs in support of exotic disease research and control activities. The countries of Europe, North America, Australia, New Zealand, and Japan are usually free of many devastating diseases of livestock such as foot-and-mouth disease, classical swine fever, African swine fever, and fowl plague that are still enzootic in other parts of the world. However, periodic incursions of these feared exotic diseases into previously free areas occur with alarming regularity and very substantial adverse economic impact. Thus it is of the utmost importance that the clinical diagnosis of a suspected high-consequence viral infection be confirmed quickly and accurately. Many countries maintain or share the use of specialized biocontainment laboratories devoted to rapid and accurate diagnosis and research on high-consequence viruses that cause economically devastating "foreign animal diseases."

Prevention of new, emerging, and re-emerging viral diseases of animals. Continuous surveillance of animal populations for evidence of new viruses, new diseases, and new epizootics is essential if new threats are to be dealt with rapidly and comprehensively. New viruses and new virus–disease associations continue to be discovered, virtually every year. Vigilance by astute veterinary clinicians as well as by diagnosticians and epidemiologists is essential for early recognition of such occurrences.

COLLECTION, PACKAGING, AND TRANSPORT OF SPECIMENS

The chance of detecting a virus depends critically on the attention given by the attending veterinarian to the collection of specimens. Clearly, such specimens must be taken from the right site, from the most appropriate animal, and at the right time. The right time for virus detection is as soon as possible after the animal first develops clinical signs, because maximal amounts (titers) of virus are usually present at the onset of signs and often then decrease rapidly during the ensuing days. Specimens for virus detection taken as a last resort when days or weeks of empirical therapy have failed are almost invariably a useless endeavor and a waste of consumer and laboratory resources. Similarly, the incorrect collection and storage of specimens, and the submission of inappropriate specimens, will diminish the likelihood of accurate diagnostic laboratory success.

The site from which the specimen is collected will be influenced by the clinical signs and knowledge of the pathogenesis of the suspected agent(s) (Table 5.2). In viral respiratory infection in cattle, for example, the most important diagnostic specimens that should be collected include nasal or throat swabs or transtracheal wash fluid from live animals, and lung tissue and lymph nodes from dead animals; whole-blood samples from this type of case are often useless because the causative viral agents (bovine respiratory syncytial virus, bovine herpesvirus 1, bovine coronavirus, etc.) may not produce detectable concentrations of virus in blood samples (viremia). Likewise, for routine enteric cases (diarrhea), feces would be the primary sample in calves with rotavirus, coronavirus, or torovirus infections, with whole-blood being useful only if bovine virus diarrhea virus was a likely cause. Timing of sample collection is also critical, particularly with enteric cases, as detection of rotavirus may not be possible more than 48 hours after the onset of clinical signs. PCR tests do extend the sampling period because of their high analytical sensitivity and their ability to detect viral nucleic acids even if the causative virus is already complexed with neutralizing antibodies, but this longer detection period does not eliminate the need to be attentive to timing.

TABLE 5.2 Specimens Appropriate for Laboratory Diagnosis of Various Clinical Syndromes in the Live Animal

Syndrome	Specimen
Respiratory	Nasal or throat swab; nasopharyngeal aspirate, tracheal wash fluid
Enteric	Feces
Genital	Genital swab
Eye	Conjunctival swab
Skin	Vesicle swab or scraping; biopsy of solid lesion
Central nervous system	Cerebrospinal fluid
Generalized	Nasal swab[a], feces[a], blood leukocytes[a], serum, urine
Biopsy	Relevant organ
Any disease	Blood for serology[b]

[a]Depending on presumed pathogenesis.
[b]Blood allowed to clot, serum kept for assay of antibody.

Furthermore, the extended detection of viral nucleic acid by PCR assays increases the likelihood of false-positive results, wherein a virus detected by PCR is not the actual cause of the affected animal's disease.

Tissue specimens should always be taken from any part of the body where lesions are observed, either by surgical biopsy or at necropsy of dead animals, as it is critical that laboratory findings be reconciled with lesions that are manifest in the affected animal. Thus separate samples should be split between material that will be fixed (formalin or other fixative) and material that will remain unfixed for virus detection assays such as immunohistochemical staining, PCR testing, or virus isolation.

Because of the lability of many viruses, specimens intended for virus isolation must always be kept cold and moist, which requires preparation ahead of time. In collection of specimens such as swabs, the discussion immediately turns to viral transport media. The various transport media consist of a buffered salt solution to which has been added protein (e.g., gelatin, albumin, or fetal bovine serum) to protect the virus against inactivation and antimicrobials to prevent the multiplication of bacteria and fungi. A transport medium designed for bacteria or mycoplasma should not be used for virus sampling unless it has been proven not to be inhibitory for the intended test. Separate samples should be collected for bacterial testing. In general, specimens correctly collected and maintained for virus isolation

will be acceptable for antigen and nucleic acid detection testing. An example of a kit containing materials suitable for the collection and transportation of specimens is shown in Figure 5.1.

Specimens should be forwarded to the testing laboratory as soon as possible. With courier services increasingly available throughout the world, overnight delivery services have greatly decreased the time interval required for agent detection, and also greatly increased the rate of diagnostic success (pathogen detection rate). Specimens should not be frozen but should be kept cold (refrigeration temperature), if delivery to the laboratory will be within several days. While viability is not necessary for PCR assays and direct antigen detection, maintaining the specimens under optimum condition for virus isolation will also enhance detection by these other techniques. Specimens should never be sent to the diagnostic laboratory without a detailed clinical history of the animal and/or herd from which the specimens are derived. Clinical histories assist diagnosticians in selecting the most appropriate tests for the specimens received and permit a dialogue with the clinician over additional specimens if needed. Similarly, a detailed and accurate description of the nature and distribution of the lesions in affected animals is critical if samples are to be submitted for histopathological evaluation, regardless of whether the tissue specimens were obtained at necropsy or at surgical biopsy.

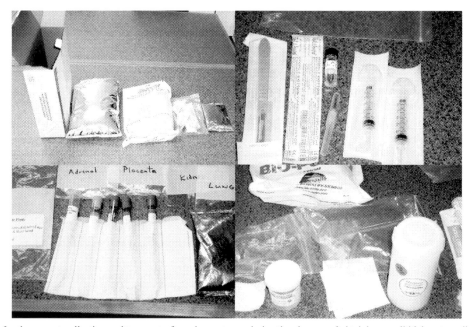

FIGURE 5.1   Kit for the correct collection and transport of specimens to maximize the chances of obtaining a valid laboratory diagnosis of a clinical case. The diagnostic laboratories can provide such kits, which contain materials both for collecting specimens and for proper shipping of the specimens that meet transportation standards. Items that may be included are: kit shipping box; insulated pouch, freezer packs, 95-kPa-rated specimen pouch; 95-kPa-rated formalin jars (1 small, 1 large); sealable plastic bags (small- and medium-sized); absorbent material sufficient to absorb all fluid in the shipment; serum blood collection tubes: ethylenediamine tetra-acetic acid (EDTA) blood collection tubes; blood collection needles; syringes; scalpels; buffered saline; alcohol swabs; history form; mailing label; formalin shipping label; shipping declaration forms as defined by the country of origin. (*Courtesy of B. Thompson, Animal Health Diagnostic Center, College of Veterinary Medicine, Cornell University.*)

Packaging and specimen labeling and identification may be a mundane topic, but attention to these details maximizes the likelihood of safe arrival of the specimens at the laboratory and prevents legal sanctions over incorrectly shipped hazardous materials. The submitter should have an understanding of local transport regulations, which in most instances mirror international air transport regulations, and pack diagnostic specimens accordingly. Although specimens may have been dispatched locally by land transport, often shipments will be partially transported by air over even short to moderate distances, without the knowledge of the shipper. The specimens should be protected from breaking in transit and should be sent refrigerated (but not frozen), with "cold packs." Wherever possible, sampling should include specimens that allow the use of several diagnostic tests, as no single test will provide an unambiguous diagnosis in all cases.

DIAGNOSIS OF VIRAL INFECTIONS BY GROSS EVALUATION AND HISTOPATHOLOGY

The gross and histological evaluation of tissues from animals with presumptive viral diseases is still a useful and important diagnostic method. If biopsy/necropsy samples are collected for possible histopathological diagnosis of viral infections, then the appropriate tissue specimens in the appropriate fixative—routinely formalin—are required. If special procedures are to be requested, such as electron microscopy or frozen sections for immunohistochemical staining, the receiving laboratory should be consulted for procedural and material details. It is critical that a thorough, accurate history and description of the lesions in affected animals accompany the submitted specimens.

The great benefit of pathology is that it can provide unambiguous confirmation of specific viral diseases, especially when done in conjunction with appropriate laboratory virological testing. In contrast, the mere demonstration of a particular virus, or seroconversion of an animal to that virus, is not necessarily proof of disease causality. Thus laboratory demonstration of a specific virus combined with compatible clinical signs and lesions in the affected animal strongly reinforces confidence in a specific diagnosis. Similarly, the identification of characteristic lesions in an animal without associated detection of the relevant virus should stimulate additional laboratory efforts to confirm or refute the tentative diagnosis.

METHODS OF DETECTION OF VIRUSES

Detection of Viruses by Electron Microscopy

Perhaps the most obvious method of virus detection/identification is direct visualization of the virus itself (Figure 5.2).

The morphology of most viruses is sufficiently characteristic to identify the image as a virus and to assign an unknown virus to the correct family. In the context of the particular case (e.g., detection of parapoxvirus in a scraping from a pock-like lesion on a cow's teat), the method may provide an immediate definitive diagnosis. Non-cultivable viruses may also be detectable by electron microscopy. Beginning in the late 1960s, electron microscopy was the means to the discovery of several new families of previously non-cultivable viruses, notably rotaviruses, noroviruses, astroviruses, and toroviruses, and unknown members of recognized families such as adenoviruses and coronaviruses. Even today, non-cultivable viruses such as those in the genus *Anellovirus* (torque teno viruses) have been identified by electron microscopy in samples from humans and a variety of animals.

Two general procedures can be applied to virus detection by electron microscopy: negative-stain electron microscopy and thin-section electron microscopy. For the negative stain procedure, virus particles in a fluid matrix are applied directly to a solid support designed for the procedure.

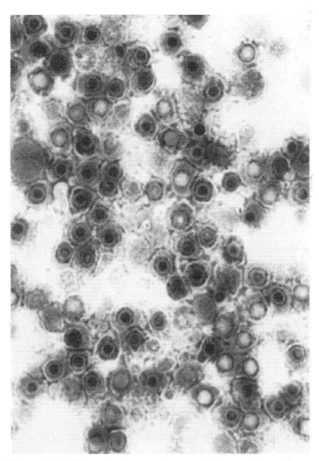

FIGURE 5.2 Diagnostic electron microscopy. The morphology of most viruses is sufficiently characteristic to assign an unknown virus to the correct family. In this case, direct negative staining of vesicular fluid revealed large numbers of herpesvirus particles, allowing a presumptive diagnosis of infectious bovine rhinotracheitis. Magnification: ×10,000.

Contrast stains are applied and the virus particles are directly visualized by electron microscopy. Thin-section electron microscopy can be used directly on fixed tissue samples, usually containing "viral" inclusions from the affected animal or on cell cultures growing an unidentified virus. Low sensitivity is the biggest limitation of electron microscopy as a diagnostic tool, followed by the need for expensive equipment and a highly skilled microscopist. To detect virus particles by negative-stain electron microscopy, the fluid matrix must contain approximately 10^6 virions per ml. Such concentrations are often surpassed in clinical material such as feces and vesicle fluid, or in virus-infected cell cultures, but not in respiratory mucus, for instance. Aggregation of virus particles by specific antiserum (immunoelectron microscopy) can enhance sensitivity and provide provisional identity of the agent. For thin-section electron microscopy, most of the cells in the tissue sample must contain virus if virions are likely to be visualized. Routine electron microscopy procedures have been largely replaced with more sensitive and less expensive procedures such as antigen-capture tests or immunostaining techniques, but because electron microscopy is an agent-independent test, it still has use in specialized cases and in facilities with the necessary equipment and expertise.

Detection of Viruses by Isolation

Despite the explosion of new techniques for "same-day diagnosis" of viral disease by demonstration of viral antigen or viral nucleic acid in specimens, virus isolation in cell culture remains an important procedure. Theoretically at least, a single viable virion present in a specimen can be grown in cultured cells, thus expanding it to produce enough material to permit further detailed characterization. Virus isolation remains the "gold standard" against which newer methods must be compared, but nucleic acid detection tests, particularly quantitative PCR assays, are challenging that paradigm.

There are several reasons why virus isolation remains as a standard technique in many non-commercial laboratories. Until recently it was the only technique that could detect the unexpected—that is, identify a totally unanticipated virus, or even discover an entirely new agent. Accordingly, even those laboratories well equipped for rapid diagnosis may also inoculate cell cultures in an attempt to isolate a virus. Metagenomic and "deep sequencing" techniques can detect unknown agents (so-called pathogen mining), but few laboratories outside subsidized research programs have the resources to routinely apply this technology. Culture is the easiest method of producing a supply of live virus for further examination by molecular methods (genome sequencing, antigenic variation, etc.). Research and reference laboratories, in particular, are always on the lookout for new viruses within the context of emerging diseases; such viruses require comprehensive characterization, as recently shown by the quickly evolving strains of influenza virus. Moreover, large quantities of virus must be grown in cultured cells to produce diagnostic antigens and reagents such as monoclonal antibodies. Until recently, vaccine development has also been reliant on the availability of viruses grown in culture, although this may quickly change in the future with the increasing sophistication of recombinant DNA technology.

The choice of cell culture strategy for the primary isolation of an unknown virus from clinical specimens is largely empirical. Primary cells derived from fetal tissues of the same species usually provide the most sensitive cell culture substrates for virus isolation. Continuous cell lines derived from the homologous species are, in many cases, an acceptable alternative. As interest in wildlife diseases increases, most laboratories are challenged to have the necessary cell cultures to "match" with the affected species. Testing strategies for challenging cases tend to reflect the creativity and bias of the diagnostic virologist and the particular laboratory, although the clinical signs exhibited by the affected animals will often suggest which virus might be present. Most laboratories also select a cell line that is known to grow many types of viruses, in case an unanticipated agent is present. Arthropod cell cultures are used frequently as a parallel system for isolating "arboviruses." Even with the best cell culture systems available, some viruses such as papillomaviruses will not grow in traditional cell culture conditions. Special culture systems such as organ cultures and tissue explants can be of value, but contact should be made with the testing laboratory to determine their capabilities before requesting such specialized and sophisticated diagnostic expertise.

Historically, when standard methods had failed to diagnose what appeared to be an infectious disease, inoculation of the putative natural host animal was used to define the infectious nature of the problem and to aid in the eventual isolation of the agent. This practice has largely been abandoned, as a result of costs and animal welfare concerns. Some specialized laboratories still have the capability to inoculate suckling mice, a system that has been valuable for isolating arboviruses that resist cultivation in cell cultures. Embryonated hens' eggs are still used for the isolation of influenza A viruses, even though cell cultures [Madin–Darby canine kidney (MDCK) cells] are now more commonly used. Many avian viruses also replicate much better in eggs than in cell cultures derived from chick embryo tissues, and there is a lack of widely available avian cell lines for routine virus isolation procedures. According to the virus of interest, the diagnostic specimen is inoculated into the amniotic cavity, or the allantoic cavity, the yolk sac, onto the chorioallantoic membrane or, in rare instances, intravenously into the vessels of the shell membrane and embryo. Evidence of viral growth may be seen on the chorioallantoic membrane (e.g., characteristic pocks caused by poxviruses), but otherwise other means are used to detect viral growth (e.g., death of the embryo, hemagglutination, immunofluorescence or immunohistochemical staining of viral antigens, or antigen-capture ELISA).

Attempts to isolate viruses require stringent attention by the clinician to the details of sample collection and transport, because success depends on the laboratory receiving a specimen containing viable virus. Contact with the testing laboratory before specimen collection is strongly advised in order to clarify the sampling strategy, assess shipping requirements, and alert the laboratory to the number and type of specimens being shipped. Having cell cultures available on the day of arrival of a specimen can enhance the success of isolation. There is no such thing as an emergency ("stat") virus isolation; each virus has its own biological clock and no amount of concern will speed up the replication cycle. For viruses such as the alphaherpesviruses, a successful isolation can be evident as cytopathic effect in the inoculated cell cultures within 2–3 days, whereas others are considerably slower and require repeated serial passage. In general, the time for detection will depend on the laboratory's procedures for identifying virus in the culture system. For instance, non-cytopathic bovine viral diarrhea virus can be detected by virus isolation as early as 3 days postinoculation or as late as 3 weeks, depending on laboratory procedures. Procedures for routinely detecting and identifying virus in inoculated cell cultures include immunofluorescence or immunohistochemical staining of the infected monolayer, antigen-capture ELISA, nucleic acid detection tests such as PCR, hemadsorption, or even negative-stain electron microscopy for unknown isolates.

Detection of Viral Antigens

The direct detection of viral antigens in a clinical sample can be achieved in as little as 15 minutes with some immunoassays, or the procedure can take several days if extensive sample preparation and staining is involved. Viable virus is generally not required in the specimen for a positive antigen detection test result, but the timing of sample collection is as important with these assays as it is for virus isolation. Analytical sensitivity varies across the various test modalities, ranging from detection of a single infected cell to assays that require as much as 10^5 antigen units. The advance that revolutionized this type of testing was the development of monoclonal antibodies. These reagents are highly specific in their binding to antigen and, once developed, provide a virtually inexhaustible supply of the same material for test consistency.

The downside to antigen detection tests is that many antigens are altered or masked by tissue fixation. Furthermore, they are agent specific, thus a test for canine parvovirus cannot detect the presence of canine coronavirus in the specimen, which would require a separate and additional agent-specific test.

Immunofluorescence Staining

Immunofluorescence or fluorescent antibody staining is an antigen-detection test that is used primarily on frozen tissue sections, cell "smears," or cultured cells; formalin-fixed tissue samples are generally not useful with this procedure. Antigen is detected through the binding to the sample matrix of specially modified, agent-specific antibodies. The modification is the "tagging" of the antibody with a fluorochrome that absorbs ultraviolet light of a defined wavelength, but emits light at a higher wavelength. The emitted light is detected optically with a special microscope equipped with filters specific for the emission wavelength of the fluorochrome. The fluorochrome can be bound directly to the agent-specific antibody (direct immunofluorescence) or it can be attached to an anti-immunoglobulin molecule that recognizes the agent-specific antibody (indirect immunofluorescence) (Figure 5.3A). The indirect method enhances the sensitivity of the test, but may also increase background.

Immunofluorescence staining does require specialized equipment, including a cryostat for sectioning frozen tissue along with a fluorescent microscope for detecting the bound antibody. Immunofluorescence has proven to be of

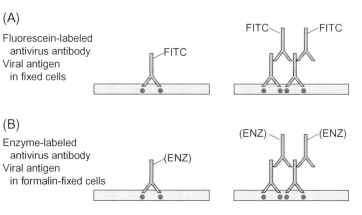

(A)

Fluorescein-labeled antivirus antibody
Viral antigen in fixed cells

FITC

FITC — FITC

Fluorescein-labeled goat anti-rabbit antibody
Antivirus antibody (rabbit)
Viral antigen in fixed cells

(B)

Enzyme-labeled antivirus antibody
Viral antigen in formalin-fixed cells

(ENZ)

(ENZ) — (ENZ)

Enzyme-labeled goat anti-rabbit antibody
Antivirus antibody (rabbit)
Viral antigen in formalin-fixed cells

FIGURE 5.3 (A) Immunofluorescence. Left: Direct method. Right: Indirect method. (B) Immunohistochemistry. Left: Direct method. Right: Indirect method.

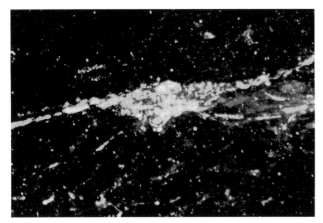

FIGURE 5.4 Direct fluorescent antibody stain of brain tissue for rabies virus. Frozen tissue sections from the brain of a bovine showing abnormal neurological signs were fixed in cold acetone and stained with a commercial reagent containing three monoclonal antibodies specific for the nucleocapsid of rabies virus. Antibodies were labeled with fluorescein. Positive staining is noted in a Perkinje cell. (*Courtesy of J. Galligan, New York State Department of Health.*)

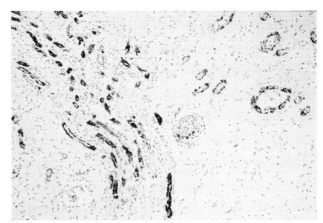

FIGURE 5.5 Immunohistochemical staining of bovine viral diarrhea virus (BVDV)-infected tissue. A formalin-fixed kidney specimen from an acutely ill calf was reacted with monoclonal antibody 15.c.5. Binding was detected using goat-antimouse serum tagged with horseradish peroxidase. Substrate for the enzyme was 3-amino-9-ethyl carbazole. Dark staining cells are positive for BVDV antigen.

great value in the identification of viral antigens in infected cells taken from animals or in cultured cells inoculated with specimens from infected animals. For certain viral diseases, specimens that include virus-infected cells can easily be collected from the mucous membrane of the upper respiratory tract, genital tract, eye, or skin, simply by swabbing or scraping the infected area with reasonable firmness. Cells are also present in mucus aspirated from the nasopharynx or in fluids from other sites, including tracheal and bronchial lavages, or pleural, abdominal, or cerebrospinal fluids. Respiratory infections with parainfluenzaviruses, orthomyxoviruses, adenoviruses, and herpesviruses are particularly amenable to rapid diagnosis (less than 3 hours test time) by immunofluorescence staining. The method can also be applied to tissue—for example, biopsies for the diagnosis of herpesvirus diseases, or at necropsy on brain tissue from a raccoon showing neurological signs as a result of infection with canine distemper virus or rabies virus (Figure 5.4).

Immunohistochemical (Immunoperoxidase) Staining

In principle, immunohistochemical staining is very similar to immunofluorescence staining of viral antigens, but with several key differences (Figure 5.3B). The "tag" used in immunohistochemical staining is an enzyme, generally horseradish peroxidase. The enzyme reacts with a substrate to produce a colored product that can be visualized in the infected cells with a standard light microscope. The tissue sample will often be formalin fixed, which permits testing of the specimen days to weeks after sampling, without the need for low-temperature storage. Another major advantage

for the immunohistochemical staining technique is that it involves an amplification process wherein the product of the reaction increases with increasing incubation, whereas immunofluorescence staining generates a real-time signal that does not get stronger with a longer incubation period. Furthermore, immunohistochemically stained slides can be kept for extended periods of time for several observations, whereas the immunofluorescence slides deteriorate more rapidly. Immunofluorescence does have the advantage of speed; immunohistochemical staining on formalin-fixed tissues requires more than 24 hours to give results. Perhaps the greatest benefit of immunohistochemical staining is that it readily facilitates comparison of virus distribution and cellular localization in tissue sections to determine whether or not viral antigen distribution coincides with that of any lesions that are present (Figure 5.5).

Enzyme Immunoassay—Enzyme-Linked Immunosorbent Assay

Enzyme immunoassays (EIAs)—often referred to as enzyme-linked immunosorbent assays (ELISAs)—have revolutionized diagnostic testing procedures. Assays can be designed to detect antigens or antibodies. Although EIAs have high relative sensitivity, samples may still require more than 10^5 virus particles/ml for positive reactions with many tests. This level of sensitivity still makes these tests highly valuable, particularly in group settings, where any positive animal defines the herd status. Assays may be conducted on a single sample in the veterinarian's clinic or on many hundred samples at the same time, using automated systems in centralized laboratories. Some commonly used antigen detection test kits include those specific for feline leukemia virus, canine parvovirus, bovine viral diarrhea

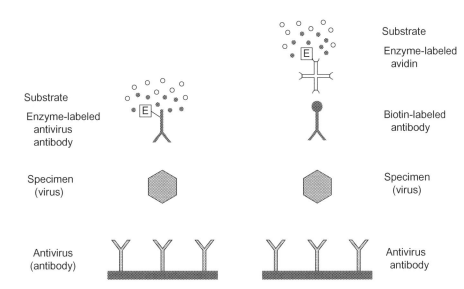

FIGURE 5.6 Enzyme immunoassay (EIA, also called enzyme-linked immunosorbent assay—ELISA) for the detection of virus and/or viral antigen. Left: Direct method. Right: Indirect method using biotinylated antibody, enzyme (e.g., peroxidase)-labeled avidin, and an enzyme substrate and chromogen for color reaction.

virus, rotavirus, and influenza virus. There are many different types of EIA tests that differ in their geometric properties, detector systems, amplification systems and sensitivity. Not all possible tests will be discussed, as the basic test principles apply to all.

Most EIAs are solid-phase enzyme immunoassays; the "capture" antibody is attached to a solid substrate, typically the wells of polystyrene or polyvinyl microtiter plates. The simplest format is a direct EIA (Figure 5.6). Virus and/or soluble viral antigens from the specimen are allowed to bind to the capture antibody. After unbound components are washed away, an enzyme-labeled antiviral antibody (the "detector" antibody) is added; various enzymes can be linked to the antibody, but horseradish peroxidase and alkaline phosphatase are the most commonly used. After a washing step, an appropriate organic substrate for the particular enzyme is added and readout is based on the color change that follows. The colored product of the reaction of the enzyme on the substrate can be detected visually or read by a spectrophotometer to measure the amount of enzyme-conjugated antibody bound to the captured antigen. The product of the enzyme reactions can be modified to produce a fluorescent or chemiluminescent signal to enhance sensitivity. With all such assays, extensive validation testing must be carried out to determine the cut-off values of the test, which define the diagnostic sensitivity and diagnostic specificity of the test.

Indirect EIAs are widely used because of their greater analytical sensitivity, but the increase in sensitivity is usually accompanied by a loss of specificity. In this test format, the detector antibody is unlabeled and a second labeled (species-specific) anti-immunoglobulin is added as the "indicator" antibody (Figure 5.6). Alternatively, labeled staphylococcal protein A, which binds to the Fc moiety of IgG of many mammalian species, can be used as the indicator in indirect immunoassays. Monoclonal antibodies

have especially facilitated the development of EIA tests, because they provide a consistent supply of highly sensitive and specific reagents for commercial tests. However, any variation (antigenic variation of the virus target) in the specific epitopes recognized by specific monoclonal antibodies can lead to loss of binding and loss of test sensitivity because of false-negative results.

EIAs have been adapted to formats for use in veterinary clinics on single animal specimens (Figure 5.7).

Immunochromatography

Immunochromatography simply refers to the migration of antigen or antigen–antibody complexes through a filter matrix or in a lateral flow format—for example, using nitrocellulose strips. In most formats, a labeled antibody binds to the antigen of interest. The antigen–antibody complexes are then immobilized in the support matrix by an unlabeled antibody bound to the matrix. All controls are included in the membrane as well, and results are seen as colored spots or bands, as one of the test reagents is conjugated to colloidal gold or a chromogenic substance. This test format is especially convenient for point-of-care testing, as the test process is simple and each test unit contains both positive and negative controls to assess test validity.

Detection of Viral Nucleic Acids

Developments in the area of nucleic acid technology in the past few years have relegated some (earlier) techniques to the annals of history with respect to their use in diagnostic testing. For example, classic hybridization techniques are not typically amenable to use for routine testing, especially with the requirement for rigorous quality-control standards. The most dramatic changes in nucleic acid detection

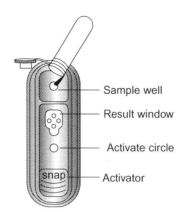

Sample well
Result window
Activate circle
Activator

Interpreting test result

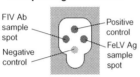

FIV Ab sample spot

Positive control

Negative control

FeLV Ag sample spot

To determine test result, read the reaction spots in the result window. Color development in sample spots is proportional to the concentration of FeLV antigen or FIV antibody in the sample. If no color develops in the positive control spot, repeat the test.

Negative result

Only positive control spot develops color.

Positive result

FeLV Antigen   **FeLV antigen and FIV antibody**   **FIV antibody**

1)   2)    3)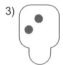

Positive control spot and FeLV Ag sample spot develop color.

Positive control spot and both sample spots develop color.

Positive control spot and FIV Ab sample spot develop color.

Reaction with negative control

The negative control spot serves as a safeguard against false positives.

1)

Positive result
If color in the FIV Ab or FeLV Ag sample spot is darker than negative control spot, result is positive for that spot.

2)

Invalid result
If color in the negative control spot is equal to or darker than FIV Ab or FeLV Ag sample spot, the test is invalid for that sample spot.

Invalid results

1. Background
If the sample is allowed to flow past the activate circle, background color may result. Some background color is normal. However, if colored background obscures test result, repeat the test.

2. No color development
If positive control does not develop color, repeat the test.

FIGURE 5.7 Commercial enzyme immunoassay device for clinical use on a single animal. This kit is for the simultaneous detection of feline leukemia virus (FeLV) antigen (Ag) and feline immunodeficiency virus (FIV) antibody (Ab) in feline serum, plasma, or whole blood. The detection of FeLV group-specific antigen is diagnostic of FeLV infection, and the detection of specific antibody to FIV is indicative of infection. The test utilizes a monoclonal antibody to FeLV p27, inactivated FIV antigen, and positive and negative controls. A conjugate mixture contains enzyme-conjugated antibody to p27 and enzyme-conjugated antigen. When the conjugate and the test sample are mixed, conjugated monoclonal antibody will bind to p27 antigen (if present). The sample–conjugate mixture is then added to the "Snap" device and flows across the spotted matrix. The matrix-bound p27 antibody (FeLV spot) will capture the p27-conjugated antibody complex, whereas the matrix-bound FIV antigen (FIV spot) will capture the FIV antibody-conjugated antigen complex. The device is then activated (snapped), releasing wash, and substrate reagents stored within the device. Color development in the FeLV antigen sample spot indicates the presence of FeLV antigen, whereas color development in the FIV antibody sample spot indicates the presence of FIV antibody. (*Courtesy of Idexx Laboratories, Inc.*)

technology have been in the evolution of *polymerase chain reaction* (PCR) testing, and the equally important standardization of nucleic acid extraction procedures. In addition, the rapid advances in nucleotide sequencing technology, oligonucleotide synthesis, and development of genetic databases permit inexpensive sequence analysis that has replaced less rigorous procedures for comparing genetic changes in virus strains and isolates. Current technology permits PCR amplification of virus "populations" with direct sequencing of the amplified products from the clinical specimen without the potential introduction of cell culture selection bias. More recent developments permit the detection and characterization of unknown agents (viral metagenomics). With the developments in nanotechnology, one could anticipate the future advent of inexpensive nucleic acid detection units that could reliably detect infectious agents when used in the clinician's office or in the field, without the need for highly trained personnel.

Nucleic acid detection methods are invaluable when dealing with: (1) viruses that cannot be cultured readily; (2) specimens that contain inactivated virus as a result of prolonged storage, fixation of tissue, or transport; (3) latent infections in which the viral genome lies dormant and infectious virus is absent; (4) virus complexed with antibody as would be found in the later stages of an acute infection or during some persistent viral infections. However, the added sensitivity provided by amplification of viral nucleic acid can actually create new problems. Unlike the situation with bacterial pathogens, it has usually been the case that merely detecting a pathogenic virus in a lesion, or from a clinically ill animal, has been considered evidence of its etiologic role (causal relationship). As detection methods have become increasingly sensitive and testing includes more agents, questions of viral "passengers" become more pertinent. Indeed, with viruses such as bluetongue virus, viral nucleic acid can be detected in the blood of previously infected ruminants several months after infectious virus has been cleared. Furthermore, with bovine herpesvirus 1 as an example, detection of viral nucleic acid does not address whether it is present as a consequence of acute infection, reactivation of a latent infection, or vaccination.

Polymerase Chain Reaction

The PCR assay is an *in-vitro* method for the enzymatic synthesis of specific DNA sequences using two oligonucleotide primers, usually of about 20 residues (20-mers), that hybridize to opposite strands and flank the region of interest in the target DNA; the primer pairs are sometimes referred to as forward and reverse primers (Figure 5.8). Primers are necessary to provide the DNA polymerase with a substrate upon which to add new nucleotides, and to direct the reaction to the specific region of the DNA for amplification. Primers can also be designed to provide "tags" on the amplified

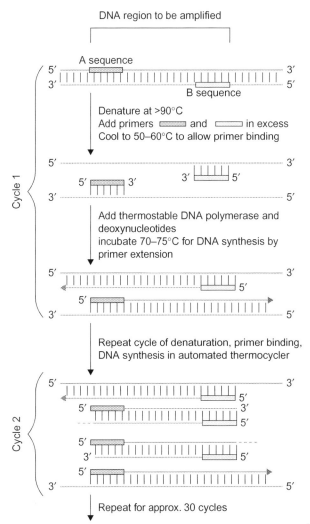

FIGURE 5.8 Amplification of part of a DNA sequence by the polymerase chain reaction. Oligonucleotide primers must first be made according to the sequences of either end of the portion of DNA to be amplified. After the DNA has been denatured by heating, the primers can hybridize to the complementary sequences on the opposite strand. In the presence of heat-resistant DNA polymerase and deoxynucleotide triphosphates, two new copies of the desired region are produced. The cycles of melting, annealing, and extension are repeated rapidly; each time, the amount of target DNA sequence doubles. After the first few cycles, virtually all the templates consist of just the short region chosen for amplification. After 30 cycles, taking about 3 hours, this region bounded by the chosen primers has been amplified many millionfold. (*Courtesy of I. H. Holmes and R. Strugnell.*)

products for purposes of detection. Computer programs are used for the design of optimum primer sets and to predict the parameters (time/temperature) for the reactions. Where there are either known mismatched bases or anticipated mismatches between the primer and target sequences, the primers can be made to be degenerate—sets of primers with different bases at a given location. This can increase the diagnostic sensitivity of the test, as more genetic variants can be detected. For PCR, reactions are carried out in a thermocycler under carefully controlled conditions of ionic strength, temperature, primer concentration, and nucleotide concentration. Repetitive cycles involving template denaturation by heating, primer annealing, and extension of the annealed primers by DNA polymerase result in the exponential accumulation of a specific DNA fragment the termini of which are defined by the 5′ ends of the primers. The primer extension products synthesized in one cycle serve as templates in the next, hence the number of target DNA copies approximately doubles every cycle; 20 cycles yields about a millionfold amplification.

Since the introduction of the concept of PCR in 1983, there have been numerous changes to virtually every facet of the process. Incorporation of a thermostable DNA polymerase permitted high temperature denaturation and strand separation of the synthesized products, which eliminated the need to replenish the polymerase at each cycle. The use of a thermostable polymerase also increased the specificity of the reaction, as cycling could be done under more stringent annealing conditions; specifically, higher annealing temperatures reduce mismatch base pairing which can lead to false-positive results. In order to increase the sensitivity of the test, a "nested" PCR procedure was developed. In this procedure, one set of primers was used to do an initial amplification of a target area and the product of the first reaction became the template for a second PCR test in which new primers targeted a region internal to the first set of primers. This amplification of amplified product greatly increased the sensitivity of the test, but greatly increased the chances for false-positive results through contamination of test materials by the initial amplified product. Further developments in quantitative PCR technology have markedly reduced the use of nested procedures.

The development of reverse transcriptase polymerase chain reaction (RT-PCR) methods to detect RNA sequences was a major advance in cell biology and viral diagnostics. For RT-PCR, the RNA is first transcribed into cDNA using a DNA polymerase capable of using RNA as a template, such as retrovirus reverse transcriptase. Newer reverse transcriptase enzymes have been developed that permit synthesis of the cDNA strand at higher temperatures, which increases the analytical sensitivity and specificity of the reaction. In single-tube RT-PCR tests, all components for both reactions are placed in the reaction tube at the onset of the testing. The cDNA synthesis step is followed immediately by the PCR reaction. In this test format, there is no opportunity for products of one reaction to cross contaminate another, because the reaction tube is never opened until the end of the testing protocol. Advances such as the single-tube test greatly increased the reliability of PCR test results by virtually eliminating laboratory contamination problems.

Methods for Detection of Amplified Products

In the initial era of PCR testing, the amplified products were detected by analyzing the reaction products by gel separation. Amplified products of a defined sized were visualized by using fluorescent dyes that bound to the oligonucleotides separated in agarose gels. A "band" at the appropriate size was taken as a positive test for the presence of an agent in a sample. Methods were developed to increase the sensitivity of detecting bands in the gels, but even with enhanced sensitivity, this detection procedure had one major flaw—the reaction tube had to be opened in order to assess the status of the sample. Many laboratory areas became contaminated with the amplified reaction products, with false-positive results frequently obtained from subsequent samples run in the facility. Heroic efforts were made to avoid the false-positive problem, but suspicion of positive test results became prevalent and still linger. Fortunately, technology provided an answer that has come to dominate PCR testing: *real-time PCR* testing (Figure 5.9). This major technology advance was facilitated by the development of a thermocycler with a fluorimeter that could accurately measure (quantify) the accumulation of PCR product (amplicons) in the reaction tube as it was being made—that is, in real-time. Product is measured by increases in fluorescence intensity generated by several different fluorescent reporter molecules, including non-specific DNA binding dyes (SYBR Green I), TaqMan® probes (Figure 5.9A), and molecular beacons as examples. Once reactants are added to the reaction tubes, the tubes need never to be opened again, thus preventing any opportunity for laboratory contamination. The real-time detection systems are also more sensitive than standard gel systems, and added assay specificity is achieved through the use of reaction detection probes, because signal is generated only if the probe sequence is also able to bind to the target sequence.

Another advantage of the real-time system is that the process can be quantitative. Under optimum conditions, the amount of the amplicon increases by a factor of 10 with each 3.3 amplification cycle (Figure 5.9B). With real-time systems, the generation of product is recorded at each cycle. The amount of product generated in a test reaction can be compared with a copy number control and, with proper extraction controls in the system, a direct measure of the amount of starting sequence can be determined. In humans, for example, this feature has particular value in monitoring responses over time to drug treatments for infections with hepatitis C and human immunodeficiency viruses.

A further variation in PCR testing that is becoming more commonly used is multiplex PCR. In this method, two or more primer pairs specific for different target sequences are included in the same amplification reaction. In this manner, testing can be done for several agents at the same time and in the same assay tube, thereby saving time and costs. With real-time, multiplex PCR assays, several probes with different fluorescent molecules can be detected simultaneously. This type of application is useful in evaluation of samples from disease complexes, such as acute respiratory disease in dogs. Issues of test sensitivity

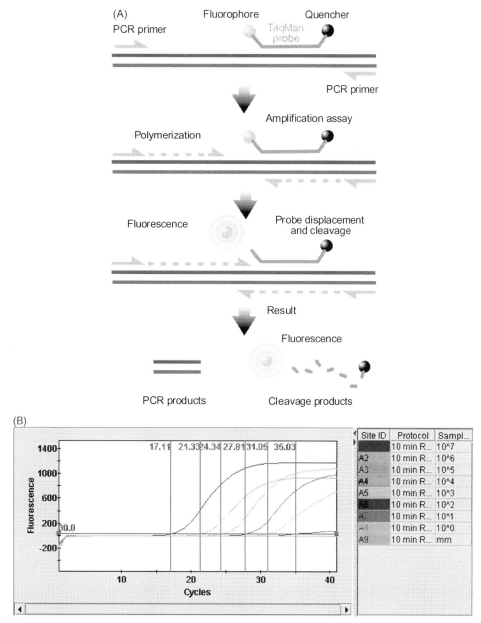

FIGURE 5.9 (A) TaqMan® probe chemistry mechanism. These probes rely on the 5′-3′ nuclease activity of Taq DNA polymerase to cleave a dual-labeled probe during hybridization to the complementary target sequence. (B) Real-time quantitative PCR data. Reaction curves for a test run to assess assay conditions using dilutions of an RNA transcript (copy number control) of a cloned segment of canine pneumovirus. The vertical lines represent the Ct value, which is the number of PCR cycles required for the fluorescent signal to cross the threshold value. TaqMan© probe was labeled with FAM (6-carboxy fluorescein; the reporter dye) at the 5′ end and BHQ (Black Hole Quencher; the quencher) at the 3′ end.

must be addressed in this format, because several reactions must compete for common reagents in the reaction, thus an agent in high copy number might mask the presence of one at low copy number.

Advantages and Limitations of the Polymerase Chain Reaction Technology

Given the explosion in use and availability of PCR assays in virological testing, consideration should be given to the potential benefits and limitations of these assays. The PCR assay is especially useful in the detection of viruses that are difficult to grow in culture, such as certain enteric adenoviruses, papillomaviruses, astroviruses, coronaviruses, noroviruses, and rotaviruses. PCR can be used on any sample that is appropriate for virus isolation; the decision to do PCR as opposed to other virus detection tests is based on speed, cost, and laboratory capability. PCR tests also may be preferred for the initial identification of zoonotic viruses such as rabies virus, certain poxviruses, or influenza viruses, to minimize the risk of exposure for laboratory personnel as amplification of infectious virus is not necessary for detection.

A limitation of PCR or any nucleic acid amplification technique can be the matrix in which the target sample is embedded. Material in the sample matrix can inhibit the enzymes on which the assay is based, which has been a constant source of concern when dealing with fecal samples and, to some extent, milk samples. Extraction controls need to be included in these types of sample in order to detect problems with the amplification process itself (rather than lack of specific template). Furthermore, PCR and simple nucleic acid amplification tests are agent specific, thus no signal will be generated if the primers do not match the sequence of any virus contained in the sample. With earlier direct PCR assays, and especially with nested PCR assays, false-positive test results were a very significant concern as a result of the ease of laboratory contamination with amplified product. With the availability of single-tube real-time PCR testing formats and real-time PCR tests, this problem has largely been eliminated, although correct performance of PCR assays remains a technically challenging process. Performance of real-time PCR assays is being continually improved with standardized reagent kits, robust instrumentation, standardized extraction protocols, and defined laboratory operating procedures, and this nucleic acid detection test format has become the mainstay of testing laboratories. However, test interpretation still requires evaluation of whether or not a particular test result (either positive or negative) is biologically relevant, which in turn requires a global assessment of history, clinical signs, and lesions in the particular animal from which the sample was obtained.

Microarray (Microchip) Techniques

Another technological advance that is impacting the field of diagnostics is the advent of *microarrays* or *microchips*. The microchip for nucleic acid detection is a solid support matrix onto which have been "printed" spots, each containing one of several hundred to several thousand oligonucleotides. Increasingly, these oligonucleotides can represent conserved sequences from virtually all viruses represented in the various genetic databases, or can be customized to represent only viruses from a given species involved in a specific disease syndrome, such as acute respiratory disease in cattle. The basis of the test is the capture by these oligonucleotides of randomly amplified labeled nucleic acid sequences from clinical specimens. The binding of a labeled sequence is detected by laser scanning of the chip and software programs assess the strength of the binding. From the map position of the reacting oligonucleotides, the software identifies the species of virus in the clinical sample. This type of test was used to determine that the virus responsible for severe acute respiratory syndrome (SARS) was a coronavirus. With knowledge of the oligonucleotide sequences that bound the unknown agent, primers can be made to eventually determine the entire nucleotide sequence

of a new species of virus. The low cost of oligonucleotides synthesis, development of laser scanning devices, nucleic acid amplification techniques, and software development have made this technology available in specialized laboratories. A variation of this technique is the re-sequencing microarray. These arrays consist of a set of overlapping probes, which may differ from each other at a single base. The strength of binding to the individual probes in the family provides information on the genetic sequence of the amplified product. With current technology, the microarray approach is only available in specialized reference laboratories and it would not be used for routine diagnostic testing. In the standard format, this technique would probably not detect a new virus family not represented in a current database, because oligonucleotides for the new agent would not be included on the microchip.

Gene Amplification by Isothermal Amplification

For nucleic acid amplification, it is necessary to continually displace the newly synthesized product so that another copy of the sequence can be made. With PCR, the strand displacement is achieved with temperature: the 95°C temperature maximum melts (separates) the DNA strands, permitting binding of new primers. Isothermal amplification is a technique that does not require the temperature cycling and accompanying equipment used in PCR. Two techniques using different polymerases to achieve sequence amplification have been developed for isothermal amplification: nucleic acid sequence-based amplification (NASBA) and loop-mediated isothermal amplification (LAMP). If these techniques show significant advantages over PCR, one would expect the availability of an expanding array of available tests.

NUCLEIC ACID (VIRAL GENOMIC) SEQUENCING

Perhaps no area in molecular biology has advanced so rapidly as nucleic acid sequencing. With speed and capacity has come low cost, so that direct sequencing of complete viral genomes is now commonplace. Older techniques such as restriction mapping and oligonucleotide fingerprinting that were used to detect genetic differences among virus isolates have been displaced by sequencing methodology. In the area of diagnostics, new viruses are being discovered by techniques that take advantage of random nucleic acid amplification and low-cost sequencing. There are several basic techniques with numerous modifications that are too detailed to discuss individually. In general, the process involves random amplification of enriched nucleic acid samples or total nucleic acid samples, followed by sequencing of all the amplified products. The process works best if host-cell nucleic acids can be eliminated from the samples by nuclease treatment or subtraction of host sequences by hybridization to normal cell sequences immobilized on solid supports. No prior knowledge of the viral sequence is needed, and there is no need for any virus-specific reagents. Computer analysis of the sequenced material can identify sequences that are closely or distantly related to those of specific virus families. The method used to construct the entire genome, if this is desired, is somewhat dependent upon the number and size of sequences identified, but methods are available to "walk" down the entire genome from a single viral sequence. With these types of nucleic acid detection protocols, unknown viruses can be discovered and characterized without the requirement that they first be propagated in cell culture.

DETECTION AND QUANTITATION OF VIRUS-SPECIFIC ANTIBODIES (SEROLOGIC DIAGNOSIS)

The detection of an immune response to an infectious agent has, for the most part, relied on determining the antibody response of the host to the agent of interest. This approach measures only one limb of the adaptive immune response (humoral immunity); techniques for reliably measuring the cell-mediated responses have not been routinely available or cost effective. For many situations, measurement of antibody responses remains a valuable technique for defining the infection status of animals. Serological tests can be used to: (1) define whether an animal has ever been infected by a particular virus; (2) determine if a specific virus (or other pathogen) is linked to a clinical event; (3) determine if an animal has responded to a vaccination. For the serologic diagnosis of an acute viral disease in an individual animal, the classic approach has been to test paired sera—that is, an acute and a convalescent serum from the same animal, for a change in titer (fourfold or greater) of virus-specific antibody. The acute-phase serum sample is taken as early as possible in the illness; the convalescent-phase sample usually at least 2 weeks later. Given this time line, diagnosis based on this approach is said to be "retrospective." In recent years this approach has been complemented by serologic methods for detecting virus-specific IgM antibodies—in many viral diseases a presumptive diagnosis may be made on the basis of detecting IgM antibody in a single acute-phase serum specimen—for example, West Nile virus infection of horses.

To assess whether an animal has ever been infected with certain viruses, serological testing can be more reliable than trying to detect the virus itself. For example, serological testing is used to screen horses for exposure to equine infectious anemia virus, cattle for bovine leukemia virus, and goats for caprine arthritis encephalitis virus. In these instances, the number of infected cells in chronically infected animals may be too low for even PCR detection, but infection generally stimulates an antibody response that is readily detected by various tests. Serological testing is also widely used both during virus eradication programs and in the certification of animals for movement and trade.

Use of serological tests to assess vaccine efficacy can be an important aspect of an infectious disease management program. In many countries, purchase of vaccine can be done by the animal owner. Antibody testing of selected animals can provide the practitioner with valuable insight as to whether the immunization program of the producer is being performed correctly. As eradication programs expand for diseases of production animals, marker vaccines are more frequently being used and so-called DIVA serological assays can distinguish whether a given antibody response is caused by vaccine or natural infection. For herpesvirus infections such as bovine herpesvirus 1, it is essential to determine whether an antibody response is the result of infection, because infection invariably leads to latency. Movement of a latently infected animal into a negative herd can result in an outbreak of disease, thus gene deletion "marker" vaccines were developed to facilitate differentiation of vaccinated and naturally infected cattle.

Serum Specimens for Serologic Assays

For most serological tests, serum is the sample of choice. However, some tests have been validated using plasma as well as serum. Communication with the testing laboratory is necessary when fluids other than serum are being collected, in order to avoid having to re-sample the animal when serum is the only acceptable test material. Antibodies in serum are very stable to moderate environmental conditions. Standard protocols call for serum to be kept cold, but freezing of the sample is not necessary unless several weeks will elapse between collection and testing. Antibodies can even be detected from blood samples dried onto filter paper and stored for months before testing.

As with other aspects of diagnostic testing, technological advances continue to modify how antibodies to specific viruses are detected. In most cases, the newer technologies are applied to those tests that have some commercial potential. In veterinary medicine, there are many tests for agents that may be of minor importance but useful in certain situations. Tests available for these agents may be the first ones developed with older testing technology. As viruses of wildlife species assume greater importance through public awareness, it will be necessary to develop additional serological tests, because species-specific tests for domestic species cannot be used. All serological test types will not be discussed in detail (below), but readers should be aware that other test formats may become available and continuing communication with their testing laboratory is the most efficient way to learn about the tests available for each species and for each virus.

Enzyme Immunoassay—Enzyme-Linked Immunosorbent Assay

Enzyme immunoassays (EIAs, ELISA) are the serologic assays of choice for the qualitative (positive or negative) or quantitative determination of viral antibodies because they are rapid, relatively cost effective, and may not require the production of infectious virus for antigen if recombinant antigens are used. In the EIA test format for antibody detection, viral antigen is bound to a solid matrix. Serum is added and, if antibodies to the antigen are present in the sample, they bind to it. In direct EIA tests, the bound antibody is detected by an anti-species antibody tagged with an enzyme. With addition of the enzyme substrate, a color reaction develops that can be assessed either visually or with a spectrophotometer. Controls run with the sample define whether the test is acceptable and which samples in the test are positive. Kinetics-based EIAs offer the advantage that quantitative assays can be based on a single dilution of serum. The product of the enzyme reaction is determined several times over a short interval. Software programs convert the rate of product development to the amount of antibody bound to the antigen.

A disadvantage of direct EIA tests is that they are species specific. A test developed for canine distemper virus antibodies in a dog cannot be used to determine the presence or absence of antibodies to the same virus in a lion. To obviate this problem, competitive or blocking EIA tests have been developed. In this test format, an antibody that binds to the antigen of interest (usually a monoclonal antibody) is tagged with the enzyme. Unlabeled antibody that can bind to the same site as the monoclonal antibody will compete with the labeled monoclonal antibody for that site. A reduction in the binding of the labeled monoclonal antibody indicates that the sample did contain antibody (Figure 5.10). In this test format, the species of the unlabeled antibody is not a factor. The diagnostic sensitivity and specificity of EIA tests, whether direct or indirect, have been greatly enhanced by the development of monoclonal antibodies and the production of recombinant antigens.

In a widely used format for test kits that can be run in a practitioner's office, the test serum flows through a membrane filter that has three circular areas impregnated with antigen, two of which have already interacted with a positive and a negative serum, respectively (Figure 5.7). After the test serum flows through the membrane and a washing step is completed, a second anti-species antibody with an enzyme linked to it is added and the membrane is again rinsed before the addition of the enzyme substrate. The result is read as a color change in the test sample circle, which is compared against the color change in the positive control and no change in the negative control. Such single-patient tests are relatively expensive compared with the economies of testing hundreds of sera in a single run

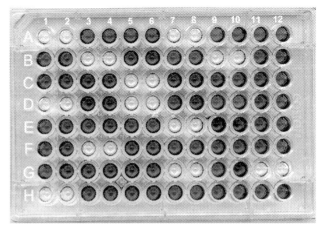

FIGURE 5.10 Competitive enzyme-linked immunosorbent assay (cELISA) for caprine arthritis encephalitis viral (CAEV) antibodies. Undiluted serum samples in duplicate are added to antigen-coated wells of a commercial cELISA test for CAEV antibodies. After removal of the test sera, an antibody specific for CAEV antigen and coupled to horseradish peroxidase is added. The detector antibody is removed after incubation, and a substrate is added to detect the presence of bound detector antibody. If there are antibodies specific for CAEV in the test sera, these antibodies bound to antigen will prevent the detector antibody from binding. A positive sample will therefore show less enzyme product (color) than the negative controls. Cut-off values are determined by reading the intensity of the reaction with a spectrophotometer, although visual inspection can usually detect positive samples. Wells A1–2 and G11–12: positive controls; wells B1–2 and H11–12: negative controls; wells D1–2, H1–2, B3–4, F3–4, C5–6, D5–6, A7–8, E7–8, G7–8, and B9–10: samples positive for antibodies to CAEV.

in a fully automated laboratory. The great savings in time and effort to send samples to the laboratory, in addition to the fact that decisions can be made while both client and patient are still in the consulting room, make single tests attractive and useful in the immediate clinical management of critically ill animals.

Serum (Virus) Neutralization Assay

As virus isolation is considered the gold standard for the detection of virus against which other assays must be compared, the serum (virus) neutralization test has historically been the gold standard, when available, for the detection and quantitation of virus-specific antibodies. Neutralizing antibody also attracts great interest because it is considered a direct correlate of protective antibody *in vivo*. For the assay of neutralizing antibody, two general procedures are available: the constant-serum–variable-virus method and the constant-virus–variable-serum method. Although the constant-serum–variable-virus method may be a more sensitive assay, it is rarely used because it utilizes relatively large amounts of serum, which may not be readily available. The basis of the neutralization assay is the binding of antibody to infectious virus, thus preventing the virus from initiating an infection in a susceptible cell. The growth of the virus is detected by its ability to kill the cell (cytopathic effect) or by its ability to produce antigen in the infected cells that is detected by immunofluorescence or immunohistochemistry. The amount of antibody in a sample is determined by serial dilution of the sample and "challenging" each of these dilutions with a standard amount of virus (constant-virus–variable-serum method). The last dilution that shows neutralization of the virus is defined as the endpoint and the *titer* of the serum is the reciprocal of the endpoint dilution; for example, an endpoint of 1:160 equates to a titer of 160. The disadvantages of serum neutralization tests are that they are relatively slow to generate a result, require production of infectious virus for the test, and have a constant high overhead cost in maintaining cell culture facilities for the test. These assays have the benefit of being species independent and, as such, are very useful in wildlife studies. With new agents, a serum neutralization test can be operational with several weeks of isolating the virus, whereas EIA test development may take months or even years to validate.

Immunoblotting (Western Blotting)

Western blotting tests simultaneously but independently measure antibodies against several proteins of the agent of interest. There are four key steps to western blotting. First, concentrated virus is solubilized and the constituent proteins are separated into discrete bands according to their molecular mass (M_r), by sodium dodecyl sulfate–polyacrylamide gel electrophoresis (SDS-PAGE). Secondly, the separated proteins are transferred electrophoretically ("blotted") onto nitrocellulose to immobilize them. Thirdly, the test serum is allowed to bind to the viral proteins on the membrane. Fourthly, their presence is demonstrated using a radio-labeled or, most commonly, an enzyme-labeled anti-species antibody. Thus immunoblotting permits demonstration of antibodies to some or all of the proteins of any given virus, and can be used to monitor the presence of antibodies to different antigens at different stages of infection. Although this procedure is not routinely used in a diagnostic setting with viruses, western blots were central to the identification of immunogenic proteins in a variety of viruses. Similarly, the assay is used in the analysis of samples for the presence of prion proteins in ruminant tissues. Western blots are more of a qualitative test than a quantitative one, and are not easily standardized from laboratory to laboratory. For this reason, ELISAs and bead-based assays are preferred test formats.

Indirect Immunofluorescence Assay

Indirect immunofluorescence assays are used for the detection and quantitation of antibody; specifically, these are tests that use virus-infected cells (usually on glass microscope slides) as a matrix to capture antibodies specific for that virus. Serial dilutions of test serum are applied to individual wells of the cell substrate and usually an anti-species antibody with a fluorescent tag is then added as the detector of antibody binding. Slides are read with a fluorescent microscope and scored as positive if the infected cell shows a fluorescent pattern consistent with the antigen distribution of the virus used. This test is rapid (less than 2 hours) and can be used to determine the isotype of the reacting antibody if one uses an anti-isotype-specific serum such as an anti-canine IgM. Non-specific fluorescence can be an issue, particularly with animals that have been heavily vaccinated as they may contain anti-cell antibodies that will bind to uninfected cells and mask specific anti-virus fluorescence. Test slides for some agents can be purchased, so that laboratories offering this test need not have infectious virus or a cell culture facility.

Hemagglutination-Inhibition Assay

For those viruses that hemagglutinate red blood cells of one or another species, such as many of the arthropod-borne viruses, influenza viruses, and parainfluenza viruses, *hemagglutination-inhibition assays* have been widely used. For detecting and quantitating antibodies in the serum of animals, the methods are sensitive, specific, simple, reliable, and quite inexpensive. In spite of all of the technological advances, hemagglutination inhibition assays remain the mainstay for determining antibody responses to specific influenza A viruses. The principle of the assay is simple—virus binds to red blood cells through receptors on their surface. Antiviral antibodies bind to these receptors and block hemagglutination. Serum is diluted serially in the wells of the microtiter plate, usually in twofold steps, and to each well a constant amount of virus, usually four or eight hemagglutinating units, is added. The reciprocal of the highest dilution of serum that inhibits the agglutination of the red blood cells by the standardized amount of virus represents the hemagglutination-inhibition titer of the serum (Figure 5.11). Care should be taken in interpreting many prior sero-surveys based on results of hemagglutination inhibition tests, particularly for paramyxoviruses, as non-specific inhibitors of agglutination produced many false-positive test results in some of those studies.

Immunodiffusion

Historically, agar gel immunodiffusion (AGID) assays were used for the specific diagnosis of a number of viral infections and diseases, including bluetongue, hog cholera, influenza, equine infectious anemia (Coggins test), and bovine leukemia. These assays are very simple to perform, they utilize inexpensive materials, and they do not require

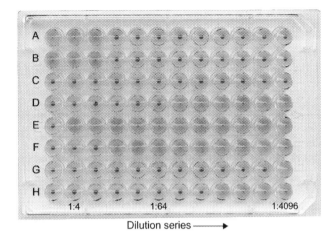

Dilution series ⟶

FIGURE 5.11 Hemagglutination inhibition (HI) test for detecting antibodies specific for canine influenza virus (H3N8). Sera treated to remove non-specific agglutinins and non-specific inhibitors of agglutination are diluted (twofold) in buffered saline in the wells of a 96-well microtiter plate. Following the dilution operation, an equal volume of canine influenza virus ($\approx$4 hemagglutinin units) is added to each well and the plate incubated for 30 minutes. An equal volume of turkey red blood cells (0.5% suspension) is then added to each well. The HI reactions are determined when the control-cell wells show complete settling (button) of the red blood cells. Rows A, B: titration of viral suspension used in test, showing correct amount of hemagglutinin added to test wells. Row C: red blood cell control. Rows D–H: test canine sera. Wells D–H1: test serum control showing no non-specific agglutination of red blood cells at lowest dilution tested. HI titers are the reciprocal of the last dilution showing inhibition of agglutination by test virus. Row D: HI titer = 64; row E: HI titer <4; row F: HI titer = 8; row G: HI titer = 2048; row H: HI titer = 256.

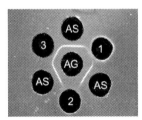

FIGURE 5.12 Agar gel immunodiffusion test for antibody detection for viral agents such as BTV, EIA, EHD, and influenza A viruses. Spatially defined wells are produced in a semi-solid matrix such as agar or agarose. Into the central well is placed the test antigen (AG). Serum containing antibodies (AS) to the virus of interest is placed in alternating wells around the central antigen well. Test sera (1,2,3) are placed in the remaining wells. Plates are incubated for 24–48 hrs to allow the development of visible precipitin lines between the antigen and the test sera. Well 1 = weak positive; well 2 = negative; well 3 = strong positive.

production of infectious material by the testing laboratory. Often crude cell extracts or even tissue extracts from infected animals can be used as the test antigen. AGID tests are relatively fast, easily controlled, but lacked sensitivity as compared with later developed EIA tests. Furthermore, they are strictly qualitative (providing a simple yes/no answer) and cannot be automated (Figure 5.12). Thus most of these tests have been replaced with EIA tests.

IgM Class-Specific Antibody Assay

A rapid antibody-based diagnosis of a viral infection or disease can be made on the basis of a single acute-phase serum by demonstrating virus-specific antibody of the IgM class. Because IgM antibodies appear early after infection but drop to low levels within 1–2 months and generally disappear altogether within 3 months, they are usually indicative of recent (or chronic) infection.

The most common method used is the IgM antibody capture assay, in which the viral antigen is bound on a solid-phase substrate such as a microtiter well. The test serum is allowed to react with this substrate and the IgM antibodies "captured" by the antigen are then detected with labeled anti-IgM antibody matched to the species from which the specimen was obtained.

New Generation Technologies

As with nucleic acid technologies, technological developments for analyte detection are rapidly evolving, and a substantial number of potentially novel platforms for serological assays have been developed that have not yet been fully validated for routine diagnostic use. It is beyond the scope of this text to provide an exhaustive catalog of these technologies, many of which will never find their way into routine diagnostic use. However, one technology that has demonstrated particular promise in both the clinical and research arena is xMAP®, developed by Luminex. The success of this testing platform probably reflects the maturity of existing technologies that were combined to provide a versatile analyte detection system. xMAP® combines a flow cytometry platform, uniquely labeled microspheres, digital signal processing, and standard chemical coupling reactions to provide a system that can be used to detect either proteins or nucleic acids (Figure 5.13). The microspheres carry unique dyes (up to 100 different ones) that emit fluorescent signals that identify the individual beads coupled with a specific ligand. For antibody detection tests, the antigen of interest is coupled to a specific bead. The beads are exposed to the test serum and the bound antibody is detected with an anti-species antibody tagged with a reported dye. The microspheres are analyzed in a flow cytometer in which lasers excite both the bead dyes and the reporter dyes. Multiple beads for each antigen are analyzed in each test, providing independent readings of the reaction.

One distinct advantage of this system is its multiplex capability. Theoretically, 100 or more different antigens can be assessed for antibody reactivity in a single assay. For maximum sensitivity and specificity, recombinant antigens are needed to eliminate extraneous proteins that would reduce specific antigen density on the beads and increase non-specific background reactivity that can confuse test interpretation. Advantages of this bead-based system

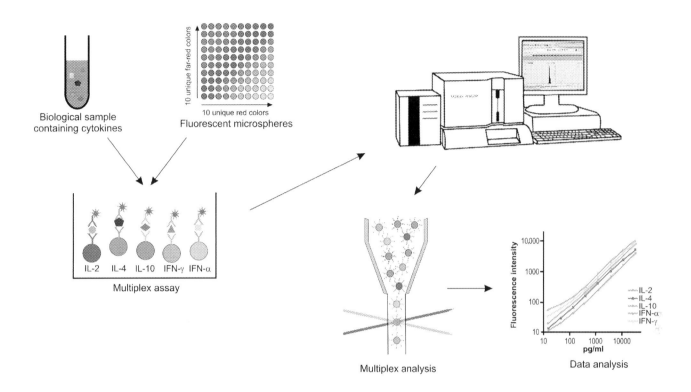

FIGURE 5.13 Multiplex assay for the detection of cytokines. The feasibility of this type of multiplex assay resides in the ability to make microspheres with unique fluorescent signatures and with surface-reactive groups that can be used to bind various ligands. For the cytokine assay, sets of microspheres are individually coated with antibodies specific for cytokines in the screening panel. The microspheres are mixed together and reacted with the test specimen. The binding is detected by anti-cytokine antibodies with a fluorescent tag. The fluorescent signature of the individual microspheres and the fluorescent signal from the bound antibodies are read in a cell-sorting device using lasers for excitation of the dyes. The unique signatures of the microspheres permit a quantitative analysis of up to 100 different reactants in a single specimen. *(Courtesy of B. Wagner, Cornell University.)*

are: (1) it utilizes small sample volumes; (2) it can be multiplexed; (3) it has been reported to be more sensitive than standard ELISA tests; (4) it can be less expensive than many serology tests; (5) it can be more rapid than ELISA tests, particularly when testing for antibodies to several antigens. As an example, this test platform is ideal for the antibody screening tests that are necessary for maintaining research rodent colonies in which antibody responses to several agents are monitored and for which sample volumes are often limiting. This platform can also provide DIVA testing as would be applied for control of important regulatory disease such as foot-and-mouth disease. As an example, recombinant antigens representing the capsid proteins present in inactivated foot-and-mouth disease virus vaccines along with non-structural viral protein can be coupled to different beads to analyze the antibody profile of a suspect animal. In a single assay, the test can provide evidence of vaccination—response to capsid antigen only—or of a natural infection—response to both types of proteins. One could envision this type of bead-based assay

as a quantitative western blot, in that reactivity to several antigens can be assessed. As eradication programs progress for viral diseases of production animals, it is very likely that the requirement for this type of DIVA testing will only increase. The disadvantage for antibody detection is the need for recombinant antigens to achieve acceptable sensitivity, and high validation costs associated with multiplex reactions.

INTERPRETATION OF LABORATORY FINDINGS

As with any laboratory data, the significance of specific results obtained from the virology laboratory must be interpreted in light of the clinical history of the animal from which the sample was collected. To some extent, the significance of any result is also influenced by the type of virus that was detected. A fluorescent-antibody positive test for rabies virus on a bat found in a child's bedroom will elicit a public health response in the absence of clinical data, whereas a positive serological test for bovine leukemia virus from the dam of an aborted fetus is likely to be an irrelevant finding if the animal is from an enzootic region. With multiplex PCR testing, it may be possible to detect several different viruses, bacteria, and mycoplasma species in a single dog with acute respiratory disease, raising the obvious question, "what is significant?" Are the virus signals due to a recent vaccination, reactivation of a herpesvirus, or "footprints" of the etiological agent? Clearly, several sources of data must be integrated by the clinician to arrive at a coherent treatment strategy. However, it is also clear that the speed, the number, and the reliability of virus detection tests have changed the way in which clinicians use laboratory test results, and these results are having greater impact on treatment and management decisions. When attempting to interpret the significance of the detection of a specific virus in a clinical specimen, one may be guided by the following considerations.

The site from which the virus was isolated. For example, one would be quite confident about the etiological significance of equine herpesvirus 1 detected in the tissues of a 9-month-old aborted equine fetus with typical gross and microscopic lesions. However, recovery of an enterovirus from the feces of a young pig may not necessarily be significant, because such viruses are often associated with inapparent infections.

The epidemiologic circumstances under which the virus was isolated. Interpretation of the significance of a virus isolation result is much more meaningful if the same virus is isolated from several cases of the same illness in the same place and time.

The pathogenetic character of the virus detected. Knowledge that the virus detected is nearly always etiologically associated with frank disease—that is, rarely is found as a "passenger"—engenders confidence that the finding is significant.

The identity of the specific virus. The detection of foot-and-mouth disease virus in any ruminant in a virus-free country would, in and of itself, be the cause for great alarm. Similarly, the identification of mouse hepatitis virus in a free colony, or koi herpesvirus amongst highly valuable ornamental fish, would trigger a substantial response.

Interpretation of Serologic Laboratory Findings

A significant (conventionally, fourfold or greater) increase in antibody titer between acute and convalescent samples is the basis, albeit in retrospect, for linking a specific virus with a clinical case of a particular disease. However, one must always be aware of the vaccination status of the animal, as sero-responses to vaccines, especially live-attenuated virus vaccines, may be indistinguishable from those that occur after natural infections. The demonstration of antibody in a single serum sample can be diagnostic of current infection in an unvaccinated animal (e.g., with retroviruses and herpesviruses), because these viruses establish life-long infections. However, in such circumstances there is no assurance that the persistent virus was responsible for the disease under consideration. Assays designed to detect IgM antibody provide evidence of recent or current infection. A summary of the major strengths and limitations of the several alternative approaches to the serological diagnosis of viral infections is given in Table 5.1.

Detection of antiviral antibody in pre-suckle newborn cord or venous blood provides a basis for specific diagnosis of *in-utero* infections. This approach was used, for example, to show that Akabane virus was the cause of arthrogryposis-hydranencephaly in calves. Because transplacental transfer of immunoglobulins does not occur in most domestic animals, the presence of either IgG or IgM antibodies in pre-suckle blood is indicative of infection of the fetus.

Sensitivity and Specificity

The interpretation and value of a particular serologic test is critically dependent on an understanding of two key parameters: *diagnostic sensitivity* and *diagnostic specificity*. The diagnostic sensitivity of a given test is expressed as a percentage and is the number of animals with the disease (or infection) in question that are identified as positive by that test, divided by the total number of the animals that have the disease (or infection) (Table 5.3). For example, a particular EIA used to screen a population of cattle for antibody to bovine leukemia virus may have a diagnostic sensitivity of 98%—that is, of every 100 infected cattle tested, 98 will be diagnosed correctly and 2 will be missed (the false-negative rate = 2%). In contrast, the diagnostic specificity of a test is a measure of the percentage of those without the disease (or infection) who yield a negative result. For example, the same EIA for bovine leukemia virus antibody may have a diagnostic specificity of 97%—that is, of every 100 uninfected cattle, 97 will be diagnosed correctly as negative, but 3 will be diagnosed incorrectly as infected (the false-positive rate = 3%). Whereas diagnostic sensitivity and diagnostic specificity are fixed percentages intrinsic to the particular diagnostic assay and the population of animals used to validate the test, the *predictive value* of an assay is affected greatly by the prevalence of the disease (or infection) in the test population. Thus, if the same EIA is used to screen a high-risk population with a known bovine leukemia prevalence of 50%, the predictive value of the assay will be high, but if it is used to screen a population with a known prevalence of 0.1%, the great majority of the 3.1% of animals that test positive will in fact be false-positives and will require follow-up with a confirmatory test of much higher specificity. This striking illustration draws attention

TABLE 5.3 Calculations of Accuracy of Serologic Testing

Test Table

		Reference Test Results	
		+	−
New Test Results	+	TP	FP
	−	FN	TN

Sensitivity	The sensitivity of a test is the probability that it will produce a true positive result when used on an infected population (as compared to a reference or "gold standard"). After inserting the test results into a table set up like the Test Table above, the sensitivity of a test can be determined by calculating: $\dfrac{TP}{TP + FN}$
Specificity	The specificity of a test is the probability that a test will produce a true negative result when used on a noninfected population (as determined by a reference or "gold standard"). After inserting the test results into a table set up like the Test Table above, the specificity of a test can be determined by calculating: $\dfrac{TN}{TN + FP}$
Positive Predictive Value	The positive predictive value of a test is the probability that a person is infected when a positive test result is observed. In practice, predictive values should only be calculated from cohort studies or studies that legitimately reflect the number of people in that population who are infected with the disease of interest at that time. This is because predictive values are inherently dependent upon the prevalence of infection. After inserting results into a table set up like the Test Table above, the positive predictive value of a test can be determined by calculating: $\dfrac{TP}{TP + FP}$
Negative Predictive Value	The negative predictive value of a test is the probability that a person is not infected when a negative test result is observed. This measure of accuracy should only be used if prevalence is available from the data. (See note in positive predictive value definition.) After inserting test results into a table set up like the Test Table above, the negative predictive value of a test can be determined by calculating: $\dfrac{TN}{TN + FN}$

FP, number of false positive specimens; FN, number of false negative specimens; TP, number of true positive specimens; TN, number of true negative specimens.

to the importance of selecting diagnostic assays with a particular objective in mind. An assay with high diagnostic sensitivity is required when the aim is to screen for a serious infection or when eradication of the disease is the aim, in which case positive cases must not be missed. An assay (usually based on an independent technology) with very high diagnostic specificity is required for confirmation that the diagnosis is correct.

The *analytic sensitivity* of a given immunoassay is a measure of its ability to detect small amounts of antibody (or antigen). For instance, EIAs and serum neutralization assays generally display substantially higher analytical sensitivity than AGID tests. Improvements in analytical sensitivity may be obtained by the use of purified reagents and sensitive instrumentation. However, the analytical specificity of an immunoassay is a measure of its capacity to discriminate the presence of antibody directed against one virus versus another. This quality is influenced mainly by the purity of the key reagents, especially the antigen when testing for antibody and the antibody when testing for antigen.

Chapter 6

Epidemiology and Control of Viral Diseases

Chapter Contents

EPIDEMIOLOGY OF VIRAL INFECTIONS

Fundamental to the understanding of the occurrence of viral diseases are delineation of the mechanisms whereby viruses are spread and how they cause disease (see Chapter 3), how viruses survive in nature, how they evolve and how this potentially alters properties such as their virulence, how diseases caused by viruses continue to emerge and re-emerge, and how new viral diseases arise, often seemingly from nowhere. Epidemiology is the study of the determinants, dynamics, and distribution of diseases in populations. The risk of infection and/or disease in an animal or animal population is determined by characteristics of the virus (e.g., genetic variation from evolution), the host and host population (e.g., passive, innate, and acquired resistance), and behavioral, environmental, and ecological factors that affect virus transmission from one host to another. Epidemiology, which is part of the science of population biology, attempts to meld these factors into a unified population-based perspective.

Although originally derived from the root term *demos*, meaning people, the word "epidemiology" is widely used now no matter what host is concerned; the words endemic, epidemic, and pandemic are used to characterize disease states in human populations, and enzootic, epizootic and panzootic are their equivalents in animal populations. By introducing quantitative measurements of disease trends, epidemiology has come to have a major role in advancing our understanding of the nature of diseases, and in alerting and directing disease-control activities. Epidemiologic study is also effective in clarifying the role of viruses in the etiology of diseases, in understanding the interaction of viruses with environmental determinants of disease, in determining factors affecting host susceptibility, in unraveling modes of transmission, and in large-scale testing of vaccines and drugs.

Terms and Concepts Used in Epidemiology

The term *enzootic (endemic) disease* refers to the presence of several or continuous chains of transmission resulting in

Fenner's Veterinary Virology. DOI: 10.1016/B978-0-12-375158-4.00006-7

the continuous occurrence of disease in a population over a period of time.

Epizootic (epidemic) disease refers to peaks in disease incidence that exceed the endemic/enzootic baseline or expected incidence of disease. The size of the peak required to constitute an epidemic/epizootic is arbitrary and is influenced by the background infection rate, the morbidity rate, and the anxiety that the disease arouses because of its clinical severity or potential economic impact. Thus a few cases of velogenic Newcastle disease in a poultry flock might be regarded as an epizootic, whereas a few cases of infectious bronchitis would not be.

Pandemic (panzootic) disease refers to a very extensive, typically worldwide epidemic/epizootic, such as that recently associated with H1N1 influenza virus and previously with canine parvovirus, amongst others.

Incubation period refers to the interval between infection and the onset of clinical signs. In many diseases there is a period during which animals are infectious before they become sick.

Period of contagiousness refers to the time during which an infected animal sheds virus. This period varies depending on the disease concerned. For example, in lentivirus infections such as feline immunodeficiency virus infection, animals shed virus for a very long period before showing clinical signs. In such infections the amount of virus shed may be very small, but because the period of infectivity is so long, the virus is maintained readily in the population.

Seroepidemiology simply denotes the use of serological data as the basis of epidemiological investigation, as determined by diagnostic serological techniques (see Chapter 5). Seroepidemiology is extremely useful in veterinary disease control operations and in veterinary research. Because of the expense of collecting and storing sera properly, advantage is often taken of a wide range of sources of representative serum samples, such as abattoirs, culling operations (especially useful for assessment of wildlife populations), and vaccination programs. Such sera can be used to determine the prevalence or incidence of particular infections, to evaluate eradication and immunization programs, and to assess the impact, dynamics, and geographic distribution of new, emerging, and re-emerging viruses. By detecting antibodies to selected viruses in various age groups of the population, it is possible to determine how effectively viruses have spread or how long it has been since the last appearance of a particular virus in the population. Correlation of serologic data with clinical observations makes it possible to determine the ratio of clinical to subclinical infections.

Molecular epidemiology denotes the use of molecular biological data as the basis of epidemiological investigation (see Chapter 5). Quantitative polymerase chain reaction (PCR) assays and nucleotide sequence data are increasingly used for such studies, as they respectively facilitate rapid detection of viruses and direct genetic comparison of individual virus strains, for example in tracking the introduction and relative prevalence of different viral genotypes in animal populations.

COMPUTATIONS AND DATABASES

Calculations of Rates and Proportions

The comparison of disease experience in different populations is expressed in the form of rates and proportions. Multipliers (e.g., rates per 10^n) are used to provide rates that are manageable whole numbers—the most common rate multiplier used is 100,000—that is, the given rate is expressed per 100,000 of the given population per unit of time. Four rates or proportions are most widely used to describe disease occurrence in populations: the *incidence rate*, the *morbidity rate*, the *mortality rate*, and *prevalence*, which is a proportion, since it represents a snapshot of disease status of the population at a single time-point.

In all four measures, the denominator (total number of animals at risk) may be as general as the total population in a herd, state, or country, or as specific as the population known to be susceptible or at risk (e.g., the number of animals in a specified population that lack antibodies to the virus of interest). In each situation it is imperative that the nature of the denominator is made clear—indeed, epidemiology has been called "the science of the denominator." Each of these measures may be affected by various attributes that distinguish one individual animal from another: age, sex, genetic constitution, immune status, nutrition, pregnancy, and various behavioral parameters. The most widely applicable attribute is age, which may encompass, and can therefore be confounded by, the animal's immune status in addition to various physiologic variables.

The case definition (numerator) is a critical component of rates and proportions that should be standardized to allow comparison of disease occurrence in different populations and subpopulations. Criteria can be specified for confirmed, probable, and possible cases, depending on whether the selected criteria are pathognomonic for the viral disease of interest and whether laboratory results are available for all cases. Different case definitions can be specified at the individual animal and at the aggregate level.

Determining the occurrence of a particular disease in a given animal population is more difficult than the computation of the rates described below. The denominator—that is, the number of animals in the population at risk—is often impossible to calculate or estimate accurately. Determining the number of cases of the disease may also prove impossible, depending on the case definition that is selected. Where such information is regarded as essential, government regulations may declare a disease to be *notifiable*, requiring veterinarians to report all cases to authorities. For example, suspicion of the presence of foot-and-mouth disease is notifiable in virtually all developed countries.

Incidence Rate

Incidence rate

$$= \frac{\text{number of cases} \times 10^n}{\text{population at risk}} \text{ in a specified period of time}$$

The incidence rate, or *attack rate*, is a measure of the occurrence of infection or disease in a population over time—for example, a month or a year, and is especially useful for describing acute diseases of short duration. For acute infections, several parameters determine the incidence of infection or disease in a population, including: (1) the percentage of susceptible animals; (2) the percentage of susceptible animals that are infected; (3) the percentage of infected animals that suffer disease; (4) the contact rate for those diseases transmitted by contact, which is affected by animal housing density, housing time, and related factors. The percentage of animals susceptible to a specific virus reflects their past history of exposure to that virus and the duration of their immunity. The percentage infected during a year or a season may vary considerably, depending on factors such as animal numbers and density, season, and—for arbovirus infections—the vector population. Of those infected, only some may develop overt disease; the ratio of clinical to subclinical (inapparent) infections varies greatly with different viruses.

The *secondary attack rate*, when applied to comparable, relatively closed groups such as herds or flocks, is a useful measure of the "infectiousness" of viruses transmitted by aerosols or droplets. It is defined as the number of animals in contact with the primary or *index* case(s) that become infected or sick within the maximum incubation period as a percentage of the total number of susceptible animals exposed to the virus.

Prevalence

Prevalence

$$= \frac{\text{number of cases} \times 10^n}{\text{population at risk}} \text{ at a particular time}$$

It is difficult to measure the incidence of chronic diseases, especially when the onset is insidious, and for such diseases it is customary to determine the prevalence—that is, the ratio, at a particular point in time, of the number of cases currently present in the population divided by the number of animals in the population; it is a snapshot of the occurrence of infection or disease at a given time, and hence a proportion rather than a rate. The prevalence is thus a function of both the incidence rate and the duration of the disease.

Seroprevalence relates to the occurrence of antibody to a particular virus in a population, thus seroprevalence rates usually represent the cumulative experience of a population with a given virus, because neutralizing antibodies often last for many years, or even for life.

Morbidity Rate

The morbidity rate is the percentage of animals in a population that develop clinical signs attributable to a particular virus over a defined period of time (commonly the duration of an outbreak).

Mortality Rate

Mortality from a disease can be categorized in two ways: the cause-specific mortality rate (the number of deaths from the disease in a given year, divided by the total population at mid-year), usually expressed per 100,000 population, or the case-fatality rate (the percentage of animals with a particular disease that die from the disease).

TYPES OF EPIDEMIOLOGIC INVESTIGATION

Conceptual Framework

The *case–control study*, the *cohort study*, the *cross-sectional study*, and the *long-term herd study* provide the conceptual framework upon which can be determined the relationships between cause and effect, the incidence and prevalence of disease, the evaluation of risk factors for disease, the safety and efficacy of vaccines, and the therapeutic value of vaccines and drugs.

Case–Control Studies

Case–control studies are *retrospective*—that is, investigation starts after the disease episode has occurred. In human disease epidemiology, this is the most common type of study, often used to identify the cause of a disease outbreak. Advantages of retrospective studies are that they make use of existing data and are relatively inexpensive to carry out. In many instances they are the only practical method of investigating rare occurrences. Although case–control studies do not require the creation of new data or records, they do require careful selection of the control group, carefully matched to the case (subject) group, so as to avoid bias. The unit of interest might be individual animals or aggregates of animals such as herds/flocks but, because necessary records are generally not available in most animal disease outbreaks, this can present irresolvable difficulties in veterinary medicine.

Cohort Studies

Cohort studies are prospective or longitudinal—investigation starts with a presumed disease episode, say a suspected viral disease outbreak, and with a population exposed to the suspected causative virus. The population is monitored for evidence of the disease. This type of study requires the creation of new data and records. It also requires careful selection of the control group, designing it to be as similar as possible to the exposed group, except for the absence of contact with the presumed causative virus. Cohort studies do not lend themselves to quick analysis, because groups must be followed until disease is observed, often for long periods of time. This makes such studies expensive. However, when cohort studies are successful, proof of cause–effect relationships is usually strong. Once the causal agent is identified, and serological and other diagnostic tests have been developed, case–control and cohort studies can progress to cross-sectional and long-term herd studies.

Cross-Sectional Studies

When the cause of a specific disease is known, a cross-sectional study can be carried out relatively quickly using serology and/or virus identification. This provides data on the prevalence of the particular disease/infection in a population in a specific area.

Long-Term Herd Studies

Long-term herd studies are another kind of epidemiologic investigation that can provide unique information about the presence and continued activity (or lack of activity) of a given virus in an area. They can be regarded as a series of cross-sectional studies. They can also be designed to provide information on the value of vaccines or therapeutic drugs. Despite automation of diagnostic methods and computerization of data files, such studies are still expensive and labor intensive. When used for evaluating vaccines or therapeutic agents, long-term herd studies have the advantage that they include all the variables attributable to the entire husbandry system.

When used to determine the introduction of a particular virus into a population in a given area, such investigations are referred to as sentinel studies. For example, sentinel studies are widely used for determining the initial introduction of zoonotic arboviruses into high-risk areas—sentinel animals, usually chickens, are bled regularly and sera are tested serologically for the first evidence of virus activity, so that appropriate vector control actions can be initiated. For animal viruses, other animal species are frequently used as sentinels, such as sentinel cattle for bluetongue virus infection.

Examples of How Various Kinds of Epidemiological Investigation are Used in Prevention and Control of Viral Diseases

Investigating Causation of Disease

The original investigations of the production of congenital defects in cattle by Akabane virus provide examples of both case–control and cohort studies. Case–control studies of epizootics of congenital defects in calves, characterized by deformed limbs and abnormal brain development, were carried out in Australia in the 1950s and 1960s, but the cause of the disease was not identified. During the summer and early winter months from 1972 to 1975, more than 40,000 calves were born with these same congenital defects in central and western Japan. Japanese scientists postulated that the disease was infectious, but were unable to isolate a virus from affected calves. However, when pre-colostral sera from such calves were tested for antibody to a number of viruses, antibody to Akabane virus, a bunyavirus that was first isolated from mosquitoes in Akabane Prefecture in Japan in 1959, was present in almost all sera. A retrospective serologic survey indicated a very strong association between the geographic distribution of the disease and the presence of antibody to the virus, suggesting that Akabane virus was the etiologic agent of the congenital arthrogryposis-hydranencephaly in cattle. Cohort (prospective) studies were then organized. Sentinel herds were established in Japan and Australia, and it was soon found that the virus could be isolated from fetuses obtained by slaughter or cesarean section for only a short period after infection, thus explaining earlier failures in attempts to isolate virus after calves were born. Experimental inoculation of pregnant cows with Akabane virus during the first two trimesters resulted in congenital abnormalities in calves similar to those seen in natural cases of the disease; clinical signs were not seen in the cows. Following these studies and estimates of the economic impact of the disease, a vaccine was developed and ongoing control programs were started.

Investigating Geographical Distribution and Genetic Variation of Viruses

The global epidemiology of bluetongue virus infection was defined using cross-sectional and long-term herd studies, and the application of both seroepidemiology and molecular epidemiology. Bluetongue virus is enzootic throughout tropical and temperate regions of the world but, before 1998, the virus had only transiently incurred in Europe. Since 1998, several serotypes and strains of bluetongue virus have spread throughout extensive portions of Europe, precipitating a massive disease epizootic, predominantly in sheep. The extensive use of long-term sentinel herd studies coupled with entomological surveillance in several European countries, notably Italy, has definitively established the distribution of the virus and important aspects of its transmission cycle. Furthermore, molecular analyses of the virus serotypes and strains that invaded Europe has led in some instances to determination of their precise geographic origin by comparison with bluetongue viruses isolated elsewhere in the world. Molecular techniques have also been used to monitor the evolution of the viruses within each region, and to determine the contribution of live-attenuated vaccine viruses to the evolution of field strains of the virus. International trade regulations have been substantially modified to reflect the findings from these studies, in addition to data from similar studies in other regions of the world such as North America, Australia, and Southeast Asia, where bluetongue virus infection of ruminants is also enzootic.

Vaccine Trials

The immunogenicity, potency, safety, and efficacy of vaccines are first studied in laboratory animals, followed by small-scale closed trials in the target animal species, and finally by large-scale open field trials. In the latter, epidemiologic methods like those employed in cohort studies are used. There is no alternative way to evaluate new vaccines, and the design of randomized controlled field trials has now been developed so that they yield maximum information with minimum risk and cost. Even with this system, however, a serious problem may be recognized only after a vaccine has been licensed for commercial use. This occurred after the introduction of live-attenuated virus vaccines for infectious bovine rhinotracheitis (caused by bovine herpesvirus 1) in the United States in the 1950s. Surprisingly, the vaccines had been in use for 5 years before it was recognized that abortion was a common sequel to vaccination. Case–control and cohort studies confirmed the causal relationship.

Mathematical Modeling

From the time of William Farr, who studied both medical and veterinary problems in the 1840s, mathematicians have been interested in "epidemic curves" and secular trends in the incidence of infectious diseases. With the development of mathematical modeling using the computer, there has been a resurgence of interest in the dynamics of infectious diseases within populations. Because modeling involves predictions about future occurrences of diseases, models carry a degree of uncertainty; skeptics have said that "for every model there is an equal and opposite model," but in recent years models have played an increasing role in directing disease-control activities.

Mathematical models have been developed to predict various epidemiologic parameters, such as: (1) critical population sizes required to support the continuous transmission of animal viruses with short and long incubation periods; (2) the dynamics of endemicity of viruses that establish persistent infection; (3) the important variables in age-dependent viral pathogenicity. Computer modeling also provides insights into the effectiveness of disease control programs. In this regard, most attention has been given to the potential national and international spread of exotic viral diseases. Models bring a number of issues into focus. The results are often unexpected, pointing to the need for better data and different strategies for disease control. They are also dependent on detailed information on the mechanisms of virus transmission and virus survival in nature, as is discussed next.

VIRUS TRANSMISSION

Viruses survive in nature only if they can be transmitted from one host to another, whether of the same or another species (Table 6.1). Transmission cycles require virus entry into the body, replication, and shedding with subsequent spread to another host (see Chapter 3). Aspects relevant to the spread of viruses in populations are covered here.

Virus transmission may be horizontal or vertical. Vertical transmission describes transmission from dam to offspring. However, most transmission is horizontal—that is, between animals within the population at risk, and can

occur via direct contact, indirect contact, or a common vehicle, or may be airborne, vector-borne, or iatrogenic. Some viruses are transmitted in nature via several modes, others exclusively via a single mode.

Horizontal Transmission

Direct-Contact Transmission

Direct-contact transmission involves actual physical contact between an infected animal and a susceptible animal (e.g., licking, rubbing, biting). This category also includes sexual contact, which, for example, is important in the transmission of some herpesviruses.

Indirect-Contact Transmission

Indirect-contact transmission occurs via *fomites*, such as shared eating containers, bedding, dander, restraint devices, vehicles, clothing, improperly sterilized surgical equipment, or improperly sterilized syringes or needles (the latter also comes under the heading of iatrogenic transmission).

Common-Vehicle Transmission

Common-vehicle transmission includes fecal contamination of food and water supplies (fecal–oral transmission) and virus-contaminated meat or bone products [e.g., for the transmission of vesicular exanthema of swine, classical swine fever (hog cholera) and bovine spongiform encephalopathy].

Airborne Transmission

Airborne transmission, resulting in infection of the respiratory tract, occurs via droplets and droplet nuclei (aerosols) emitted from infected animals during coughing or sneezing (e.g., influenza) or from environmental sources such as dander or dust from bedding (e.g., Marek's disease). Large droplets settle quickly, but microdroplets evaporate, forming droplet nuclei (less than 5μm in diameter) that remain suspended in the air for extended periods. Droplets may travel only a meter or so, but droplet nuclei may travel long distances—many kilometers if wind and other weather conditions are favorable.

Arthropod-Borne Transmission

Arthropod-borne transmission involves the bites of arthropod vectors (e.g., mosquitoes transmit equine encephalitis viruses, ticks transmit African swine fever virus, *Culicoides* spp. transmit bluetongue and African horse sickness viruses) (see section on Arthropod-Borne Virus Transmission Pattern later in this chapter).

Other terms are used to describe transmission by mechanisms that embrace more than one of the just-described routes.

TABLE 6.1 Common Modes of Transmission of Viruses of Animals

Virus Family	Mode of Transmission
Poxviridae	Contact (e.g., orf, cowpox viruses) Arthropod (mechanical, e.g., myxoma virus, fowlpox virus) Respiratory, contact (e.g., sheeppox virus)
Asfarviridae	Respiratory, arthropod (ticks), ingestion of garbage (infected meat)
Herpesviridae	Sexual (e.g., equine coital exanthema virus) Respiratory (e.g., infectious bovine rhinotracheitis virus) Transplacental (e.g., pseudorabies virus)
Adenoviridae	Respiratory, fecal–oral
Papillomaviridae	Direct contact, skin abrasions
Parvoviridae	Fecal–oral, respiratory, contact, transplacental (e.g., feline panleukopenia virus)
Circoviridae	Fecal–oral, respiratory, contact
Retroviridae	Contact, in ovo (germ line), ingestion, mechanically by arthropods
Reoviridae	Fecal–oral (e.g., calf rotavirus) Arthropod (e.g., bluetongue viruses)
Birnaviridae	Fecal–oral, water
Paramyxoviridae	Respiratory, contact, formites
Rhabdoviridae	Animal bite (e.g., rabies virus) Arthropod and contact (e.g., vesicular stomatitis viruses)
Filoviridae	Unknown in nature; human-to-human spread is by direct contact
Bornaviridae	Unknown in nature; animal-to-animal spread is by direct contact
Orthomyxoviridae	Respiratory, formites
Bunyaviridae	Arthropod (e.g., Rift Valley fever virus)
Arenaviridae	Contact with contaminated urine, respiratory
Coronaviridae	Fecal–oral, respiratory, contact
Arteriviridae	Direct contact, fomites; vertical transmission in semen
Picornaviridae	Fecal–oral (e.g., swine enteroviruses) Respiratory (e.g., equine rhinoviruses) Ingestion of garbage (infected meat) (e.g., foot-and-mouth disease viruses in swine)
Caliciviridae	Respiratory, fecal–oral, contact
Togaviridae	Arthropod (e.g., Venezuelan equine encephalitis virus)
Flaviviridae	Arthropod (e.g., Japanese encephalitis virus) Respiratory, fecal–oral, transplacental (e.g., bovine viral diarrhea virus)
Prions	Contaminated pastures (scrapie); contaminated feedstuff (e.g., bovine spongiform encephalopathy); unknown (e.g., chronic wasting disease of deer and elk)

Iatrogenic Transmission

Iatrogenic ("caused by the doctor") transmission occurs as a direct result of some activity of the attending veterinarian, veterinary technologist, or other person in the course of caring for animals, usually via non-sterile equipment, multiple-use syringes, or inadequate handwashing. Iatrogenic transmission has been important in the spread of equine infectious anemia virus via multiple-use syringes and needles. Similarly, chickens have been infected with reticuloendotheliosis virus via contaminated Marek's disease vaccine.

Nosocomial Transmission

Nosocomial transmission occurs while an animal is in a veterinary hospital or clinic. During the peak of the canine parvovirus epidemic in the 1980s, many puppies became infected in veterinary hospitals and clinics. In some hospitals, the disinfectants in routine use were found to be ineffective against the virus. Feline respiratory infections are also acquired nosocomially. In human medicine, the Ebola virus episodes in Zaire (now Democratic Republic of Congo) in 1976 and 1995 were classic examples of iatrogenic nosocomial epidemics.

Zoonotic Transmission

Because most viruses are host restricted, the majority of viral infections are maintained in nature within populations of the same or closely related species. However, a number of viruses are spread naturally between several different species of animals—for example, rabies and the arboviral encephalitides. The term *zoonosis* is used to describe infections that are transmissible from animals to humans. Zoonoses, whether involving domestic or wild animal reservoirs, usually occur only under conditions in which humans are engaged in activities involving close contact with animals, or where viruses are transmitted by arthropods (Tables 6.2 and 6.3).

Vertical Transmission

The term "vertical transmission" is usually used to describe infection that is transferred from dam to embryo, or fetus, or newborn before, during, or shortly after parturition, although some authorities prefer to restrict the term to situations in which infection occurs before birth. Certain retroviruses are transmitted vertically via the integration of proviral DNA directly into the DNA of the germ line of the fertilized egg. Cytomegaloviruses are often transmitted to the fetus via the placenta, whereas other herpesviruses are transmitted during passage through the birth canal. Yet other viruses are transmitted via colostrum and milk (e.g., caprine arthritis-encephalitis virus and maedi-visna virus of sheep). Vertical transmission of a virus may cause early embryonic death or abortion (e.g., several lentiviruses) or may be associated with congenital disease (e.g., bovine viral diarrhea virus, border disease virus, porcine enterovirus), or the infection may be the cause of congenital defects (e.g., Akabane virus, bluetongue virus, feline parvovirus).

MECHANISMS OF SURVIVAL OF VIRUSES IN NATURE

Perpetuation of a virus in nature depends on the maintenance of serial infections—that is, a chain of transmission;

TABLE 6.2 Major Arthropod-Borne Viral Zoonoses

Family	Genus	Virus	Reservoir Host	Arthropod Vector
Togaviridae	*Alphavirus*[a]	*Eastern equine encephalitis virus*[a]	Birds	Mosquitoes
		Western equine encephalitis virus	Birds	Mosquitoes
		Venezuelan equine encephalitis virus[a]	Mammals, horses	Mosquitoes
		Ross River virus[a]	Mammals	Mosquitoes
Flaviviridae	*Flavivirus*	*Japanese encephalitis virus*	Birds, pigs	Mosquitoes
		St. Louis encephalitis virus	Birds	Mosquitoes
		West Nile virus	Birds	Mosquitoes
		Murray Valley encephalitis virus	Birds	Mosquitoes
		Yellow fever virus[b]	Monkeys, humans	Mosquitoes
		Dengue viruses[b]	Humans, monkeys	Mosquitoes
		Kyasanur Forest disease virus	Mammals	Ticks
		Tick-borne encephalitis viruses	Mammals, birds	Ticks
Bunyaviridae	*Phlebovirus*	*Rift Valley fever virus*	Mammals	Mosquitoes
		Sandfly fever viruses[a]	Mammals	Sandflies
	Nairovirus	*Crimean-Congo hemorrhagic fever virus*	Mammals	Ticks
	Bunyavirus	*California encephalitis virus*	Mammals	Mosquitoes
		La Crosse encephalitis virus	Mammals	Mosquitoes
		Tahyna virus	Mammals	Mosquitoes
		Oropouche virus	? Mammals	Mosquitoes, midges
Reoviridae	*Coltivirus*	*Colorado tick fever virus*	Mammals	Ticks

[a]*In certain episodes, virus is transmitted by insects from human to human.*
[b]*Usually transmitted by mosquitoes from human to human.*

TABLE 6.3 Major Non-Arthropod-Borne Viral Zoonoses

Family	Virus	Reservoir Host	Mode of Transmission to Humans
Poxviridae	Cowpox virus	Rodents, cats, cattle	Contact, abrasions
	Monkeypox virus	Squirrels, monkeys	Contact, abrasions
	Pseudocowpox virus	Cattle	Contact, abrasions
	Orf virus	Sheep, goats	Contact, abrasions
Herpesviridae	B virus	Monkey	Animal bite
Paramyxoviridae	Henipah viruses (Nipah, Hendra)	Fruit-eating bats	Uncertain
Rhabdoviridae	Rabies virus and bat lyssaviruses	Various mammals	Animal bite, scratch, respiratory
	Vesicular stomatitis viruses	Cattle	Contact with secretions[a]
Filoviridae	Ebola, Marburg viruses	Bats, monkeys	Contact; iatrogenic (injection)[b]
Orthomyxoviridae	Influenza A viruses[c]	Birds, pigs	Respiratory
Bunyaviridae	Hantaviruses	Rodents	Contact with rodent urine
Arenaviridae	Lymphocytic choriomeningitis, Junin, Machupo, Lassa, Guanarito viruses	Rodents	Contact with rodent urine
Coronaviridae	Severe acute respiratory disease syndrome (SARS) coronavirus	Bats and wild mammals (Palm civets, etc.)	Respiratory

[a]May be arthropod borne.
[b]Also human-to-human spread.
[c]Usually maintained by human-to-human spread; zoonotic infections occur only rarely, but reassortants between human and avion influenza viruses (perhaps arising during coinfection of pigs) may result in human pandemics due to antigenic shift.

the occurrence of disease is neither required nor necessarily advantageous (Table 6.4). Indeed, although clinical cases may be somewhat more productive sources of virus than inapparent infections, the latter are generally more numerous and more important, because they do not restrict the movement of infectious individuals and thus provide a better opportunity for virus dissemination. As our knowledge of the different features of the pathogenesis, species susceptibility, routes of transmission, and environmental stability of various viruses has increased, epidemiologists have recognized four major patterns by which viruses maintain serial transmission in their host(s): (1) the acute self-limiting infection pattern, in which transmission is always affected by host population size; (2) the persistent infection pattern; (3) the vertical transmission pattern; (4) the arthropod-borne virus transmission pattern.

The physical stability of a virus affects its survival in the environment; in general, viruses that are transmitted by the respiratory route have low environmental stability, whereas those transmitted by the fecal–oral route have a higher stability. Thus stability of the virus in water or fomites, or on the mouthparts of mechanical arthropod vectors, favors transmission; this is particularly important in small or dispersed animal communities, for example, the parapox virus that causes orf in sheep survives for months in pastures. During the winter, myxoma virus, which causes myxomatosis in rabbits, can survive for several weeks on the mouthparts of mosquitoes.

Most viruses have a principal mechanism for survival, but if this mechanism is interrupted—for example, by a sudden decline in the population of the host species—a second or even a third mechanism may exist as a "backup." For example, in bovine viral diarrhea there is a primary, direct animal to animal transmission cycle; however, long-term infection in herds is maintained by the less common persistent shedding of virus by congenitally infected cattle. An appreciation of these mechanisms for virus perpetuation is valuable in designing and implementing control programs.

Acute Self-Limiting Infection Pattern

The most precise data on the importance of population size in acute, self-limiting infections come from studies of measles, which is a cosmopolitan human disease. Measles has long been a favorite disease for modeling epidemics, because it is one of the few common human diseases in which subclinical infections are rare, clinical diagnosis is easy, and postinfection immunity is life-long. Measles virus is related closely to rinderpest and canine distemper viruses, and many aspects of the model apply equally well to these two viruses and the diseases they cause. Survival of measles virus in a population requires a large continuous supply of susceptible hosts. Analyses of the incidence of measles in large cities and in island communities have

TABLE 6.4 Modes of Survival of Viruses in Nature

Family	Example	Mode of Survival
Poxviridae	Orf virus	Virus stable in environment
Asfarviridae	African swine fever virus	Acute self-limiting infection; persistent infection in soft ticks and chronically infected swine
Herpesviridae	Bovine herpesvirus 1	Persistent infection, intermittent shedding
Adenoviridae	Canine adenovirus 1	Persistent infection; virus stable in environment
Papovaviridae	Papillomaviruses	Persistent in lesions; virus stable in environment
Parvoviridae	Canine parvovirus	Virus stable in environment
Circoviridae	Psittacine beak and feather disease virus	Virus stable in environment
Retroviridae	Avian leukosis viruses	Persistent infection; vertical transmission
Reoviridae	Calf rotaviruses	Acute self-limiting infection; very high yield of virus from infected animals
	Bluetongue viruses	Arthropod borne
Birnaviridae	Infectious bursal disease virus	Acute self-limiting infection
Paramyxoviridae	Newcastle disease virus	Acute self-limiting infection; vertical with velogenic strains
Rhabdoviridae	Rabies virus	Long incubation period
	Vesicular stomatitis viruses	Virus stable, arthropod borne
Filoviridae	Ebola virus	Possibly in bats
Bornaviridae	Borna disease virus	Persistent infection
Orthomyxoviridae	Influenza viruses	Acute self-limiting infection
Bunyaviridae	Rift Valley fever virus	Arthropod borne; vertical transmission in flood-water mosquitoes
Arenaviridae	Lassa virus	Persistent infection
Coronaviridae	Feline enteric coronavirus (formerly feline infectious peritonitis virus)	Persistent infection with enteric virus
Arteriviridae	Equine arteritis virus	Persistent infection in carrier stallions
Picornaviridae	Foot-and-mouth disease viruses	Acute self-limiting infection; sometimes persistent infection
Caliciviridae	Feline calicivirus	Persistent infection with continuous shedding
Togaviridae	Equine encephalitis viruses	Arthropod borne
Flaviviridae	Japanese encephalitis virus	Arthropod borne
	Bovine viral diarrhea virus	Acute self-limiting infection; persistent after congenital infection
Prions	Scrapie prion	Prion stable in environment

shown that a population of about half a million persons is needed to ensure a large enough annual input of new susceptible hosts, by birth or immigration, to maintain the virus in the population. Because infection depends on respiratory transmission, the duration of epidemics of measles is correlated inversely with population density. If a population is dispersed over a large area, the rate of spread is reduced and the epidemic will last longer, so that the number of susceptible persons needed to maintain the transmission chain is reduced. However, in such a situation a break in the transmission chain is much more likely.

When a large percentage of the population is susceptible initially, the intensity of the epidemic builds up very quickly and attack rates are almost 100% (*virgin-soil epidemic*). There are many examples of similar transmission patterns among viruses of domestic animals, but quantitative data are not as complete as those for measles. *Exotic viruses*—that is, those that are not present in a particular country or region—represent the most important group of viruses with a potential for causing virgin-soil epidemics, as graphically illustrated recently with the epizootic of bluetongue in Europe.

The history of rinderpest in cattle in Africa in the early 20th century shows many parallels with measles in isolated human populations. When it was first introduced into cattle populations the initial impact was devastating. Cattle and wild ruminants of all ages were susceptible, and the mortality was so high that in Tanzania the ground was so littered with the carcasses of cattle that a Masai tribesman commented that "the vultures had forgotten how to fly." The development of vaccines beginning in the 1920s changed the epidemiology of rinderpest, leading to a period in the 1960s when its global eradication was anticipated. Unfortunately, in the 1970s, vaccination programs in West Africa were maintained poorly and by the 1980s the disease had once again become rampant and the cause of major losses in many parts of Africa. This prompted renewed vaccination and control campaigns in Africa and the Indian subcontinent, so that there is now real optimism that rinderpest has been eradicated entirely.

The cyclical nature of the occurrence of such diseases is determined by several variables, including the rate of build-up of susceptible animals, introduction of the virus, and environmental conditions that promote virus spread.

Persistent Infection Pattern

Persistent viral infections, whether they are associated with acute initial disease or with recurrent episodes of clinical disease, play an important role in the perpetuation of many viruses. For example, recurrent virus shedding by a persistently infected animal can reintroduce virus into a population of susceptible animals all of which have been born since the last clinically apparent episode of infection. This transmission pattern is potentially important for the survival of bovine viral diarrhea virus, classical swine fever (hog cholera) virus, and some herpesviruses, and such viruses have a much smaller critical population size than occurs in acute self-limited infections; indeed the sustaining population for some herpesviruses may be as small as a single farm, kennel, cattery, or breeding unit.

Sometimes the persistence of infection, the production of disease, and the transmission of virus are dissociated; for example, togavirus and arenavirus infections have little adverse effect on their reservoir hosts (arthropods, birds, and rodents) but transmission is very efficient. However, the persistence of infection in the central nervous system, as with canine distemper virus, is of no epidemiologic significance, as no infectious virus is shed from this site; infections of the central nervous system may have a severe effect on the dog, but is of no consequence for survival of the virus.

Vertical Transmission Pattern

Transmission of virus from the dam to the embryo, fetus, or newborn can be important in virus survival in nature: all arenaviruses, several herpesviruses, parvoviruses, pestiviruses, and retroviruses, some togaviruses, and a few bunyaviruses and coronaviruses may be transmitted in this way. Indeed, if the consequence of vertical transmission is life-long persistent infection, as in the case of arenaviruses and retroviruses, the long-term survival of the virus is assured. Virus transmission in the immediate perinatal period, by contact or via colostrum and milk, is also important.

Arthropod-Borne Virus Transmission Pattern

Several arthropod-borne diseases are discussed in appropriate chapters of Part II of this book; this chapter considers some common features that will be useful in understanding their epidemiology and control. More than 500 arboviruses are known, of which some 40 cause disease in domestic animals and many of the same cause zoonotic diseases (Table 6.2). Sometimes arthropod transmission may be mechanical, as in myxomatosis and fowlpox, in which mosquitoes act as "flying needles." More commonly, transmission involves replication of the virus in the arthropod vector, which may be a tick, a mosquito, a sandfly (*Phlebotomus* spp.), or a midge (*Culicoides* spp.).

The arthropod vector acquires virus by feeding on the blood of a viremic animal. Replication of the ingested virus, initially in the insect gut, and its spread to the salivary gland take several days (the *extrinsic incubation period*); the interval varies with different viruses and is influenced by ambient temperature. Virions in the salivary secretions of the vector are injected into new animal hosts during blood meals. Arthropod transmission provides a way for a virus to cross species barriers, as the same arthropod may bite birds, reptiles, and mammals that rarely or never come into close contact in nature.

Most arboviruses have localized natural habitats in which specific receptive arthropod and vertebrate hosts are involved in the viral life cycle. Vertebrate reservoir hosts are usually wild mammals or birds; domestic animals and humans are rarely involved in primary transmission cycles, although the exceptions to this generalization are important (e.g., Venezuelan equine encephalitis virus in horses, yellow fever, and dengue viruses in humans). Domestic animal species are, in most cases, infected incidentally—for example, by the geographic extension of a reservoir vertebrate host and/or a vector arthropod.

Most arboviruses that cause periodic epidemics or epizootics have ecologically complex enzootic cycles, which often involve arthropod and vertebrate hosts that are different from those involved in epidemic/epizootic cycles. Enzootic cycles, which are often poorly understood and inaccessible to effective control measures, provide for the amplification of virus and therefore are critical in dictating the magnitude of epidemics or epizootics.

When arthropods are active, arboviruses replicate alternately in vertebrate and invertebrate hosts. A puzzle that has concerned many investigators has been to understand what happens to these viruses during the winter months in temperate climates when the arthropod vectors are inactive. Important mechanisms for "overwintering" are *transovarial* and *trans-stadial transmission*. Transovarial transmission occurs with the tick-borne flaviviruses, and has been shown to occur with some mosquito-borne bunyaviruses and flaviviruses. Some bunyaviruses are found in high northern latitudes where the mosquito breeding season is too short to allow virus survival by horizontal transmission cycles alone; many of the first mosquitoes to emerge each summer carry virus as a result of transovarial and trans-stadial transmission, and the pool of virus is amplified rapidly by horizontal transmission in mosquito–vertebrate–mosquito cycles.

Vertical transmission in arthropods may not explain overwintering of all arboviruses, but other possibilities are still unproven or speculative. For example, hibernating vertebrates have been thought to play a role in overwintering. In cold climates, bats and some small rodents, as well as snakes and frogs, hibernate during the winter months. Their low body temperature has been thought to favor persistent infection, with recrudescent viremia occurring when the temperature increases in the spring. Although demonstrated in the laboratory, this mechanism has never been proven to occur in nature. Similarly, in temperate climates, individual insects can survive for extended periods during the winter months, and initiate a low-level cycle of vertebrate–invertebrate virus transmission that sustains viruses during the interseasonal transmission period.

Many human activities disturb the natural ecology and hence the natural arbovirus life cycles, and have been incriminated in the geographic spread or increased prevalence of the diseases caused by these viruses:

1. Population movements and the intrusion of humans and domestic animals into new arthropod habitats have resulted in dramatic epidemics. Some have had historic impact: the Louisiana Purchase came about because of the losses Napoleon's army experienced from yellow fever in the Caribbean. Several decades later, the same disease markedly and adversely affected the building of the Panama Canal. Ecologic factors pertaining to unique environments and geographic factors have contributed to many new, emergent disease episodes. Remote eco niches, such as islands, free of particular species of reservoir hosts and vectors, are often particularly vulnerable to an introduced virus.

2. Deforestation has been the key to the exposure of farmers and domestic animals to new arthropods—there are many contemporary examples of the importance of this kind of ecological disruption.

3. Increased long-distance travel facilitates the carriage of exotic arthropod vectors around the world. The carriage of the eggs of the Asian mosquito, *Aedes albopictus*, to the United States in used tires represents an unsolved problem of this kind. The increased long-distance transportation of livestock facilitates the carriage of viruses and arthropods (especially ticks) around the world.

4. Ecologic factors pertaining to water usage—that is, increasing irrigation and the expanding re-use of water, are becoming very important factors in the emergence of viral disease. The problem with primitive water and irrigation systems, which are developed without attention to arthropod control, is exemplified in the emergence of Japanese encephalitis in new areas of southeast Asia.

5. New routes of long-distance bird migrations brought about by new man-made water impounds represent an important yet still untested new risk of introduction of arboviruses into new areas. The extension of the geographical range of Japanese encephalitis virus into new areas of Asia has probably involved virus carriage by birds.

6. Ecologic factors pertaining to environmental pollution and uncontrolled urbanization are contributing to many new, emergent disease episodes. Arthropod vectors breeding in accumulations of water (tin cans, old tires, etc.) and sewage-laden water are a worldwide problem. Environmental chemical toxicants (herbicides, pesticides, residues) can also affect vector–virus relationships directly or indirectly, including fostering the development of mosquito resistance to licensed insecticides.

7. Climate change, affecting sea level, estuarine wetlands, fresh water swamps, and human habitation patterns, may be affecting vector–virus relationships throughout the tropics; however, definitive data are lacking and many programs to study the effect of global warming on emergence of infectious diseases have failed to adequately address the potential importance of other environmental and anthropogenic factors in the process.

The history of the European colonization of Africa is replete with examples of new arbovirus diseases resulting from the introduction of susceptible European livestock into that continent—for example, African swine fever, African horse sickness, Rift Valley fever, Nairobi sheep disease, and bluetongue. The viruses that cause these diseases are now feared in the industrialized countries as exotic threats that may devastate their livestock, with recent poignant examples of events such as the emergence of bluetongue throughout Europe. Another example of the importance of ecologic factors is the infection of horses in the eastern part of North America with eastern equine encephalitis virus, when their pasturage is made to overlap the natural swamp-based mosquito–bird–mosquito cycle of this virus. Similarly, in Japan and southeastern Asian countries, swine may become infected with Japanese encephalitis virus and become important amplifying hosts when they are bitten by mosquitoes that breed in rice fields.

Tick-borne flaviviruses illustrate two features of epidemiologic importance. First, transovarial infection in ticks is often sufficient to ensure survival of the virus independently of a cycle in vertebrates; vertebrate infection amplifies the population of infected ticks. Secondly, for some of these viruses, transmission from one vertebrate host to another, once initiated by the bite of an infected tick, can also occur by mechanisms not involving an arthropod. Thus, in central Europe and the eastern part of Russia, a variety of small rodents may be infected with tick-borne encephalitis viruses. Goats, cows, and sheep are incidental hosts and sustain inapparent infections, but they excrete virus in their milk. Adult and juvenile ungulates may acquire virus during grazing on tick-infested pastures, and newborn animals may be infected by drinking infected milk. Humans may be infected by being bitten by a tick or by drinking milk from an infected goat.

Variations in Disease Incidence Associated with Seasons and Animal Management Practices

Many viral infections show pronounced seasonal variations in incidence. In temperate climates, arbovirus infections transmitted by mosquitoes or sandflies occur mainly during the months of late summer and early fall (autumn), when vectors are most numerous and active. Infections transmitted by ticks occur most commonly during the spring and early summer months. Other biologic reasons for seasonal disease include both virus and host factors. Influenza viruses and poxviruses survive better in air at low rather than at high humidity, and all viruses survive better at lower temperatures in aerosols. It has also been suggested that there are seasonal changes in the susceptibility of the host, perhaps associated with changes in the physiological status of nasal and oropharyngeal mucous membranes.

More important in veterinary medicine than any natural seasonal effects are the changes in housing and management practices that occur in different seasons. Housing animals such as cattle and sheep for the winter often increases the incidence of respiratory and enteric diseases. These diseases often have a complex pathogenesis with an obscure primary etiology, usually viral, followed by secondary infections with other pathogens, often bacteria. In such cases, diagnosis, prevention, and treatment of infectious diseases must be integrated into an overall system for the management of facilities as well as husbandry practices. In areas where animals are moved—for example, to feedlots or seasonally to distant pasturage—there are two major problems: animals are subjected to the stress of transportation, and they are brought into contact with new populations carrying and shedding different infectious agents.

In areas of the world where livestock are moved annually over vast distances, such as in the Sahel zone of Africa, viral diseases such as pestes des petits ruminants

are associated with the contact between previously separate populations brought about by this traditional husbandry practice. In southern Africa, the communal use of waterholes during the dry season promotes the exchange of viruses such as foot-and-mouth disease virus between different species of wildlife and, potentially, between wildlife and domestic animals.

Epidemiologic Aspects of Immunity

Immunity acquired from prior infection or from vaccination plays a vital role in the epidemiology of viral diseases; in fact, vaccination (see Chapter 4) is the single most effective method of controlling most viral diseases. For example, vaccination against canine distemper and infectious canine hepatitis has sharply decreased the incidence of both diseases in many countries. For some viruses, immunity is relatively ineffective because of the lack of neutralizing of antibodies at the site of infection (e.g., the respiratory or intestinal tract). Respiratory syncytial viruses cause mild to severe respiratory tract disease in cattle and sheep. Infections usually occur during the winter months when the animals are housed in confined conditions. The virus spreads rapidly by aerosol infection, and reinfection of the respiratory tract is not uncommon. Pre-existing antibody, whether derived passively by maternal transfer or actively by prior infection, does not prevent virus replication and excretion, although clinical signs are usually mild when the antibody titer is high. Not surprisingly, vaccination is not always effective.

EMERGING VIRAL DISEASES

An emerging viral disease is one that is newly recognized or newly evolved, or that has occurred previously but shows an increase in incidence or expansion in geographical, host, or vector range. By this definition, numerous viral diseases in this book currently qualify as emerging diseases. Tables 6.5 and 6.6 list some of these diseases and the viruses that cause them. Constant changes in demographic, ecological, and anthropogenic factors ensure that new and recurring diseases will continue to emerge, but virological and host determinants also contribute to the emergence of some viral diseases, and the emergence of new diseases in particular.

VIROLOGICAL DETERMINANTS OF THE EMERGENCE OF VIRAL DISEASES

Viruses exist, not as individuals of a single genotype, but rather as populations of genetically distinct but related virus strains. The number of individual virus species continues to grow (currently more than 3600), particularly with the evaluation of wildlife and other "non-traditional" species such as reptiles and fish. With the advent of molecular technologies such as PCR and rapid sequencing, the

TABLE 6.5 Some Important New, Emerging, and Re-Emerging Animal Viruses

African horse sickness viruses (mosquito borne; a historic problem in southern Africa; recently active in sub-Saharan Africa a major threat to horses worldwide)

African swine fever virus (tick borne and also spread by contact; an extremely pathogenic virus; recently present in Russia, Georgia and adjacent countries; a potential threat to commercial swine industries)

Avian influenza viruses (highly pathogenic H5N1 in Asia, Africa, and Europe; major threat to commercial poultry industries of all countries)

Bluetongue viruses (*Culicoides* spp. borne; epizootic in Europe forced revision of European Union protocols)

Bovine spongiform encephalopathy prion (the cause of a major epidemic in cattle in the United Kingdom, resulting in major economic loss and trade embargo)

Canine influenza virus (H3N8 equine influenza virus that spread to greyhound dogs in Florida in 2004, causing fatal hemorrhagic pneumonia; virus now circulates in dogs, often causing asymptomatic infection)

Canine parvovirus (a new virus, that quickly spread throughout the world causing a panzootic of severe disease in dogs)

Chronic wasting disease of deer and elk prion (a spongiform encephalopathy of captive and wild cervids in North America)

Hendra virus (recognized in Queensland, Australia, in 1994; the cause of fatal acute respiratory distress syndrome in horses and humans; bats serve as reservoir host)

Feline calicivirus (variant of FCV that is associated with a highly virulent systemic infection of cats)

Feline immunodeficiency virus (a recently recognized (since 1987) cause of morbidity and mortality in cats globally)

Foot-and-mouth-disease viruses (still considered the most dangerous exotic viruses of animals in the world because of their capacity for rapid transmission and great economic loss; still entrenched in Africa, the middle East, and Asia; still capable of emergence in any commercial cattle industry): outbreaks most recently in South Korea and Japan

Malignant catarrhal fever virus (the African form is an exotic, lethal herpesvirus of cattle; its presence is an important non-tariff trade barrier issue)

Marine mammal morbilliviruses (epidemic disease first identified in 1988 in European seals; now realized as several important emerging viruses, endangering several species of marine mammals)

Porcine circovirus 2 (recognized as the cause of several important disease syndromes of swine worldwide)

Porcine reproductive and respiratory syndrome virus (also called Lelystad virus—rather recently recognized as an important cause of disease in swine in Europe, Asia, and the United States)

Simian immunodeficiency virus (significance of these viruses increasingly recognized as important models in acquired immunodeficiency syndrome research)

West Nile virus (the cause of neurological disease in horses and high mortality in birds in North America and portions of Europe)

numbers of distinct virus strains within individual virus species continues to grow even more rapidly. The importance of this genetic diversity is that specific strains of the same virus species can have profoundly different biological properties, including such critical determinants as host range, tissue tropism, and virulence. Thus new diseases continue to emerge as a consequence of evolution of novel viruses that arise from enzootic viruses. An appreciation of viral genetics and evolution, therefore, is central to the understanding of the emergence of viral diseases.

In nature, viruses undergo an ongoing series of replication cycles as they are transmitted from host to host. During this process, genetic variants are continually generated, some of which will have different biological properties (such as virulence, tropism, or host range) than the parent virus from which they arise. Many viruses, particularly RNA viruses, have short generation times and relatively high mutation rates, whereas other viruses evolve through more drastic genetic changes, including the exchange of entire gene segments (reassortment), gene deletion or acquisition, recombination, and translocation. Selective pressures exerted by their animal hosts or insect vectors can favor the selection of certain of these biological variants, primarily because of their preferential ability to be

TABLE 6.6 Some Important New, Emerging, and Re-Emerging Zoonotic Viruses

Bovine spongiform encephalopathy prion (recognized in 1986; the cause of a major epidemic in cattle in the United Kingdom, resulting in major economic loss and trade embargo; identified as the cause of human central nervous system disease: new-variant Creutzfeldt–Jakob disease)

Crimean-Congo hemorrhagic fever virus[a] (tick borne; reservoir in sheep; severe human disease with 10% mortality; widespread across Africa, the Middle East, and Asia)

Eastern equine encephalitis virus (increase in number of human cases in eastern United States, in areas where rarely detected previously)

Ebola[a] and Marburg[a] viruses (bats and nonhuman primates appear to be natural reservoir hosts; Ebola and Marburg viruses are the causes of the most lethal hemorrhagic fevers known)

Hendra virus (recognized in Queensland, Australia, in 1994; the cause of fatal acute respiratory distress syndrome in horses; spread to humans causing similar, also fatal, disease; bats serve as reservoir host)

Guanarito virus[a] (rodent borne; the newly discovered cause of Venezuelan hemorrhagic fever)

Hantaviruses[a] (rodent borne; the cause of important rodent-borne hemorrhagic fever in Asia and Europe; Sin Nombre virus and related viruses are the cause of hantavirus pulmonary syndrome in the Americas)

Influenza viruses (reservoir in birds, especially waterfowl birds, with intermediate evolution in swine, and virus species jumping, bringing new viruses to human populations each year; the cause of the single most deadly human epidemic ever recorded—the pandemic of 1918 in which 25–40 million people died; the cause of panic in Hong Kong in 1997 as an H5N1 avian influenza virus for the first time appeared in humans, causing severe disease and several deaths; the cause of thousands of deaths every winter in the elderly)

Japanese encephalitis virus (mosquito borne; swine serve as amplifying reservoir hosts; very severe, lethal encephalitis in humans; now spreading across southeast Asia; great epidemic potential)

Junin virus[a] (rodent borne; the cause of Argentine hemorrhagic fever)

Lassa virus[a] (rodent borne; a very important, severe disease in West Africa)

Machupo virus[a] (rodent borne; the cause of Bolivian hemorrhagic fever)

Rabies virus (transmitted by the bite of rabid animals; raccoon epizootic still spreading across the northeastern United States; thousands of deaths every year in India, Sri Lanka, the Philippines, and elsewhere)

Rift Valley fever virus[a] (mosquito borne; sheep, cattle, and wild mammals serve as amplifying hosts; the cause of one of the most explosive epidemics ever seen when the virus first appeared in 1977 in Egypt); recent epidemics in southern and eastern Africa, and the Arabian Peninsula

Ross River virus (mosquito borne; cause of human epidemic arthritis; has moved across the Pacific region several times)

Sabiá virus[a] (rodent borne; cause of severe, even fatal, hemorrhagic fever in Brazil)

Severe acute respiratory disease syndrome (SARS) coronavirus (reservoir in bats, spread to humans by palm civets, raccoon dogs, etc. in live animal markets in Asia; severe respiratory disease in affected humans

Yellow fever virus[a] (mosquito borne; monkeys serve as reservoir hosts; one of the most deadly diseases in history, potential for urban re-emergence)

[a]*Viruses that cause hemorrhagic fevers in humans.*

transmitted serially. Properties important in the survival and evolutionary progression of viruses in nature can include:

1. *The capacity to replicate rapidly.* In many instances, the most virulent strains of a virus replicate faster than more temperate strains. However, if replication is too rapid, it can be self-defeating—extremely rapid viral growth may not allow time enough for transmission before the host is removed by death or severe illness.

2. *The capacity to replicate to high titer.* A very high vertebrate host viremia titer is employed as a survival

mechanism by arthropod-borne viruses, to favor infection of the next arthropod. The same viruses produce very high titers in the salivary glands of their arthropod hosts in order to favor infection of the next vertebrate host. Such high virus titers can be associated with silent infections in some natural vertebrate hosts (e.g., reservoir avian hosts), but in vertebrate hosts the evolution of this capacity is most often associated with severe, even fatal, illness.

3. *The capacity to replicate in certain key tissues.* This quality is often important for the completion of the

virus transmission cycle. For example, the evolution of virus tropisms and the employment of specific host-cell receptors define many disease patterns. Further, the evolution of the capacity to grow in immunologically sequestered sites or in cells of the immune system itself provides great survival advantage (see Chapter 3).

4. *The capacity to be shed for long periods of time.* The evolution of the capacity for chronic shedding offers exceptional opportunity for virus survival and entrenchment. Recrudescence and intermittent shedding add additional survival advantages to the virus (e.g., herpesvirus infections in all animals).

5. *The capacity to elude host defenses.* Animals have evolved elaborate immune systems to defend themselves against the viruses, but the viruses in turn have evolved equally elaborate systems to evade host defenses (see Chapter 4). Viruses, particularly those with large genomes, have genes that encode proteins that interfere with specific host antiviral activities. The capacity to cause fetal infection and persistent postnatal viral infection represents an evolutionary progression that gives the virus an extreme survival advantage (e.g., bovine viral diarrhea virus infection in calves or lymphocytic choriomeningitis virus infection in mice).

6. *The capacity to survive after being shed into the external environment.* All things being equal, a virus that has evolved a capsid that is environmentally stable must have an evolutionary advantage. For example, because of its stability, canine parvovirus was transported around the world within 2 years of its emergence, mostly by carriage on fomites (human shoes and clothing, cages, etc.).

7. *The capacity to be transmitted vertically.* Viruses that employ vertical transmission and survive without ever confronting the external environment represent another evolutionary progression.

Evolution of Viruses and Emergence of Genetic Variants

A simple question that can be posed is: "how important is genetic diversity to the survival of viruses?" Predictably, however, the answer is not simple. Viruses that cause sudden epidemics or epizootics of disease, such as outbreaks of foot-and-mouth disease, influenza, and severe acute respiratory syndrome (SARS) frequently attract great public interest and concern. It is to be stressed, however, that these viruses emerge from some endemic/enzootic niche, and it is clear that, as a group, those viruses that are constantly present in populations (endemic or enzootic) often exact a greater ongoing toll than emerging or new diseases. Thus an understanding of virus evolution is prerequisite to the understanding of both emergence of viral diseases and the maintenance of endemic/enzootic ones.

Viruses have evolved with variable reliance on the generation of genetic diversity. Viruses such as rinderpest virus

(and close relatives such as measles and canine distemper) have limited genetic and antigenic diversity, and infection or vaccination generates long-term immunity. Thus viruses of this type are reliant on continued access to susceptible animal populations for their maintenance, with periodic and regular epidemic or epizootic spread. Control and potential global eradication of rinderpest have been achieved using appropriate management strategies coupled with vaccination of susceptible livestock. In contrast, viruses such as rotaviruses that are constantly enzootic in livestock populations are reliant on genetic diversity and transient host immunity to ensure their perpetuation. These viruses continually circulate and typically cause disease in only some individuals—those that are infected at critical stages when they are most susceptible to infection because of lack of immune protection and other physiological and environmental factors.

Viruses evolve through a variety of mechanisms, but it is to be stressed that the key biological properties of individual virus strains are rarely determined by single nucleotide substitutions. Rather, important differences in the phenotypic properties of individual virus strains (e.g., virulence, tropism, host range) are usually determined by multiple genes as polygenic traits.

Mutation

In productive virus infections of animals, a few virions gain entry and replicate through many cycles, to generate millions or billions of progeny. During such replication cycles, errors in copying the viral nucleic acid inevitably occur, leading to accumulation of mutations. Most mutations involve single nucleotide changes (*syn.* point mutations), but deletions or insertions of several contiguous nucleotides also occur. Mutations are lethal typically because the mutated virus has lost some vital information and can no longer replicate or compete with the wild-type virus. Whether a particular nonlethal mutation survives depends on whether the resultant phenotypic change in its gene product is disadvantageous, neutral, or affords the mutant virus some selective advantage.

Replication of cellular DNA in eukaryotic cells is subject to *proofreading*, an error-correction mechanism involving exonuclease activity. Because the replication of those DNA viruses that replicate in the nucleus is subject to the same proofreading, their mutation rates are probably similar to that of host-cell DNA (a rate of 10^{-10} and 10^{-11} per incorporated nucleotide, i.e., per nucleotide per replication cycle). Error rates during the replication of viral RNAs are much higher than those of viral DNA, in part because of the absence of a cellular proofreading mechanism. For example, the nucleotide substitution rate in the 11-kb genome of the vesicular stomatitis virus is 10^{-3} to 10^{-4} per nucleotide per replication cycle, so that in an infected cell nearly every progeny genome will be different from the parental genome and from every other progeny genome in at least one nucleotide. This rate of nucleotide substitution is about one million times greater than the average rate in eukaryotic DNA. Of course, most of the nucleotide substitutions are deleterious and the genomes containing them are lost. However, non-lethal mutations in the genome of RNA viruses accumulate very rapidly.

Viral Quasispecies Concept of Virus Evolution

Every virus species, as defined by conventional phenotypic properties, exists as a genetically dynamic, diverse population of virions in which individual genotypes have only a fleeting existence. Most individual viral genomes differ, in one or more nucleotides, from the consensus or average sequence of the population; over relatively short times, genotypic drift occurs as particular variants gain advantage. Genotypic drift over longer times leads to the evolution of substantially different viruses. Manfred Eigen, John Holland, and others introduced the term "quasispecies" to describe such diverse, rapidly evolving, and competing virus populations.

The evolution of quasispecies would be expected to be most conspicuous in viruses with large RNA genomes, in which non-lethal changes may accumulate rapidly. Indeed, the genomes of coronaviruses, the largest RNA genomes known, are fraught with "genetic defects." At the mutation rates noted earlier, 1 out of 3000 nucleotides in every coronavirus genome would be changed in every round of replication; because coronavirus genomes contain about 30,000 nucleotides, every genome must differ from the next by at least one nucleotide. Further, coronavirus genomes undergo other more substantial mutations, including large deletions, which affect their pathogenicity. From this, one might wonder how coronaviruses or other RNA viruses can maintain their identities as pathogens over any evolutionarily significant period of time; why have these viruses not mutated out of existence? The answer lies in the quasispecies concept, which is now well accepted for many viruses.

If viral nucleic acid replication was without error, all progeny would be the same and there would be no evolution of phenotypes. If the error rate was too high, mutants of all sorts would appear and the virus population would lose its integrity. However, at an intermediate error rate such as occurs with RNA viruses, the virus population becomes a coherent, self-sustaining entity that resembles a metaphorical cloud of variants centered around a consensus sequence, but capable of continuous expansion and contraction in different directions as new mutants continue to emerge and others disappear within the population. Darwinian selection limits the survival of the most extreme mutants—extreme outliers do not survive—and favors variants near the center of the cloud, as these best achieve environmental "fit." Just as the center of a cloud is unclear, so the consensus sequence at the heart of the quasispecies is inscrutable. Any published viral genomic nucleotide sequence reflects a random choice of starting material: one biological clone among many, more or less representative of the consensus

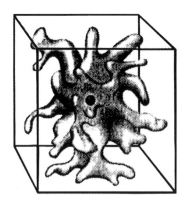

FIGURE 6.1   Depiction of the quasispecies concept of Manfred Eigen. The box represents "sequence space," i.e., the confines of all possible variants that might occur when a virus replicates through many infection cycles. The central spot represents the lack of variance that would follow if the replication process of the virus was perfectly accurate and environmental selective pressures were constant. The *cloud* (also called the *swarm*) represents the viral population diversity that actually follows on an intermediate error rate in replication. The population, overall, becomes a coherent, self-sustaining entity that metaphorically resembles a cloud in that its center, the original consensus sequence, is inscrutable, whereas its edges represent probes pushing into the environment seeking a better-and-better "fit." Viral evolution operates at the level of the quasispecies as a whole, not individual genotypes, and the result is the continuing emergence of new viral phenotypes, some of which cause new or more severe disease. (*Courtesy of C. A. Mims.*)

sequence of the genome of the population as a whole, the cloud as a whole. In Eigen's metaphor, the cloud is the quasispecies—a graphic depiction has been used to try to make this concept more understandable (Figure 6.1).

Genetic Recombination between Viruses

When two different viruses simultaneously infect the same cell, genetic recombination may occur between the nucleic acid molecules during or after their synthesis; this may take the form of intramolecular recombination, reassortment, or reactivation (the latter if one of the viruses had been inactivated).

Intramolecular Recombination

Intramolecular recombination involves the exchange of nucleotide sequences between different, but usually closely related, viruses during replication (Figure 6.2). It occurs with all double-stranded DNA viruses, presumably because of template switching by the polymerase. Intramolecular recombination also occurs among RNA viruses (e.g., picornaviruses, coronaviruses, and togaviruses); western equine encephalitis virus probably arose as a result of intramolecular recombination between an ancient Sindbis-like virus and eastern equine encephalitis virus. Such phenomena are likely to be more widespread among RNA viruses than was appreciated previously. Under experimental conditions, intramolecular recombination may even occur between viruses belonging to different families, as exemplified

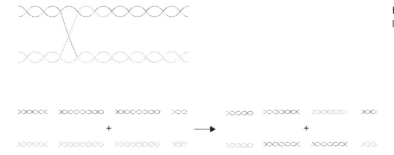

FIGURE 6.2   Genetic recombination: intramolecular recombination, as occurs with double-stranded DNA viruses.

by the now classical discovery of recombination between SV40 (a papovavirus) and adenoviruses.

Recombination between viral and cellular genetic information has been established and, for at least some viruses, is also important in virus evolution. After all, viruses have access to the almost unlimited gene pool of their host cells, and they certainly have the capacity to incorporate and exploit genes that favor their growth and survival. The presence of cellular genes or "pseudogenes" within the genomes of retroviruses is well established, and the same has now been found for other RNA viruses. For example, in influenza virus infections, proteolytic cleavage of the viral hemagglutinin by cellular proteases is essential for the production of infectious progeny. During the adaptation of non-virulent influenza virus strains to chicken cells (which are non-permissive for hemagglutinin cleavage), a pathogenic variant was isolated that contained an insertion of 54 nucleotides that was complementary to a region of host-cell 28S ribosomal RNA. This suggests template switching by the viral polymerase during viral RNA replication. This insertion seems to have changed the conformation of the viral gene product, the hemagglutinin, rendering it accessible to cellular proteases and thereby producing infectious virions in previously non-permissive cells.

The pathogenetic consequences of cellular information being inserted into viruses by intramolecular recombination can be dramatic. The discovery that Marek's disease virus, an oncogenic herpesvirus of chickens, had been misclassified because it carries extra genes was particularly surprising. This virus had been previously considered to be a gammaherpesvirus, partly because all other oncogenic herpesviruses are members of this subfamily. Subsequently, as the genome of the virus was partially sequenced, it was realized that it is an alphaherpesvirus—oncogenic strains of the virus had acquired oncogenic genes either from avian retroviruses or from the cellular homologs of retrovirus genes.

Equally surprising was the discovery of the molecular basis for the progression of bovine viral diarrhea to mucosal disease. When a cellular ubiquitin gene (or various other cell sequences) is inserted into the non-structural gene *NS2-3* of non-cytopathic bovine viral diarrhea virus strains, they become cytopathic in cell culture. Severe disease—that is, mucosal disease—occurs when such mutant viruses develop in the persistently infected animals that are produced through infection of the fetus with non-cytopathic virus strains during the first 80–125 days of gestation. This complex pattern of infection and mutation explains the sporadic occurrence of universally fatal mucosal disease in calves and, in some cases, older animals.

Unlike other RNA viruses, retroviruses have no replicating pool of viral RNA. Although the genome of retroviruses is positive-sense, single-stranded RNA, replication does not occur until the genomic RNA is transcribed into DNA by the virion-associated reverse transcriptase and the resultant double-stranded DNA is integrated into the DNA of the host cell. However, both negative-strand and positive-strand recombinations occur between the two DNA copies of the diploid retrovirus genome, as well as between the DNA provirus and cellular DNA. In the latter instance, the retrovirus may pick up a cellular oncogene; such oncogenes are then incorporated into the viral genome to become viral oncogenes, which confer the property of rapid oncogenicity on the retrovirus concerned (see Chapter 4).

Reassortment

Reassortment is a form of genetic recombination that occurs in RNA viruses with segmented genomes, whether these be single- or double-stranded and whether these involve few or many segments. Reassortment has been documented in families with 2 (*Arenaviridae* and *Birnaviridae*), 3 (*Bunyaviridae*), 6, 7, or 8 (*Orthomyxoviridae*), or 10, 11, or 12 (family *Reoviridae*) genome segments. In a cell infected with two related viruses within each of these families, an exchange of segments may occur, with the production of viable and stable reassortants. Such reassortment occurs in nature and is an important source of genetic variability; for example, bluetongue virus strains are often reassortants, sometimes containing genes similar or identical to those of live-attenuated vaccine viruses.

HOST AND ENVIRONMENTAL DETERMINANTS OF THE EMERGENCE OF VIRAL DISEASES

In order for a new viral disease to emerge, the causative virus must infect and successfully invade its host, bypassing the complex and sophisticated antiviral defenses that have evolved in all animals (see Chapter 4). It is to be stressed that necessary host, virological, and environmental factors must typically coincide for a disease to emerge.

Crossing the Species Barrier— "Species-Jumping"

Genetic variation in viruses (as described earlier) can lead to the emergence of viruses with altered host tropism, either to new animal species or humans. For example, it is proposed that porcine reproductive and respiratory syndrome virus arose from lactate dehydrogenase-elevating virus, presumably after a species-jumping event of the latter virus from mouse to pig. Similarly, phocid distemper, which affects seals, probably originated from a seal that contracted infection from a dog that was shedding canine distemper virus. Influenza A typifies a virus capable of inter-species transmission as a consequence of rapid genetic change as a result of reassortment of gene segments. In addition to the regular and highly publicized transmission of novel influenza A viruses from birds to humans, similar exchange can occur between other animal species—such as the recent transmission of equine influenza virus to dogs.

Zoonotic agents are those that are transmitted from animals to humans, and the majority of new infectious diseases of humans discovered in the past half century or more are zoonoses. Examples include the transmission to humans of a genetic variant of simian immunodeficiency virus that entered and spread amongst the human population as human immunodeficiency virus (HIV); both HIV-1 and HIV-2 are believed to have arisen in humans within the past 100 years, HIV-1 from the chimpanzee and HIV-2 from the sooty mangabey. Although these viruses can experimentally infect non-human primates, they cause no disease. Other important examples include the henipah viruses (Hendra and Nipah), hantaviruses and arenaviruses, flaviviruses such as West Nile and Japanese B encephalitis viruses, the encephalitic equine alphaviruses, and bunyaviruses such as Rift Valley fever virus. In many instances, humans are dead-end hosts that play no part in the natural cycle of virus transmission, whereas in others such as Dengue, influenza A, and HIV, transmission between humans continues after the initial incursion of the virus into the human population.

It is increasingly apparent that bats harbor a number of zoonotic viruses with the potential to cause devastating diseases in humans. Bats are virtually ubiquitous throughout the world, and they frequently co-exist within or adjacent to human populations. Furthermore, bats typically reside in densely populated colonies that readily facilitate animal-to-animal transmission of viruses. Examples of viruses transmitted from bats to humans include rabies and related zoonotic bat lyssaviruses, Nipah and Hendra viruses, SARS coronavirus, and Ebola and Marburg viruses. It is likely that bats also harbor other potentially zoonotic viruses.

Rodents, like bats, occur in virtually every corner of the planet, which they co-inhabit with humans. Rodents are important reservoirs of the hantaviruses that cause hemorrhagic fever with renal syndrome in the Far East and eastern Europe, and hantavirus pulmonary syndrome in the Americas. Similarly, rodents are the asymptomatic reservoir hosts of several arenaviruses that cause viral hemorrhagic fevers of people in portions of South America—for example, Lassa fever, Bolivian hemorrhagic fever, and Argentine hemorrhagic fever. Rodents also serve as reservoir hosts of some arboviruses (e.g., louping ill virus, Venezuelan equine encephalitis virus) that can be transmitted to humans or other animals by the bites of infected vectors (respectively, ticks and mosquitoes).

Birds are also important reservoir hosts of a number of zoonotic viruses, most notably influenza A viruses. Furthermore, birds are the reservoir hosts of a variety of arboviruses, including alphaviruses such as eastern and western equine encephalitis viruses, and flaviviruses such as West Nile virus. Viruses are transmitted from infected birds to humans and animals by the bites of vector mosquito insects. Some of these viruses can cause disease in their bird reservoir hosts, whereas others invariably do not.

Environmental Factors

Ecological change inevitably alters the occurrence and distribution of viral diseases, especially those transmitted by arthropods. Human activities will continue to alter the distribution of viral diseases, both directly through translocation of viruses and their vectors and indirectly through anthropogenic changes such as altered population demographics in response to climate change, the increasing blurring of the urban–rural interface, and destruction of long established ecosystems such as the tropical rain forests of South America.

Bioterrorism

The new world order has led to revised attitudes to biological warfare. In comparison with nuclear weapons and, to a lesser extent, chemical agents of mass destruction, biological agents combine relatively easy availability with maximum potential for destruction and terror. Economic and/or ecological catastrophes in animal populations are possible through the orchestrated and intentional use of several viruses discussed in this book.

SURVEILLANCE, PREVENTION, CONTROL, AND ERADICATION OF VIRAL DISEASES

PRINCIPLES OF DISEASE PREVENTION, CONTROL, AND ERADICATION

The prevention, control, and eradication of veterinary and zoonotic diseases are increasingly more complex in an era of global trade and intertwined political systems (e.g., the European Union, North American Free Trade Agreement, Association of Southeast Asian Nations). Similarly, food production, processing, and distribution systems are also increasingly complex and intertwined, as exemplified by international trade in meat and poultry, dairy products, and seafood and shellfish. With these changes has come increased public awareness of disease risks, and an increasing public expectation of the veterinary medical profession as the global steward of animal health and the related areas of environmental quality, food safety and security, animal welfare, and zoonotic disease control. All these responsibilities will require the application of the principles of preventive medicine, meaning that surveillance and time-honored investigative and disease prevention and control actions will increasingly be required.

Good preventive medicine starts with the local practitioner, on the farm, ranch, feedlot, or poultry house and in the veterinary clinic. In this respect, little has changed: the basic principles of good husbandry, knowledge of the prevalence of specific diseases and how they are transmitted, and the best methods for disinfection, vaccination, and vector control still apply. However, the requisite depth of knowledge of the scientific base underpinning preventive medicine practice is advancing rapidly—in many instances it will be the prevention and control of viral diseases that will lead the way for other veterinary medical risk assessment and risk management activities.

Nowhere in veterinary medicine is the adage "an ounce of prevention is better than a pound of cure" more appropriate than in viral diseases. Apart from supportive therapy such as the administration of fluids for hydration of animals with viral diarrhea or the use of antibiotics to prevent secondary bacterial infections after viral respiratory diseases, there are no effective or practical treatments for most viral diseases of domestic animals, especially for livestock (see Chapter 4). Nevertheless, there are well-proven approaches to the prevention, control, and even the eradication of important viral diseases of animals.

Viral disease prevention and control are based on diverse strategies, each chosen in keeping with the characteristics of the virus, its transmission pattern(s) and environmental stability, and its pathogenesis and threat to animal health, productivity and profitability, zoonotic risk, and so on. Exclusion is increasingly practiced for many pathogenic viruses of production animals, and comprehensive use of vaccines is also widely utilized—not solely for the protection of the individual animal, but to build up a level of population immunity sufficient to break chains of transmission. Hygiene and sanitation measures are especially important in the control of enteric (fecal–oral) infections in kennels and catteries, on farms and ranches, and in commercial aquaculture facilities. Arthropod vector control is the key to regional prevention of several arthropod-borne viral diseases. Test-and-removal programs continue to be used to eradicate important viral diseases of livestock and poultry. The importation of exotic diseases (syn. foreign animal diseases) into countries or regions is prevented by surveillance and quarantine programs. Lastly, following the lead taken in human medicine for the global eradication of smallpox, there is optimism that rinderpest also has been eradicated, and perhaps other diseases can follow.

DISEASE SURVEILLANCE

The implementation of disease control programs and regulatory policy is critically dependent on accurate intelligence on disease incidence, prevalence, transmission, enzootic presence, epizootic spread, and so on. Surveillance of viral diseases provides this basic information; it is the systematic and regular collection, collation, and analysis of data on disease occurrence. Its main purpose is to detect trends—changes in the distribution of diseases.

The need for data on the occurrence of infectious diseases has led to the concept of "notifiable" diseases: veterinary practitioners are required to report to central authorities such as state or national veterinary authorities. In turn, through regional or international agreement such as the World Organization for Animal Health [Office International des Epizooties (OIE)], national authorities may elect, or be obliged, to inform other countries immediately of even the suspicion, let alone confirmation, of disease in their country. Clearly the list of notifiable diseases must be appropriate; if not, notification will be ignored. However, data provided by a system of notification influence decisions on resource allocation for the control of diseases and the intensity of follow-up.

Many countries collect data on diseases that are not notifiable, providing useful data that can be used to develop strategies of prevention, especially by allowing calculations of cost:benefit ratios and indices of vaccine efficacy. Dependent on the characteristics of the disease, the availability of effective vaccines, and sensitivity and specificity of the diagnostic tests, progressive eradication programs can also be planned and implemented, such as the relatively recent eradication of pseudorabies and classical swine fever from many countries.

Sources of Surveillance Data

The methods of surveillance used commonly for animal diseases are: (1) notifiable disease reporting; (2) laboratory-based surveillance; (3) population-based surveillance. The key to surveillance is often the veterinary practitioner. Although any one practitioner may see only a few cases of a particular disease, data from many practitioners can be accumulated and analyzed to reveal spatial and temporal trends in the occurrence of diseases. One key to effective surveillance, especially for exotic or unusual animal diseases, is a sense of heightened awareness among veterinary practitioners—"when you hear hoofbeats, think horses, not zebras" may be good diagnostic advice to clinicians in general, but heightened awareness means that one should not totally dismiss the possibility that the hoofbeats may, indeed, be zebras.

Each country has its own system for collecting and collating data. International agencies such as the World Organization for Animal Health coordinate information exchange between countries. There are several sources of information on disease incidence that are used by veterinary authorities in most countries, not all of which are pertinent in any particular disease:

1. Morbidity and mortality data assessed through information submitted to national, state, and local diagnostic laboratories and made available, with varying degrees of access, through national, regional, and international agencies. Some of these data are published through annual reports, scientific journals, and so on.
2. Information from case and outbreak investigations, again often linked to diagnostic laboratories and state and national veterinary investigations units.
3. Monitoring of virus activity by clinical, pathologic, serologic, and virologic examination of animals presented for slaughter at abattoirs, tested for legal movement, examined in pathology laboratories, or exposed as sentinels to detect virus activity.
4. Monitoring of arthropod populations and viral infection rates and monitoring of sentinel animals to detect arbovirus activity.
5. Specific serologic and virologic surveys.
6. Analyses of vaccine manufacture and use.
7. Reviews of local media reports of disease.
8. List servers, special interest group communications, and other Internet resources.

Having collected data, it is important that they should be analyzed quickly enough to influence necessary follow-up measures. For example, data available from national databases are likely to be reliable and annotated, but often reflect information collected several weeks or even several months earlier. In contrast, information gleaned from reviews of local media and from individual reports of unconfirmed disease on the internet may represent the earliest warning of an impending epizootic or epidemic. However, such sources may provide well-intended, but false, information. Quick action when necessary and dissemination of information, particularly to local veterinary practitioners, is a vital component of effective surveillance systems. Caution must be exercised, however, to avoid unnecessary public alarm.

INVESTIGATION AND ACTION IN DISEASE OUTBREAKS

When there is a disease outbreak, it must first be recognized, frequently at the level of primary veterinary care.

This is not always easy when a new disease occurs or a disease occurs in a new setting. Investigation and actions may be described in the form of a "discovery-to-control continuum." The continuum involves three major phases, each with several elements.

Early Phase

Initial investigation at the first sign of an unusual disease episode must focus on practical characteristics such as mortality, severity of disease, transmissibility, and remote spread, all of which are important predictors of epizootic potential and risk to animal populations. Clinical and pathologic observations often provide key early clues.

Discovery. The precise recognition of a new disease in its host population is the starting point. For diseases that are identified as enzootic or present sporadically in a given animal population, outbreaks are usually handled by veterinary practitioners working directly with producers and owners. For diseases that are identified as exotic or as having epizootic potential, further investigation and action depends on specialized expertise and resources.

Epidemiologic field investigation. Many of the early investigative activities surrounding a disease episode must be carried out in the field, not in the laboratory. This is the world of "shoe-leather epidemiology."

Etiologic investigation. Identification of the etiologic virus is crucial—it is not enough to find a virus; its causative role in the episode must be established.

Diagnostic development. It can be difficult after identifying a causative virus to develop and adapt appropriate diagnostic tests (to detect virus or virus-specific antibodies—see Chapter 5) that can be used in epidemiologic investigations. This requires tests that are accurate (sensitive and specific), reproducible, reliable, and cost-effective, as well as proof-testing of diagnostics in the field in the setting of the specific disease episode.

Intermediate Phase

The continuum progresses to the general area of risk management, the area represented not by the question, "What's going on here?", but by the question, "What are we going to do about it?" This phase may include expansion of many elements.

Focused research. The importance of focused research, aimed at determining more about the etiologic virus, the pathogenesis and pathophysiology of the infection, and related immunologic, ecologic (including vector biology, zoonotic host biology, etc.), and epidemiologic sciences, plays a major role in disease-control programs.

Training, outreach, continuing education and public education. Each of these elements requires professional expertise and adaptation to the special circumstances of the disease locale.

Communications. Risk communications must be of an appropriate scope and scale, utilizing the technologies of the day, including newspapers, radio, television, and the Internet.

Technology transfer. Diagnostics development, vaccine development, sanitation and vector control, and many veterinary care activities require the transfer of information and specialized knowledge to those in need. This is especially true regarding transfer from national centers to local disease-control units.

Commercialization or governmental production. Where appropriate, the wherewithal for the production of diagnostics, vaccines, and so on must be moved from research-scale sites to production-scale sites. This differs in different countries and with different viral diseases.

Late Phase

Actions become increasingly complex as more expensive, specialized expertise and resources come into play.

Animal health systems development. This includes rapid case/herd reporting systems, ongoing surveillance systems, and records and disease registers. It also includes staffing and logistical support such as facilities, equipment, supplies, and transport. Often, the development of legislation and regulation is required. These elements are illustrated by the systems needed to control an outbreak of foot-and-mouth disease in an otherwise free country or region.

Special clinical systems. In some cases, isolation of cases by quarantine (usually requiring legal authorization and enforcement) and special clinical care and herd/flock management are necessary.

Public infrastructure systems. In some cases, new or additional sanitation and sewage systems, clean water supplies, environmental control, and reservoir host and vector control are required, which of necessity involves government or regulatory bodies. The largest epizootics may require substantial resources—for example, limiting the movement of animals on a national or regional scale, test-and-slaughter programs—and similar actions often require special new funding and the involvement of international agencies.

Of course, not all these elements are appropriate in every episode of viral disease; rather, outbreaks of serious or exotic or zoonotic diseases typically evoke the greatest response.

STRATEGIES FOR CONTROL OF VIRAL DISEASES

Disease Control through Hygiene and Sanitation

Intensive animal husbandry leads to accumulation in the local environment of feces, urine, hair, feathers, and so on that may be contaminated with viruses; this is especially problematic

with viruses that are resistant to environmental desiccation. To avoid this, intensive livestock units operate an "all in, all out" management system, by which the animal houses are emptied, cleaned, and disinfected between cohorts of animals. Hygiene and disinfection are most effective in the control of fecal–oral infections; they have much less effect on the incidence of respiratory infections. Efforts to achieve "air sanitation" are generally unsuccessful, especially in intensive animal production systems with high population densities.

Nosocomial Infections

Nosocomial infections are less common in large animal veterinary practices, where animals are usually treated on the farm, than in companion-animal practices. Appropriate management can reduce the likelihood of nosocomial viral infections, and veterinary clinics usually require that all inpatients have current immunization. Clinics should be designed for easy disinfection, with wash-down walls and flooring and as few permanent fixtures as possible. They should also have efficient ventilation and air conditioning, not only to minimize odors, but also to reduce the aerosol transmission of viruses. Frequent hand washing and decontamination of contaminated equipment are essential.

Disinfection and Disinfectants

Disinfectants are chemical germicides formulated for use on inanimate surfaces, in contrast to *antiseptics*, which are chemical germicides designed for use on the skin or mucous membranes. Disinfection of contaminated premises and equipment plays an important part in the control of diseases of livestock.

Viruses of different families vary greatly in their resistance to disinfectants, with enveloped viruses usually being much more sensitive than non-enveloped viruses. Most modern disinfectants inactivate viruses, but their effectiveness is greatly influenced by access and time of exposure: viruses trapped in heavy layers of mucus or fecal material are not inactivated easily. There are special problems when surfaces cannot be cleaned thoroughly or where cracks and crevices are relatively inaccessible, as in old timber buildings or the fence posts and railings of cattle and sheep yards. New data on the effectiveness of standard disinfectants or the release of new products requires access to updated information on the correct use of disinfectants. An excellent resource in this regard is the Center for Food Security & Public Health at Iowa State University (www.cfsph.iastate.edu).

Disease Control through Eliminating Arthropod Vectors

Control of arbovirus infections relies, where possible, on the use of vaccines, because the large areas and extended periods over which vectors may be active make vector control difficult. However, surveillance of vector populations (e.g., mosquito larval counts) and/or the climatic conditions conducive to vector transmissions over wider geographical areas (e.g., remote sensing by satellite imagery for Rift Valley fever in East Africa) provide the justification for local vector control, both as a preventive and as a control strategy. For example, aerial spraying with ultra-low-volume insecticides has been used to prevent the establishment of mosquito populations carrying encephalitis viruses in some parts of North America, although there are issues pertaining to increasing mosquito resistance and environmental objections. Some countries have based their emergency arbovirus control program plans on aerial insecticide spraying. This strategy is aimed at rapid reduction of the adult female mosquito population in a defined area for a very short time.

Organophosphorus insecticides such as malathion or fenitrothion are delivered as an ultra-low-volume (short-acting) aerosol generated by spray machines mounted on backpacks, trucks, or low-flying aircraft. Spraying of the luggage bays and passenger cabins of aircraft with insecticides reduces the chances of intercontinental transfer of exotic arthropods, whether infected or non-infected.

Exclusion of ticks has proven successful in the control of African swine fever in enzootic regions; however, control is difficult in free-ranging animals.

Disease Control through Quarantine

Movement of domestic animals across international and even state borders can be regulated in countries where there are appropriate veterinary services and regulatory infrastructure. Quarantine remains a cornerstone in many animal disease control programs. A period of quarantine, with or without specific etiologic (e.g. PCR) or serologic testing (see Chapter 5), is usually a requirement for the importation of animals from another country and similar requirements may be enforced within a country or region for the control or eradication of specific infectious agents.

As international movement of live animals for breeding purposes and exhibition has increased, so has the risk of introducing disease. Before the advent of air transport, the duration of shipment usually exceeded the incubation period of most diseases, but this is no longer the case. With the ever-increasing value of livestock, national veterinary authorities have tended to adopt stricter quarantine regulations to protect their livestock industries. Complete embargoes on importation are imposed for some animals by some countries. The concept of quarantine (Italian, *quarantina*: originally 40 days during which, in medieval times, ships arriving in port were forbidden to land freight or passengers if there was a suspicion of a contagious disease), whereby animals were simply isolated and observed for clinical signs of disease for a given period of time, is now augmented by extensive laboratory testing designed to detect previous exposure to selected viruses or a carrier state. Laboratory testing requirements are set down in detailed protocols and are supported by national legislation.

Historically the quarantine of animals has been a successful method for preventing the introduction of many diseases; however, other diseases may be introduced in animal products (e.g., foot-and-mouth disease in meat products) or by virus-infected arthropods (e.g., bluetongue). It must also be recognized that most countries have land boundaries with their neighbors and cannot control human and wildlife movement easily, thus countries are expected to confirm their disease status to the World Organization for Animal Health, which is the responsible international body. In addition to its central role in the reporting of livestock diseases globally, this organization also is responsible for harmonizing diagnostic testing and the creation of internationally agreed criteria for the safe movement of animals and animal products. However, problems persist that reflect problems that are often social, economic, and political rather than scientific—for example, smuggling of exotic birds may play a significant role in the introduction of Newcastle disease and fowl plague (highly pathogenic avian influenza) viruses.

Disease Control through Vaccination

Each of the foregoing methods of control of viral diseases is focused on reducing the chances of infection, whereas vaccination is intended to render animals resistant to infection with specific viruses. Furthermore, immunized animals cannot participate in the transmission and perpetuation of such viruses in the population at risk. Thus vaccination can reduce the circulation of virus in the population at risk, as confirmed in countries where there is widespread vaccination of dogs against canine distemper and infectious canine hepatitis. Relaxation of vaccine usage, however, can have devastating consequences, as for example in Finland in the 1990s, when canine distemper virus re-emerged into a dog population in which vaccine usage had declined.

Safe and effective vaccines are available for many common viral diseases of animals. They are especially effective in diseases with a necessary viremic phase, such as canine distemper and feline panleukopenia. It has proved much more difficult to immunize effectively against infections that localize only in the alimentary or respiratory tracts.

Vaccination has been utilized extensively, and with varying success, in programs for the control and/or eradication of certain diseases. For instance, vaccination was key to eradication of rinderpest, but cattle no longer are immunized in previously enzootic regions, so that serological surveillance can be used to detect any re-emergence of the virus. Vaccination has widely been used in efforts to control foot-and-mouth disease in portions of South America and Asia, in conjunction with other disease control activities. The use of genetically engineered vaccines with accompanying serological tests that distinguish vaccinated from naturally infected animals (DIVA) are especially useful in control programs (see Chapter 4).

Influence of Changing Patterns of Animal Production on Disease Control

Relatively recent changes in systems of food animal management and production have had profound effects on disease patterns and control. Systems of animal production for food and fiber are extensive in much of the world, typified by the grazing of sheep and cattle across grasslands as in the Americas and Australia, or by the movement of small herds of cattle or goats across the Sahel by nomadic tribes in Africa. Chickens and swine were penned and housed centuries ago, but intensive animal production systems, particularly for chickens and swine and, to a lesser extent, for cattle and sheep, were established only relatively recently. Concern over the welfare of animals in these intensive units has led to the reintroduction of more traditional husbandry in many countries.

Infectious diseases, particularly viral diseases, have often been the rate- and profit-limiting step in the development of intensive systems. Significant aspects of intensive animal production include the following:

1. The bringing together of large numbers of animals, often from diverse backgrounds, and confining them to limited spaces, at high density.
2. Asynchronous removal of animals for sale and the introduction of new animals.
3. The care of large numbers of animals by few, sometimes inadequately trained, personnel.
4. Elaborate housing systems with complex mechanical systems for ventilation, feeding, waste disposal, and cleaning.
5. Limitation of the husbandry system to one species.
6. Manipulation of natural biologic rhythms (artificial daylight, estrus synchronization, etc.).
7. Use of very large batches of premixed, easily digestible foodstuffs.
8. Improved hygienic conditions.
9. Isolation of animal populations.

Intensive animal production units such as cattle feedlots, swine units, dry-lot dairies, and broiler chicken houses co-localize extraordinarily large numbers of animals in very close proximity. Three consequences follow upon these situations:

1. The conditions favor the emergence and spread of enzootic infectious diseases, as well as opportunistic infections.

2. The introduction of non-enzootic viruses poses a great risk to such populations; although many farms are designed to provide reliable barriers against such introductions, many others are not.
3. These conditions favor several infections working synergistically, further complicating diagnosis, prevention, and therapy.

Disease is a component of the current concerns over welfare in intensive systems, but viral diseases are unlikely to change these intensive livestock production systems because of their economic efficiency. Nevertheless, there is great merit in improving these production systems by minimizing disease losses, thereby increasing yields and lowering costs. The chief constraint is management, with the solution requiring the introduction of modern epidemiologic methods into the training and experience of veterinarians and other animal scientists concerned with livestock production.

The increased adoption of organic farming methods and the traditional extensive farming of livestock that is practiced in many countries increases the possibility of interaction of livestock with other species, and wildlife in particular, e.g. free-range poultry with wild water fowl. Frequent and extensive movement of domestic livestock, wildlife species, and people exacerbates the spread of infectious diseases, especially in regions where wildlife harbor viruses that are contagious to livestock or humans. These are matters of national and international concern, not only for humanitarian reasons, but because of the risk of the international transfer of exotic viruses of livestock.

The situation with companion animals is very different, but the risk of infectious diseases varies greatly between the single, mature-age household dog, cat, or pony and the large, sometimes disreputable, breeding establishments for these species ("puppy farms," for example) in which several hundred animals, of all ages, are kept and bred. Similarly, the movement of horses for athletic events, breeding, and commerce greatly increases the risk of translocation of viral diseases to free regions or countries, as confirmed by recent outbreaks of equine influenza in both Australia and South Africa.

ERADICATION OF VIRAL DISEASES

Disease control, whether by vaccination alone or by vaccination plus the various other methods described earlier, is a continuing process that must be maintained as long as the disease is of economic importance. Successful eradication of a disease that is enzootic often requires a sustained and substantial financial commitment. If a disease can be eradicated within a country so that the virus is no longer present anywhere except in secure laboratories, control measures within that country are no longer required and costs are decreased permanently. Surveillance to prevent the reintroduction of the disease into the country is still necessary. Close cooperation between veterinary services and agricultural industries is essential, which requires that disease eradication programs be justified politically and by cost–benefit and risk–benefit analyses. As programs proceed, they must ensure feedback of information on progress (or problems) directly to those involved and to the public via the media.

Foot-and-mouth disease has now been eradicated from a number of countries in which it was once important, but outbreaks of the disease in previously free countries continue to occur regularly, often with devastating economic consequences. An outbreak in Taiwan in 1997 illustrates vividly the impact of this disease on the agricultural exports of a small country, and is a salient reminder of the importance of this disease. Capitalizing on its geographical advantage of being an island, Taiwan had been free of foot-and-mouth disease since 1929, while most neighboring countries of continental Asia remained enzootic. Before the outbreak, Taiwan had a robust export market of pork to Japan (6 million pigs per year), which represented 70% of its pork exports and approximately 60% of its pig production. The presence of foot-and-mouth disease on the island went unnoticed initially, and when the extent of the epizootic became apparent all exports of pork ceased and international markets were lost. Factors that contributed to the very rapid spread of the virus included high density of pigs and ineffective control of animal and product movement until the epizootic was well into its course. There was no legislation against the feeding of waste food, and several outbreaks probably originated from infected pig products. The procedures used for the disposal of pigs were chaotic, and probably resulted in the dissemination of virus. During the first 100 days of the epizootic, some 60 outbreaks were reported each day—quite a challenge for any veterinary service!

A similar but even more economically devastating outbreak of foot-and-mouth disease occurred in the United Kingdom in 2001, some 34 years after the last such outbreak. The 2001 outbreak precipitated a crisis that led to the slaughter of more than 10 million cattle and sheep, and which had a devastating impact on British agriculture, tourism and the economy: this event is estimated to have cost the British economy up to US$16 billion. Similarly, foot-and-mouth disease very recently has occurred in both South Korea and Japan.

So far, *global* eradication has been achieved for only one disease, and that a disease of humans. The last endemic case of smallpox occurred in Somalia in October 1977. Global eradication was achieved by an intensified effort led by the World Health Organization, which involved a high level of international cooperation and made use of a potent, inexpensive, and very stable vaccine. However, mass vaccination alone could not have achieved eradication of the disease from the densely populated tropical countries, where it remained endemic in the 1970s, because it was impossible to achieve the necessary very high level of vaccine coverage in many remote settings. A revised strategy was implemented in the last years of the eradication campaign, involving surveillance and containment: cases and niches where transmission was current were actively sought out and "ring vaccination" (vaccination of everyone in the area, first in the household and then at increasing distances from the index case) was implemented. The global smallpox eradication campaign was a highly cost-effective operation, especially in light of the ongoing cost for vaccination, airport inspections, and suchlike made necessary by the existence of smallpox, to say nothing of the deaths, misery, and costs of smallpox itself or of the complications of vaccination.

The first animal disease targeted for global eradication is rinderpest. Rinderpest was a devastating disease of cattle in Europe before it was finally eliminated in 1949. It has been a scourge in sub-Saharan Africa ever since livestock farming was introduced in the late 1800s; remarkably, it was very nearly eliminated from Africa in the 1980s by massive cattle vaccination programs, but regional wars and violence interceded, programs were stopped, and the disease made a rapid comeback in many areas. The lessons learned from these vaccination programs, additional lessons from the success in eradicating smallpox and polio, the availability of an effective vaccine and the technology to maintain a cold chain for assuring vaccine potency, and renewed commitment have led to the point that global eradication of rinderpest is now anticipated.

Successful regional/country eradication of velogenic Newcastle disease, fowl plague, classical swine fever, foot-and-mouth disease, infectious bovine rhinotracheitis, pseudorabies, equine influenza, bovine leukemia and even bovine viral diarrhea raises the question of whether there are other animal diseases that might one day be eradicated globally. The viruses that cause diseases most amenable to eradication typically have no uncontrollable reservoirs, they exist as one or few stable serotypes, and safe and efficacious vaccines are available to prevent infection with them.

Part II

Veterinary and Zoonotic Viruses

Poxviridae

Chapter Contents

The family *Poxviridae* includes numerous viruses of veterinary and/or medical importance. Poxviruses are large DNA viruses that are capable of infecting both invertebrates and vertebrates. Poxvirus diseases occur in most animal species, and are of considerable economic importance in some regions of the world. Sheeppox, for example, has been eradicated in many countries, whereas it remains enzootic in Africa, the Middle East, and Asia. A characteristic of many of these viruses is their common ability to induce characteristic "pox" (pockmark) lesions in the skin of affected animals.

The history of poxviruses has been dominated by smallpox. This disease, once a worldwide and greatly feared disease of humans, has now been eradicated by use of the vaccine that traces its ancestry to Edward Jenner and the cowsheds of Gloucestershire in England. Prior to Jenner's innovations, immunization of humans required the dangerous practice of "variolation"—specifically, the deliberate exposure to infectious smallpox virus. Although Jenner's first vaccines probably came from cattle, the origins of modern vaccinia virus, the smallpox vaccine virus, are unknown. In his *Inquiry* published in 1798, Jenner described the clinical signs of cowpox in cattle and humans and how human infection provided protection against smallpox. Jenner's discovery soon led to the establishment of vaccination programs around the world. However, it was not until Pasteur's work nearly 100 years later that the principle was used again—in fact it was Pasteur who suggested the general terms *vaccine* and *vaccination* (from *vacca*, Latin for cow) in honor of Jenner. Other important discoveries came from early research on myxoma virus, an important cause of disease and high mortality in domestic rabbits, described first by Sanarelli in 1896. Myxoma virus is the cause of myxomatosis in European rabbits (*Oryctolagus cuniculus*) and was the first viral pathogen of a laboratory animal to be described. Rabbit fibroma virus was first described in 1932 by Shope, as the cause of large wart-like tumors of the face, feet, and legs of affected North American *Sylvilagus* spp. rabbits, the first virus shown to cause tissue hyperplasia.

With the eradication of smallpox in the second half of the 20th century, use of the smallpox vaccine was discontinued throughout the world. However, vaccinia and other poxviruses are now used as vectors for delivering a wide range of microbial antigens in recombinant DNA vaccines. For example, a vaccinia virus vectored rabies vaccine has been widely used in some enzootic areas, to control rabies in

Fenner's Veterinary Virology. DOI: 10.1016/B978-0-12-375158-4.00007-9

wildlife. Similarly, canarypox virus vectored vaccines have been developed for canine distemper, West Nile, and equine influenza viruses, amongst others, as have recombinant raccoonpox virus vectored vaccines for rabies and feline panleukopenia. Additional potential future uses for poxviruses include gene therapy and tissue-targeted oncolytic viral therapies for cancer treatment.

PROPERTIES OF POXVIRUSES

Classification

The family *Poxviridae* is subdivided into two subfamilies: *Chordopoxvirinae* (poxviruses of vertebrates) and *Entomopoxvirinae* (poxviruses of insects). The subfamily *Chordopoxvirinae* is subdivided into eight genera (Table 7.1). Each of the genera, includes species that cause diseases in domestic or laboratory animals. Because of the large size and distinctive structure of poxvirus virions, negative-stain electron microscopic examination of lesion material is used in many veterinary and zoonotic virology laboratories for diagnosis—this method allows rapid visualization of poxviruses in various specimens, but it does not allow specific verification of virus species or variants. Hence, diagnostic specimens are frequently left with a diagnosis of "poxvirus," "orthopoxvirus," or "parapoxvirus," with further identification only pertaining to the species of origin. Characterization of these viruses with molecular methods will identify additional pathogenic poxvirus species; for example, a poxvirus was recently associated with proliferative gill disease in farmed salmon, and preliminary evaluation is suggestive it is a member of *Entomopoxvirinae*.

Virion Properties

Most poxvirus virions are pleomorphic, typically brick-shaped (220–450 nm × 140–260 nm) wide with an irregular surface of projecting tubular or globular structures, whereas those of the genus *Parapoxvirus* are ovoid (250–300 nm long and 160–190 nm in diameter) with a regular surface (Figure 7.1; Table 7.2). Virions of the members of the genus *Parapoxvirus* are covered with long thread-like surface tubules, which appear to be arranged in crisscross fashion, resembling a ball of yarn. Virions of some ungrouped viruses from reptiles are brick shaped but have a surface structure similar to that of parapoxviruses (Figure 7.1). The virion outer layer encloses a dumbbell-shaped core and two lateral bodies. The core contains the viral DNA, together with several proteins. There is no isometric nucleocapsid conforming to either icosahedral or helical symmetry that is found in most other viruses; hence poxviruses are said to have a "complex" structure. Virions that are released from cells by budding, rather than by cellular disruption, have an extra envelope that contains cellular lipids and several virus-encoded proteins.

The genome of poxviruses consists of a single molecule of linear double-stranded DNA varying in size from 130 kbp (parapoxviruses), to 280 kbp (fowlpox virus), up to 375 kbp (entomopoxviruses). Poxvirus genomes have cross-links that join the two DNA strands at both ends; the ends of each DNA strand have long inverted tandemly repeated nucleotide sequences that form single-stranded loops. Poxviruses have more than 200 genes in their genomes, and as many as 100 of these encode proteins that are contained in virions. Many of the viral proteins with known functions are enzymes involved in nucleic acid synthesis and virion structural components. Examples of the former are DNA polymerase, DNA ligase, RNA polymerase, enzymes involved in capping and polyadenylation of messenger RNAs, and thymidine kinase. The genomes of members of the *Poxviridae* also include a remarkable number of genes encoding proteins that specifically counteract host adaptive and innate immune responses. The activities of these immunomodulating proteins are diverse, and include complement and serine protease inhibitors, proteins that modulate chemokine and cytokine activity, and those that specifically target innate immune pathways such as toll-like receptor complex signaling and interferon-induced antiviral resistance. As an example, poxviruses encode a variety of proteins that modulate chemokine activity by functioning as: (1) chemokine receptor homologs that bind chemokines, (2) biologically inactive chemokine homologs that block authentic cellular receptors, or (3) chemokine binding proteins that neutralize chemokine activity. By interfering with normal chemokine responses and activity, these poxvirus-encoded immunomodulatory proteins inhibit the migration of leukocytes into areas of infection or injury. These proteins have no known mammalian homologs.

Poxviruses are transmitted between animals by several routes: by introduction of virus into skin abrasions, or directly or indirectly from a contaminated environment. Several poxviruses, including sheeppox, swinepox, fowlpox, and myxoma virus, are transmitted mechanically by biting arthropods. Poxviruses are generally indigenous to specific host niches, but, in many cases, they are not species-specific. Poxviruses are resistant in the environment under ambient temperatures, but can survive for many years in dried scabs or other virus-laden material.

Virus Replication

Replication of poxviruses occurs predominantly, if not exclusively, in the cytoplasm. To achieve this independence from the cell nucleus, poxviruses, unlike other DNA viruses, have evolved to encode the enzymes required for

TABLE 7.1 Poxviruses: Host Range and Geographic Distribution

Genus	Virus	Major Hosts	Host Range	Geographic Distribution
Orthopoxvirus	Variola (smallpox) virus	Humans	Narrow	Eradicated globally
	Vaccinia virus	Numerous: humans, cattle,[a] buffalo,[a] swine,[a] rabbits[a]	Broad	Worldwide
	Cowpox virus	Numerous: rodents, domestic cats and large felids, cattle, humans, elephants, rhinoceros, okapi, mongoose	Broad	Europe, Asia
	Camelpox virus	Camels	Narrow	Asia, Africa
	Ectromelia virus	Mice, voles	Narrow	Europe
	Monkeypox virus	Numerous: squirrels, monkeys, anteaters, great apes, humans	Broad	Western and central Africa
	Uasin Gishu disease virus	Horses	Broad	Eastern Africa
	Tatera poxvirus	Gerbils (*Tatera kempi*)	?	Western Africa
	Raccoon poxvirus	Raccoons	Broad	North America
	Volepox virus	Voles (*Microtus californicus*)	?	California
	Skunkpox virus	Skunks (*Mephitis mephitis*)	?	North America
Capripoxvirus	Sheeppox virus	Sheep, goats	Narrow	Africa, Asia
	Goatpox virus	Goats, sheep	Narrow	Africa, Asia
	Lumpy skin disease virus	Cattle, Cape buffalo	Narrow	Africa
Suipoxvirus	Swinepox virus	Swine	Narrow	Worldwide
Leporipoxvirus	Myxoma virus, rabbit fibroma virus	Rabbits (*Oryctolagus* and *Sylvilagus* spp.)	Narrow	Americas, Europe, Australia
	Hare fibroma virus	European hare (*Lepus europaeus*)	Narrow	Europe
	Squirrel fibroma virus	Eastern and western gray (*Sciurus carolinensis*), red (*Tamaiasicuris hudsonicus*), and fox (*S. niger*) squirrels	Narrow	North America
Molluscipoxvirus	Molluscum contagiosum virus	Humans, non-human primates, birds, kangaroos, dogs and equids	Broad	Worldwide
Yatapoxvirus	Yabapox virus and tanapox virus	Monkeys, humans	Narrow	West Africa
Avipoxvirus	Fowlpox virus, canarypox, crowpox, juncopox, mynahpox, pigeonpox, psittacinepox, quailpox, sparrowpox, starlingpox, turkeypox (etc.) viruses	Chickens, turkeys, many other bird species	Narrow	Worldwide
Parapoxvirus	Orf virus	Sheep, goats, humans (related viruses of camels and chamois)	Narrow	Worldwide
	Pseudocowpox virus	Cattle, humans	Narrow	Worldwide
	Bovine papular stomatitis virus	Cattle, humans	Narrow	Worldwide
	Ausdyk virus	Camels	Narrow	Africa, Asia
	Sealpox virus	Seals, humans	Narrow	Worldwide
	Parapoxvirus of red deer	Red deer	Narrow	New Zealand
Currently unclassified	Poxviruses of fish—carp edema and proliferative gill disease viruses	Koi (*Cyprinus carpio*), Atlantic salmon (*Salmo salar*)	Narrow Narrow	Japan, Norway
	Squirrel Poxvirus	Red and gray squirrels	Narrow	Europe and North America

[a]*Infected from humans; now that smallpox vaccination has been discontinued for the civilian populations of all countries, such infections are unlikely to be seen.*

transcription and replication of the viral genome, several of which must be carried in the virion itself. Virus replication begins after fusion of the extracellular enveloped virion with the plasma membrane, or after endocytosis, and the virus core is then released into the cytoplasm where it "uncoats" (Figure 7.2).

Transcription is characterized by a cascade in which the transcription of each temporal class of gene ("early," "intermediate," and "late" genes) requires the presence of specific transcription factors that are transcribed from the preceding temporal class of genes. Intermediate gene transcription factors are encoded by early genes, whereas late

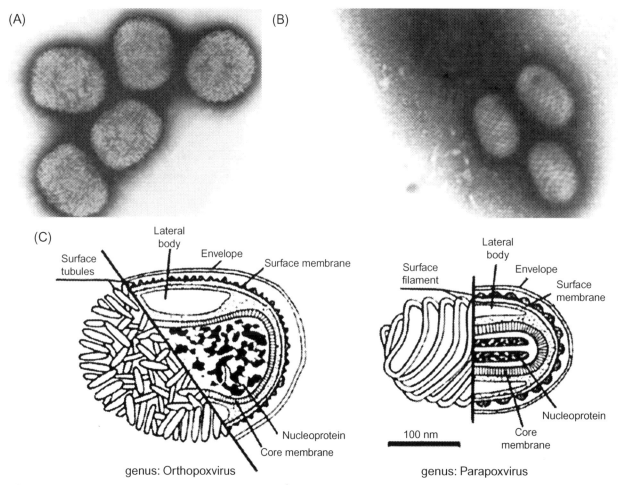

FIGURE 7.1 *Poxviridae* (bar = 100 nm). (A) Negatively stained vaccinia virus virions showing surface tubules characteristic of member viruses of all genera except the genus *Parapoxvirus*. (B) Negatively stained orf virus showing characteristic surface tubules of the member viruses of the genus *Parapoxvirus*. (C, left) Schematic diagram, genus *Orthopoxvirus* (and all other vertebrate poxvirus genera except the genus *Parapoxvirus*). (C, right) Schematic diagram, genus *Parapoxvirus*. Part of the two diagrams shows the surface structure of an unenveloped virion, whereas the other part shows a cross-section through the center of an enveloped virion.

TABLE 7.2 **Properties of Poxviruses**

Virions in most genera are brick-shaped (220–450 × 140–260 nm), with an irregular arrangement of surface tubules. Virions of members of the genus *Parapoxvirus* are ovoid (250–300 × 160–190 nm), with regular spiral arrangement of surface tubules.

Virions have a complex structure with a core, lateral bodies, outer membrane, and sometimes an envelope.

Gernome is composed of a single molecule of linear double-stranded DNA, 170–250 kbp (genus *Orthopoxvirus*), 300 kbp (genus *Avipoxvirus*), or 130–150 kbp (genus *Parapoxvirus*) in size.

Genomes have the capacity to encode about 200 proteins, as many as 100 of which are contained in virions. Unlike other DNA viruses, poxviruses encode all the enzymes required for transcription and replication, many of which are carried in the virion.

Cytoplasmic replication, enveloped virions released by exocytosis; non-enveloped virions released by cell lysis.

transcription factors are encoded by intermediate genes. Transcription is initiated by the viral transcriptase and other factors carried in the core of the virion that mediate the production of messenger RNAs within minutes after infection. These early transcripts are synthesized from both DNA strands, and extruded from the virus core particle before translation by host-cell ribosomes. Proteins produced by translation of these messenger RNAs complete the uncoating of the core and transcription of about 100 early genes; all this occurs before viral DNA synthesis begins. Early

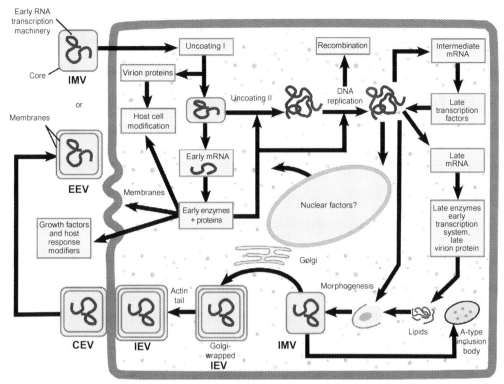

FIGURE 7.2 The infectious cycle of vaccinia virus. IEV, intracellular enveloped virus; EEV, extracellular enveloped virus; CEV, cell-associated enveloped virions; IMV, intracellular mature virus. [*From* Virus Taxonomy: Eighth Report of the International Committee on Taxonomy of Viruses *(C. M. Fauquet, M. A. Mayo, J. Maniloff, U. Desselberger, L. A. Ball, eds.), p. 120. Copyright © Elsevier (2005), with permission.]*

proteins include DNA polymerase, thymidine kinase, and several other enzymes required for replication of the genome. Some viral proteins require post-translational modification by proteolytic cleavage, phosphorylation, glycosylation, etc. Host macromolecular synthesis is inhibited with the production of viral proteins.

Poxvirus DNA replication involves the synthesis of long concatameric intermediates, which are subsequently cut into unit-length genomes that are ultimately covalently linked. With the onset of DNA replication there is a dramatic shift in gene expression. Transcription of "intermediate" and "late" genes is controlled by binding of specific viral proteins to promoter sequences in the viral genome. Some early gene transcription factors are made late in infection, packaged in virions, and used in the subsequent round of infection.

Because poxvirus virions are composed of a very large number of proteins, it is not surprising that virus assembly is a complex process that requires several hours to be completed. Virion formation involves coalescence of DNA within crescent-shaped immature core structures, which then mature by the addition of outer coat layers. Replication and assembly occur in discrete sites within the cytoplasm (called *viroplasm* or virus factories), and virions are released by budding (enveloped virions), by exocytosis, or by cell lysis (non-enveloped virions). Most virions are not enveloped and

are released by cell lysis. Both enveloped and non-enveloped virions are infectious, but they apparently infect cells by different pathways; enveloped virions are taken up by cells more readily and appear to be more important in the spread of virions through the body of the animal.

MEMBERS OF THE GENUS *ORTHOPOXVIRUS*

VACCINIA VIRUS AND BUFFALOPOX VIRUS

Because of its widespread use and its wide host range, vaccinia virus sometimes has caused naturally spreading diseases in domestic animals (e.g., teat infections of cattle) and also in laboratory rabbits ("rabbitpox"). Outbreaks of disease associated with "vaccinia-like" viruses (Aracatuba and Cantagalo viruses) have been reported among dairy cattle and humans in Brazil, and genetic analyses of selected viral genes showed these viruses to be related most closely to vaccinia virus. Before human vaccination against smallpox had been discontinued, putative instances of cowpox were frequently caused by vaccinia virus infection.

Outbreaks of buffalopox affecting buffalos, cows, and humans have been recorded regularly in the Indian subcontinent and Egypt. The causative agent is an orthopoxvirus that is related so closely to the vaccinia virus that it is considered a clade. The disease is characterized by pustular lesions on the teats and udders of milking buffalo. Lesions also can occur at the base of the ear and in the inguinal region. Rarely, especially in calves, a generalized disease occurs. Outbreaks still occur in India (even though vaccinia virus is not used for any type of vaccination in the country), sometimes producing lesions on the hands and face of milkers who are no longer protected by vaccination against smallpox.

COWPOX VIRUS

Inappropriately named, cowpox virus has as its reservoir hosts rodents, from which the virus occasionally spreads to domestic cats, cows, humans, and zoo animals, including large felids (especially cheetahs, ocelots, panthers, lynx, lions, pumas, and jaguars), anteaters, mongooses, rhinoceroses, okapis, and elephants. Cowpox virus infection is enzootic in Europe and adjacent regions of Russia. During an outbreak at the Moscow zoo, the virus was also isolated from laboratory rats used to feed the big cats, and a subsequent survey demonstrated infection in wild susliks (*Spermophilus citellus* and *S. suslicus*) and gerbils (*Rhombomys opimus*) in Russia. In Germany, transmission of cowpox virus occurred from rat to elephant to human. The elephant exhibited disseminated ulcerative lesions of the skin and mucosal membranes. In the United Kingdom, the reservoir species are bank voles (*Clethrionomys glareolus*), field voles (*Microtus agrestis*), and wood mice (*Apodemus sylvaticus*). Zoonotic transmission of cowpox virus from pet rats has been reported with increasing frequency from several countries in Europe. Lesions in humans usually appear as single maculopapular eruptions on the hands or the face with minimal systemic reaction, except in immunosuppressed patients.

Clinical cowpox disease in cattle is extremely rare, but occurs sporadically in enzootic areas. Cowpox virus produces lesions on the teats and the contiguous parts of the udder of cows, and is spread through herds by the process of milking. Cowpox virus infection in domestic cats is often a more severe disease than in cattle or humans. There is typically a history of a single primary lesion manifest as necrotizing dermatitis, generally on the head or a forelimb, but by the time the cat is presented for veterinary attention, widespread skin lesions have usually developed. Pulmonary infection and even disseminated systemic infection sometimes occur in cats, typically with fatal consequences.

Cowpox virus, like smallpox, monkeypox and other pathogenic orthopoxviruses, encodes a unique family of ankyrin repeat-containing proteins that inhibit the nuclear factor κB (NF-κB) signaling pathway and so inhibit inflammation at the sites of viral infection.

CAMELPOX VIRUS

Camelpox virus infection causes a severe generalized disease in camels and dromedaries that is characterized by extensive skin lesions. It is an important disease, especially in countries of Africa, the Middle East, and southwestern Asia, where the camel is used as a beast of burden and for milk. The more severe cases usually occur in young animals, and in epizootics the case-fatality rate may be as high as 25%. The causative virus is a distinctive orthopoxvirus species, and comparative genome analysis shows camelpox virus to be closely related to other orthopoxviruses, including variola virus (smallpox virus). Genomic differences that distinguish camelpox from other orthopoxviruses occur in genes that probably determine either host range or virulence. Camelpox virus has a narrow host range, and despite the frequent exposure of unvaccinated humans to florid cases of camelpox, human infection has not been described. A parapoxvirus (Ausdyk virus) also infects camels, producing a disease that can be confused with camelpox (Table 7.1).

ECTROMELIA VIRUS (MOUSEPOX VIRUS)

Ectromelia virus, the cause of mousepox, has been spread around the world inadvertently in shipments of laboratory mice and mouse products, and has been repeatedly reported from laboratories in the United States, Europe, and Asia. Outbreaks in mouse colonies in the United States have resulted from importation of infected mice or products from other countries—for example, via mouse tumor material and commercial sources of mouse serum from China. The origin of ectromelia virus remains a mystery. It first appeared in a laboratory mouse colony in England, involving mice with amputation of limbs and tails. The name is derived from the Greek designations *ectro*, which means abortion, and *melia*, which means limb (Figure 7.3). The disease has since spread throughout the world, but its occurrence is sporadic and rare.

There are several named strains of ectromelia virus that vary in virulence, including NIH-79, Wash-U, Moscow,

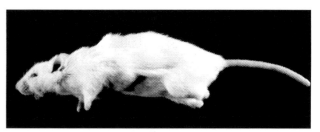

FIGURE 7.3 Ectromelia: healed amputating lesions of the distal extremities of a mouse that survived natural ectromelia virus infection. [*From* Pathology of Laboratory Rodents and Rabbits, *D. H. Percy, S. W. Barthold, 3rd ed., p. 127. Copyright © Wiley-Blackwell (2007), with permission.*]

Hampstead, St. Louis-69, Bejing-70, and Ishibashi I–III. Disease severity is determined by virus strain, but mouse genotype and age are also important determinants. Susceptible mouse strains include C3H, A, DBA, SWR, CBA, and BALB/c. Resistant mouse strains include AKR and C57BL/6. Infection is acquired primarily through skin abrasions and direct contact. Virus may be shed from skin, respiratory secretions, feces, and urine. Highly susceptible genotypes of mice develop disseminated infection, but die rapidly within hours and shed little virus. Highly resistant genotypes of mice develop more limited infections and recover before shedding virus. Mice with intermediate susceptibility are therefore critical for outbreaks of disease, in that they develop disseminated infections and survive long enough to spread virus to other animals. Under these circumstances, such mice develop multifocal necrotizing lesions in all organs, particularly liver, lymphoid tissues, and spleen, as well as disseminated rash and gangrene of limbs. Necrosis of Peyer's patches in the intestine may result in intestinal hemorrhage. Colonies that contain mice of various genotypes and immune perturbations are most at risk for high mortality, in that they may contain semi-susceptible mice that sustain infection, and highly susceptible mice that contribute to high mortality. Under these circumstances, the typical clinical picture within the population is a spectrum of clinical disease, ranging from subclinical infections to high mortality.

The consequences of the introduction of ectromelia virus into a mouse colony are sufficiently serious that rapid and definitive diagnosis is required. Mousepox can be diagnosed by the histopathologic examination of tissues of suspected cases, its diagnostic features being the typical clinical signs and gross lesions and, histologically, the presence of multifocal necrosis of many tissues, with distinctive eosinophilic cytoplasmic inclusion bodies in epithelial cells at the edges of skin lesions and mucosa. Electron microscopy is also a valuable diagnostic adjunct: distinctive virions may be seen in any infected tissue. Virus may be isolated in mouse embryo cell cultures and identified by immunological means.

Because mice are infected readily by inoculation, virus-contaminated mouse serum, hybridoma lines, transplantable tumors, or tissues constitute a risk to laboratory colonies previously free of infection. Prevention and control of mousepox are based on quarantine and regulation of the importation and distribution of ectromelia virus, mice, and materials that may be carrying the virus. However, because such precautions offer no protection against unsuspected sources of infection, regular serologic testing (enzyme-linked immunosorbent assay) is performed in many colonies housing valuable animals. In immunocompetent strains of mice, infection is acute and animals recover with no carrier status. Thus seropositive animals can be quarantined, held without breeding for a few weeks, and then used to re-establish breeding colonies. Vaccination with vaccinia virus (IHD-T strain) has been used to protect valuable colonies against severe clinical disease, but vaccination will not prevent ectromelia virus infection or transmission. Vaccination, however, will also obscure serosurveillance, because vaccinia virus is transmissible among mice and may remain enzootic within the population.

MONKEYPOX VIRUS

Monkeypox virus is a zoonotic agent with a broad host range that includes humans. Outbreaks of human disease occur in villages in the tropical rain forests of west and central Africa, especially in the Democratic Republic of Congo. The virus was discovered in 1958, when it was isolated from pox lesions of cynomolgus macaques imported into Denmark. The first human cases were recognized in the 1970s. The signs and symptoms are very like those of smallpox, with a generalized pustular rash, fever, and lymphadenopathy. Monkeypox virus is acquired by humans by direct contact with wild animals killed for food, especially squirrels and monkeys. The virus is maintained in rodents and non-human primate species.

The human disease is relatively uncommon, although more than 500 human cases were reported in the Congo in 1996–1997, the largest reported outbreak of the disease. In 2003, a widely publicized outbreak of monkeypox virus infection occurred in the United States. In this outbreak, monkeypox virus was transmitted from imported African rodents [*Funisciurus* spp. (rope squirrel), *Cricetomys* spp. (giant pouched rat), and *Graphiurus* spp. (African dormouse)] to co-housed prairie dogs (*Cynomys* spp.). Infected prairie dogs then transmitted the virus to humans. A total of 82 infections in children and adults occurred during the outbreak, which subsequently resulted in a ban on the importation of African rodents into the United States.

MEMBERS OF THE GENUS *CAPRIPOXVIRUS*

SHEEPPOX VIRUS, GOATPOX VIRUS, AND LUMPY SKIN DISEASE (OF CATTLE) VIRUS

Although the geographic distribution of sheeppox, goatpox, and lumpy skin disease is very different, suggesting that they are caused by distinct viruses, the causative viruses are indistinguishable by conventional serological assays and are genetically very similar. The African strains of sheeppox and lumpy skin disease viruses are related more closely to each other than sheeppox virus is to goatpox virus. Although sheeppox and goatpox are considered to be host specific, in parts of Africa where sheep and goats are herded together, both animal species may show clinical signs during an outbreak, indicating that some virus strains may infect both sheep and goats.

Sheeppox, goatpox and lumpy skin diseases are considered to be the most important of all pox diseases of domestic animals, because they cause significant economic loss and high mortality in young and/or immunologically naïve animals. Furthermore, these viruses are currently expanding their distribution, with recent outbreaks of sheeppox or goatpox in Vietnam, Mongolia, and Greece, and outbreaks of lumpy skin disease in Ethiopia, Egypt, and Israel (Figure 7.4).

Lumpy skin disease affects cattle breeds derived from both *Bos taurus* and *Bos indicus*, and was first recognized in an extensive epizootic in Zambia in 1929. An epizootic in 1943–1944 that involved other countries, including South Africa, emphasized the importance of this disease, which remained restricted to southern Africa until 1956, when it spread to central and eastern Africa. Since the 1950s, the virus has continued to spread progressively throughout Africa, first north to the Sudan and subsequently westward, to appear by the mid-1970s in most countries of western Africa. In 1988, the disease was confirmed in Egypt, and in 1989 a single outbreak occurred in Israel, the first report outside the African continent.

Clinical Features and Epidemiology

In common with most poxviruses, environmental contamination can lead to the introduction of sheep or goat poxvirus into small skin wounds. Scabs that have been shed by infected sheep remain infective for several months. The common practice of herding sheep and goats into enclosures at night in countries where the disease occurs provides sufficient exposure to maintain enzootic infection. During an outbreak, the virus is probably transmitted between sheep by respiratory droplets; there is also evidence that mechanical transmission by biting arthropods, such as stable flies, may

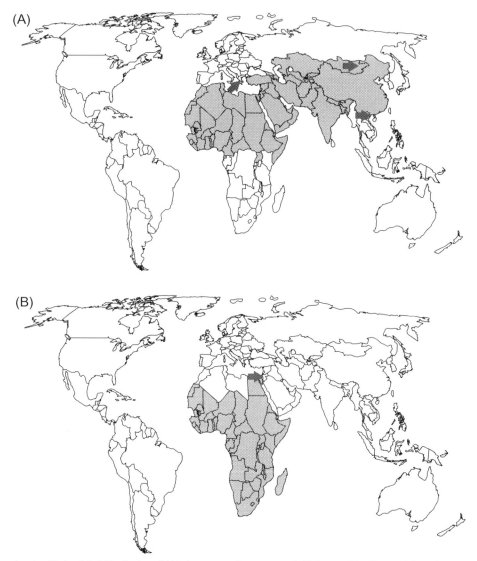

FIGURE 7.4 Map showing likely global distribution of (A) sheeppox and goatpox, and (B) lumpy skin disease (LSD) viruses. Recent outbreaks are marked with arrows. *[From S. L. Babiuk, T. R. Bowden, S. B. Boyle, D. B. Wallace, R. P. Kitchen. Capripoxviruses: an emerging worldwide threat to sheep, goats and cattle.* Transbound. Emerg Dis. **55**, *263–272 (2008), with permission.]*

be important. Lumpy skin disease has shown the potential to spread outside continental Africa. It is likely that the virus is transmitted mechanically between cattle by biting insects, with the virus being perpetuated in a wildlife reservoir host, possibly the African Cape buffalo. Because it is transmitted principally by insect vectors, the importation of wild ruminants to zoos could establish new foci of infection, if suitable vectors were available.

Clinical signs vary in different hosts and in different geographical areas, but the signs of sheeppox, goatpox, and lumpy skin disease of cattle are similar. Sheep and goats of all ages may be affected, but the disease is generally more severe in young and/or immunologically naïve animals. An epizootic in a susceptible flock of sheep can affect over 75% of the animals, with mortality as high as 50%; case-fatality rates in young and/or naïve sheep may approach 100%. After an incubation period of 4–8 days, there is an increase in temperature, an increase in respiratory rate, edema of the eyelids, and a mucous discharge from the nose. Affected

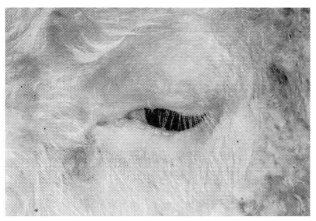

FIGURE 7.5 Sheeppox, with characteristic raised skin lesions. *(Courtesy of D. Rock, University of Illinois.)*

sheep may lose their appetite and stand with an arched back. One to 2 days later, cutaneous nodules about 1 cm in diameter develop; these may be distributed widely over the body (Figure 7.5). These lesions are most obvious in the areas of skin where the wool hair is shortest, such as the head, neck, ears, axillae, and under the tail. These lesions usually scab and persist for 3–4 weeks, healing to leave a permanent depressed scar. Lesions within the mouth affect the tongue and gums, and ulcerate. Such lesions constitute an important source of virus for infection of other animals. In some sheep, lesions that develop in the lungs progress to multicentric areas of pulmonary fibrosis and consolidation. Goatpox is similar clinically to sheeppox.

Lumpy skin disease of cattle is characterized by fever, followed shortly by the development of nodular lesions in the skin that subsequently undergo necrosis (Figure 7.6). Generalized lymphadenitis and edema of the limbs are common. During the early stages of the disease, affected cattle show lacrimation, nasal discharge, and loss of appetite. The skin nodules involve the dermis and epidermis; they are raised and later ulcerate, and may become infected secondarily. Ulcerated lesions may be present in the mouth and nares. Healing is slow and affected cattle often remain debilitated for several months (Figure 7.6). Morbidity in susceptible herds can be as high as 100%, but mortality is rarely more than 1–2%. The economic importance of the disease relates to the prolonged convalescence and, in this respect, lumpy skin disease is similar to foot-and-mouth disease.

Pathogenesis and Pathology

Sheeppox, goatpox, and lumpy skin disease viruses all have tropism for epithelial cells. Sheeppox and goatpox virus infection in immunologically naïve animals leads to concurrent fever and skin papules, followed by rhinitis,

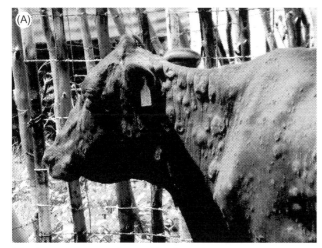

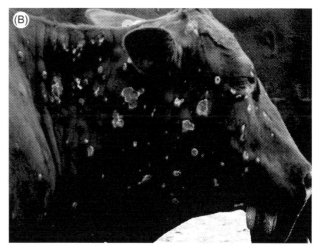

FIGURE 7.6 (A) Acute lumpy skin disease in cattle. (B) Animal approximately 2 months after infection with lumpy skin disease virus. *(Courtesy of M. Scacchia, Namibia.)*

conjunctivitis, and hypersalivation. Although pox lesions can be widespread, the more common presentation is a few nodules beneath the tail. Pox lesions also develop in the lungs and gastrointestinal tract. High viral loads occur in the skin and viremia is probably cell associated. Lesions seen at necropsy include tracheal congestion and patchy discoloration of the lungs. The spleen and lymph nodes are enlarged, with multifocal to coalescing areas of necrosis. The essential histological lesion is necrosis, with depletion of lymphocytes in the paracortical regions and absence of germinal centers in the spleen and lymph nodes.

Lumpy skin disease is most commonly recognized by widespread skin lesions. Disease is characterized by fever, lymphadenopathy, and skin nodules that persist for many months. Certain breeds of cattle such as Jersey and Guernsey have enhanced susceptibility.

Diagnosis

Apart from occasional outbreaks in partly immune flocks—in which the disease may be mild—or when the presence of orf (contagious ecythema) complicates the diagnosis, sheeppox and goatpox present little difficulty in clinical diagnosis. For presumptive laboratory diagnosis, negative-contrast electron microscopy can be used to demonstrate virions in clinical material, as the virions are indistinguishable from those of vaccinia virus. The viruses can be isolated in various cell cultures derived from sheep, cattle, or goats; the presence of virus is indicated by cytopathology and cytoplasmic inclusion bodies. The clinical diagnosis of lumpy skin disease also presents few problems to clinicians familiar with it, although the early skin lesions can be confused with generalized skin infections of pseudo lumpy skin disease, caused by bovine herpesvirus 2.

Immunity, Prevention, and Control

Control of sheeppox, goatpox, and lumpy skin disease in free countries is by exclusion; these are notifiable diseases in most countries of the world, with any suspicion of disease requiring disclosure to appropriate authorities. Control in countries where the diseases are enzootic is by vaccination; attenuated virus and inactivated virus vaccines are used. Two vaccines are currently available: in South Africa an attenuated virus vaccine (Neethling) is used, and in Kenya a strain of sheep/goatpox virus propagated in tissue culture has been used.

MEMBERS OF THE GENUS *SUIPOXVIRUS*

SWINEPOX VIRUS

Swinepox virus is the sole member of the *Suipoxvirus* genus within the subfamily *Chordopoxvirinae*. Swinepox-virus-induced disease occurs worldwide and is associated with poor sanitation. Comparative genetic analyses indicate that swinepox virus is most closely related to lumpy skin disease virus, followed by yatapoxvirus and leporipoxviruses. Many outbreaks of poxvirus disease in swine have been caused by vaccinia virus, but swinepox virus is now the primary cause of the disease. Swinepox is most severe in pigs up to 4 months of age, in which morbidity may approach 100%, whereas adults usually experience a mild disease with lesions restricted to the skin. The typical "pox" lesions may occur anywhere, but are most obvious on the skin of the abdomen. A transient low-grade fever may precede the development of papules which, within 1–2 days, become vesicles and then umbilicated pustules, 1–2 cm in diameter. The pocks crust over and scab by 7 days; healing is usually complete by 3 weeks. The clinical picture is characteristic, so laboratory confirmation is seldom required.

Swinepox virus is transmitted most commonly between swine by the bite of the pig louse, *Hematopinus suis*, which is common in many herds; the virus does not replicate in the louse, but sporadic vertical transmission has been reported. No vaccines are available for swinepox, which is controlled most easily by elimination of the louse from the affected herd and by improved hygiene. As with other poxviruses of livestock, swinepox virus is being developed as a recombinant vaccine vector for expression of heterologous genes.

MEMBERS OF THE GENUS *LEPORIPOXVIRUS*

MYXOMA VIRUS, RABBIT FIBROMA VIRUS, AND SQUIRREL FIBROMA VIRUS

Myxoma virus causes localized benign fibromas in its natural hosts, wild rabbits in the Americas (*Sylvilagus* spp.); in contrast, it causes a severe generalized disease in European rabbits (*Oryctolagus cuniculus*), with a very high mortality rate. Myxoma virus originated in the Americas, but is now enzootic on four continents: North and South America, Europe, and Australia. The characteristic early signs of myxomatosis in the European rabbit are blepharoconjunctivitis and swelling of the muzzle and anogenital region, giving animals a leonine appearance (Figure 7.7). Infected rabbits become febrile and listless, and often die within 48 hours of onset of clinical signs. This rapid progression and fatal outcome are seen especially with the California strain of myxoma virus. The myxoma virus genome encodes a number of immunomodulatory proteins that target host cytokines, host-cell signaling cascades, and apoptosis, and these probably contribute to the virulence of individual virus strains. In rabbits that survive longer, subcutaneous gelatinous swellings (hence the name *myxomatosis*) appear all over the body within 2–3 days. The vast majority of rabbits (over 99%) infected from a wild (*Sylvilagus* spp.) source of myxoma virus die within 12 days of infection. Transmission

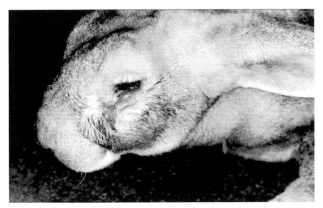

FIGURE 7.7 Myxomatosis in a laboratory rabbit (*Oryctolagus cuniculus*), showing generalized facial lesions. (*Courtesy of S. Barthold and D. Brooks, University of California.*)

can occur via respiratory droplets, but more often via mechanical transmission by arthropods (mosquitoes, fleas, black flies, ticks, lice, mites).

Diagnosis of myxomatosis in European rabbits can be made by the clinical appearance or virus isolation in rabbits, on the chorioallantoic membrane of embryonated hens' eggs, or in cultured rabbit or chicken cells. Electron microscopy of exudates or smear preparations from lesions reveals virions morphologically indistinguishable from those of vaccinia virus.

Laboratory or hutch rabbits can be protected against myxomatosis by inoculation with the related rabbit fibroma virus or with attenuated myxoma virus vaccines developed in California and France.

Myxoma virus was the first virus ever introduced into the wild with the purpose of eradicating a vertebrate pest, namely the feral European rabbit in Australia in 1950, and in Europe 2 years later. History confirms the long-term failure of this strategy.

Although myxoma virus receives the most attention, there are many antigenically distinct but related poxviruses of wild *Oryctolagus* and *Sylvilagus* rabbits and *Lepus* spp. hares in Europe and the Americas, including rabbit fibroma virus (or Shope fibroma virus), hare fibroma virus, and myxoma virus. Myxoma virus is considered a variant of rabbit fibroma virus; indeed, California myxoma virus is also termed "California rabbit fibroma virus." Myxoma and rabbit fibroma viruses originated in the Americas, whereas hare fibroma virus was originally indigenous to Europe. All leporid species are susceptible to infection with these various leporipoxviruses. Less virulent viruses and those that infect their natural hosts tend to produce localized fibromatous lesions, whereas virulent isolates tend to produce myxomatous lesions in aberrant *Oryctolagus* hosts.

American gray squirrels (*Sciurus* spp.) and red squirrels (*Tamiasciurus* spp.) develop natural outbreaks of squirrel fibromatosis as a result of a virus that is closely related to myxoma and rabbit fibroma leporipoxviruses. The animals develop multifocal to coalescing, nodular, tan cutaneous lesions, often involving the head, and disseminated lesions in internal organs, characterized by focal proliferation of mesenchymal cells with cytoplasmic inclusions. Natural outbreaks of squirrel fibromatosis occur periodically in some regions of the United States, resulting in declines in squirrel populations.

MEMBERS OF THE GENUS *MOLLUSCIPOXVIRUS*

MOLLUSCUM CONTAGIOSUM VIRUS

Molluscum contagiosum virus is a human pathogen, but it has been documented as naturally producing similar lesions in birds (chickens, sparrows, and pigeons), chimpanzees, kangaroos, dogs, and horses, among other species. Infection is characterized by multiple discrete nodules 2–5 mm in diameter, limited to the epidermis, and occurring anywhere on the body except on the soles and palms. The nodules are pearly white or pink in color and painless. The disease may last for several months before recovery occurs. Cells in the nodule are hypertrophied greatly and contain pathognomonic large hyaline acidophilic cytoplasmic masses called molluscum bodies. These consist of a spongy matrix divided into cavities, in each of which are clustered masses of virus particles that have the same general structure as those of vaccinia virus. The disease is seen most commonly in children and occurs worldwide, but is much more common in some localities—for example, parts of the Democratic Republic of Congo and Papua New Guinea. The virus is transmitted by direct contact, perhaps through minor abrasions and sexually in adults. In developed countries, communal swimming pools and gymnasiums have been sources of contagion. Infection in animals is rare, and is typically associated with human contact.

MEMBERS OF THE GENUS *YATAPOXVIRUS*

YABAPOX AND TANAPOX VIRUSES

Yabapox and tanapox occur naturally only in tropical Africa. The yabapox virus was discovered because it produced large benign tumors on the hairless areas of the face, on the palms and interdigital areas, and on the mucosal surfaces of the nostrils, sinuses, lips, and palate of Asian monkeys (*Cercopithecus aethiops*) kept in a laboratory in Nigeria. Subsequent cases occurred in primate colonies in California, Oregon, and Texas. Yabapox is believed to cause epizootic infection in African and Asian monkeys. The virus is zoonotic, spreading to humans in contact with diseased monkeys and causing similar lesions as in affected monkeys.

Tanapox is a relatively common skin infection of humans in parts of Africa, extending from eastern Kenya to the Democratic Republic of Congo. It appears to be spread mechanically by insect bites from an unknown wild animal reservoir, probably a species of monkey. In humans, skin lesions start as papules that progress to vesicles. There is usually a febrile illness lasting 3–4 days, sometimes with severe headache, backache, and prostration.

MEMBERS OF THE GENUS *AVIPOXVIRUS*

FOWLPOX AND OTHER AVIAN POXVIRUSES

Serologically related poxviruses that specifically infect birds have been recovered from lesions in all species of poultry and many species of wild birds, with natural pox virus infections having been described in 232 species in 23 orders of birds. Viruses recovered from various species of birds are given names pertaining to their respective hosts, such as fowlpox (chickens), canarypox, turkeypox, pigeonpox, magpiepox, etc. Differences in the genome sequences and biological properties of individual viruses confirm that there are several different species of avian poxviruses. Mechanical transmission by arthropods, especially mosquitoes, provides a mechanism for transfer of the viruses between different species of birds.

Fowlpox is a serious disease of poultry that has occurred worldwide for centuries. Fowlpox virus is highly infectious for chickens and turkeys, rarely so for pigeons, and not at all for ducks and canaries. In contrast, turkeypox virus is virulent for ducks. There are two forms of fowlpox, probably associated with different routes of infection. The most common form, the *cutaneous form*—which probably results from infection by biting arthropods or mechanical transmission to injured or lacerated skin—is characterized by small papules on the comb, wattles, and around the beak; lesions occasionally develop on the legs and feet and around the cloaca. The nodules become yellowish and progress to a thick dark scab. Multiple lesions often coalesce. Involvement of the skin around the nares may cause nasal discharge, and lesions on the eyelids can cause excessive lacrimation and predispose poultry to secondary bacterial infections. In uncomplicated cases, healing occurs within 3 weeks. The second form of fowlpox is probably caused by droplet infection and involves infection of the mucous membranes of the mouth, pharynx, larynx, and sometimes the trachea (Figure 7.8A). This is often referred to as the *diphtheritic* or *wet form* of fowlpox because the lesions, as they coalesce, result in a necrotic pseudomembrane, which can cause death by asphyxiation. The prognosis for this form of fowlpox is poor. Extensive infection in a flock may cause a slow decline in egg production. Cutaneous infection causes little mortality, and these flocks return to normal production on recovery. Recovered birds are immune.

Under natural conditions there may be breed differences in susceptibility; chickens with large combs appear to be

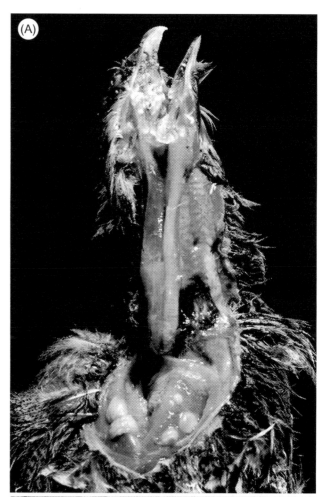

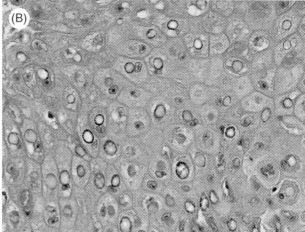

FIGURE 7.8 Avian poxvirus disease. (A) Avian pox affecting the oral cavity and stomach. (B) Histological appearance of avian pox disease; epidermal hyperplasia with characteristic eosinophilic (red) intracytoplasmic inclusion bodies. *(A: Courtesy of L. Woods, University of California.)*

more affected than those with small combs. The mortality rate is low in healthy flocks, but in laying flocks and in chickens in poor condition or under stress the disease may assume serious proportions with mortality rates of 50% or even higher, although such mortality is rare.

The cutaneous form of fowlpox seldom presents a diagnostic problem. The diphtheritic form is more difficult to diagnose, because it can occur in the absence of skin lesions and may be confused with vitamin A, pantothenic acid, or biotin deficiency, T-2 mycotoxicosis-induced contact necrosis, and several other respiratory diseases caused by viruses such as infectious laryngotracheitis herpesvirus. Histopathology and electron microscopy are used to confirm the clinical diagnosis. Typical lesions include extensive, local hyperplasia of the epidermis and underlying feather follicle epithelium, with accompanying ulceration and scabbing. Histologically, the hyperplastic epithelium contains cells with characteristic large, intracytoplasmic eosinophilic inclusion bodies (Figure 7.8B). The virus can be isolated by the inoculation of avian cell cultures or the chorioallantoic membrane of embryonated eggs.

Fowlpox virus is extremely resistant to desiccation: it can survive for long periods under the most adverse environmental conditions in exfoliated scabs. The virus is transmitted within a flock through minor wounds and abrasions, by fighting and pecking, mechanically by mosquitoes, lice, and ticks, and possibly by aerosols.

Several types of vaccine are available. Non-attenuated fowlpox virus and pigeonpox virus vaccines prepared in embryonated hens' eggs and attenuated virus vaccines prepared in avian cell cultures are widely used for vaccination. Vaccines are applied by scarification of the skin of the thigh. One vaccine can be administered in drinking water. In flocks with enzootic infection, birds are vaccinated during the first few weeks of life and again 8–12 weeks later. Recombinant vaccines for poultry have been developed using either fowlpox or canarypox viruses as vectors. In poultry, fowlpox-vectored vaccines have been licensed with gene inserts for Newcastle disease virus (paramyxovirus), H5 and H7 avian influenza virus (orthomyxoviruses), infectious laryngotracheitis (herpesvirus), infectious bursal disease virus (birnavirus), and *Mycoplasma* spp. These viruses have also been utilized as vaccine vectors in mammals.

Other than fowlpox, the most economically significant reports of pox have been canarypox, turkeypox, quailpox, and psittacinepox in Amazon parrots. These poxvirus infections are typically the cutaneous form, but in canaries the cutaneous form is rare and the systemic form is common and may produce 80–90% mortality. In canaries, the systemic disease presents with hepatic necrosis and pulmonary nodules. Vaccination is practiced in canary aviaries.

MEMBERS OF THE GENUS *PARAPOXVIRUS*

Parapoxviruses infect a wide range of species, generally causing only localized cutaneous lesions. Disease in sheep, cattle, goats, and camels can be of economic significance. Parapoxviruses also infect several species of terrestrial and

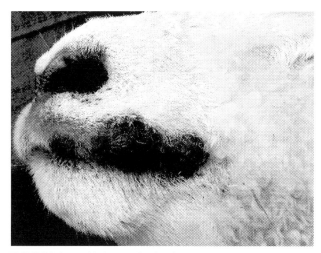

FIGURE 7.9 Orf lesion on the lip of a lamb. *(Courtesy K. Thompson, Massey University.)*

marine wildlife (e.g., chamois, red and black-tailed deer, seals, and reindeer), but their clinical importance in these species is more conjectural. These viruses are zoonotic; farmers, sheep shearers, veterinarians, butchers, and others who handle infected livestock or their products are especially at risk and can develop localized lesions, usually on the hand. The lesions, which are identical irrespective of the source of the virus and resemble those in the animal host, begin as an inflammatory papule, and then enlarge before regressing. They may persist for several weeks. If the infection is acquired from milking cows, the lesion is known as "milker's nodule;" if from sheep, it is known as "orf."

ORF VIRUS (CONTAGIOUS ECTHYEMA/CONTAGIOUS PUSTULAR DERMATITIS VIRUS)

Orf (*syn.* contagious pustular dermatitis, contagious ecythema, scabby mouth) is an important disease in sheep and goats, and is common throughout the world wherever sheep and goats are raised. Orf, which is Old English for "rough," commonly involves only the muzzle and lips, although lesions within the mouth affecting the gums and tongue can occur, especially in young lambs and kids. The lesions can also affect the eyelids, feet, and teats. Human infection can occur among persons exposed occupationally.

Lesions of orf progress from papules to pustules and then to thick crusts (Figure 7.9). The scabs are often friable and mild trauma causes the lesions to bleed. Orf may prevent lambs from suckling. Severely affected animals may lose weight and be predisposed to secondary infections. Morbidity is high in young sheep, but mortality is usually low. Clinical differentiation of orf from other diseases seldom presents a problem, but electron microscopy can be used, if necessary, to confirm the diagnosis.

Sheep are susceptible to reinfection and chronic infections can occur. These features, and the resistance of the virus to desiccation, explain how the virus, once introduced to a flock, can be difficult to eradicate. Spread of infection can be by direct contact or through exposure to contaminated feeding troughs and similar fomites, including wheat stubble and thorny plants.

Ewes can be vaccinated several weeks before lambing, using commercial non-attenuated virus vaccines derived from infected scabs collected from sheep or from virus grown in cell culture—in a manner analogous to pre-Jennerian vaccination for smallpox. Vaccines are applied to scarified skin, preferably in the axilla, where a localized lesion develops. A short-lived immunity is generated; ewes are thus less likely to develop orf at lambing time, thereby minimizing the risk of an epizootic in the lambs.

Orf virus is zoonotic; however, infections are frequent in humans, especially when they are in contact with sheep (e.g., during shearing, docking, drenching, slaughtering) or wildlife. In humans, after an incubation period of 2–4 days, the following stages may be observed: (1) macular lesions; (2) papular lesions; (3) rather large nodules, becoming papillomatous in some cases. Lesions are, as a rule, solitary, although multiple lesions have been described. The duration of lesions ranges from 4 to 9 weeks. Healing takes place without scarring, but secondary infections may retard healing. Severe complications, such as fever, regional adenitis, lymphangitis, or blindness when the eye is affected, are seen only rarely.

PSEUDOCOWPOX VIRUS

Pseudocowpox occurs as a common enzootic infection in cattle in most countries of the world. It is a chronic infection in many milking herds and occasionally occurs in beef herds. The lesions of pseudocowpox are characterized by "ring" or "horseshoe" scabs, the latter being pathognomonic for the disease. Similar lesions can occur on the muzzles and within the mouths of nursing calves. Infection is transmitted by cross-suckling of calves, improperly disinfected teat clusters of milking machines, and probably by the mechanical transfer of virus by flies. Attention to hygiene in the milking shed and the use of teat dips reduce the risk of transmission.

BOVINE PAPULAR STOMATITIS VIRUS

Bovine papular stomatitis is usually of little clinical importance, but occurs worldwide, affecting cattle of all ages, although the incidence is higher in animals less than 2 years of age. The development of lesions on the muzzle, margins of the lips, and the buccal mucosa is similar to that of pseudocowpox (Figure 7.10). Immunity is of short duration, and cattle can become reinfected. Demonstration by electron microscopy of the characteristic parapoxvirus virions in lesion scrapings is used for diagnosis.

POXVIRUSES OF FISH

Two poxviruses of significance to the culture of fish have been reported: the first associated with disease in koi (*Cyprinus carpio*) that is characterized by edema, and the second with a proliferative gill disease in Atlantic salmon (*Salmo salar*). Although the viruses involved in both disease syndromes are only partially characterized, they share similarities in their virion morphogenesis and genetic makeup that are more similar to those of viruses in the subfamily *Entomopoxvirinae* than those of viruses in the subfamily *Chordopoxvirinae*. This association of the fish poxviruses with entomopoxviruses may reflect the long evolutionary co-existence of fish with aquatic insects.

The disease syndrome associated with the carp edema virus has been designated as "sleepy disease" as, before death, affected fish lie on their sides on the pond bottom. The disease was first recognized in 1974 among cultured koi populations in Japan. Affected fish developed swollen bodies and proliferation of the gill epithelium, the latter beginning from the most distal tips and preceding to the base of the lamella.

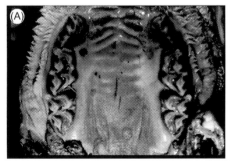 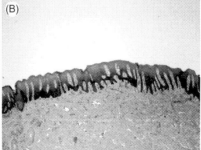 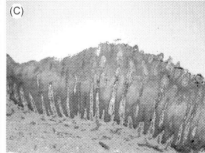

FIGURE 7.10   Bovine papular stomatitis. (A) Gross appearance of hard palate. (B) Histologic appearance of normal buccal epithelium. (C) Histologic appearance of affected buccal mucosal epithelium. *(A: Courtesy of M. Anderson, University of California.)*

Electron microscopy of the affected gill epithelium revealed pleomorphic mulberry-like virions of $335 \times 265\,nm$, with an envelope and surface membrane surrounding the core. In severe outbreaks, mortality ranged from 80 to 100% among juvenile koi at water temperatures in the range 15–25°C. The virus has not been isolated in cell culture, but the disease can be transmitted to naïve koi by injections with filtrates from the gills of infected koi. Current diagnostic methods include the characteristic clinical signs in juvenile koi, and electron microscopic examination of tissues from affected fish. A polymerase chain reaction (PCR) assay has been developed to detect viral DNA in fish. Control is currently reliant upon extended treatment of the water of affected ponds with the addition of 0.5% NaCl, a process that prevents virus-induced mortality but probably does not affect infection of carrier fish.

An emerging proliferative gill disease first recognized in 1998 has continued to increase in prevalence such that 35% of Atlantic salmon farms in Norway reported the condition in 2003. The disease is most frequent shortly after juvenile fish are transferred to sea water, and it occurs at water temperatures from 8.5 to 16°C, with mortality ranging from 10 to 50%. Protozoa (amoeba) and bacteria (chlamydia) may contribute to disease expression, but a recently described poxvirus is likely to be the true causative agent. The hyperplasia and hypertrophy of the gill epithelium in Atlantic salmon are similar to those described in koi with carp edema virus infection. Virions with a similar morphology but smaller in size than those from koi have been identified in the gill epithelium of affected Atlantic salmon. Although a PCR has been developed to detect this virus, it has not been widely used, and control measures for the disease have not been described to date.

OTHER POXVIRUSES

Poxvirus infections also have been described in raccoons, skunks, voles, and various species of deer, seals, horses, donkeys, and other animal species. The number of species of poxviruses will unquestionably grow as additional viruses are characterized and new viruses are isolated.

SQUIRREL POXVIRUS

Squirrelpox is a fatal disease of red squirrels in the United Kingdom. It is a highly significant wildlife disease, in that the mortality rate is nearly 100%, and is responsible for local extinctions of red squirrel populations. The virus is carried by an introduced non-native species, the gray squirrel from North America. Gray squirrels develop only mild disease when infected with the virus. The historical origins of the virus have not been determined. Although the virus is considered to have been introduced by gray squirrels, serological evidence of infection of gray squirrels in North America has been only recently identified, and the virus has not been identified among gray squirrels introduced to other parts of Europe. Although squirrel poxvirus initially was classified as a member of the genus *Parapoxvirus*, subsequent genetic studies have shown it to be distinct from other poxviruses and that it belongs in its own clade. The virus is notable in that it encodes homologs of both protein kinase (PKR) and 2′–5′ oligoadenylate synthetase, which are host-cell enzymes that mediate interferon-induced antiviral resistance. These viral homologs disrupt host innate antiviral immunity (see Chapter 4); for example, the three enzymatically active sites of authentic oligoadenylate synthetase enzyme are all inactivated in the viral homolog.

Chapter 8

Asfarviridae and *Iridoviridae*

Chapter Contents

Viruses in the families *Asfarviridae* and *Iridoviridae* are taxonomically and biologically distinct, but both families include large viruses with highly complex genomes of double-stranded DNA that are distantly related to one another, as well as to other large DNA viruses in the family *Poxviridae* and the order *Herpesvirales* (Figure 8.1). African swine fever virus in the family *Asfarviridae* is the cause of African swine fever, an important disease that remains a serious threat to swine industries throughout the world. The family *Iridoviridae* includes numerous viruses in several genera that have been isolated from poikilothermic animals, including fish, arthropods, mollusks, amphibians, and reptiles. Many iridovirus infections are subclinical or asymptomatic, but individual viruses are the cause of important and emerging diseases of fish and amphibians.

MEMBERS OF THE FAMILY *ASFARVIRIDAE*

PROPERTIES OF ASFARVIRUSES

Classification

African swine fever virus is a large enveloped DNA virus that is the sole member of the genus *Asfivirus* within the family *Asfarviridae* (Asfar = African swine fever and related viruses). African swine fever virus is the only known DNA arbovirus and is transmitted by soft ticks of the genus *Ornithodoros*. Virus strains are distinguished by their virulence to swine, which ranges from highly lethal to subclinical

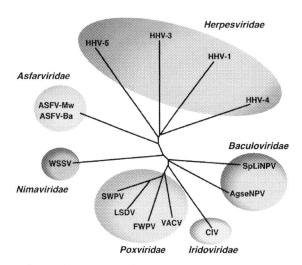

FIGURE 8.1 Phylogenetic tree comparing the dUTPase proteins encoded by African swine fever virus (AFSV) with those of other DNA viruses. Sequences were aligned using ClustalW and the tree displayed using Treeview. Sequences shown are from: ASFV_Mw and -Ba, Malawi and Ba71V isolates of African swine fever virus, WSSV white spot syndrome virus, SWPV swinepox virus, LSDV lumpy skin disease virus, FWPV fowlpox virus, VACV vaccinia virus, CIV chilo iridescent virus, AgseNPV Agrotis segetum granulosis virus, SpLiNPV spodoptera liturna nucleopolyhedron virus, HHV-1 human herpesvirus 1, HHV-3 human herpesvirus 3, HHV-4 human herpesvirus 4, HHV-5 human herpesvirus 5. *(Provided by Dr. D. Chapman, IAH, Pirbright.) [From* Virus Taxonomy: Eighth Report of the International Committee on Taxonomy of Viruses *(C. M. Fauquet, M. A. Mayo, J. Maniloff, U. Desselberger, L. A. Ball, eds), p. 142. Copyright © Elsevier (2005), with permission.]*

disease. Strains can also be differentiated by their genetic sequences, and the virus-encoded *p72* (also referred to as *p73*) gene can be used for genotyping the virus; however, the genomic diversity of the virus in nature remains to be thoroughly characterized. The genome of African swine fever virus contains a unique complement of multigene families.

Virion Properties

Asfarvirus virions are enveloped, approximately 200 nm in diameter, and possess a nucleocapsid core that is surrounded by internal lipid layers and a complex icosahedral capsid (Figure 8.2; Table 8.1). The capsid consists of a hexagonal arrangement of structural units, each of which appears as a hexagonal prism with a central hole. The genome consists of a single molecule of linear double-stranded DNA, 170–190 kbp in size, depending on the virus strain. The DNA has covalently closed ends with inverted terminal repeats and hairpin loops, and includes approximately 150 open reading frames that are closely spaced and read from both DNA strands. More than 50 proteins are present in virions, including a number of enzymes and factors required for early messenger RNA (mRNA) transcription and processing.

African swine fever virus is thermolabile and sensitive to lipid solvents. However, the virus is very resistant to a wide range of pH (several hours at pH 4 or pH 13), and survives for months and even years in refrigerated meat.

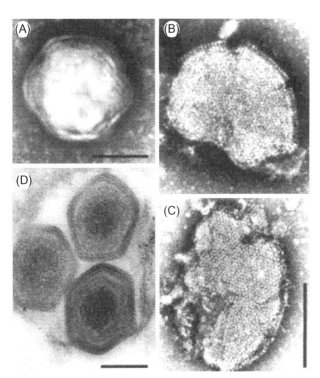

FIGURE 8.2 Family *Asfarviridae*, genus *Asfivirus*, African swine fever virus. (A) Negatively stained virion showing the hexagonal outline of the capsid enclosed within the envelope. (B and C) Negatively stained damaged capsids showing the ordered arrangement of the very large number of capsomers (between 1892 and 2172 structural units) that make up the capsid. (D) Thin section of three virions showing multiple layers surrounding their cores. Bars: 100 nm. *(Courtesy of J. L. Carrascosa.)*

Virus Replication

Primary isolates of African swine fever virus replicate in swine monocytes and macrophages. After adaptation, some isolates can replicate in certain mammalian cell lines. Replication occurs primarily in the cytoplasm, although the nucleus is needed for viral DNA synthesis and viral DNA is present in the nucleus soon after infection. Virus enters susceptible cells by receptor-mediated endocytosis, and cell binding and neutralization studies suggest that the viral p72 and p54 proteins are involved in virus attachment, and p30 in virus internalization. Like that of poxviruses, virion genomic DNA includes genes for all the machinery necessary for transcription and replication: after entry into the cytoplasm, virions are uncoated and their DNA is transcribed by a virion-associated, DNA-dependent RNA polymerase (transcriptase). DNA replication is similar to that of poxviruses: parental genomic DNA serves as the template for the first round of DNA replication, the product of which then serves as a template for the synthesis of large replicative complexes that are cleaved to produce mature virion DNA. Late in infection, African swine fever virus produces paracrystalline arrays of virions in the cytoplasm. Infected cells form many microvillus-like projections through which virions bud; however, acquisition of an envelope is not necessary for viral infectivity.

AFRICAN SWINE FEVER VIRUS

African swine fever was considered a disease of only sub-Saharan Africa until 1957, when an outbreak occurred on the Iberian Peninsula. Sporadic outbreaks subsequently occurred in the 1970s in some Caribbean islands, including Cuba and the Dominican Republic, and the virus appeared

---

TABLE 8.1　Properties of Asfarviruses and Iridoviruses

Asfarvirus virions are enveloped, approximately 200 nm in diameter, and contain a complex icosahedral capsid, approximately 180 nm in diameter

The genome of African swine fever virus is a single molecule of linear double-stranded DNA, approximately 170–190 kbp in size. It has covalently closed ends with inverted terminal repeats and hairpin loops, and encodes approximately 150 proteins, more than 50 of which are included in virions

Vertebrate iridovirus virions are similar in morphology to those of asfarviruses: the genome is a single molecule of linear double-stranded DNA, 140–200 kbp in size, that encodes up to 200 proteins. It is permuted circularly and has terminally redundant ends and methylated bases

The nucleus is involved in DNA replication; late functions and virion assembly occur in the cytoplasm

in France, Belgium, and other European countries in the 1980s. Since 2007, African swine fever virus has spread throughout portions of Georgia, Armenia, Azerbaijan, and Russia. The disease remains enzootic in sub-Saharan Africa and Sardinia. The presence of wild boar and extensive pig farming sustain enzootic African swine fever in Sardinia.

African swine fever virus infects domestic swine and other members of the family *Suidae*, including warthogs (*Potamochoerus aethiopicus*), bush pigs (*P. porcus*), and wild boar (*Sus scrofa ferus*). All efforts to infect other animals have been unsuccessful. The virus may have originated as a virus of ticks: in Africa, numerous isolates have been made from the soft tick *Ornithodoros moubata* collected in warthog burrows. When African swine fever virus was believed to be confined to sub-Saharan Africa, it was assumed that this was because of its natural cycle in argasid ticks and wild swine; however, the virus has spread on occasion beyond this traditional range and invaded portions of Europe, where the soft tick *Ornithodoros erraticus* can potentially serve as a vector.

Clinical Features and Epidemiology

The acute or hyperacute form of African swine fever in susceptible swine is characterized by a severe, hemorrhagic disease with high mortality. After an incubation period of 5–15 days, swine develop fever (40.5–42°C), which persists for about 4 days. Starting 1–2 days after the onset of fever, there is inappetence, diarrhea, incoordination, and prostration. Swine may die at this stage without other clinical signs. In some swine there is dyspnea, vomiting, nasal and conjunctival discharge, reddening or cyanosis of the ears and snout, and hemorrhages from the nose and anus. Pregnant sows often abort. Mortality is often 100%, with domestic swine dying within 1–3 days after the onset of fever. In prior epizootic geographic extensions of African

swine fever virus infection, the disease was usually severe and fatal at first, but diminished quickly until cases were predominantly subclinical and persistent. Infected adult warthogs do not develop clinical disease.

Two distinct patterns of transmission occur: a sylvatic cycle in warthogs and ticks in Africa, and epizootic and enzootic cycles in domestic swine (Figure 8.3).

Sylvatic Cycle

In its original ecologic niche in southern and eastern Africa, African swine fever virus is maintained in a sylvatic cycle involving asymptomatic infection in wild pigs (warthogs and, to a lesser extent, bush pigs) and argasid ticks (soft ticks, genus *Ornithodoros*), which occur in the burrows used by these animals. Ticks are biological vectors of the virus. Most tick populations in southern and eastern Africa are infected, with infection rates as high as 25%. After feeding on viremic swine, the virus replicates in the gut of the tick and subsequently infects its reproductive system, which leads to transovarial and venereal transmission of the virus (primarily male to female tick). The virus is also transmitted between developmental stages of the tick (trans-stadial transmission), and is excreted in tick saliva, coxal fluid, and Malpighian excrement. Infected ticks may live for several years, and are capable of transmitting disease to swine at each blood meal.

Serologic studies indicate that many warthog populations in southern and eastern Africa are infected. After primary infection, young warthogs develop viremia sufficient to infect at least some of the ticks feeding on them. Older warthogs are persistently infected, but are seldom viremic; it is therefore likely that the virus is maintained in a cycle involving young warthogs and ticks. The primary source of virus in epizootics of African swine fever in southern and eastern Africa are infected ticks that are transported by live warthogs or their carcasses.

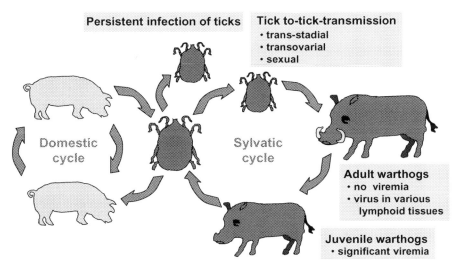

Persistent infection of ticks

Tick to-tick-transmission
• trans-stadial
• transovarial
• sexual

Domestic cycle

Sylvatic cycle

Adult warthogs
• no viremia
• virus in various lymphoid tissues

Juvenile warthogs
• significant viremia

FIGURE 8.3 Patterns of transmission of African swine fever virus. [*From E. R. Tulman, G. A. Delhon, B. K. Ku, D. L. Rock. African swine fever virus.* Curr. Top. Microbiol. Immunol. *328, 43–87 (2009), with permission.*]

Domestic Cycle

Primary outbreaks of African swine fever in domestic swine in Africa probably result from the bite of an infected tick, although tissues of acutely infected warthogs, if eaten by domestic swine, can also cause infection. Introduction of the virus into a previously non-infected country may result in transmission amongst swine, as well as infection of indigenous ticks. Several species of soft tick found in association with domestic and feral swine in the western hemisphere have been shown in experimental studies to be capable of biological transmission of the virus, although there is no evidence that they became infected during the epizootics in the Caribbean islands and South America.

Once the virus has been introduced into domestic swine, either by the bite of infected ticks or through infected meat, infected animals constitute the most important source of virus for susceptible swine. High titers of virus are present in nasopharyngeal excretions during onset of clinical signs, and virus is also present in other excretions, including high amounts in feces during acute disease. Disease spreads rapidly by contact and within buildings by aerosol. Mechanical spread by people, vehicles, and fomites is possible because of the stability of the virus in swine blood, feces, and tissues.

The international spread of African swine fever virus has been linked to feeding scraps of uncooked meat from infected swine. When the virus appeared in Portugal in 1957 and in Brazil in 1978, it was first reported in the vicinity of international airports, among swine fed on food scraps. Virus spread to the Caribbean and Mediterranean islands in 1978 may have arisen from the unloading of infected food scraps from ships. The source of the virus responsible for the outbreak in Georgia in 2007 is uncertain, although food waste from ships in Black Sea ports is suspected.

Pathogenesis and Pathology

African swine fever virus infection of domestic swine results in leukopenia, lymphopenia, thrombocytopenia, and apoptosis of both lymphocytes and mononuclear phagocytic cells. The ability of African swine fever virus to efficiently induce cytopathology in macrophages is a critical factor in viral virulence. In infected macrophages, the virus effectively inhibits the expression of pro-inflammatory cytokines such as tissue necrosis factor (TNF), type 1 interferon (IFN), and interleukin-8, but induces expression of transforming growth factor β. In contrast, increased expression of TNF has been also reported after African swine fever virus infection *in vitro* and *in vivo*. Importantly, African swine fever virus strains with different virulence phenotypes differ in their ability to induce (or inhibit) expression of pro-inflammatory cytokines or IFN-related genes early in infection of macrophages (Figure 8.4). Inhibition of

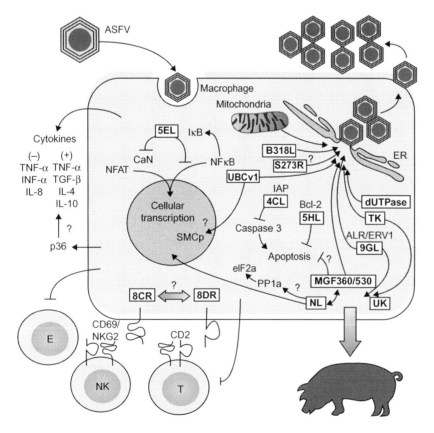

FIGURE 8.4 African swine fever virus (ASFV) – macrophage interactions in the swine host. ASFV contains several genes (white boxes) that interact or potentially interact with cellular regulatory pathways in macrophages, the primary target cells infected by ASFV. A viral homologue of IκB (5EL) inhibits both NFκB and calcineurin (CaN)/NFAT transcriptional pathways. The SMCp DNA-binding domain protein is a possible substrate for viral ubiquitin conjugating enzyme (UBCv1), and viral Bcl-2 and IAP homologues (5HL and 4CL, respectively) exhibit anti-apoptotic properties. ASFV infection affects host immune responses through induction of apoptosis in uninfected lymphocytes, through modulation of cytokine expression, and potentially through 8CR and 8DR, which are virally encoded homologues of immune cell proteins such as CD2 and CD69/NKG2. Efficient virus assembly and viral production in macrophages requires or may utilize viral genes similar to cellular ALR/ERV1 (9GL), nucleotide metabolism enzymes (dUTPase and thymidine kinase, TK), SUMO-1-specific protease (S273R) and *trans*-geranylgeranyl-diphosphate synthase (B318L). ASFV genes that affect viral virulence in domestic swine include NL, UK, and members of the MGF360 and MGF530 multigene families. *[From E. R. Tulman, D. L. Rock. Novel virulence and host range genes of African swine fever virus.* Curr. Opin. Microbiol. *4, 456–461 (2001), with permission.]*

inflammation is mediated at least in part by the viral gene *A238L*, which encodes a protein that is similar to an inhibitor of the cellular transcription factor, nuclear factor κB (NFκB). This viral protein has been shown to inhibit activation of NFκB and thus downregulate the expression of all of the antiviral cytokines that are controlled by NFκB. Mechanistically, the A238L protein acts as an analog of the immunosuppressive drug cyclosporin A, which represents a novel viral immune evasion strategy. Furthermore, this protein may be central to expression of fatal hemorrhagic disease in domestic pigs but mild, persistent infection in its natural host, the African warthog. Additional proteins encoded by African swine fever virus also modulate host immune responses; these include 8DR (pEP402R), a viral homolog of cellular CD2 involved in T lymphocyte activation and mediation of hemadsorption by cells infected with African swine fever virus.

If infection is acquired via the respiratory tract, the virus replicates first in the pharyngeal tonsils and lymph nodes draining the nasal mucosa, before being disseminated rapidly throughout the body via a primary viremia in which virions are associated with both erythrocytes and leukocytes. A generalized infection follows, with very high virus titers (up to 10^9 infectious doses per ml of blood or per gram of tissue), and all secretions and excretions contain large amounts of infectious virus.

Swine that survive the acute infection may appear healthy or chronically diseased, but both groups may remain persistently infected. Indeed, swine may become persistently infected without ever showing clinical signs. The duration of the persistent infection is not known, but low levels of virus have been detected in tissues more than a year after exposure.

In acutely fatal cases in domestic swine, gross lesions are most prominent in the lymphoid and vascular systems (Figure 8.5). Hemorrhages occur widely, and the visceral lymph nodes may resemble blood clots. There is marked petechiation of all serous surfaces, lymph nodes, epicardium and endocardium, renal cortex, and bladder, and edema and congestion of the colon and lungs. The spleen is often large and friable, and there are petechial hemorrhages in the cortex of the kidney. The chronic disease is characterized by cutaneous ulcers, pneumonia, pericarditis, pleuritis, and arthritis.

Diagnosis

The clinical signs of African swine fever are similar to those of several diseases, including bacterial septicemias such as erysipelas and acute salmonellosis, but the major diagnostic problem is in distinguishing it from classical swine fever (hog cholera). Any febrile disease in swine associated with disseminated hemorrhage (hemorrhagic diathesis) and high mortality should raise suspicion of African swine fever. Diagnosis of chronic infections is problematic as the clinical signs and lesions in affected pigs are highly variable.

Laboratory confirmation is essential, and samples of blood, spleen, kidney, visceral lymph nodes, and tonsils, in particular, should be collected for virus isolation, detection of antigen, or polymerase chain reaction (PCR) for detection of the *p72* gene. Virus isolation is done in swine bone marrow or peripheral blood leukocyte cultures, in which hemadsorption can be demonstrated and a cytopathic effect is manifest within a few days after inoculation. After initial isolation, the virus can be adapted to grow in various cell lines, such as Vero cells. Antigen detection is achieved by immunofluorescence staining of tissue smears or frozen

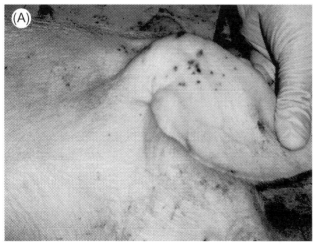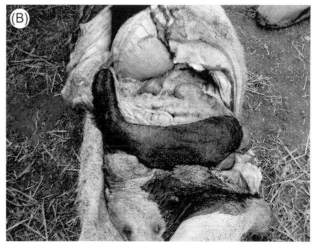

FIGURE 8.5 Lesions of acute African swine fever. (A) Subcutaneous hemorrhages in the ear. (B) Splenomegaly. *(Courtesy of R. Harutynan, State Veterinary and Epizootic Diagnostic Center, Yerevan, Armenia and W. Laegried, University of Illinois.)*

sections, by immunodiffusion using tissue suspensions as the source of antigen, and by enzyme immunoassay.

Immunity, Prevention and Control

Both humoral and cellular (including virus-specific CD8$^+$ lymphocyte) components contribute to the protective immune response of swine to African swine fever virus. Antibody responses to African swine fever virus have been shown to protect pigs from lethal challenge; however, neutralizing antibodies to virion proteins p30, p54, and p72 are not sufficient to confer antibody-mediated protection.

The prevention and control of African swine fever can be complicated by several factors, including the lack of an effective vaccine, the transmission of virus in fresh meat and some cured pork products, the existence of persistent infection in some swine, diagnostic confusion with agents that cause similar disease syndromes such as classical swine fever (hog cholera), and (in some parts of the world) the participation of soft ticks in virus transmission. The presence of the virus in ticks and warthogs in many countries of sub-Saharan Africa makes it difficult, if not impossible, to break the sylvatic cycle of the virus. However, domestic swine can be reared in Africa if the management system avoids feeding uncooked waste food scraps and prevents the access of ticks and contact with warthogs, usually by double fencing with a wire mesh perimeter fence extending beneath the ground.

Elsewhere in the world, countries that are free of African swine fever maintain their virus-free status by prohibiting the importation of live swine and swine products from infected countries, and by monitoring the destruction of all waste food scraps from ships and aircraft involved in international routings.

If disease does occur in a previously non-infected country, control depends first on early recognition and rapid laboratory diagnosis. The virulent forms of African swine fever cause such dramatic mortality that episodes are brought quickly to the attention of veterinary authorities, but the disease caused by less virulent strains that has occurred outside Africa in the past can cause confusion with other diseases and therefore may not be recognized until the virus is well established in the swine population.

Once African swine fever is confirmed in a country that has hitherto been free of disease, prompt action is required to control and then eradicate the infection. All non-African countries that have become infected have elected to attempt eradication. The strategy for eradication involves slaughter of infected swine and swine in contact with them, and disposal of carcasses, preferably by burning. Movement of swine between farms is controlled, and feeding of waste food prohibited. Where soft ticks are known to occur, infested buildings are sprayed with acaricides. Re-stocking of farms is allowed only if sentinel swine do not become infected. Elimination has been widely successful using this approach, except in Sardinia.

MEMBERS OF THE FAMILY *IRIDOVIRIDAE*

The family *Iridoviridae* is large and complex; viruses within this family infect arthropods, fish, amphibians, and reptiles. Iridoviruses in the genera *Ranavirus*, *Megalocytivirus*, and *Lymphocystivirus* are the cause of a range of disorders in fish, including systemic lethal diseases (genera *Ranavirus*, *Megalocytivirus*) and tumor-like skin lesions (*Lymphocystivirus*). Ranaviruses are considered as a potential cause of the global decline in amphibian populations. Viruses in all three genera are capable of long-term persistence in their fish or amphibian hosts, following recovery from acute or inapparent infections.

PROPERTIES OF IRIDOVIRUSES

Members of the *Iridoviridae* are generally 120–200 nm diameter, but are sometimes even larger DNA viruses, with virions that are similar morphologically to those of the *Asfarviridae*. Virions exhibit icosahedral symmetry, with a virus core and outer capsid that are separated by an internal lipid membrane (Figure 8.6). Up to 36 proteins are contained in the virions. A viral envelope is present on virions that bud from infected cells, but is not necessary for infectivity. The genomes of iridoviruses consist of a single linear double-stranded DNA molecule that ranges from 140 to 200 kbp in size, and individual viruses encode between approximately 100 and 200 proteins. Termini are different from those of African swine fever virus, being circularly permuted and terminally redundant. The family is segregated into two groups on the basis of levels of genomic methylation: a methyltransferase present in the iridoviruses of fish facilitates methylation of up to 20% of cytosine residues in the genomic DNA, similar to that in bacterial genomic DNA.

The family *Iridoviridae* includes five genera, specifically *Iridovirus*, *Chloriridovirus*, *Ranavirus*, *Megalocytivirus*, and *Lymphocystivirus* (Table 8.2). Viruses in this family are of emerging significance, as several are important pathogens in commercial fish production and others cause mortality in captive and wild amphibians. Iridoviruses also cause disease among reptiles, including chelonians (turtles and tortoises), snakes, and lizards. Interestingly, although viruses in the genera *Iridovirus* and *Chloriridovirus* are considered to be viruses of arthropods, these viruses recently have been identified in several species of lizards and scorpions. The genetic similarity of viruses isolated from insects and reptiles suggests they may be transmitted to the lizards from their insect prey.

Most information concerning the iridovirus replication cycle is derived from studies of frog virus 3, the type

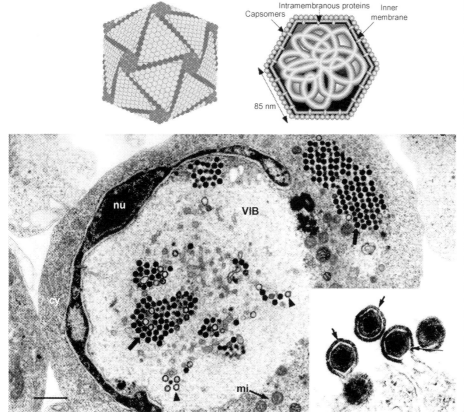

FIGURE 8.6 (Top left) Outer shell of invertebrate iridescent virus 2 (IIV-2) (From Wrigley, *et al.* (1969). *J. Gen. Virol.*, **5**, 123. With permission). (Top right) Schematic diagram of a cross-section of an iridovirus particle, showing capsomers, transmembrane proteins within the lipid bilayer, and an internal filamentous nucleoprotein core (From Darcy-Triper, F. *et al.* (1984). *Virology*, **138**, 287. With permission). (Bottom left) Transmission electron micrograph of a fat head minnow cell infected with an isolate of European catfish virus. Nucleus (Nu); virus inclusion body (VIB); paracrystalline array of non-enveloped virus particles (arrows); incomplete nucleocapsids (arrowheads); cytoplasm (cy); mitochondrion (mi). The bar represents 1 μm. (From Hyatt *et al.* (2000). *Arch. Virol.* **145**, 301, with permission). (insert) Transmission electron micrograph of particles of frog virus 3 (FV-3), budding from the plasma membrane. Arrows and arrowheads identify the viral envelope (Devauchelle *et al.* (1985). *Curr. Topics Microbiol. Immunol.*, **116**. 1, with permission). The bar represents 200 nm. [*From Virus Taxonomy: Eighth Report of the International Committee on Taxonomy of Viruses* (C. M. Fauquet, M. A. Mayo, J. Maniloff, U. Desselberger, L. A. Ball, eds), p. 145. Copyright © Elsevier (2005), with permission.]

TABLE 8.2 Taxonomy of the Family *Iridoviridae*

Genus	Virus Species
Iridovirus	Invertebrate iridescent virus 6 (IIV-6) and IIVs-1, -2, -9, -16, -21, -22, -23, -24, -29, -30, and -31
Chloriridovirus	Invertebrate iridescent virus 3
Ranavirus	Frog virus 3 (tadpole edema virus, tiger frog virus) Ambystoma tigrinum virus (regina ranavirus) Epizootic hematopoietic necrosis virus European catfish virus (European sheatfish virus) Santee-Cooper ranavirus (largemouth bass virus, doctor fish virus, guppy virus 6) Singapore grouper iridovirus
Megalocytivirus	Infectious spleen and kidney necrosis virus (red sea bream iridovirus, African lampeye iridovirus, orange spotted grouper iridovirus, rock bream iridovirus)
Lymphocystivirus	Lymphocystis disease virus 1 (LCDV-1) and LCDV-2
Unclassified	White sturgeon iridovirus

species for the genus *Ranavirus* (Figure 8.7). The iridoviruses of vertebrates grow in a wide variety of cells of piscine, amphibian, avian, and mammalian origin at temperatures between 12 and 32°C. Their replication is similar to that of African swine fever virus; however, the viruses do not encode an RNA polymerase, but instead use cellular RNA polymerase II, which their structural proteins modify to favor viral mRNA synthesis. Like African swine fever virus, there is a limited round of initial replication in the nucleus, followed by extensive cytoplasmic replication. Late in infection, vertebrate iridoviruses produce paracrystalline arrays of virions in the cytoplasm. Infected cells form many microvillus-like projections through which virions bud; however, acquisition of an envelope is not necessary for viral infectivity, and infectious, naked virus particles are released after lysis of infected cells.

RANAVIRUSES

Since the initial detection of frog virus 3 in the 1960s, an increasing number of related viruses have been associated with diseases in amphibians and fish in their freshwater environments. Frog virus 3 was initially isolated from leopard frogs in the eastern United States, during an

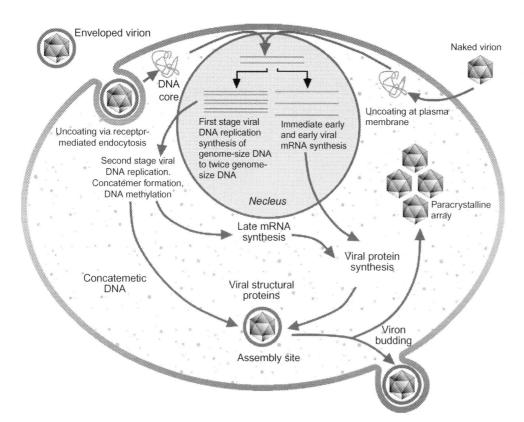

Enveloped virion

Naked virion

DNA core

Uncoating via receptor-mediated endocytosis

Uncoating at plasma membrane

First stage viral DNA replication synthesis of genome-size DNA to twice genome-size DNA

Immediate early and early viral mRNA synthesis

Second stage viral DNA replication. Concatemer formation, DNA methylation

Necleus

Late mRNA synthesis

Paracrystalline array

Concatemetic DNA

Viral protein synthesis

Viral structural proteins

Viron budding

Assembly site

FIGURE 8.7 Replication cycle of frog virus 3 (FV-3) (From Chinchar *et al.*, (2002). *Arch. Virol.*, **147**, 447, with permission). *[From Virus Taxonomy: Eighth Report of the International Committee on Taxonomy of Viruses (C. M. Fauquet, M. A. Mayo, J. Maniloff, U. Desselberger, L. A. Ball, eds), p. 148. Copyright © Elsevier (2005), with permission.]*

investigation into causes of naturally occurring renal carcinomas that was later traced to infection with an oncogenic alloherpesvirus, ranid herpesvirus 1. Although ranaviruses such as frog virus 3 were initially considered to be relatively benign, by the mid-1980s it was increasingly apparent that ranaviruses were associated with severe and widespread disease epizootics amongst wild amphibian populations in North America, Europe, and Asia. Infected tadpoles, which are most susceptible, and frogs may exhibit localized cutaneous hemorrhage and/or ulceration or severe systemic disease with edema, hemorrhage, and necrosis in numerous organs. Subclinical infections occur in apparently normal wild and captive populations of frogs, in which ranavirus is detected in kidney tissues, including macrophages, which serve as a site for virus persistence.

Ambystoma tigrinum virus is a ranavirus that causes mortality in both larval and adult salamanders in western North America from late summer to early autumn. Mortality that can exceed 90% occurs within 7–14 days of exposure to virus in the water or by direct contact with diseased salamanders. Diseased animals may exhibit any combination of necrosis and hemorrhage within the spleen, liver, kidney, and gastrointestinal tract, sloughing of the skin, development of skin polyps, and discharge of inflammatory exudate from the vent. Environmental temperature plays an important role in the pathogenesis of infection,

as most salamanders infected at 26°C survive, whereas at 18°C most die of the infection. The role of vertical transmission from infected adults to eggs is unknown, and the virus does not appear to have an alternate reservoir host.

Ranavirus-associated diseases of fish were first reported in Australia in 1986, initially amongst lake populations of redfin perch that had a systemic disease characterized by extensive necrosis of the liver, pancreas, and hemopoietic cells of the kidney and spleen. This disease, termed "epizootic hemopoietic necrosis," was later identified in farmed populations of rainbow trout in the same water systems as the affected redfin perch. The causative virus was transmitted experimentally to seven additional fish species found in Australia. Fingerling and juvenile fish are commonly affected; however, when epizootic hematopoietic necrosis virus is newly introduced, adults are also susceptible. In general, the ranaviruses of fish can be readily detected by isolation from internal organs (kidney, spleen, liver) on a range of cell lines, usually of fish origin, which are incubated at 20–25°C. The virus can be distinguished from other ranaviruses by DNA-based diagnostic procedures.

Additional ranaviruses have recently been detected during disease episodes among cultured freshwater populations of silurid and ictalurid catfish in Europe and Atlantic cod fry in a hatchery in Denmark. Largemouth bass virus (*syn.* Santee–Cooper virus) is a ranavirus that has been associated with substantial seasonal loss of wild adult largemouth bass in lakes in the United States. The virus affects a variety of internal tissues, including the swim bladder, which becomes reddened and enlarged and contains a yellow exudate. Involvement of the swim bladder results in moribund fish that float to the surface, which is often the first indication of disease in wild fish. In experimental studies, the virus caused only low-grade mortality in largemouth bass, which suggests that the epizootic mortality that occurs during disease outbreaks among wild fish is probably due to additional contributing factors. As in amphibians, ranaviruses can often be isolated from asymptomatic fish, a feature that contributes to the unintentional dispersal of virus with the international trade of live amphibians and fish. Transmission of ranaviruses between amphibian and fish has been demonstrated in both natural and experimental settings.

Ranaviruses are increasingly recognized as the cause of disease among wild and captive reptiles. Ranavirus infections have been identified among chelonians (turtles and tortoises), lizards, and snakes on several continents, sometimes in association with disease syndromes similar to those encountered in ranavirus-infected amphibians.

MEGALOCYTIVIRUSES

The emerging and significant impact of megalocytiviruses on the commercial production of both food and ornamental fish has become increasingly apparent since their initial detection in 1990 among cultured populations of red sea bream in Japan. Over 30 species of marine and freshwater fish from Japan, the South China Sea, and several Southeast Asian countries are now documented as potential hosts of megalocytiviruses. The viruses all share significant homology, with 97% or greater identity at the deduced amino acid level for the major capsid protein. The entire genome sequence has been determined for at least three megalocytiviruses, namely infectious spleen and kidney necrosis virus, rock bream iridovirus, and orange spotted grouper iridovirus. Mortality of up to 100% has been described during epizootics in captive fish populations, and after experimental infection. Signs exhibited by diseased fish include lethargy, severe anemia, and branchial hemorrhages. At necropsy, the spleen may be greatly enlarged. On microscopic evaluation, numerous large, basophilic, "cytomegalic" cells that have a subendothelial location are typically present in internal organs such as spleen, kidney, intestine, eye, pancreas, liver, heart, gill, brain, and intestine; these characteristic cells are reflected in the genus name for these viruses. The enlarged cells contain abundant numbers of developing and complete virions. In contrast to ranaviruses, the megalocytiviruses are often difficult to isolate in cell culture, and thus diagnosis has traditionally been reliant on histologic evaluation followed by confirmation with electron microscopy. DNA-based diagnostic methods such as PCR are now routinely used to detect and distinguish megalocytiviruses in captive and wild fish populations.

Control methods include the use of pathogen-free fish, improved sanitation on fish farms and husbandry practices that minimize stress (lower fish densities, good water quality, etc.). A formalin-killed virus vaccine administered by injection has proven efficacious in the control of the red sea bream iridovirus in Japan. The megalocytiviruses are horizontally transmitted among fish in the water, and there is no evidence to date for vertical transmission from adults to progeny. The broad host range and detection of megalocytiviruses in many ornamental fish species shipped from enzootic areas create a major concern for the control of this important group of fish pathogens.

LYMPHOCYSTIVIRUSES

Lymphocystis is a benign and self-limiting disease described in a broad range of freshwater and marine fish species. The condition is caused by a group of iridoviruses that infect and then transform fibroblasts of the skin and gills and internal connective tissues, resulting in remarkable hypertrophy of the affected cells (Figure 8.8). These cells, termed "lymphocysts," appear as raised pearl-like lesions and can be observed readily with the naked eye. Infections occur in over 125 species and 34 families of fish from warm, temperate, and cold, and marine or freshwater environments. Lymphocysts, which may reach 100,000 times the normal cell size, are a result of virus-mediated arrest of cell division but not cell growth, which leads to the formation of megalocytes. Lymphocysts possess a distinct hyaline-like capsule, an enlarged nucleus, and bizarre and segmented cytoplasmic inclusions that contain developing virions. The characteristic histologic appearance of lymphocysts is pathognomonic for lymphocystis disease, although electron microscopy is often used to confirm the presence of typical iridovirus virions.

Lymphocystis disease virus 1 is associated with infections in two marine fish species, flounder and plaice, whereas lymphocystis disease virus 2 occurs in a third marine fish, dab. There are many additional and related viruses associated with lymphocystis that occur in other fish species in marine and freshwater habitats, but these have not been fully characterized. Infections with lymphocystis disease virus are seldom fatal and most often fish recover by sloughing external lymphocysts. The most important impact of the virus is the loss of commercial value as a result of cosmetic effects that occur in cultured or wild-caught fish sold as food. In addition to the cosmetic effects with ornamental fish, heavy infections in the oral region may inhibit feeding, and the effects of the viral infections may result in entry points for secondary pathogens. Transmission from fish to fish is probably via contact with virus released from ruptured lymphocysts that spreads

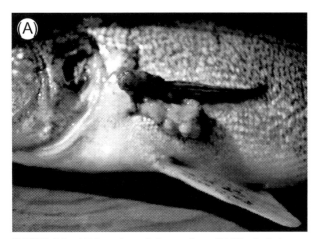 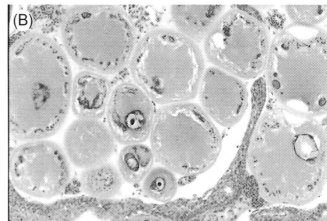

FIGURE 8.8 (A) Lymphocystis in a walleye. (B) Histological appearance of lymphocystis, depicting cellular hypertrophy. *(Courtesy of P. Bowser, Cornell University and R. Hedrick, University of California.)*

the virus among crowded fish populations. Separation and quarantine of infected fish until lymphocysts resolve are the means to reduce infections in captive fish populations. Genetic analyses of Japanese flounder with lymphocystis suggest a genetic basis for susceptibility to the virus, a finding that may eventually aid in selective breeding to reduce the prevalence of disease.

OTHER IRIDOVIRUSES OF FISH

Erythrocytic necrosis virus is a group of unassigned iridoviruses that share morphologic features with members of the family *Iridoviridae*. Virions are present in the cytoplasm of immature hemopoietic cells or mature erythrocytes of a range of marine fish (e.g., herring and cod) and some species of salmonid fish found in the North Pacific and North Atlantic oceans. Heavy infections result in significant anemia and losses among both wild and farmed populations of fish. Infected erythrocytes contain a distinct circular cytoplasmic inclusion(s) as seen in stained blood smears. Viral infections in erythrocytes are confirmed by the presence of iridovirus-like virions in the cytoplasm by electron microscopy. Viruses associated with erythrocytic necrosis have also been observed in reptiles and amphibians. The viruses found in fish have not been isolated, presumably because of the absence of suitable cell lines of hemopoietic origin. Fish erythrocytic necrosis virus can be transmitted experimentally by intraperitoneal injections with infected erythrocytes. Many features of the disease remain uncharacterized.

The white sturgeon iridovirus, a currently unassigned virus in the family *Iridoviridae*, was first recognized as the cause of epizootic mortality of farmed juvenile sturgeon in the 1980s in California. Infection with this virus results in destruction of the epithelium of the skin and gills,

compromising both respiration and osmotic balance. White sturgeon iridovirus disease is considered the most problematic viral disease of white sturgeon cultured for meat or caviar. The virus has been identified in wild and captive populations of white sturgeon throughout the Pacific Northwest of North America. It has also been moved beyond its original range through the export of live white sturgeon. Infections are detected by histologic examination that reveals the presence of characteristic enlarged amphophilic to basophilic-staining cells in the epithelium, often associated with necrosis of surrounding cells. Virions can be identified by electron microscopic examination of enlarged cells. More recently, specific PCR tests have been developed to assist in confirming infections with the white sturgeon iridovirus. Virus transmission occurs in contaminated water, and there is strong evidence of vertical transmission of the virus with gametes from infected adult fish. Separation of year classes of sturgeon and segregation of infected lots of juvenile fish are the principal control methods. Infections and significant losses of several different species of juvenile sturgeon with viruses related to the white sturgeon iridovirus have now been reported in wild and captive populations of shovelnose, pallid, and lake sturgeon in the United States, and Italian and Russian sturgeon in Europe.

IRIDOVIRUSES OF MOLLUSKS

Iridovirus or iridovirus-like agents associated with mortality of larval and adult oysters have been described in both Europe and North America. Catastrophic losses of the Portuguese oyster cultured along the Atlantic coast of France during the early 1970s were attributed to iridovirus infection that caused severe necrosis of the gill epithelium, or that infected hemocytes. A subsequent outbreak of the hemocytic disease occurred among Pacific oysters in

France in 1977, suggesting that this introduced oyster species was the potential source of the virus that infected the resident oyster populations. Oyster velar virus disease was first described in the late 1970s as the cause of mortality—that approached 100%—among larval stages of the Pacific oyster in hatcheries in the state of Washington. The target tissue of this virus is the velum, a ciliated structure responsible for locomotion and feeding of the larvae. Infection results in the formation of blisters and sloughing of the ciliated epithelium and then death. Virions in infected cells share morphologic properties with those in affected adult oysters in France, although they are slightly smaller in size (228 nm diameter). Control measures for iridovirus infections in mollusks rely upon early detection and destruction of infected groups, followed by vigorous disinfection, particularly in hatchery settings.

Herpesvirales

Chapter Contents

Herpesviruses have been found in insects, fish, reptiles, amphibians, and mollusks as well as in virtually every species of bird and mammal that has been investigated. It is likely that every vertebrate species is infected with several herpesvirus species. At least one major disease of each domestic animal species, except sheep, is caused by a herpesvirus, including such important diseases as infectious bovine rhinotracheitis, pseudorabies, and Marek's disease. Herpesviruses are adapted to their individual hosts, probably as a consequence of prolonged co-evolution. Thus, with

Fenner's Veterinary Virology. DOI: 10.1016/B978-0-12-375158-4.00009-2

some exceptions—notably some members of the subfamily *Alphaherpesvirinae* in particular—herpesvirus infections typically produce severe disease only in neonates, fetuses, immunocompromised individuals, or in alternate host species (so-called species-jumping).

Herpesvirus virions are easily inactivated and do not survive well outside the body. In general, transmission requires close contact, particularly mucosal contact (e.g., coitus, licking and nuzzling, as between mother and offspring or between neonates). In large, closely confined populations, such as found in cattle feedlots, modern swine farrowing units, animal shelters, catteries, or broiler facilities, sneezing and short-distance droplet spread are major modes of transmission. However, moist, cool environmental conditions provide opportunity for transmission over longer distances, as shown with ovine herpesvirus 2, the causative agent of sheep-associated malignant catarrhal fever of cattle. Similarly, during active herpesvirus outbreaks in fish, virus shed into the water may spread rapidly between individuals in densely stocked ponds. In addition, vertical transmission from adults to progeny may be the major mode by which herpesviruses are maintained in wild and captive fish populations.

An important aspect of herpesvirus pathogenesis is latency. Latency is defined as persistent life-long infection of a host with restricted but recurrent virus replication. Recurrent virus replication can lead to shedding, transmission, and the maintenance of detectable antiviral immune responses. Therefore, latent infections in clinically normal hosts provide a potentially undiagnosed reservoir for virus transmission.

PROPERTIES OF HERPESVIRUSES

Classification

The classification of herpesviruses is complex. All herpesviruses share a common morphology and have genomes of linear, double-stranded DNA (dsDNA) but, with the recent increased availability of genomic sequence data, it is apparent that the herpesviruses segregate into three distinct genetic groupings that are related only tenuously to each other. Thus the herpesviruses were recently assigned to the new order *Herpesvirales*, with three distinct families: the *Herpesviridae* that includes herpesviruses of mammals, birds, and reptiles; the *Alloherpesviridae* that includes the herpesviruses of fish and frogs, and the *Malacoherpesviridae* that contains a virus of oysters (bivalve). The family *Herpesviridae* is further subdivided into three subfamilies: *Alphaherpesvirinae*, *Betaherpesvirinae*, and *Gammaherpesvirinae*, and the various families and subfamilies are subdivided into genera. A substantial number of viruses have not yet been assigned to specific genera, and further taxonomic subdivision and reclassification of individual viruses will unquestionably occur as additional herpesviruses are characterized in detail,

particularly those isolated from evolutionarily distant host species.

Antigenic relationships among the herpesviruses are complex; there are some shared antigens within the order, but different species have distinct envelope glycoproteins.

Family Herpesviridae

The recently designated family *Herpesviridae* includes the herpesviruses of birds, mammals, and reptiles. The family includes three subfamilies, a grouping that reflects common genetic and biological properties of the viruses within each subfamily.

Subfamily *Alphaherpesvirinae*

The subfamily is subdivided into four genera: *Simplexvirus*, *Varicellovirus*, *Mardivirus*, and *Iltovirus*. Prototypic viruses of the genera of this subfamily are human herpesvirus 1 (herpes simplex virus 1; genus *Simplexvirus*), human herpesvirus 3 (varicella-zoster virus; genus *Varicellovirus*), gallid herpesvirus 2 (Marek's disease virus; genus *Mardivirus*), and gallid herpesvirus 1 (infectious laryngotracheitis virus; genus *Iltovirus*). Most alphaherpesviruses grow rapidly, lyse infected cells, and establish latent infections primarily in sensory ganglia. Some alphaherpesviruses such as pseudorabies virus (suid herpesvirus 1) have a broad host range, whereas most are highly restricted in their natural host range, suggesting that individual alphaherpesviruses evolve in association with a single host.

Subfamily *Betaherpesvirinae*

This subfamily comprises four genera: *Cytomegalovirus*, *Muromegalovirus*, *Proboscivirus*, and *Roseolovirus*, with human herpesvirus 5 (cytomegalovirus), murid herpesvirus 1, elephantid herpesvirus (elephant endotheliotropic herpesvirus), and human herpesvirus 6 serving respectively as the prototypes of each genus. Individual betaherpesviruses have a highly restricted host range. Their replicative cycle is slow and cell lysis delayed. The viruses may remain latent in secretory glands, the kidneys, and lymphoreticular and certain other tissues.

Subfamily *Gammaherpesvirinae*

This subfamily comprises four genera: *Lymphocryptovirus*, *Macavirus*, *Percavirus*, and *Rhadinovirus*. Viruses in this subfamily have a narrow host range, are lymphotropic, and become latent in lymphocytes; some are linked to oncogenic transformation of lymphocytes, notably human herpesvirus 4 (Epstein–Barr virus), which is the cause of Burkitt's lymphoma and nasopharyngeal carcinoma in humans, and some also cause cytocidal infections in epithelial and fibroblastic cells. The non-human primate and ungulate gammaherpesviruses are not generally recognized as significant causes of disease in their natural hosts unless they are immunocompromised, but they can cause very severe lymphoproliferative disease in heterologous, but related hosts.

Family Alloherpesviridae

The family includes herpesviruses of fish and frogs, with only a single assigned genus, *Ictalurivirus*, although there are proposals for at least five additional genera. The genus *Ictalurivirus* contains channel catfish virus, which serves as a prototype for approximately 30 alloherpesviruses that represent a genetically distinct and diverse virus lineage. The only other assigned species is cyprinid herpesvirus 3 that contains the herpesvirus that occurs in koi and common carp. Additional alloherpesviruses have been isolated or identified from frogs and several types of fish, including goldfish, carp, sturgeon, pike, flounder, cod, smelt, sharks, angelfish, pilchards, walleye, turbot, and salmonids.

Family Malacoherpesviridae

This family currently includes the single herpesvirus from an invertebrate host, specifically ostreid herpesvirus 1, which was recovered from an oyster.

Virion Properties

Herpesvirus virions are enveloped and include a core, capsid, and tegument (Figure 9.1). The core consists of the viral genome packaged as a single, linear dsDNA molecule within the protein capsid that in human herpesviruses has an external diameter of approximately 125 nm and is composed of 162 hollow capsomers—150 hexons and 12 pentons. The DNA genome is wrapped around a fibrous spool-like core, which has the shape of a torus and appears to be suspended by fibrils that are anchored to the inner side of the surrounding capsid and pass through the hole of the torus. Surrounding the capsid is a layer of globular material, known as the tegument, which is enclosed by a typical lipoprotein envelope with numerous small glycoprotein spikes. Because of the variable size of the envelope, virions can range in diameter from 120 to 250 nm (Table 9.1).

The genome consists of a single linear molecule of dsDNA that is infectious under appropriate experimental conditions. There is a remarkable degree of variation in the composition, size, and organization of the genomes of the herpesviruses: (1) the percentage of guanine plus cytosine (G + C ratio) varies substantially more than that of eukaryote DNA; (2) the size of herpesvirus genomes varies

TABLE 9.1 Properties of Herpesviruses

Virions are enveloped and variably sized (approximately 120–250 nm in diameter), containing an icosahedral nucleocapsid composed of 162 capsomers

Genome is linear double-stranded DNA, 125–290 kbp in size

Replication occurs in the nucleus, with sequential transcription and translation of immediate early (α), early (β), and late (γ) genes producing α, β, and γ proteins, respectively; the earlier genes and their gene products regulate the transcription of later genes

DNA replication and encapsidation occur in the nucleus; the envelope is acquired by budding through the inner layer of the nuclear envelope

Infection results in characteristic eosinophilic intranuclear inclusion bodies

Infection becomes latent, with recrudescence and intermittent or continuous virus shedding

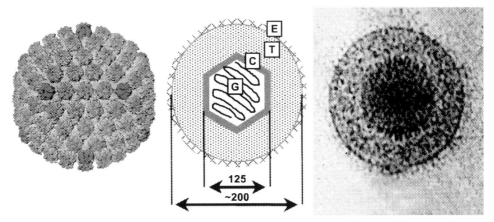

FIGURE 9.1 Herpesvirus morphology. (Left) Reconstruction of a human herpesvirus 1 (HHV-1) capsid generated from cryo-electron microscope images, viewed along the 2-fold axis. The hexons are shown in blue, the pentons in red, and the triplexes in green. (Courtesy of W. Chiu and H. Zhou). (Center) Schematic representation of a virion with diameters in nm. (G) genome, (C) capsid, (T) tegument, (E) envelope. (Right) Cryo-electron microscope image of a HHV-1 virion. (Reproduced from Rixon (1993) with permission from Elsevier). *[From* Virus Taxonomy: Eighth Report of the International Committee on Taxonomy of Viruses *(C. M. Fauquet, M. A. Mayo, J. Maniloff, U. Desselberger, L. A. Ball, eds), p. 193. Copyright © Elsevier (2005), with permission.]*

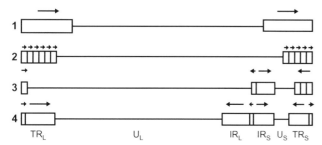

FIGURE 9.2 Examples of four different strategies utilized by individual herpesviruses. Alphaherpesvirus genomes comprise two regions, designated long (L) and short (S). Terminal repeat (TR) and internal repeat (IR) sequences may bracket unique sequences (U_L, U_S) of both L and S or only S. Repeat sequences are shown as boxes and are encoded as indicated by the direction of the arrows. *[From Virus Taxonomy: Eighth Report of the International Committee on Taxonomy of Viruses (C. M. Fauquet, M. A. Mayo, J. Maniloff, U. Desselberger, L. A. Ball, eds), p. 195. Copyright © Elsevier (2005), with permission.]*

between 125 and 290 kbp; (3) the organization of genomes varies in complex fashion amongst the various herpesviruses, both in order and in orientation (Figure 9.2), which is reflected in turn by the complex taxonomic classification of these viruses. Reiterated DNA sequences generally occur at both ends (and in some viruses also internally), dividing the genome into two unique sections, designated large (U_L) and small (U_S). When these reiterated sequences are inverted in their orientation, the unique L and S components can invert relative to one another during replication, giving rise to two or four different isomers of the genome that are present in equimolar proportions. Further, intragenomic and intergenomic recombination events can alter the number of any particular reiterated sequence polymorphism.

Herpesvirus genes fall into three general categories: (1) those encoding proteins concerned with regulatory functions and virus replication (immediate early and early genes); (2) those encoding structural proteins (late genes); (3) a heterologous set of "optional" genes, in the sense that they are not found in all herpesviruses and are not essential for replication in cultured cells. Herpesvirus virions contain more than 30 structural proteins, of which six are present in the nucleocapsid, two being DNA associated. The glycoproteins, of which there are about 12, are located in the envelope, from which most project as spikes (peplomers). One of the spike glycoproteins found in some of the alphaherpesviruses (gE) possesses Fc receptor activity and binds immunoglobulin G (IgG). Some of the growth-regulating and immunomodulatory proteins that are not necessary for virus replication and maturation in cultured cells are homologs of cellular genes that encode key regulatory proteins involved in growth regulation and modulation of the immune response. Examples include virus-encoded chemokine receptor homologs or chemokine-binding proteins that alter immune responsiveness through mimicry. Viral-encoded chemokines show a

considerable diversity in their pharmacological properties—from agonistic to antagonistic. For instance, Marek's disease virus encodes an interleukin-8 homolog (vIL-8) that shares homology with mammalian and avian IL-8, a prototype CXC chemokine. Similarly, IL-10 homologs have been identified in most primate cytomegaloviruses, equid herpesvirus 2, and in at least one herpesvirus of fish. It is likely that these virus-encoded proteins play a significant role in the pathogenesis of herpesvirus infections. Furthermore, as they are clustered at the initiation site for viral DNA replication, it has been proposed that the genes encoding these proteins were acquired from host cells, with the viruses acting as natural cloning vectors for the capture of cellular genes. Latent herpesvirus genomes are primarily maintained in host cells in a circular episomal (extrachromosomal) form or, less often, through chromosomal integration.

Virus Replication

Herpesvirus replication has been studied most extensively with human herpesviruses (herpes simplex virus 1) and, in light of the genetic diversity of viruses in the family, it is likely that there is considerable variation in the replication strategy utilized by individual herpesviruses. Cellular attachment of herpesviruses occurs via the binding of virion glycoprotein spikes to one of several host-cell receptors. Following attachment, the viral envelope fuses with the cell plasma membrane, the nucleocapsid enters the cytoplasm, and the DNA–protein complex is then freed from the nucleocapsid and enters the nucleus, quickly shutting off host-cell macromolecule synthesis.

Three classes of mRNA—α, β, and γ—are transcribed in sequence by cellular RNA polymerase II (Figure 9.3). Thus α (immediate early) RNAs, when processed appropriately to become mRNAs, are translated to form α proteins, which initiate transcription of β (early) mRNAs, the translation of which produces β (early) proteins and suppresses the transcription of further α mRNAs. Viral DNA replication then commences, utilizing some of the viral α and β proteins, in addition to host-cell proteins. The transcription program then switches again, and the resulting γ (late) mRNAs, which are transcribed from sequences situated throughout the genome, are translated into γ proteins. Over 70 virus-encoded proteins are made during the cycle, with many of the α and β proteins being enzymes and DNA-binding proteins, whereas most of the γ proteins are structural. Intricate controls regulate expression at the level of both transcription and translation. Viral DNA is replicated in the nucleus and newly synthesized DNA is spooled into preformed immature capsids.

Maturation involves the completion of encapsidation of virion DNA into nucleocapsids and the association of nucleocapsids with altered patches of the inner layer of the nuclear envelope. Complete envelopment occurs by budding through the nuclear membrane (Figure 9.4). Mature

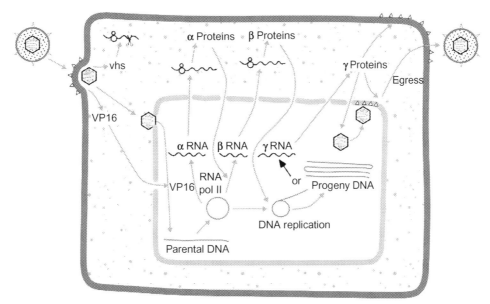

FIGURE 9.3 Diagram representing transcription, translation, and DNA replication of a typical herpesvirus. Transcription and post-transcriptional processing occur in the nucleus, translation in the cytoplasm; some of the α and β proteins are involved in further transcription, and some β proteins are involved in DNA replication. vhs is a tegument protein encoded by the UL41 gene, and inhibits host cell protein synthesis; VP16, encoded by the UL48 gene, is another tegument protein that is a transcription factor that enters the nucleus and activates immediate early viral genes. [*From* Virus Taxonomy: Eighth Report of the International Committee on Taxonomy of Viruses *(C. M. Fauquet, M. A. Mayo, J. Maniloff, U. Desselberger, L. A. Ball, eds), p. 197. Copyright © Elsevier (2005), with permission.*]

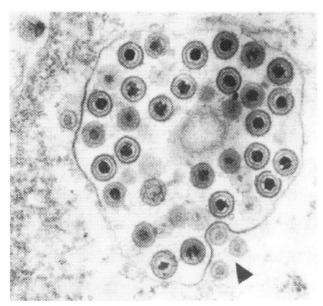

FIGURE 9.4 Thin-section electron microscopy of a herpesvirus-infected cell showing the formation of capsids and their primary envelopment by budding through the nuclear envelope (arrow). Magnification: ×65,000.

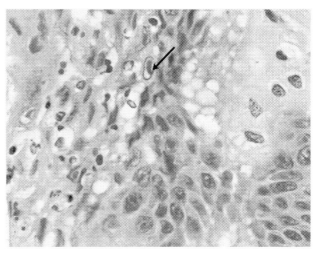

FIGURE 9.5 Histologic appearance of feline viral rhinotracheitis (felid herpesvirus 1). Lesion in the tongue of an infected cat showing epithelial necrosis and an infected cell with an intranuclear inclusion body (arrow). *(Courtesy P. Pesavento, University of California.)*

Intranuclear inclusion bodies are characteristic of herpesvirus infections, both in animals and in cell cultures (Figure 9.5).

Characteristics Common to Many Herpesvirus Infections

The herpesviruses exhibit many extraordinary infection characteristics that make them versatile pathogens. Transmission is

virions accumulate within vacuoles in the cytoplasm and are released by exocytosis or cytolysis. Virus-specific proteins are also found in the plasma membrane, where they are involved in cell fusion, may act as Fc receptors, and are presumed to be targets for immune cytolysis.

generally associated with mucosal contact, but droplet infection is also common. Moist, cool environmental conditions promote extended survival of herpesviruses, and windy conditions can promote aerosol transmission over longer distances. Many alphaherpesviruses produce localized lesions, particularly in the skin or on the mucosae of the respiratory and genital tracts, whereas generalized infections characterized by foci of necrosis in almost any organ or tissue are typical of infection of very young or immunocompromised animals. In pregnant animals, a mononuclear-cell-associated viremia may result in the transfer of virus across the placenta, leading to abortion, characteristically with multifocal areas of necrosis in several fetal organs. Infections with the beta- and gammaherpesvirus infections are often, but not invariably, clinically silent.

Persistent infection with periodic or continuous shedding occurs in all herpesvirus infections. In alphaherpesvirus infections, multiple copies of viral DNA are demonstrable, either as episomes or—more rarely—integrated into the chromosomal DNA of latently infected neurons. The latent genome is essentially silent, except for the production of a latency-related gene. This RNA transcript is not known to code for any protein; however, a small open reading frame (ORF-E) located within the latency-related gene appears to be expressed and inhibits apoptosis; the precise mechanisms responsible for the establishment, maintenance, and reactivation of latent infection are not fully characterized. Reactivation is usually associated with stress caused by intercurrent infections, shipping, cold, crowding, or by the administration of glucocorticoid drugs. Shedding of virus in nasal, oral, or genital secretions provides the source of infection for other animals, including transfer from dam to offspring. In domestic animals, reactivation is usually not noticed, in part because lesions on nasal or genital mucosae are not seen readily. Some betaherpesviruses and gammaherpesviruses are shed continuously from epithelial surfaces.

MEMBERS OF THE FAMILY *HERPESVIRIDAE*, SUBFAMILY *ALPHAHERPESVIRINAE*

BOVINE HERPESVIRUS 1 (INFECTIOUS BOVINE RHINOTRACHEITIS AND INFECTIOUS PUSTULAR VULVOVAGINITIS VIRUSES)

The rapid expansion of cattle feedlots in the United States during the 1950s quickly led to the recognition of several new disease syndromes, including a distinctive rhinotracheitis syndrome from which a herpesvirus was isolated. At the time, comparison of the herpesvirus isolated from cases of rhinotracheitis and from cases of vulvovaginitis in dairy cattle in the eastern United States indicated that the viruses were indistinguishable. It is now clear that the causative agent, bovine herpesvirus 1, is the causative agent of a variety of diseases in cattle, including rhinotracheitis, vulvovaginitis, balanoposthitis, conjunctivitis, abortion, enteritis, and a generalized disease of newborn calves. Encephalitis previously associated with bovine herpesvirus 1 infection is now known to be caused by a distinct virus, bovine herpesvirus 5.

Clinical Features and Epidemiology

Bovine herpesvirus 1 is the cause of both infectious bovine rhinotracheitis and infectious pustular vulvovaginitis. Infectious bovine rhinotracheitis occurs as a subclinical, mild, or severe disease. Morbidity approaches 100% and mortality may be substantial, particularly if complications occur. Initial signs include fever, depression, inappetence, and a profuse nasal discharge, initially serous and later mucopurulent. The nasal mucosa is hyperemic and lesions within the nasal cavity, which may be difficult to see, progress from focal necrosis with associated purulent inflammation to large areas of shallow, hemorrhagic, ulcerated mucosa covered by a cream-colored diphtheritic membrane. The breath may be fetid. Dyspnea, mouth breathing, salivation, and a deep bronchial cough are common. Acute, uncomplicated cases can last for 5–10 days.

Unilateral or bilateral conjunctivitis, often with profuse lacrimation, is a common clinical sign in cattle with infectious bovine rhinotracheitis, but may occur in a herd as an almost exclusive clinical sign. Gastroenteritis may occur in adult cattle and is a prominent finding in the generalized disease of neonatal calves, which is often fatal. Abortion may occur at 4–7 months gestation, and the virus has also been reported to cause mastitis.

Infectious pustular vulvovaginitis is recognized most commonly in dairy cows. Affected cows develop fever, depression, anorexia, and stand apart, often with the tail held away from contact with the vulva; micturition is frequent and painful. The vulval labia are swollen, there is a slight vulval discharge, and the vestibular mucosa is reddened, with many small pustules (see Figure 9.6 for comparable lesions in a goat). Adjacent pustules usually coalesce to form a fibrinous pseudomembrane that covers an ulcerated mucosa. The acute stage of the disease lasts 4–5 days and uncomplicated lesions usually heal by 10–14 days. Many cases are subclinical or go unnoticed.

Lesions of infectious balanoposthitis in bulls and the clinical course of disease are similar to the above equivalent in cows. Semen from recovered bulls may be contaminated with virus as a result of periodic shedding. However, cows may conceive to servicing or artificial insemination by infected bulls, from which they acquire infectious pustular vulvovaginitis, and pregnant cows that develop the infection rarely abort. Bovine herpesvirus 1 has been isolated occasionally from cases of vaginitis and balanitis in swine, from stillborn piglets, and from aborted equine fetuses.

Genital and respiratory diseases are rarely diagnosed simultaneously in the same herd. Infectious bovine rhinotracheitis is an uncommon disease in free-range cattle, but is of major significance in feedlots. Primary infection often coincides with transport and introduction to a feedlot of young, fully susceptible cattle from diverse sources. Adaptation from range to feedlot conditions and dietary changes, including the high protein diet, contribute to a stressful environment that may potentiate disease. Virus-induced injury to the mucosal lining of the respiratory tract predisposes to bacterial infection, especially in stressed cattle, and contributes to the complex syndrome called shipping fever (bovine respiratory disease complex) that culminates in severe pneumonia caused by *Mannheimia haemolytica*. The virus can be mechanically transmitted between bulls in artificial insemination centers, and virus may also be spread by artificial insemination.

Life-long latent infection with periodic virus shedding occurs after bovine herpesvirus 1 infection; the sciatic and trigeminal ganglia are the sites of latency following genital and respiratory disease, respectively. The administration of corticosteroids results in reactivation of the virus and has been used as a means of detecting and eliminating carrier bulls in artificial insemination centers.

Bovine herpesvirus 1 and the diseases it causes occur worldwide, although several countries within the European Union have recently eradicated the virus (including Denmark, Finland, Sweden, Switzerland, and Austria), and eradication is under way in several other countries. Control measures in breeding farms within eradication zones preclude the purchase of virus-positive animals, the use of live-attenuated or whole-virus vaccines, and the insemination of cows with semen from positive bulls. Successful eradication prompts strict import restrictions on cattle, semen, and embryos because the reintroduction of the virus into these immunologically naïve populations is likely to have serious consequences and lead to severe economic losses. Cattle are the primary reservoir, and infection is transmitted during initial clinical disease or from reactivation of latent infections, with subsequent virus shedding.

Pathogenesis and Pathology

Genital disease may result from coitus or artificial insemination with infective semen, although some outbreaks, particularly in dairy cows, may occur in the absence of coitus. Respiratory disease and conjunctivitis result from droplet transmission. Within the animal, dissemination of the virus from the initial focus of infection probably occurs via a cell-associated viremia.

In both the genital and the respiratory forms of the disease, the lesions are focal areas of epithelial cell necrosis in which there is ballooning of epithelial cells; typical herpesvirus inclusions may be present in nuclei at the periphery of necrotic foci. There is an intense inflammatory response within the necrotic mucosa, frequently with formation of an overlying accumulation of fibrin and cellular debris (pseudomembrane). Gross lesions are frequently not observed in aborted fetuses, but microscopic necrotic foci are present in most tissues and the liver and adrenal glands are affected most consistently.

Diagnosis

The clinical presentation of infectious bovine rhinotracheitis and infectious pustular vulvovaginitis are characteristic; however, many bovine herpesvirus 1 infections are subclinical, especially in free-ranging cattle. Rapid diagnostic methods for detection of bovine herpesvirus 1 include virus-specific polymerase chain reaction (PCR), electron microscopy of vesicular fluid or scrapings, and immunofluorescence staining of smears or tissue sections. Virus isolation and characterization provide a definitive diagnosis. Herpesviruses are grown most readily in cell cultures derived from their natural host. As with other alphaherpesviruses, there is a rapid cytopathic effect, with syncytia and characteristic eosinophilic intranuclear inclusion bodies. Bovine herpesvirus 1 specific PCR for virus detection and specific enzyme immunoassays for antibody detection (serology) are now routinely used in reference laboratories in many countries.

For aborted fetuses, histopathologic evaluation coupled with immunohistochemical staining is diagnostic and the presence of bovine herpesvirus 1 can be further confirmed using PCR or virus isolation.

Immunity, Prevention, and Control

Bovine herpesvirus 1 infections are especially important in feedlot cattle, where control strategies are directed at management practices and vaccination. Bovine herpesvirus 1 vaccines are used extensively, alone or in combination as multiple virus formulations. Inactivated and live-attenuated vaccines are available and recombinant DNA vaccines have been constructed in which the thymidine kinase and other glycoprotein "marker" genes have been deleted. Although they do not prevent infection, vaccines significantly reduce the incidence and severity of disease. Importantly, breeding animals in enzootic countries, except those for export to countries free of bovine herpesvirus 1, should be vaccinated before coitus, to prevent the virus inducing abortion. In enzootic regions, vaccination to maintain population immunity is best done prior to stressful situations such as weaning or transport. Experimental vaccines produced by recombinant methods have been tested: they are based on single glycoprotein genes, particularly *gD*, that have been expressed in various expression systems or have been placed in plasmid vectors for delivery as DNA vaccines.

Whole-virus vaccines were not used in the successful bovine herpesvirus 1 eradication programs in some countries within the European Union, because of an inability to differentiate vaccinated from latently infected animals. Within the European Union eradication program, vaccination can only be authorized by veterinary authorities and is compulsory in farms with recent evidence of virus transmission. Live marker vaccines can be used only for immunological priming of young cattle. Serologically negative and positive cattle can be held in the same barn, but positive animals must be immunized with an inactivated marker vaccine before leaving. Immunization before departure is thought to increase antibody titers and decrease transmission risk should virus reactivation occur.

BOVINE HERPESVIRUS 2 (MAMMILLITIS/PSEUDO-LUMPY SKIN DISEASE VIRUS)

Two clinical forms of bovine herpesvirus 2 infections are described: one in which lesions are localized to the teats, occasionally spreading to the udder (bovine mammillitis), and a second, more generalized skin disease (pseudo-lumpy skin disease). Bovine herpesvirus 2 was first isolated in 1957 from cattle in South Africa with a generalized lumpy skin disease. The disease was mild and its major significance lay in the need to differentiate it from a more serious lumpy skin disease found in South Africa caused by a poxvirus (see Chapter 7). The benign nature of pseudo-lumpy skin disease, the characteristic central depression on the surface of the skin nodules, the superficial necrosis of the epidermis, and the shorter course of the disease are all helpful in differentiating the condition from true lumpy skin disease. Elsewhere in Africa, a similar herpesvirus was isolated from cattle with extensive erosions of the teats; it was subsequently isolated from similar lesions in cattle in many countries of the world. Bovine herpesvirus 2 is both antigenically and genetically related to human herpes simplex virus.

Clinical Features and Epidemiology

As is generally true for members of the subfamily *Alphaherpesvirinae*, serologic surveys indicate a higher incidence of infection than disease. Pseudo-lumpy skin disease has an incubation period of 5–9 days and is characterized by a mild fever, followed by the sudden appearance of skin nodules: a few, or many, on the face, neck, back, and perineum. The nodules have a flat surface with a slightly depressed center, and involve only the superficial layers of the epidermis, which undergo necrosis. Within 7–8 days, the local swelling subsides and healing, without scar formation, is complete within a few weeks.

In many countries, bovine herpesvirus 2 is recognized only as a cause of mammillitis, but virus isolated experimentally from cases of mammillitis can cause generalized skin disease. Lesions usually occur only on the teats, but in severe cases most of the skin of the udder may be affected. Occasionally, heifers may develop fever, coinciding with the appearance of lesions. Milk yield may be reduced by as much as 10% as a result of difficulty in milking the affected cows, and intercurrent mastitis.

Pseudo-lumpy skin disease occurs most commonly in southern Africa, in moist low-lying areas, especially along rivers, and has its highest incidence in the summer months and early fall. Susceptible cattle cannot be infected by placing them in contact with diseased cattle if housed in insect-proof accommodation. It is therefore assumed that mechanical transmission of the virus occurs by arthropods, but the specific vector remains uncharacterized. Buffalo, giraffe, and other African wildlife may be naturally infected with bovine herpesvirus 2.

Although milking machines were initially believed to be responsible for the transmission of mammillitis in dairy herds, there is evidence that this is rarely the case. The infection may spread rapidly through a herd, but in some outbreaks disease is confined to newly calved heifers or pregnant cattle in late gestation.

Pathogenesis and Pathology

The distribution of lesions in mammillitis suggests restricted, local spread, whereas the generalized distribution of lesions in pseudo-lumpy skin disease suggests viremic spread. However, viremia is difficult to demonstrate.

Diagnosis

Demonstration of virus in scrapings or vesicular fluid by electron microscopy, coupled with virus isolation, is used for confirming a diagnosis.

Immunity, Prevention, and Control

Because of the possibility of transmission from clinically normal but persistently infected cattle through reactivation of latent virus, infected cattle should not be introduced into naïve populations. The clinical differentiation of the various conditions that affect the teats of cattle can be difficult; other viral infections that can produce similar teat lesions are warts, cowpox, pseudocowpox, vesicular stomatitis, and foot-and-mouth disease viruses. For this reason it is advisable to examine the whole herd, as a comparison of the early developmental stages helps considerably in the diagnosis. Advanced lesions are often similar, irrespective of the cause.

BOVINE HERPESVIRUS 5 (BOVINE ENCEPHALITIS VIRUS)

Subtypes of bovine herpesvirus 1 were previously associated with encephalitis, particularly amongst cattle in Argentina, Brazil, and Australia. Subtype bovine herpesvirus 1.3 has been renamed bovine herpesvirus 5. Encephalitis caused by bovine herpesvirus 5 has been recognized in several countries as a fatal meningoencephalitis in calves. The disease is thought to result from direct neural spread from the nasal cavity, pharynx, and tonsils via the maxillary and mandibular branches of the trigeminal nerve. Lesions initially occur in the midbrain and later involve the entire brain. Because of the close antigenic relationship of bovine herpesviruses 1 and 5, bovine herpesvirus 1 vaccines are likely to be protective against bovine herpesvirus 5 infection.

CANID HERPESVIRUS 1

Canid herpesvirus 1 is the cause of a rare but highly fatal, generalized hemorrhagic disease of pups under 4 weeks of age. The prevalence of the virus, based on antibody surveys, is low (<20%). It probably occurs worldwide. In sexually mature dogs, canid herpesvirus 1 causes genital disease, although this is rarely diagnosed clinically.

The incubation period varies from 3 to 8 days and in fatal disease the course is brief, just 1–2 days. Signs in affected pups include painful crying, abdominal pain, anorexia, and dyspnea. In older dogs there may be vaginal or preputial discharge and, on careful examination, a focal nodular lesion of the vaginal, penile, and preputial epithelium may be identified. The virus may also cause respiratory disease and may be part of the canine respiratory disease complex (so called "kennel cough" syndrome).

Pups born to presumably seronegative bitches are infected oronasally, either from their dam's vagina or from other infected dogs. Pups less than 4 weeks old that become hypothermic develop the generalized, often fatal disease. There is a cell-associated viremia, followed by virus replication in vascular endothelium lining small blood vessels. The optimal temperature for virus replication is about 33°C—that is, the temperature of the outer genital and upper respiratory tracts. The hypothalamic thermoregulatory centers of the pup are not fully operative until about 4 weeks of age. Accordingly, in the context of canine herpesvirus 1 infection, the pup is critically dependent on ambient temperature and maternal contact for the maintenance of its normal body temperature. The more severe the hypothermia, the more severe and rapid is the course of the disease, so raising the body temperature early in the course of infection may have therapeutic value.

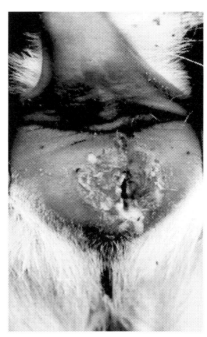

FIGURE 9.6 Caprine herpesvirus-induced vulvovaginitis. *(Courtesy of K. Thompson, Massey University.)*

Gross necropsy findings, particularly ecchymotic hemorrhages throughout the kidney and gastrointestinal tract of affected pups, are characteristic. Inclusion bodies may be present in hepatocytes, and the causative virus can be isolated readily in canine cell cultures. An inactivated (killed virus) vaccine is available in Europe.

CAPRINE HERPESVIRUS 1

Herpesviruses have been isolated from goats in much of the world, in association with a variety of clinical signs, including conjunctivitis and disease of the respiratory, digestive, and genital tracts, including abortion and a disease identical to infectious pustular vulvovaginitis of cattle (Figure 9.6). Caprine herpesvirus 1 is both genetically and antigenically related to bovine herpesvirus 1; although the goat virus can infect cattle, its ability to cause disease appears restricted to goats.

CERCOPITHECINE HERPESVIRUS 1 (B VIRUS DISEASE OF MACAQUES)

Macaques are frequently infected with cercopithecine herpesvirus 1 (*syn.* B virus). The natural history of this infection is very similar to that of herpes simplex type 1 infection in humans, and, like herpes simplex, it causes generally mild disease in macaques. B virus is a significant zoonotic hazard. Although zoonotic transmission to humans is relatively rare, the consequences are profound. A number of fatal cases of ascending paralysis and encephalitis in humans have occurred, with infection being transmitted directly by monkey bite or indirectly by monkey saliva. Most cases have occurred among animal handlers and biomedical researchers with occupational exposure to macaques, although transmission has also been documented among laboratory workers handling macaque central nervous system and kidney tissues. The risk presented to owners by pet macaques and to tourists visiting exotic wild-animal parks where there are free-ranging macaques has also been recognized.

Cercopithecine herpesvirus 1 infection is common in all macaques (*Macaca spp.*), with rhesus, Japanese, cynomolgus, pig-tailed, and stump-tailed macaques being the species used most commonly in biomedical research. Neutralizing antibodies are found in 75–100% of adult macaques in captive populations. The virus is transmitted among free-ranging or group-housed monkeys, primarily through sexual activity and bites. These biologic features lend themselves to eliminating enzootic infection in captive macaques by isolating young, uninfected animals from older infected monkeys. Through this process, growing numbers of captive-bred research macaques are becoming free of B virus. Like many herpes simplex virus infections in humans, primary B virus infection in monkeys is often minor, but is characterized by life-long latent infection in trigeminal and lumbosacral ganglia, with intermittent reactivation and shedding of the virus in saliva or genital secretions, particularly during periods of stress or immunosuppression. Infected animals, especially acutely infected juveniles, may develop oral vesicles and ulcers.

B virus disease in humans usually results from macaque bites or scratches. Incubation periods may be as short as 2 days, but more commonly are 2–5 weeks. In some cases, the first clinical signs are the formation of vesicles, pruritus, and hyperesthesia at the bite site. This is followed quickly by ascending paralysis, encephalitis, and death. In some case there are no characteristic clinical symptoms before the onset of encephalitis. In a series of 24 reported human cases, 19 (79%) were fatal and most surviving patients have had moderate to severe neurologic impairment, sometimes requiring life-long institutionalization; however, the use of antiviral drugs (aciclovir or related agents) can be of benefit, and the rapid diagnosis and initiation of therapy are of paramount importance in preventing death or permanent disability in surviving patients.

In most developed countries, there are strict regulations regarding the importation, breeding, and handling of non-human primates, in many cases prohibiting their ownership as pets. However, macaque and other primate species continue to be marketed and kept as pets, despite evidence that all macaque species are inherently dangerous because of the risk of B virus transmission, as well as the likelihood of serious physical injury from bite wounds. Following occupational exposure of a human to a macaque

monkey by bite, scratch, or needle-stick injury, the macaque should be evaluated for possible B virus shedding: (1) the monkey is examined for any signs of ulceration of oral and genital mucosa or neurologic abnormalities; (2) oral swab specimens are collected for viral antigen and/or nucleic acid testing and blood/serum is collected for serology at a special reference laboratory (enzyme immunoassays and immunoblot assays have replaced virus isolation and serum neutralization in these laboratories); (3) a physician specializing in such occupational risks is contacted to treat the person.

HERPES SIMPLEX VIRUS 1 IN ANIMALS

Herpes simplex virus 1 can be a significant anthropozoonotic agent. It has been associated with outbreaks of severe generalized disease with high mortality in New World primates, particularly marmosets and owl monkeys, and is a hazard for pet New World primates also. A wide variety of New World species are experimentally susceptible. Old World primates tend not to be as susceptible to severe disease. Epizootics of multisystemic disease with high mortality have been documented in rabbitries that are attributable to a virus that is genetically related to, if not the same as, herpes simplex virus. Transmission of herpes simplex virus from human owners to pet rabbits, resulting in encephalitis, occurs sporadically.

CERCOPITHECINE HERPESVIRUS 9 (SIMIAN VARICELLA VIRUS)

Simian varicella is a naturally occurring disease of Old World monkeys (superfamily *Cercopithecoidea*). The disease is characterized by varicella-like (chickenpox) clinical signs, including fever, lethargy, and vesicular rash on the face, abdomen, and extremities. Disseminated infection often results in life-threatening pneumonia and hepatitis. Epizootics have occurred in captive African green (vervet) monkeys (*Cercopithecus aethiops*), patas monkeys (*Erythrocebus patas*), and several species of macaque (*Macaca* spp.). Like human varicella-zoster virus, the simian virus establishes latency in sensory ganglia and is reactivated to cause recrudescent disease and shedding. Reactivation leads to transmission of the highly contagious virus to susceptible monkeys and is the basis for epizootics.

EQUID HERPESVIRUS 1 (EQUINE ABORTION VIRUS)

Equid herpesvirus 1 is considered to be the most important viral cause of abortion in horses, and is enzootic in horse populations worldwide. The virus is also the cause of respiratory disease and encephalomyelitis.

Equid herpesvirus 1 was historically designated equine rhinopnuemonitis virus but, with the discovery of equid herpesvirus 4 as a predominantly respiratory virus, the term "equine rhinopnuemonitis virus" is now being applied to this agent. However, with regard to the scientific literature, simply equating equine rhinopnuemonitis virus to equid herpesvirus 4 will be incorrect in many instances.

Clinical Signs and Epidemiology

The principal route of equid herpesvirus 1 infection is via the respiratory tract. A small proportion of foals are infected very early in life and the virus then circulates, often inapparently, between mares and foals and, subsequently, between older foals after weaning and amongst adult horses. Viremia occurs after respiratory infection, sometimes leading to systemic infection and serious disease manifestations. In fully susceptible horses, equid herpesvirus 1 is a significant cause of abortion. Cases of abortion are usually sporadic and only affect a single mare, but if large numbers of susceptible mares are exposed to the aborted conceptus, extensive outbreaks of abortion (abortion storms) occur. Mares abort without any specific premonitory signs and the fetus is usually born dead. Although abortions may occur early in gestation, the majority occur in the last trimester of gestation. It may be difficult to definitively identify the source of virus responsible for abortion storms, as such outbreaks can occur in fully closed herds to which no new horses have been introduced for many years. In other instances, outbreaks occur following the introduction of new animals into an established herd. Systemic disease can occur in newborn foals infected immediately before parturition.

Encephalomyelitis has been recognized for many years as an uncommon clinical manifestation of systemic equid herpesvirus 1 infection. However, outbreaks of herpesvirus-induced encephalomyelitis have been reported with increased frequency in recent years, particularly in the United States. A number of large race tracks, veterinary hospitals, and other venues where horses congregate have been closed and quarantined because of outbreaks of this disease. Clinical signs vary in presentation and severity, depending on the site and extent of the lesion within the central nervous system, ranging from mild ataxia and urinary incontinence to limb paralysis and death. The prognosis for horses that do not become recumbent is generally favorable, but recumbency is associated with high mortality.

Pathogenesis and Pathology

Most cases of equid herpesvirus 1 abortion occur late in gestation and the fetus is aborted without evidence of autolysis. In contrast, fetuses aborted before 6 months of gestation may exhibit significant autolysis. Aborted fetuses may exhibit icterus, meconium staining of the integument, excessive fluid (edema) in body cavities, distention of the lungs (Figure 9.7), splenomegaly with prominent lymphoid follicles, and numerous pale foci of necrosis that are evident on the capsular or cut surfaces of the liver.

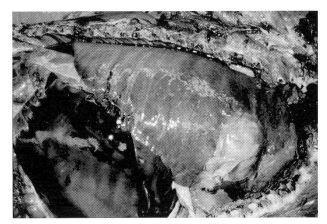

FIGURE 9.7 Equid herpesvirus abortion: interstitial pneumonia in aborted foal. *(Courtesy of H. DeCock, University of California.)*

Characteristic microscopic lesions include bronchiolitis and interstitial pneumonitis, severe necrosis of splenic white pulp, and focal necrosis of the liver and adrenal glands, and the presence of typical herpesvirus intranuclear inclusion bodies that are often abundant within these lesions. Similar lesions can be present in live-born foals infected in very late gestation.

Equid herpesvirus 1 encephalomyelitis is not a result of infection of neurons or glial cells; rather, lesions result from viral infection and replication in the endothelial cells lining arterioles of the brain and spinal cord. Lesions are characterized by vasculitis with thrombosis and ischemic necrosis of adjacent neural tissue. The lesions are focal and their identification may require thorough examination of the entire brain and spinal cord of an affected horse. Affected regions are identified by discrete, randomly distributed areas of hemorrhage within the brain and/or spinal cord of affected horses. Recently, a single nucleotide polymorphism corresponding to a single amino acid change in the polymerase enzyme (encoded by open reading frame 30) has been putatively associated with increased neurovirulence of equid herpesvirus 1; however, this change is not present in all viruses isolated from cases of encephalomyelitis and is also present in some strains of equid herpesvirus 1 that have been isolated from horses without neurological disease.

Diagnosis

The diagnosis of equid herpesvirus 1 infections typically begins with the characteristic clinical presentation of abortion. Gross and histological lesions in aborted foals are highly suggestive of equid herpesvirus 1, particularly the identification of intranuclear inclusion bodies within affected tissues. The diagnosis may be quickly confirmed by immunohistochemical staining using equid herpesvirus 1 specific antisera. Definitive diagnosis of equid herpesvirus 1 abortion relies on virus identification, either by virus-specific PCR or by virus isolation. The preferred samples for virus detection are fetal lung, thymus, and spleen. Identification of the causative virus is important because, although abortion is usually associated with equid herpesvirus 1, sporadic cases are caused by equid herpesvirus 4 infection. In contrast to alphaherpesvirus-induced encephalitis in other species, it can be difficult or impossible to isolate equid herpesvirus 1 from neural tissues of horses with encephalomyelitis, but presence of the virus within lesions can be confirmed by immunohistochemical staining or by virus-specific PCR assay. While equid herpesviruses 1 and 4 share many antigens, a recombinant antigen based on a variable region at the C terminus of glycoprotein G is available to detect antibody that is specific for each virus. When fetal tissue is not available, an increasing antibody level on enzyme-linked immunosorbent assay in the affected mare can be used to confirm equid herpesvirus 1 abortion.

Immunity, Prevention, and Control

Equid herpesvirus 1 circulates asymptomatically in herds with enzootic infection and, therefore, control of associated diseases is achieved through a combination of management practices and vaccination. Mares are generally vaccinated regularly to reduce the frequency of abortion, and a variety of inactivated and live-attenuated vaccines are available and widely used. Vaccination with inactivated vaccines is often used during abortion outbreaks in an effort to minimize losses, but management practices and adherence to well-established codes of practice are also key; specifically, the isolation of pregnant mares in small groups based on their foaling dates, as the likelihood of virus recrudescence can be reduced by not introducing new mares into established groups. The isolation of the index case (the first mare to abort) and all in-contact mares until they either abort or foal is also critical.

EQUID HERPESVIRUS 3 (EQUINE COITAL EXANTHEMA VIRUS)

A disease that was probably equine coital exanthema has long been known, but its causative agent was not shown to be an alphaherpesvirus (equid herpesvirus 3) until 1968. Equid herpesvirus 3 shows no serologic cross-reactivity with other equine herpesviruses by neutralization tests, but shares antigens with equid herpesvirus 1. Equid herpesvirus 3 grows only in cells of equine origin. The virus causes a venereal disease of horses analogous to human genital herpes caused by herpes simplex virus.

Equine coital exanthema is an acute, usually mild disease characterized by the formation of pustular and ulcerative lesions on the vaginal and vestibular mucosae and adjacent perineal skin of affected mares, and on the penis and prepuce of affected stallions. Lesions are occasionally present on the teats, lips, and respiratory mucosa. The incidence of antibody in sexually active horses is much higher

(about 50%) than the reported incidence of disease. The incubation period may be as short as 2 days and, in uncomplicated cases, healing is usually complete by 14 days. Where the skin of the vulva, penis, and prepuce is black, white depigmented spots mark for life the site of earlier lesions and identify potential carriers.

Although genital lesions may be extensive, there are no systemic signs, and unless the affected areas are examined carefully cases are missed readily. Abortion or infertility is not generally associated with equid herpesvirus 3 infection; indeed, mares usually conceive to the service in which they acquire the disease. Abortion has been described following experimental in-utero inoculation. Affected stallions show decreased libido and the presence of the disease may seriously disrupt breeding schedules. Recurrent disease is more likely to occur when stallions are in frequent use. Management of the disease consists of the removal of stallions from service until all lesions have healed, together with symptomatic treatment.

Equid herpesvirus 3 can cause subclinical respiratory infection in yearling horses, and has been isolated from vesicular lesions on the muzzles of foals in contact with infected mares.

EQUID HERPESVIRUS 4 (EQUINE RHINOPNEUMONITIS VIRUS)

Equid herpesvirus 4 is the most important of the several herpesviruses that cause acute respiratory disease of horses. Foals are often infected in the first few weeks of life and the virus circulates, often asymptomatically or subclinically, amongst the mare and foal population. Acute respiratory disease due to equid herpesvirus 4 occurs most commonly in foals over 2 months old, as passive immune protection derived from their mothers wanes. Weanlings and yearlings typically become infected and display clinical signs of respiratory disease caused by equid herpesvirus 4 as they are mixed into new social groups following weaning, or during preparation for yearling sales. There is fever, anorexia, and a profuse serous nasal discharge that later becomes mucopurulent. Recrudescence of latent virus may lead to disease episodes in later life. Live-attenuated and inactivated equine herpesvirus 1 vaccines are available, including combined products that include both equid herpesviruses 1 and 4.

EQUID HERPESVIRUSES 6, 8 AND 9

Equid herpesviruses 6 and 8 are also respectively designated as asinine herpesviruses 1 and 3, as both were originally isolated from donkeys. Asinine herpesvirus 1 causes venereal lesions similar to those of equid herpesvirus 3, whereas asinine herpesvirus 3 is closely related to equid herpesvirus 1. These viruses also infect wild equids, including asses and zebra. Equid herpesvirus 9 is most closely related to a neurotropic strain of equid herpesvirus 1. First described in Thomson's gazelles (gazelle herpesvirus), equid herpesvirus 9 has subsequently been identified in a giraffe with encephalitis and, most recently, an adult polar bear with progressive neurologic signs. Infection of domestic horses with equid herpesvirus 9 resulted in only transient fever.

FELID HERPESVIRUS 1 (FELINE VIRAL RHINOTRACHEITIS VIRUS)

Felid herpesvirus 1 causes acute disease of the upper respiratory tract, most commonly amongst cats in their first year of life. Infection and therefore disease are most common in households with several cats, animal shelters, and catteries. After an incubation period of 24–48 hours there is a sudden onset of bouts of sneezing, coughing, profuse serous nasal and ocular discharges, frothy salivation, dyspnea, anorexia, weight loss, and fever. Occasionally there may be ulcers on the tongue. Keratitis associated with punctate corneal ulcers is common (Figure 9.8). In fully susceptible kittens up to 4 weeks old, the extensive rhinotracheitis and an associated bronchopneumonia may be fatal. Clinically, the acute disease caused by felid herpesvirus 1 is very similar to that caused by feline caliciviruses, and virus detection assays are usually required for definitive identification of the specific causative virus. Felid herpesvirus 1 infection of cats older than 6 months of age is likely to result in mild or subclinical infection. Pregnant queens may abort, although there is no evidence that the virus crosses the placenta and fatally infects fetuses, and virus has not been isolated from aborted placenta or fetuses.

The characteristic histological lesions of feline rhinotracheitis include necrosis of epithelia of the nasal cavity, pharynx, epiglottis, tonsils, larynx, and trachea and, in extreme cases, in young kittens, a bronchopneumonia. Typical

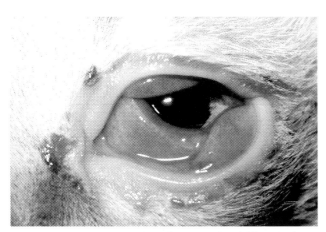

FIGURE 9.8 Feline herpesvirus disease: conjunctivitis and corneal opacity as a consequence of felid herpesvirus 1 infection. *(Courtesy of D. Maggs, University of California.)*

intranuclear inclusion bodies may be present within the affected tissues of cats that die in the course of acute disease, within 7–9 days after infection (Figure 9.5).

Inactivated virus and attenuated virus vaccines are used for the control of infections caused by felid herpesvirus 1; they reduce disease but do not prevent infection. In addition, a number of genetically engineered vaccines have been developed for felid herpesvirus 1.

GALLID HERPESVIRUS 1 (AVIAN INFECTIOUS LARYNGOTRACHEITIS VIRUS)

Identified as a specific viral disease of chickens in the United States in 1925, infectious laryngotracheitis, caused by gallid herpesvirus 1, occurs among chickens worldwide. This virus also causes disease in pheasants. Chickens of all ages are susceptible, but disease is most common in those aged 4–18 months. After an incubation period of 6–12 days, mild coughing and sneezing are followed by nasal and ocular discharge, dyspnea, loud gasping and coughing, and depression. In severe cases, the neck is raised and the head extended during inspiration—"pump handle respiration." Head shaking with coughing is characteristic, and may be associated with expectoration of bloody mucus and frank blood that appear on the beak, face, and feathers. Morbidity approaches 100%; the mortality for virulent strains may be 50–70% and that for strains of low virulence about 20%. Strains of low virulence are associated with conjunctivitis, ocular discharge, swollen infraorbital and nasal sinuses, and decreased egg production. The mild enzootic form is most common in modern poultry production, and the severe epizootic form is uncommon.

There is severe laryngotracheitis in affected birds, characterized by necrosis, hemorrhage, ulceration, and the formation of diphtheritic membranes. Extensive diphtheritic membrane formation can plug the airway at the tracheal bifurcation, resulting in death from asphyxia, which has led to the use of the term "fowl diphtheria." The virus probably persists as a latent infection, and has been recovered from tracheal explant cultures more than 3 months after infection.

Diagnosis of infectious laryngotracheitis usually is made on the basis of clinical signs and one or more confirmatory tests, such as detection of typical intranuclear inclusions in respiratory tissues, detection of virus-specific antigen by fluorescent antibody or immunohistochemical staining of smears and tissues, detection of virus-specific DNA by PCR assay, or isolation of the virus either by inoculation on the chorioallantoic membrane of embryonated eggs or by cell cultures. As an adjunct diagnostic tool, neutralizing antibody may be detected by pock or plaque reduction assays; enzyme immunoassays also have been developed.

Infectious laryngotracheitis virus is usually introduced into a flock via carrier birds; it is transmitted by droplet and inhalation to respiratory tract, droplets to conjunctiva, or, less commonly, by ingestion. Although it spreads rapidly through a flock, new clinical cases may occur over a period of 2–8 weeks; thus it spreads somewhat more slowly than acute respiratory diseases such as Newcastle disease, influenza, and infectious bronchitis. It is feasible to establish and maintain flocks free of infectious laryngotracheitis, and where management systems allow, this practice is increasingly adopted, particularly in the broiler industry where birds are harvested at 5–9 weeks of age and where "all-in–all-out" management is possible. However, for breeding and egg production flocks, vaccination is still widely practiced, using attenuated virus vaccine. This protects birds against disease, but not against infection with virulent virus or the development of a latent carrier status for either the virulent or the vaccine viruses. Outbreaks of acute disease have occurred in broilers as a result of reversion to virulence of vaccine virus strains.

GALLID HERPESVIRUS 2 (MAREK'S DISEASE VIRUS)

Jozef Marek first described the disease that now bears his name in Hungary in 1907, but the identification of the causative agent as a herpesvirus was not established until 1967. Before the introduction of vaccination in 1970, Marek's disease was the most common lymphoproliferative disease of chickens, causing substantial economic losses worldwide. Vaccination has reduced the incidence of disease dramatically, but not infection. Marek's disease remains an important disease of chickens because of continuing losses from disease and the costs of vaccination.

Clinical Features and Epidemiology

Marek's disease is a progressive disease with variable signs and several overlapping pathological syndromes. In its clinical presentation, Marek's disease can resemble avian leukosis, although there are key differences between the two diseases. Lymphoproliferative syndromes are most frequent with Marek's disease, lymphoma being most common, with involvement of several visceral organs and, usually, asymmetric paralysis of one or both legs or wings. Incoordination is a common early sign: one leg is held forward and the other backward when the bird is stationary, because of unilateral paresis or paralysis. Wing dropping and lowering of the head and neck are common. If the vagus nerve is involved, there may be dilation of the crop and gasping. Marek's disease lymphoma sometimes may occur without neurological signs, and present only as depression and comatose state, with visceral lymphomas.

Acute Marek's disease or fowl paralysis occurs in explosive outbreaks in young chickens, in which a large proportion of birds in a flock show depression followed, after a few days, by ataxia and paralysis of some birds. Significant mortality occurs without localizing neurologic signs. Visceral lymphomas are typically absent in affected birds, but nerve lesions are prominent.

Ocular lymphomatosis is a rare syndrome that leads to graying of the iris of one or both eyes as a result of infiltration of transformed lymphocytes; the pupil is irregular and eccentric, and there is partial or total blindness. Mortality is rare.

Cutaneous Marek's disease is recognized readily after plucking, when round, nodular lesions up to 1 cm in diameter occur, particularly at feather follicles of young birds. The non-feathered area of the legs may have a distinct red coloration, and Marek's disease is therefore sometimes called "redleg syndrome."

Other syndromes include lymphodegenerative syndromes, transient paralysis from transient brain edema, and atherosclerosis, all of which are rare and produce low to no mortality.

Most chickens have antibody to Marek's disease virus (gallid herpesvirus 2) by the time they are mature; infection persists and virus is released in dander from the feather follicles. Congenital infection does not occur, and chicks are refractory for the first few weeks of life because of the protected and complex process that leads to lymphoma. Birds typically are infected by the inhalation of virus in the dust. Epizootics of Marek's disease usually involve sexually immature birds 2–5 months old; a high mortality (about 80%) soon peaks and then declines sharply. Virtually all commercial chickens in the United States and other countries with intensive commercial poultry production now are vaccinated against Marek's disease at hatching, making the incidence of the disease very low.

Pathogenesis and Pathology

Marek's disease virus is slowly cytopathic and remains highly cell-associated, so that cell-free infectious virus is rare, except in dander from feather follicles. The outcome of infection of chickens by Marek's disease virus is influenced by the virus strain, dose, and route of infection and by the age, sex, immune status, and genetic susceptibility of the chickens. Subclinical infection with virus shedding is common. Infection is acquired by inhalation of dander. Epithelial cells of the respiratory tract are infected productively and contribute to a cell-associated viremia involving macrophages. Productive infection of lymphoid cells in a variety of organs, including the thymus, cloacal bursa (bursa of Fabricius), bone marrow, and spleen, results in immune suppression. During the second week after infection there is a persistent cell-associated viremia followed by a proliferation of T cells, and a week later deaths begin to occur within the flock, although regression may also occur. The discovery that the genome of Marek's disease virus has incorporated *onc* genes that resemble those found in avian retroviruses provides a very rational basis for explaining the pathogenesis of the disease. T lymphocytes are transformed by the virus to produce T-cell lymphomas, and up to 90 genome equivalents of Marek's disease virus DNA can be demonstrated in transformed cells, in both plasmid and integrated forms.

The basis for genetic resistance is not fully defined, but has been correlated with birds that carry the B21 alloantigen of the B red blood cell group. Maternal antibody may persist in newly hatched chicks for up to 3 weeks, and infection of such chicks with virulent Marek's disease virus may not produce disease but may lead to an active immune response. Chickens that are bursectomized and then actively immunized also survive challenge infection.

Many apparently healthy birds are life-long carriers and shedders of virus, but the virus is not transmitted *in ovo*. When fully susceptible 1-day-old chicks are infected with virulent virus, the minimum time for detection of microscopic lesions is 1–2 weeks, and gross lesions are present by 3–4 weeks. Maximal virus shedding occurs at 5–6 weeks after infection.

Enlargement of one or more peripheral nerve trunks is the most constant gross finding: in the vast majority of cases, a diagnosis can be made if the celiac, cranial, intercostal, mesenteric, brachial, sciatic, and greater splanchnic nerves are examined. In a diseased bird, the nerves are up to three times their normal diameter, show loss of striations, and are edematous, gray, or yellowish, and somewhat translucent in appearance. Because enlargement is frequently unilateral, it is especially helpful to compare contralateral nerves. The gross lesions of Marek's disease may be indistinguishable from those of avian leukosis.

The lesions of Marek's disease result from the infiltration and *in-situ* proliferation of T lymphocytes, which may result in leukemia, but in addition there is often a significant inflammatory cell response to the lysis of non-lymphoid cells by the virus. Lesions of the feather follicle are invariably a mixture of lymphoblasts and other inflammatory cells. Involvement of epithelial cells at the base of feather follicles is important, in that productive infection of these cells is also associated with the release of cell-free infectious virus.

Diagnosis

If sufficient numbers of birds are examined, history, age, clinical signs, and gross necropsy findings are adequate for the diagnosis, which can be confirmed by histopathology. Detection of viral antigen by immunofluorescence is the simplest reliable laboratory diagnostic procedure. Gel diffusion, indirect immunofluorescence, or virus neutralization is used for the detection of viral antibody. A variety of inoculation methods can be used for virus isolation: inoculation of cell cultures, preferably chicken kidney cells or duck embryo fibroblasts, the chorioallantoic membrane, or the yolk sac of 4-day-old embryonated eggs with suspensions of buffy coat or spleen cells. The presence of virus can be demonstrated by immunofluorescence or immunohistochemistry on tissues or cultures using monospecific

antisera to Marek's disease virus, demonstration of specific antigen in agar gel immunodiffusion tests, demonstration of parts of Marek's disease viral genome by PCR assay, or by electron microscopy to demonstrate the presence of characteristic herpesvirus virions.

Historically, Marek's disease and avian leukosis were long confused, but today they can be differentiated by clinical and pathologic features and by specific tests for each virus, or antibody to each of them.

Immunity, Prevention, and Control

Vaccination is the principal method of control. The standard method has been to vaccinate 1-day-old chicks parenterally; however, more than 80% of the 8 billion birds vaccinated annually in the United Stated are vaccinated *in ovo* at 18 days, by robotic machines. The vaccine is available as either a lyophilized cell-free preparation or a cell-associated preparation. The cell-free vaccine is not effective in immunizing chicks with maternal antibody, whereas cell-associated vaccines are. Protective immunity develops within about 2 weeks. Vaccination decreases the incidence of disease, particularly of neoplastic lesions in visceral organs, and has been most successful in the control of Marek's disease lymphoproliferative syndromes. Peripheral neurologic disease continues to occur in vaccinated flocks, but at reduced incidence.

Strains of Marek's disease virus vary considerably in their virulence and in the types of lesions they produce. Avirulent strains are recognized and have been used as vaccines, although the antigenically related turkey herpesvirus has been the preferred vaccine strain, primarily because it infects cells productively. However, with the emergence, over the past 30 years, of field strains of Marek's disease virus that can overcome turkey herpesvirus-induced immunity, there has been increasing use of new vaccine strains of low-pathogenicity Marek's disease viruses.

A further level of control can be achieved if flocks are built up with birds carrying the B21 alloantigen. It is possible to establish flocks free of Marek's disease, but commercially it is extremely difficult to maintain the disease-free status. The production of chickens on the "all-in–all-out" principle, whereby they are hatched, started, raised, and dispersed as a unit, would improve the efficacy of vaccination as a control measure. In some countries, reduction of Marek's disease virus load in the environment by removal of litter and cleaning/disinfection of the housing after each production cycle has reduced the need for vaccine use.

SUID HERPESVIRUS 1 (PSEUDORABIES OR AUJESZKY'S DISEASE VIRUS)

Pseudorabies (*syn.* Aujeszky's disease) is primarily a disease of swine, although a diverse range of secondary hosts, including horses, cattle, sheep, goats, dogs, cats, and many feral species, can become infected and develop disease.

Humans are refractory to infection. The diverse host range is also reflected *in vitro*, as cell cultures derived from almost any animal species support the replication of pseudorabies virus.

Clinical Signs and Epidemiology

Although suid herpesvirus 1 has been eradicated from domestic swine in many countries, this virus remains enzootic in wild and domestic swine in many parts of the world, causing substantial adverse economic impact to swine production in the countries where it is found. Swine are the primary host and reservoir for the virus, which causes a uniformly fatal disease when transmitted to a wide variety of secondary hosts. Virus is shed in the saliva and nasal discharges of swine, so that transmission can occur by licking, biting, and aerosols. Virus is not shed in the urine or feces. The contamination of livestock feed or the ingestion of infected carcasses by swine is common, and ingestion of virus-contaminated material, including pork, is probably the most common source of infection for secondary hosts. Rats may contribute to farm-to-farm transfer, and sick or dead rats and other feral animals are probably the source of infection for dogs and cats.

Some swine that have recovered from pseudorabies may shed virus continuously in their nasal secretions. Others from which virus cannot be isolated by conventional means may yield virus from explant cultures derived from the tonsil. Pseudorabies virus DNA can be demonstrated in the trigeminal ganglia of recovered swine by DNA hybridization and PCR assay, but there is debate about the relative significance of lymphoreticular cells and nerve cells as sites for latency.

Clinical Signs in Swine

In herds in which the disease is enzootic, reactivation of virus occurs without obvious clinical signs, but the spread of the virus within a susceptible (non-immune) herd may be rapid, with the consequences of primary infection being influenced markedly by age and, in sows, by pregnancy. Pruritus, which is such a dominant feature of the disease in secondary hosts such as cattle, is rare in swine. Importantly, in the absence of vaccination in virus-free countries, the eradication of pseudorabies virus from domestic swine provides a fully susceptible domestic swine population and intensifies the need for biosecurity.

Pregnant Sows. In fully susceptible herds, up to 50% of pregnant sows may abort over a short period of time, as a result of rapid spread of infection from an index case or carrier. Infection of a sow before the 30th day of gestation results in death and resorption of embryos, whereas infection after that time can result in abortion. Infection in late pregnancy may terminate with the delivery of a mixture of mummified, macerated, stillborn, weak, and normal swine,

and some of these pregnancies may be prolonged. Up to 20% of aborting sows are infertile on the first subsequent breeding, but do eventually conceive.

Piglets. Mortality rates among piglets born to non-immune dams depend somewhat on their age, but approach 100%. Maternal antibody is protective, and disease in piglets born to recovered or vaccinated sows is greatly diminished in severity, with recovery the usual outcome.

Weaned, Growing, and Mature Swine. The incubation period is about 30 hours in this group. In younger pigs, the course is typically about 8 days, but it may be as short as 4 days. Initial signs include sneezing, coughing, and moderate fever (40°C), which increases up to 42°C in the ensuing 48 hours. There is constipation during the fever; the feces are hard and dry, and vomiting may occur. Pigs are listless, depressed, and tend to remain recumbent. By the 5th day there is incoordination and pronounced muscle spasm, circling, and intermittent convulsions accompanied by excess salivation. By the 6th day, swine become moribund and die within 12 hours. In mature swine the mortality rate is low, usually less than 2%, but there may be significant weight loss and poor growth rates after recovery.

Clinical Signs in Secondary Hosts

Important secondary hosts include cattle ("mad itch"), dogs ("pseudorabies"), and cats. Disease in secondary hosts is sporadic and occurs where there is direct or indirect contact with swine. Infection is usually by ingestion, less commonly inhalation, and possibly via minor wounds. In cattle the dominant clinical sign is intense pruritus. Particular sites, often on the flanks or hind limbs, are licked incessantly; there is gnawing and rubbing such that the area becomes abraded. Cattle may become frenzied. There is progressive involvement of the central nervous system; following the first signs, the course leading to death may be as short as a few hours, and is never longer than 6 days.

In dogs, the frenzy associated with intense pruritus and paralysis of the jaws and pharynx, accompanied by drooling of saliva and plaintive howling, simulates true rabies; however, there is no tendency for dogs to attack other animals. In cats, the disease may progress so rapidly that frenzy is not observed.

Pathogenesis and Pathology

After primary oral or intranasal infection of swine, virus replicates in the oropharynx. There is no viremia during the first 24 hours and it is difficult to identify virus at any time. However, within 24 hours, virus can be isolated from various cranial nerve ganglia and the medulla and pons, to which virions have traveled via the axoplasm of the cranial nerves. Virus continues to spread within the central nervous system; there is ganglioneuritis at many sites, including those controlling vital functions.

The relative lack of gross lesions even in young swine is notable. Tonsillitis, pharyngitis, tracheitis, rhinitis, and esophagitis occasionally may be evident, with formation of a diphtheritic pseudomembrane overlying the affected mucosa. Similarly, discrete small white or yellow foci of necrosis may sometimes be present in the liver and spleen. Microscopically, the principal findings in both swine and secondary hosts are in the central nervous system. There is a diffuse non-suppurative (predominantly lymphocytic) meningoencephalitis and ganglioneuritis, marked perivascular cuffing, and focal gliosis associated with extensive necrosis of neuronal and glial cells. There is a correlation between the site and severity of clinical signs and the histological findings. Typical intranuclear herpesvirus inclusions are rarely found in the lesions in swine.

Diagnosis

The history and clinical signs often suggest the diagnosis, which is confirmed by histopathology and virus detection methods. Immunohistochemistry or fluorescent antibody staining of frozen tissue sections, PCR assay, virus isolation or serum neutralization assay are used for confirmation. Enzyme immunoassay has been approved as a standard test in several countries and is used in association with vaccination and eradication programs.

Immunity, Prevention, and Control

Management practices influence epidemiologic patterns of infection and disease in swine. Losses from severe disease occur when susceptible pregnant sows or swine less than 3 months old, born to non-immune sows, are infected. Such a pattern is likely to occur when the virus is newly introduced into a herd or unit within a farm. When breeding sows are immune with adequate antibody levels, overt disease in their progeny is not observed or is reduced greatly. Where breeding and growing/finishing operations are conducted separately, significant losses from pseudorabies occur when weaned swine from several sources are brought together in the growing/finishing unit, but the disease in these older swine is less severe than that in piglets. If care is taken to prevent the entry of pseudorabies virus, the move toward complete integration of swine husbandry (so-called farrow-to-finish) operations, provides an ideal situation by which to produce and maintain pseudorabies-free herds and thus avoid the costs of disease losses and the problems associated with vaccination.

Vaccination of swine in areas where the virus is enzootic can reduce losses. Recombinant DNA, deletion-mutant, live-attenuated, and inactivated vaccines are available, but they do not prevent infection or the establishment of latent infection by the wild-type virus. A pseudorabies vaccine from which both the thymidine kinase and a glycoprotein gene have been deleted, and the *E1* gene of classical swine fever (hog cholera) virus inserted, provides protection against both pseudorabies and classical swine fever in regions where both viruses are enzootic. Vaccination of secondary hosts is rarely undertaken, because of the sporadic incidence of the disease.

ALPHAHERPESVIRUS DISEASES OF OTHER SPECIES

A few species of alphaherpesviruses of other animals warrant brief mention. They have been associated with fatal diseases in hedgehogs, kangaroos, wallabies, wombats, and harbor seals. Phocid herpesvirus 1 causes significant mortalities in neonate seal pups, with generalized infection characterized by multifocal necrosis in many tissues, including the lungs and liver. Alphaherpesviruses related antigenically to bovine herpesvirus 1 have been isolated from several ruminant species, including red deer, reindeer, and buffalo. Equine herpesvirus 1 or viruses related very closely to it have not infrequently been the cause of abortion and/or encephalitis in ruminant species, including cattle, llama, alpaca, gazelles, and camels.

MEMBERS OF THE FAMILY *HERPESVIRIDAE*, SUBFAMILY *BETAHERPESVIRINAE*

Betaherpesviruses replicate more slowly than alphaherpesviruses and often produce greatly enlarged cells, hence the designation "cytomegalovirus." Their host range is narrow and, in latent infections, viral DNA is sequestered in cells of secretory glands, lymphoreticular organs, and kidney. Rather than being subject to periodic reactivation, betaherpesviruses are often associated with continuous virus excretion. The subfamily is subdivided into four genera, specifically *Cytomegalovirus*, *Muromegalovirus*, *Proboscivirus*, and *Roseolovirus*. Many of these viruses infect humans and nonhuman primates, but betaherpesviruses also infect elephant, mice (murid herpesvirus 1), rats (murid herpesvirus 2), guinea pigs (caviid herpesvirus 2), and swine.

MURID HERPESVIRUSES 1 AND 2 AND BETAHERPESVIRUSES OF LABORATORY ANIMALS

Host-specific cytomegaloviruses are frequent among the wild progenitors of laboratory mice (*Mus musculus*) and laboratory rats (*Rattus norvegicus*). The mouse virus, now termed murid herpesvirus 1, has been studied extensively as an animal model of cytomegalovirus, but the virus is not common as a natural infection in contemporary mouse colonies. It continues to be a contaminant of older mouse tumor lines. Although cytomegalovirus infection is prevalent among wild rats (murid herpesvirus 2), it is also non-existent or rare in laboratory rats. In both cases, natural infection is subclinical and associated with inclusions and cytomegaly in salivary glands. Laboratory and wild mice are also prone to infection with another, unclassified herpesvirus, which has been named murid herpesvirus 3. This agent, also known as the mouse thymic virus, is enzootic in wild mice and is a frequent co-contaminant of mouse cytomegalovirus stocks. Its classification is still in flux. Guinea pigs (*Cavia porcellus*) are universally infected with caviidherpesvirus 2, which is most often manifested as salivary gland inclusions and cytomegaly. This virus has been used as an experimental model, as it is more prone to cross the placenta than the mouse agent. Various Old and New World non-human primates also possess their own cytomegaloviruses. The rhesus cytomegalovirus has been used extensively as an animal model, and induces neurologic disease in fetuses, similar to the human disease.

ELEPHANTID HERPESVIRUS (ENDOTHELIOTROPIC ELEPHANT HERPESVIRUS)

Several related endotheliotropic herpesviruses cause either benign, localized infections or serious systemic disease in elephants, especially Asian elephants (*Elephas maximus*) in captivity.

SUID HERPESVIRUS 2 (PORCINE CYTOMEGALOVIRUS VIRUS)

First recognized in 1955, suid herpesvirus 2 is enzootic in swine herds worldwide. Within a herd, up to 90% of swine may carry the virus. Often the disease is not seen in herds in which the virus is enzootic; it is more likely to be associated with recent introduction of the virus or with environmental factors such as poor nutrition and intercurrent disease. Virus-free herds have been established.

Rhinitis occurs in affected swine up to 10 weeks of age, after which infection is subclinical, and it is most severe in swine less than 2 weeks old. There is sneezing, coughing, serous nasal and ocular discharge, and depression. The discharge becomes mucopurulent and may block the nasal passages, which interferes with suckling; such piglets lose weight rapidly and die within a few days. Survivors are stunted. A generalized disease following viremic spread is also recognized in young swine. Suid herpesvirus 2 crosses the placenta and may cause fetal death or result in generalized disease in the first 2 weeks after birth, or there may be runting and poor weight gains. Large basophilic intranuclear inclusions are found in enlarged cells of the mucous glands of the turbinate mucosa (hence the synonym "inclusion body rhinitis").

When newly introduced into a susceptible herd, virus is transmitted both transplacentally and horizontally. In herds in which the virus is enzootic, transmission is predominantly horizontal, but, because young swine are infected when maternal antibody is present, the infection is subclinical. Disease occurs when the virus is introduced into susceptible herds or if susceptible swine are mixed with carrier swine. Virus-free swine can be produced by hysterotomy; however, because the virus crosses the placenta, swine produced in this way must be monitored carefully for antibody for at least 70 days after delivery.

MEMBERS OF THE FAMILY *HERPESVIRIDAE*, SUBFAMILY *GAMMAHERPESVIRINAE*

Gammaherpesviruses are classified into four genera (*Lymphocryptovirus*, *Macavirus*, *Percavirus*, and *Rhadinovirus*). The gammaherpesviruses are characterized by replication in lymphoblastoid cells, with different members of the subfamily being specific for either B or T lymphocytes. In lymphocytes, infection is arrested frequently at a prelytic stage, with persistence and minimum expression of the viral genome. Saimiriine herpesvirus 2 (*Herpesvirus saimiri*) and human herpesvirus 8 (human Kaposi's sarcoma-associated herpesvirus) both have viral genes that encode cyclins that regulate the cell cycle at a restriction point between G_1 and S phases by phosphorylation of the retinoblastoma protein. By overriding normal cell cycle arrest, these virus-encoded proteins induce the lymphoproliferative responses that are characteristic of infections with some of these viruses. Gammaherpesviruses may also enter a lytic stage, causing cell death without production of virions. Latent infection occurs in lymphoid tissue.

Alcelaphine herpesvirus 1 and ovine herpesvirus 2 are the causative agents of malignant catarrhal fever in certain wild and domestic ruminants. These viruses were previously included in the genus *Rhadinovirus*, but have been reassigned recently to the genus *Macavirus*, along with several lymphotropic viruses of swine (suid herpesviruses 3, 4, and 5). Equid herpesviruses 2 and 5 were also included originally in the genus *Rhadinovirus*, but are now classified in the genus *Percavirus*. Leporid herpesvirus 1 (*Herpes sylvilagus*) naturally infects wild cottontail rabbits, but its experimental infection of *Sylvilagus* rabbit kits results in lymphoma, and this virus has therefore been studied as an oncogenic herpesvirus. Murid herpesvirus 4, isolated from a wild wood mouse, is a rhadinovirus that is used to experimentally infect laboratory mice, in which it produces a mononucleosis-like syndrome. Unassigned viruses in the subfamily include equid herpesvirus 7 (asinine herpesvirus 2), and phocid herpesvirus 2. Currently unclassified herpesviruses that are likely to be within this subfamily have been isolated from cell cultures and leukocytes of guinea pigs.

MALIGNANT CATARRHAL FEVER CAUSED BY ALCELAPHINE HERPESVIRUS 1 AND OVINE HERPESVIRUS 2

Malignant catarrhal fever is an almost invariably fatal, generalized lymphoproliferative disease of cattle and some wild ruminants (deer, bison, antelope), primarily affecting lymphoid tissues and the mucosal lining of the respiratory and gastrointestinal tracts. Two distinct epidemiologic patterns of infection are recognized, from only one of which has a herpesvirus been isolated. In Africa (and in and around zoos that house African ungulates, regardless of location), epizootics of the disease occur in cattle (and captive, susceptible wild ruminants) following transmission of the causative virus from wildebeest (*Connochaetes gnu* and *C. taurinus*), particularly at calving time. A herpesvirus (alcelaphine herpesvirus 1) has been isolated from this so-called African form of malignant catarrhal fever and shown experimentally to reproduce the disease.

Outside Africa and zoos, a disease designated sheep-associated malignant catarrhal fever of cattle, bison, and deer is caused by ovine herpesvirus 2 when these species are kept adjacent to carrier sheep. This sheep-associated form of malignant catarrhal fever can be transmitted by inoculation of cattle or bison with a large volume of blood from a clinically affected animal or by aerosol to cattle or bison with nasal secretions from sheep experiencing a virus-shedding episode. Climatic factors can influence the transmission efficiency of ovine herpesvirus 2 from reservoir sheep to susceptible species such as bison. Ovine herpesvirus 2 has not yet been isolated. The genome of ovine herpesvirus 2, like that of alcelaphine herpesvirus 1, has been sequenced completely, showing they are closely related herpesviruses.

Clinical Features and Epidemiology

Both ovine herpes virus 2 and alcelaphine herpesvirus 1 cause similar disease syndromes and lesions in clinically susceptible hosts. In general, after an incubation period of about 3–4 weeks, malignant catarrhal fever is characterized by fever, depression, leukopenia, profuse nasal and ocular discharges, bilateral corneal opacity that can progress to blindness (Figure 9.9), generalized lymphadenopathy, extensive mucosal erosions, and central nervous system signs. Erosions of the gastrointestinal mucosa lead to hemorrhage and melena, as well as extensive ulceration that occurs throughout the oral cavity, including the tongue.

The epidemiology of the two major types of malignant catarrhal fever viruses, specifically alcelaphine herpesvirus 1 and ovine herpesvirus 2, within their natural, well-adapted hosts differs significantly. Whereas intense virus shedding from the wildebeest occurs predominantly during the first 90 days of life, lambs do not shed virus until after 5 months of age. Wildebeest-associated malignant catarrhal

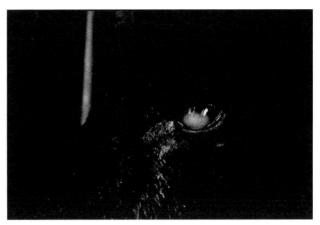

FIGURE 9.9 Corneal opacity caused by malignant catarrhal fever in a bovine. *(Courtesy of D. Knowles, Washington State University.)*

fever of cattle occurs most frequently in Africa during the wildebeest calving season, whereas the sheep-associated form of malignant catarrhal fever occurs year-round in cattle, with only a modestly increased incidence during the lambing season. In American bison, malignant catarrhal fever is typically a winter disease, with no discernible peak around the time of lambing. The sheep-associated virus is not transmitted between cattle or bison, which appear to be "dead-end" hosts. Outbreaks of the sheep-associated form of malignant catarrhal fever also have occurred amongst farmed deer, particularly red deer (*Cervus elaphus*).

Pathogenesis and Pathology

Necropsy findings in animals with malignant catarrhal fever, which are usually cattle or wild ungulates such as bison, vary according to the duration of the disease, but not the infecting virus (alcelaphine herpesvirus 1 or ovine herpesvirus 2). Affected animals often exhibit corneal opacity, and there are often extensive erosions, edema, and hemorrhage throughout the gastrointestinal tract, including the oral cavity. There is a generalized lymphadenopathy: all lymph nodes are enlarged, edematous, and sometimes hemorrhagic. Frequently there are multiple foci of interstitial inflammation in the kidney that appear grossly as discrete white streaks within the cortex, diffuse hemorrhages throughout the urinary bladder mucosa (hemorrhagic cystitis), and erosions and hemorrhages within the mucosa of the turbinates, larynx, and trachea. The epithelial lining of the muzzle may slough. Histologically, there is widespread proliferation of lymphocytes (lymphoblasts) and multifocal areas of necrosis, centered on small blood vessels, and small arteries may exhibit characteristic fibrinoid necrosis of their muscular walls. These histological lesions are present in all affected tissues, including brain and eye.

Although death characteristically occurs less than 2–7 days after the onset of clinical signs, depending on species, a small number of affected cattle and deer that develop clinical signs of disease survive, at least for a short time, with evidence of ocular disease, arteriosclerosis, and persistence of the virus as detected by PCR.

The florid lymphoproliferative and vascular lesions in animals with malignant catarrhal fever suggest that the disease is immunologically mediated. Indeed, the lesions mimic those in animals that lack IL-2, such as genetically altered (IL-2 knockout) mice or animals that lack adequate numbers of IL-2-producing $CD4^+$ lymphocytes. The vascular lesions that characterize malignant catarrhal fever are probably responsible for the necrosis and ulceration that occur in many tissues.

Diagnosis

The history and clinical signs, particularly the presence of bilateral corneal opacity coupled with the other clinical signs, suggest the diagnosis of malignant catarrhal fever. Alcelaphine herpesvirus 1 (wildebeest-associated malignant catarrhal fever) can be isolated from washed peripheral blood leukocytes in calf thyroid cells. Cell-free inocula do not yield virus. Ovine herpesvirus 2 has yet to be propagated in cell culture, but the presence of this virus can be demonstrated by virus-specific PCR assay. This assay readily can detect viral DNA in the tissues of animals ill with malignant catarrhal fever.

Immunity, Prevention, and Control

Malignant catarrhal fever is controlled by preventing contact between virus carriers and susceptible hosts. Attempts to develop a vaccine have been unsuccessful to date.

BOVINE HERPESVIRUS 4

Bovine herpesvirus 4, which has a genome organization similar to that of Epstein–Barr virus, has been isolated throughout the world from cattle suffering from a variety of diseases, including conjunctivitis, respiratory disease, vaginitis, metritis, skin nodules, and lymphosarcoma. However, there is no proven etiologic association between the diseases and the virus isolated occasionally from cases. When inoculated experimentally into susceptible cattle, these viruses produce no disease. Strains of bovine herpesvirus 4 have been isolated when cell cultures are prepared from tissues of apparently normal cattle; they have also been isolated from semen of normal bulls.

EQUID HERPESVIRUSES 2, 5, AND 7 (ASININE HERPESVIRUS 2)

Equid herpesvirus 2 can be isolated from nasal swab filtrates or from buffy coat cells of most adult horses, with rates of isolation increasing with age. Horses may be infected in the first weeks of life, even in the presence of maternal antibody.

Many antigenic types exist; more than one antigenic type may be recovered at different times, or at the same time, from the same horse. Equid herpesvirus 2 has been recovered from horses with keratoconjunctivitis, gastroesophageal ulcers, and respiratory disease characterized by coughing, swollen submaxillary and parotid lymph nodes, and pharyngeal ulceration. The role of the virus in these and other diseases is uncertain, although equine herpesvirus 2 has been incriminated as the cause of a disease syndrome in foals that resembles infectious mononucleosis of human adolescents caused by human herpesvirus 4 (Epstein–Barr virus) infection.

A second slowly growing gammaherpesvirus (equid herpesvirus 5) is also ubiquitous in horse populations worldwide. This virus has recently been incriminated as the cause of a severe, progressive syndrome of pulmonary fibrosis in horses. Horses with this disease exhibit progressive respiratory difficulty and in fulminant cases develop severe interstitial pneumonia and fibrosis. Characteristic herpesvirus inclusions are present within affected lung, but the precise role of equine herpesvirus 5 in causing this remarkable syndrome remains to be definitively characterized.

Asinine herpesvirus 2 (equid herpesvirus 7) and other poorly characterized gammaherpesviruses have been isolated from healthy equids, including donkeys and mules, and from donkeys with encephalitis or severe interstitial pneumonia.

PRIMATE GAMMAHERPESVIRUSES

Human herpesvirus 4 (Epstein–Barr virus) causes the human disease glandular fever/infectious mononucleosis and is the prototype of the genus *Lymphocryptovirus*. Several viruses of primates, including *Herpesvirus saimiri* and closely related *Herpesvirus ateles*, are members of the genus *Rhadinovirus*. *Herpesvirus saimiri* (saimiriine herpesvirus 2) is a T lymphocytotropic virus that causes subclinical latent infections in squirrel monkeys (*Saimiri sciureus*), but infection of aberrant New World monkeys (marmosets, tamarins, owl monkeys) with this virus induces rapid and fatal lymphoproliferative disease. Rhesus macaques (*Macaca mulatta*) commonly harbor two closely related rhadinoviruses—retroperitoneal fibromatosis herpesvirus and rhesus rhadinovirus—either of which may be associated with a syndrome called retroperitoneal fibromatosis, as well as B-cell lymphomas, in animals that are immunosuppressed as a result of infection with retroviruses. These agents are closely related to the rhadinovirus (human herpesvirus 8) that causes Kaposi's sarcoma in immunosuppressed humans.

UNASSIGNED MEMBERS OF THE FAMILY *HERPESVIRIDAE*

A substantial number of herpesviruses of reptiles, mammals, and birds are included in the family *Herpesviridae* without assignment to specific subfamilies or genera.

ANATID HERPESVIRUS 1 (DUCK VIRAL ENTERITIS VIRUS OR DUCK PLAGUE VIRUS)

Duck viral enteritis, historically called duck plague, occurs worldwide among domestic and wild ducks, geese, swans, and other waterfowl. Migratory waterfowl contribute to spread within and between continents, but most surveys have failed to identify the virus as enzootic in North American wild waterfowl, although major epizootics have occurred in duck farms in the United States. Ingestion of contaminated water is believed to be the major mode of transmission, but the virus may also be transmitted by contact. The incubation period is 3–7 days. There is anorexia, listlessness, nasal discharge, ruffled dull feathers, adherent eyelids, photophobia, extreme thirst, ataxia leading to recumbency with outstretched wings and with head extended forward, tremors, watery diarrhea, and soiled vents. Most ducks that develop clinical signs die, and sick wild ducks often conceal themselves and die in vegetation at the water's edge.

Clinical findings are suggestive of duck viral enteritis, and the diagnosis may be confirmed by the finding of herpesvirus inclusion bodies in tissues of affected birds, coupled with positive immunohistochemical staining for viral antigen. Virus can be isolated in 1-day-old Muscovy or white Peking ducks, or by inoculation of chorioallantoic membranes of 9–14-day-old embryonating duck eggs. Duck viral enteritis must be differentiated from hepatitis caused by picornavirus or astrovirus infections, and from Newcastle disease and influenza.

MEMBERS OF FAMILIES *ALLOHERPESVIRIDAE* AND *MALACOHERPESVIRIDAE*

Although the herpesviruses of fish, frogs, and oysters morphologically and biologically resemble other herpesviruses, their genome sequences are distinct and have almost no similarity with those of mammalian and avian herpesviruses. This obvious paradox has led to the recent creation of two new virus families within the order *Herpesvirales*. The family *Alloherpesviridae* includes a variety of viruses from fish and frogs, notably Ictalurid herpesvirus 1 (channel catfish virus), three viruses from cyprinid fish, including carp pox herpesvirus (cyprinid herpesvirus 1), hematopoietic necrosis herpesvirus of goldfish (cyprinid herpesvirus 2), and koi herpesvirus (cyprinid herpesvirus 3). The current but growing list of aquatic lower vertebrate hosts for herpesviruses includes frogs, goldfish, carp, sturgeon, pike, flounder, cod, sheatfish, smelt, sharks, angelfish, pilchards, walleye, turbot, and salmonids. The oyster (mollusk) virus (ostreid herpesvirus 1) is the sole member of the genus *Ostreavirus* in the family *Malacoherpesviridae*. The lack of sequence similarity of these viruses to herpesviruses of birds and animals

underlines the early origin and long evolutionary history of each herpesvirus with its respective host.

ICTALURID HERPESVIRUS 1 (CHANNEL CATFISH VIRUS)

Ictalurid herpesvirus 1 (channel catfish herpesvirus) was the first herpesvirus of fish to be isolated. The virus has significant adverse economic impacts on the commercial rearing of its host species in North America and, as a result, the causative virus has been studied more extensively than other herpesviruses of fish. The virus is highly virulent among young naïve populations of cultured channel catfish. The incubation period can be as short as 3 days; signs of infection include convulsive swimming, which may include a "head-up" posture, lethargy, exophthalmia, distended abdomen, and hemorrhages at the base of the fins. Mortality can approach 100% in outbreaks. Lesions in affected fish include yellow- or red-tinged fluid in the peritoneum, pale viscera, and an enlarged spleen; petechial hemorrhages on the kidney, liver, and visceral fat may be present. Microscopic lesions are characterized by edema, and severe and generalized necrosis of the hemopoietic tissues of the kidney and spleen. Necrosis and hemorrhage also occur in the liver and digestive tract.

The lack of reported virus isolations from wild channel catfish strongly indicates that factors such as dense stocking and poor environmental conditions may predispose farmed fish populations to outbreaks of disease. A key factor is temperature: most outbreaks occur in the summer months at higher water temperatures (e.g., 30°C). The acute disease occurs only in young channel catfish—usually up to about 6 months of age. The virus is transmitted readily from fish to fish; virus shedding is probably via the urine, and virus entry is probably through the gills.

Attempts to vaccinate channel catfish against channel catfish virus have shown promise. Attenuated virus vaccines prepared by serial passage of the virus in fish cells, or by thymidine kinase gene deletion, have been shown to protect recipients against lethal challenge.

CYPRINID HERPESVIRUSES 1, 2, AND 3 (CARP POX VIRUS; HEMATOPOIETIC NECROSIS HERPESVIRUS OF GOLDFISH; KOI HERPESVIRUS

Three herpesviruses have been isolated from populations of cyprinid fishes, each of which has been widely distributed via the worldwide trade in live production (aquaculture) and ornamental fish. All three viruses have been propagated in cell lines derived from cyprinid fishes, although initial isolation and propagation is challenging and histopathology, electron microscopy, and virus-specific PCR assays are used for routine diagnostic purposes. Control is reliant on exclusion of the virus whenever possible. Limited trials with the anti-herpesvirus drugs commonly used in mammals have shown little promise with the cyprinid herpesviruses.

Cyprinid herpesvirus 1 is the cause of a recurring skin disorder referred to as "carp pox," which is commonly seen during the cooler-water seasons (<25°C). Superficial papillomatous-like growths can occur over limited or extensive areas of the skin, but these are often most prominent on the fins. Although not a cause of mortality, the skin growths are cosmetically displeasing, particularly among show fish. A systemic infection with high mortality occurs in very young fish while they are still in the ponds before initial grading. Survivors of clinical or subclinical infections are probably life-long carriers, some of which later will undergo typical carp pox episodes. The cutaneous proliferations consist histologically of focal areas of extensive epidermal hyperplasia—a feature common to many herpesvirus infections of fish, although more pronounced with carp pox. The presence of virus in the skin lesions is confirmed by electron microscopy, fluorescent antibody staining, or a recently developed PCR assay. Control is principally by avoidance and segregation of fish free of recurring lesions. Although superficial skin growths can be removed by abrasion, this procedure is not recommended because of complications with other opportunistic invaders when the epidermis is disrupted.

Cyprinid herpesvirus 2 is associated with an acute systemic disease in goldfish (*Carassius auratus*) known as goldfish hemopoietic necrosis. First observed in Japan in 1992, the disease is now reported from most continents among goldfish younger than 1year, with mortality up to 90% when water temperatures are 15–25°C. Before death, affected fish may exhibit lethargy and focal pallor of the gills. Internal lesions include pallor of the kidney and spleen. Histological lesions include severe necrosis of the interstitial hemopoietic tissues in the kidney and spleen. Intranuclear inclusions within infected cells provide a presumptive diagnosis in affected goldfish populations, and the presence of the virus can be confirmed by electron microscopy, immunofluorescent staining, or PCR assay. Control of the disease has utilized artificially increased water temperatures (up to 32°C), which arrests the occurrence of disease, but does not eliminate the infection.

Cyprinid herpesvirus 3, also know as koi herpesvirus, was first detected in koi and common carp in Europe and Israel in 1996–1997. The virus has since been detected on most continents, as the cause of mortality among koi of all ages and in all settings, including production, retail, and individual hobbyist. Significant impacts of the virus have been reported on the production of common carp, a primary food fish in Israel, Europe, and Asia. The disease is generally seasonal, occurring in the spring or autumn when water temperatures are in the range 18–28°C. Mortality may approach 100% in koi and is rapid in onset—usually 7–10days following exposure to persistently infected fish that carry the virus. Hypersecretion

of mucus that may cloud the tank is often the initial sign of infection, and affected fish then develop lethargy and patchy, opaque skin lesions. Before death, affected fish develop pale, swollen, and, in severe cases, eroded gills. Internal lesions are often subtle, including swelling of the kidney and spleen. Microscopic lesions are most pronounced in the gill, and are characterized by initial epithelial hyperplasia followed by necrosis. Intranuclear inclusions occur less commonly than with the other cyprinid herpesviruses (1 and 2). Fish that survive initial outbreaks are assumed to be carriers, although this has yet to be proven experimentally. Diagnosis is based on the characteristic clinical signs in koi or common carp, and confirmed by PCR assay of pooled tissues from the gill, kidney, and spleen. Control of the koi herpesvirus disease has relied upon avoidance of seropositive fish (those with virus-specific antibodies in their serum). Vaccination with a live-attenuated virus has proven successful in Israel. Other methods of control include alteration of water temperature similar to that described for cyprinid herpesvirus 2, although this approach only reduces incidence of disease, and may not eliminate the carrier state.

SALMONID HERPESVIRUSES

Three genetically distinct salmonid herpesviruses have been associated with mortality in cultured populations of salmonid fish. Salmonid herpesvirus 1, formerly known as *Herpesvirus salmonis*, was recovered from dying adult rainbow trout (*Oncorhynchus mykiss*) in a hatchery in Washington State in the United States in the 1970s. The virus has since been identified among asymptomatic adult steelhead trout (*O. mykiss*) returning to hatcheries in California. The virus is not highly virulent, as natural or experimental infections in young salmonid fish result in low mortality, with limited clinical signs and modest internal lesions. Salmonid herpesvirus 2, or Oncorhynchus masou virus, is a more pathogenic virus that was initially isolated from several species of adult salmon and rainbow trout in Japan from 1970 to 1980. The virus is more pathogenic for young salmonids than salmonid herpesvirus 1, particularly among kokanee salmon (*O. nerka*) and cherry salmon (*O. masou*). Curiously, certain strains of salmonid herpesvirus 2 have the unique property of inducing a high prevalence of epithelial tumors in fish surviving experimental infection, although the oncogenic mechanisms involved are unknown. Before death, affected salmonid fish exhibit lethargy, darkening in color, and exophthalmia. Histologic lesions are limited but include renal tubular epithelial necrosis, syncytium formation in hemopoietic tissues, and multifocal necrosis in the liver. Lesions are most pronounced in experimentally infected juvenile chum salmon (*O. keta*). A third salmonid herpesvirus, salmonid herpesvirus 3, or epizootic epitheliotropic virus, has been described as a serious cause of mortality of hatchery-reared lake trout (*Salvelinus namaycush*) in the Great Lakes region of North America. The epidermis of the body and fins is most affected, and extensive cutaneous infections result in high mortality because of significant compromise to this important osmotic barrier. Pale patches on the skin may be the only external signs as fish progress from lethargy to death, a process dependent on water temperatures (up to 30 days at 6–9°C, but only 9–10 days at 12°C). Microscopic lesions are confined to the skin, and include hyperplasia and sloughing of epidermal cells. Both salmonid herpesviruses 1 and 2 can be isolated using appropriate salmonid cell lines and the diagnosis confirmed by virus neutralization and virus-specific PCR assays. Salmonid herpesvirus 3 has not been isolated in cell culture, and PCR assay has replaced prior confirmatory methods that relied solely upon electron microscopy. Avoidance is the principal method of control for the salmonid herpesviruses, and the screening of adult broodstocks, disinfection of fertilized eggs with iodine-containing solutions, and rearing of fish in virus-free water supplies have all helped to reduce or eliminate infection in many hatchery populations.

OTHER ALLOHERPESVIRUSES IN FISH AND FROGS

The two alloherpesviruses that originally were isolated from Japanese (*Anguilla japonica*) and European (*Anguilla anguilla*) eels are now considered to be different isolates of the same virus, anguillid herpesvirus 1. This virus is associated with a syndrome of dermal hemorrhage and mortality of farmed eels in Japan, Taiwan, and the Netherlands. The virus probably has been disseminated by the international trade and movement of both European and Japanese elvers. The presence of herpesviruses among cultured juvenile white sturgeon (*Acipenser transmontanus*) was first reported in California in 1991. Subsequently, additional alloherpesviruses have been identified as the cause of skin diseases in white and other species of sturgeon. These alloherpesviruses tend to cause insidious disease in both eels and sturgeon, probably because the skin lesions they cause predispose to infections with opportunistic pathogens. Thus, the elimination of secondary ectoparasitic diseases is central to the control of these herpesvirus infections in cultured sturgeon. Fish that survive the initial outbreaks of disease are typically resistant thereafter. Other alloherpesviruses are associated with similar skin diseases in a number of freshwater and marine fish species. Among larval stages of fish, infections can be more serious and result in significant mortality, as exemplified by cultured Japanese flounder (*Paralichthys olivaceous*), in which these viruses have greatly complicated the culture of this marine fish. Herpesviruses also have been identified in cases of dermatitis in several species of sharks, and a herpesvirus is the suspected cause of very substantial mortality among wild populations of pilchards in Australia.

Two distinct alloherpesviruses, ranid herpesviruses 1 and 2, have been identified from the leopard frog (*Rana pipiens*). Ranid herpesvirus 1 is the cause of renal adenocarcinomas that were first reported in 1932 among populations of wild leopard frogs in Vermont, United States. Cells comprising the tumor exhibit intranuclear inclusions and virions are abundant during the cold season (4–9°C) but are absent during warmer periods (20–25°C). Metastatic activity of the tumors increases during warmer periods, reaching a prevalence of up 12% in wild frogs and as great as 50% among laboratory populations of adult frogs. Ranid herpesvirus 2 was isolated from the urine of a tumor-bearing leopard frog, but was not demonstrated to have oncogenic activity. Both viruses can be detected by amplification and sequencing of specific viral genomic DNA.

MALACOHERPESVIRUSES (OSTREID HERPESVIRUS 1)

Herpesviruses were first described in 1972 among adult Eastern oysters (*Crassostrea virginica*) on the Atlantic coast of the United States that died after a regime of increased water temperature. High mortality episodes associated with herpesvirus infections among larvae and juvenile Pacific oysters (*C. gigas*) in New Zealand and European flat oysters (*Ostrea edulis*) were reported in the 1990s and later in *C. gigas* from Japan, Korea, and China. Herpesvirus infections have also been reported in two additional oyster species, adult *O. angasi* in Australia and larval *Tiostrea chilensis* in New Zealand, as well as larvae of two clam species, *Ruditapes decussatus* and *R. philippinarum*, in France. The herpesviruses involved in these outbreaks represent isolates of a newly described genus, *Ostreavirus*, and species, ostreid herpesvirus 1, in the family *Malacoherpesviridae*. Among larval oysters, the first signs of infection are a cessation of feeding, which is followed by high mortality 6–10 days later. Lesions are prominent in the connective tissues of affected oysters, where fibroblastic-like cells have enlarged nuclei with marginated chromatin and an abnormal basophilic staining to the cytoplasm. Electron microscopy confirms the presence of numerous herpesvirus virions in these cells. There is also a marked infiltration of hemocytes into affected areas of the mantle, labial palps, and digestive gland of infected oysters. Current detection methods include PCR assay, and control is reliant on exclusion of the causative herpesvirus, which may require screening of broodstocks used for larval production.

Adenoviridae

Chapter Contents

In 1953, Wallace Rowe and colleagues, having observed that explant cultures of human adenoids degenerated spontaneously, isolated a new virus that they named *adenovirus*. The next year, Cabasso and colleagues demonstrated that the etiological agent of infectious canine hepatitis was an adenovirus. Subsequently, numerous adenoviruses, most appearing to be highly host specific, were isolated from humans and many other mammals and birds, usually from the upper respiratory tract, but sometimes from feces. Indeed, it is likely that all vertebrate species, from fish to mammals, have their own unique adenovirus or adenoviruses with which they have co-evolved. Most of these viruses produce subclinical infections in their respective hosts, with occasional upper respiratory disease, but canine and avian adenoviruses are especially associated with clinically important disease syndromes.

Since their discovery, adenoviruses have been at the core of significant basic discoveries concerning virus structure, eukaryotic gene expression and organization, RNA splicing, and apoptosis. Adenoviruses are frequently used as experimental vectors for gene therapy and cancer therapy, and have been used as vectors for recombinant vaccines. They also received a brief flurry of interest shortly after their discovery, because of their oncogenic behavior in experimentally infected laboratory rodents. Specifically, some of the adenoviruses of humans, cattle, and chickens cause tumors when inoculated into newborn laboratory animals and have been used in experimental oncogenesis studies; however, none has been proven to cause tumors in their respective natural hosts.

PROPERTIES OF ADENOVIRUSES

Classification

The family *Adenoviridae* currently comprises four serologically distinct genera: (1) the genus *Mastadenovirus*, comprising viruses that infect only mammalian species; (2) the genus *Aviadenovirus*, comprising viruses that infect only birds; (3) the genus *Atadenovirus* that includes viruses that infect a broad host range, including snakes, lizards, ducks, geese, chickens, possums, and ruminants; (4) the genus *Siadenovirus*, which includes frog adenovirus 1 and turkey adenovirus 3, plus several recently described viruses of raptors, budgerigars, and tortoises. A fifth genus that includes adenoviruses of fish such as white sturgeon adenovirus is proposed. Although all adenoviruses have a similar morphology (Figure 10.1), the genomic organization differs between viruses in the various genera (Figure 10.2). Mastadenoviruses contain the unique proteins V and IX; protein V is involved in transport of viral DNA to the cell nucleus and protein IX is a transcriptional activator. Genes encoding proteins V and IX are absent in aviadenoviruses and their genomes are 20–45% larger than those of mastadenoviruses. Atadenoviruses encode a unique structural protein, p32K, and apparently lack the immunomodulatory proteins that occur in the E3 region of mastadenoviruses. The genomic structure of siadenoviruses is also unique in that genes encoding proteins V and IX are absent as well as the genes encoding early regions E1, E3, and E4 of mastadenoviruses.

Adenoviruses are designated by their host species and a serial number (e.g., canine adenovirus 1), as listed in Table 10.1. Genomic organization and relatedness, growth characteristics in cell culture, and host range have all been used for the precise categorization of virus strains and, in general, results have accorded well with previous categorizations based on serological cross-reactions. After the general structuring of the family had been re-done on the basis of molecular characteristics

of the viruses, the basis for the immunologic relationships among the viruses became clear. Specifically, antigenic determinants associated with the inner part of hexons—that is, the structural units making up the bulk of the capsid—contain the epitopes that were first used antigenically to define the two original genera. Hexons are involved in neutralization, and fibers in both neutralization and hemagglutination (Figure 10.1). Genus-specific antigen is located on the basal surface of the hexon, whereas serotype-specific antigens are located mainly on the tower region of the hexon. Serotypes are differentiated on the basis of neutralization assays; they are defined as those that include adenoviruses that exhibit no cross-reaction with other adenoviruses or show a homologous/heterologous titer ratio, in both directions, of greater than 16. The penton fibers contain other type-specific epitopes, which are also important in neutralization assays. Unexpectedly, although the distal (fiber) knobs on the penton contain the cell-binding ligands that are responsible for virus attachment to specific cellular receptors, antibody to these knobs or to the penton fibers is only weakly neutralizing. Thus the previous serologic structuring of

TABLE 10.1 Diseases of Domestic Animals Associated with Adenoviruses

Animal Species	Number of Serotypes	Disease
Dogs	2	Infectious canine hepatitis (canine adenovirus 1) Infectious canine tracheobronchitis (canine adenovirus 2)
Horses	2	Usually asymptomatic or mild upper respiratory disease. Bronchopneumonia and generalized disease in Arabian foals with primary severe combined immunodeficiency disease
Cattle	10	Usually asymptomatic or mild upper respiratory disease; occasionally severe respiratory or enteric disease in calves
Swine	4	Usually asymptomatic or mild upper respiratory disease
Sheep	7	Usually asymptomatic or mild upper respiratory disease; occasionally severe respiratory or enteric disease in lambs
Goats	2	Usually asymptomatic or mild upper respiratory disease
Deer	1	Pulmonary edema, hemorrhage, vasculitis
Rabbits	1	Diarrhea
Chickens	14	12 serotypes of aviadenovirus: fowl adenoviruses 1–11 and 8a and 8b (hydropericardium syndrome, inclusion body hepatitis) 1 serotype of atadenovirus: egg drop syndrome 1 serotype of siadenovirus: adenovirus-associated splenomegaly
Turkeys and pheasants	3	Siadenovirus: hemorrhagic enteritis (turkey); marble spleen disease (pheasant); egg drop syndrome (both) Aviadenovirus: turkey adenoviruses 1 and 2 (depressed egg production)
Quail	1	Aviadenovirus: bronchitis
Ducks	2	Atadenovirus: duck adenovirus 1 (asymptomatic or egg drop) Aviadenovirus: duck adenovirus 2 (rarely, hepatitis)
Geese	3	Aviadenovirus: isolated from liver, intestines

the family was based more on the relative dominance of certain epitopes in particular serological tests than on their location in the virion.

Virion Properties

Adenovirus virions are non-enveloped, precisely hexagonal in outline, with icosahedral symmetry, 70–90 nm in diameter (Figure 10.1; Table 10.2). Virions are composed of 252 capsomers: 240 hexons that occupy the faces and edges of the 20 equilateral triangular facets of the icosahedron and 12 pentons (vertex capsomers) that occupy the vertices. The hexons consist of two distinct parts: a pseudohexagonal base with a hollow center, and a triangular top that includes three distinct "towers." From each penton projects a penton fiber 9–77.5 nm in length, with a terminal knob. Avian adenoviruses have two fiber proteins per vertex.

The genome of adenoviruses consists of a single linear molecule of double-stranded DNA, 26–45 kbp in size, with inverted terminal repeats. The viral genome encodes approximately 40 proteins that are transcribed after complex RNA splicing. About one-third of the proteins are structural proteins, including a virus-encoded cysteine protease that is necessary for processing of some precursor proteins. Structural proteins include those that make up the hexons, pentons, and penton fibers, and others associated with the virion core.

Many adenoviruses agglutinate red blood cells, with hemagglutination occurring when the tips of penton fibers bind to cellular receptors and form bridges between cells. The optimal conditions and species of red blood cells for demonstrating this phenomenon with each adenovirus have been determined, as the hemagglutination-inhibition assay (see Chapter 5) has been a major serologic diagnostic method for many years.

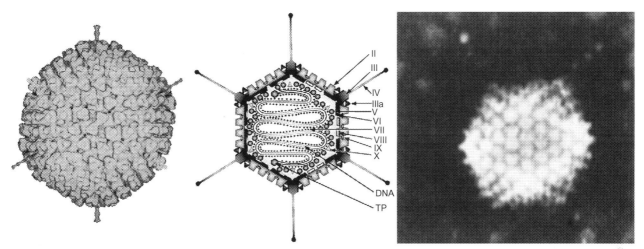

FIGURE 10.1 (Left) Cryo-electron reconstruction of a particle of an isolate of human adenovirus 2 (Stewart et al. (1991). *Cell*, **67**:145–154). (Center). Stylized section of a mastadenovirus particle showing capsid (II, III, IIIa, IV, VI, VIII, IX) and core (V, VII, X and TP (terminal protein)) proteins. As the structure of the nucleoprotein core has not been established, the polypeptides associated with the DNA are shown in hypothetical locations. (Adapted from Stewart, P.L. and Burnett, R.M. (1993). *Jpn. J. Appl. Phys.*, **32**, 1342–1347). (Right) Negative contrast electron micrograph of a particle of an isolate of human adenovirus 2 (Valentine, R.C. and Pereira, H.G. (1965). *J. Mol. Biol.*, **13**, 13–20). *[From* Virus Taxonomy: Eighth Report of the International Committee on Taxonomy of Viruses *(C. M. Fauquet, M. A. Mayo, J. Maniloff, U. Desselberger, L. A. Ball, eds.), p. 213. Copyright © Elsevier (2005), with permission.]*

TABLE 10.2 Properties of Adenoviruses

Four genera: *Mastadenovirus, Aviadenovirus, Atadenovirus,* and *Siadenovirus*

Virions are non-enveloped, hexagonal in outline, with icosahedral symmetry, 70–90 nm in diameter, with one (genus *Mastadenovirus*) or two (genus *Aviadenovirus*) fibers (glycoprotein) projecting from each vertex of the capsid

The genome consists of a single linear molecule of double-stranded DNA, 26–45 kbp in size, with inverted terminal repeats

Replication takes place in the nucleus by a complex program of early and late transcription (before and after DNA replication); virions are released by cell lysis

Intranuclear inclusion bodies are formed, containing large numbers of virions, often in paracrystalline arrays

Viruses agglutinate red blood cells

Some viruses are oncogenic in laboratory animals

Adenoviruses are relatively stable in the environment, but are inactivated easily by common disinfectants. Most of the viruses have narrow host ranges; however, canine adenovirus 1, the cause of infections canine hepatitis, has also caused epizootics in foxes, bears, wolves, coyotes, and skunks. Many adenoviruses cause acute respiratory or gastroenteric disease of varying severity.

Virus Replication

Adenoviruses replicate in the nucleus, and their replication is facilitated by extensive modulation of the host immune response. Viruses bind to host-cell receptors via their penton fiber knobs and subsequent internalization is mediated by the interaction between the penton base and cellular integrins. The outer capsid is then removed and the core comprising the viral genome with its associated histones enters the nucleus where messenger RNA (mRNA) transcription, viral DNA replication, and assembly of virions occur (see also Figure 2.10).

In the nucleus, the genome is transcribed by cellular RNA polymerase II according to a complex program involving both DNA strands (Figure 10.2). There are five early (E) transcriptional units (E1A, E1B, E2, E3, and E4), two intermediate units (IX and IVa2), and one late (L) unit from which five families of late mRNAs (L1 to L5) are transcribed. Each early region is under the control of a separate promoter, whereas the late region uses a single promoter called the major late promoter. The E1A region of the viral genome encodes proteins that are essential for three main outcomes of early adenovirus transcription: (1) induction of cell-cycle progression (DNA synthesis) to provide an optimal environment for virus replication; (2) protection of infected cells from host antiviral immune defenses, including cytokine-induced apoptosis; (3) synthesis of viral proteins necessary for viral DNA replication.

E1A and *E1B* gene products are also responsible for cell transformation and hence for the oncogenicity (experimental) of some adenoviruses. Both proteins inactivate the cellular

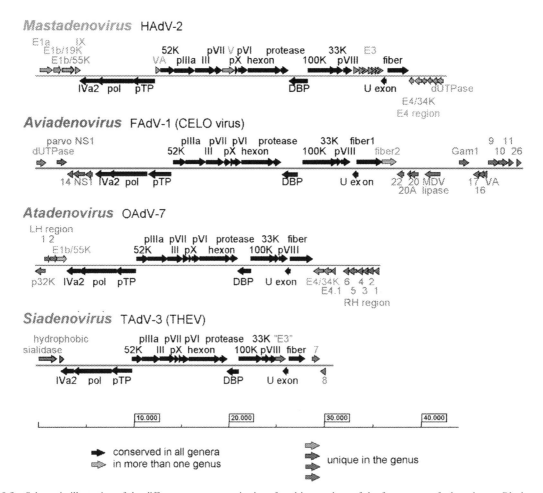

FIGURE 10.2 Schematic illustration of the different genome organizations found in members of the four genera of adenoviruses. Black arrows depict genes conserved in every genus, gray arrows show genes present in more than one genus, colored arrows shows genus-specific genes. HAdV-2, human adenovirus 2; FAdV-1, fowl adenovirus 1; OAdV-7, ovine adenovirus 7; TAdV-3, turkey adenovirus 3. *[From* Virus Taxonomy: Eighth Report of the International Committee on Taxonomy of Viruses *(C. M. Fauquet, M. A. Mayo, J. Maniloff, U. Desselberger, L. A. Ball, eds.), p. 214. Copyright © Elsevier (2005), with permission.]*

tumor suppresser gene, *p53*, and thus deregulate cell-cycle progression. Inactivation is mediated by ubiquitination of p53 and other proteins through virus-assembled E3 ligases, leading to proteasome-mediated degradation. The E3 region is not essential for adenovirus replication in cell cultures, and can be deleted or replaced without disrupting virus replication *in vitro*. It is therefore one of the insertion sites for foreign DNA when constructing adenovirus vectors. E3 proteins are known to interact with host immune defense mechanisms, thus modulating the host response to adenovirus infection. Inhibition of class I major histocompatibility antigen transport by E3/19K inhibits recognition of infected cells by cytotoxic T lymphocytes and natural killer cells. Tumor necrosis factor-induced apoptosis is inhibited by adenoviral E3/14.7K through the blocking of tumor necrosis factor receptor 1 internalization, which prevents establishment of the death-inducing signaling complex. E3/14.7K has also been shown to modulate antiviral inflammatory responses by inhibiting nuclear factor κB (NFκB) transcriptional activity.

Viral DNA replication, using the 5'-linked 55K protein as primer, proceeds from both ends by a strand-displacement mechanism. The repeat sequences form panhandle-like structures of single-stranded DNA that serve as origins of replication. After DNA replication, late mRNAs are transcribed; these are translated into structural proteins, which are made in considerable excess. All adenovirus late-coding regions are transcribed from a common promoter, the major late promoter. The primary transcript is about 29 kb; at least 18 distinct mRNAs are produced by alternative splicing of the late primary transcript. Shutdown of host-cell macromolecular synthesis occurs progressively during the second half of the replication cycle. Virions are assembled in the nucleus, where they form crystalline arrays (as shown in (Figure 2.2) Chapter 2). Many adenoviruses cause severe condensation

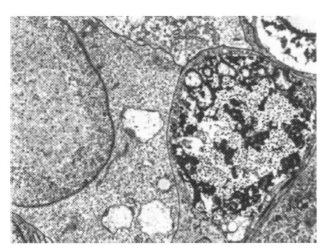

FIGURE 10.3 Avian adenovirus 1 infection in the spleen of a chick. The nucleus at the left contains dispersed virions and early margination of chromatin, whereas the nucleus at the right contains many virions and extremely condensed chromatin. Thin-section electron microscopy; magnification ×16,000. *(Courtesy of N. Cheville.)*

and margination of the host-cell chromatin, making nuclei appear abnormal; this is the basis for the inclusion bodies seen characteristically in adenovirus-infected cells (Figure 10.3). Virions are released by cell lysis.

MEMBERS OF THE GENUS *MASTADENOVIRUS*

CANINE ADENOVIRUS 1 (INFECTIOUS CANINE HEPATITIS VIRUS)

Infectious canine hepatitis, a systemic disease caused by canine adenovirus 1, is also an important pathogen of foxes, wolves, coyotes, skunks, and bears. In fact, the virus was first recognized as the cause of fox encephalitis. In dogs, as well as causing acute hepatitis, the virus may cause respiratory or ocular disease. In contrast, canine adenovirus 2 infection is localized to the respiratory tract (as described in the subsequent section).

Clinical Features and Epidemiology

Disease induced by canine adenovirus 1 is well controlled by vaccination in many countries and, therefore, most infections are asymptomatic or manifest as undifferentiated respiratory disease. In some cases, especially in the immunologically naïve host, the infection proceeds from the initial respiratory site to cause systemic disease. The systemic disease may be divided into three overlapping syndromes, which are usually seen in younger animals: (1) peracute disease in which the pup is found dead either without apparent preceding illness or after an illness lasting only 3 or 4 hours; (2) acute disease, which may be fatal, marked by fever, depression, loss of appetite, vomiting, bloody diarrhea, petechial hemorrhages of the gums, pale mucous membranes, and icterus (jaundice); (3) mild disease, which may actually be a vaccine-modified disease—that is, the result of partial immunity.

The incubation period of the acute disease is 4–9 days. Clinical signs include fever, apathy, anorexia, thirst, conjunctivitis, serous discharge from the eyes and nose, and occasionally abdominal pain and petechiae of the oral mucosa. There is tachycardia, leukopenia, prolonged clotting time, and disseminated intravascular coagulation. In some cases there is hemorrhage (e.g., bleeding around deciduous teeth and spontaneous hematomas). Although central nervous system involvement is not common, dogs affected severely may convulse. Seven to 10 days after acute signs disappear, about 25% of affected dogs develop a characteristic and diagnostically useful bilateral corneal opacity, which usually disappears spontaneously.

In foxes, canine adenovirus 1 causes primarily central nervous system disease; infected animals may exhibit intermittent convulsions during the course of their illness and, terminally, may suffer paralysis of one or more limbs.

Infection of the kidney is associated with viruria, which is a major mode of transmission, along with feces and saliva. Recovered dogs may shed virus in their urine for up to 6 months.

Pathogenesis and Pathology

The virus enters through nasopharyngeal, oral, and conjunctival routes; initial infection occurs in tonsillar crypts, spreading to regional lymph nodes and to the blood via the thoracic duct. Viremia results in dissemination to saliva, urine, feces, and infection of endothelial and parenchymal cells in many tissues, leading to hemorrhages and necrosis, especially in the liver, kidneys, spleen, and lungs. Canine adenovirus 1 is also one of the several causes of acute respiratory disease, although it is probably less important than canine adenovirus 2. The syndrome that gave the disease its name, infectious canine hepatitis, involves the extensive destruction of hepatocytes, resulting in peracute death. Invariably in such cases, histologic examination reveals characteristic inclusion bodies in hepatocytes.

In the convalescent stages of natural infection and 8–12 days after vaccination with canine adenovirus 1 attenuated-virus vaccine, corneal edema ("blue eye") is occasionally observed. Although clinically dramatic and alarming, especially after vaccination, the edema usually resolves after a few days, without consequence. The edema is caused by virus–antibody complexes (type III immune complex hypersensitivity), deposited in the small blood vessels of the ciliary body, interfering with normal fluid exchange within the cornea.

Pathologic findings depend on the clinical course of infection. A rapid clinical course results in edema and hemorrhage of superficial lymph nodes, with multifocal to diffuse petechial and ecchymotic hemorrhages on serosal surfaces. The liver and spleen are enlarged, with mottling of the splenic parenchyma, and accumulation of fibrin on the serosal surfaces of the abdominal viscera. The wall of the gallbladder is characteristically thickened and edematous. Gross lesions in other organs may include cortical renal hemorrhages and multiple areas of pulmonary consolidation. Ocular lesions may include diffuse corneal edema and opacity. Histologic hepatic findings in acutely infected puppies include multifocal hepatocellular necrosis, and sometimes centrilobular hepatic necrosis as a consequence of disseminated intravascular coagulation. Intranuclear inclusions may be present within Kupffer's cells and hepatocytes. Viral inclusions also occur in endothelial cells within the kidney of affected dogs. There is typically widespread hemorrhage and necrosis associated with intravascular thrombosis in dogs that develop disseminated intravascular coagulation.

Diagnosis

Diagnosis of canine adenovirus infections is achieved by either virus isolation or serology using an enzyme immunoassay, hemagglutination-inhibition, or neutralization assay. Viral DNA can be detected directly by polymerase chain reaction (PCR) assay. Virus isolation is performed in any of several cell lines of canine origin (e.g., Madin–Darby canine kidney cells). Cytopathology occurs in most cases in 24–48 hours and, in addition to the characteristic intranuclear inclusions, canine adenovirus 1 can be identified by immunohistochemistry and/or immunofluorescence. Virus persists in renal tubular epithelium cells and therefore can be isolated from urine for months after resolution of clinical signs.

Immunity, Prevention, and Control

Both inactivated and attenuated canine adenovirus 1 vaccines have been widely used for many years. The antigenic relationship between canine adenoviruses 1 and 2 is sufficiently close for canine adenovirus 2 vaccine to be cross-protective; it has the advantage that it does not cause corneal edema. Annual revaccination is recommended by many manufacturers. Maternal antibody interferes with active immunization until puppies are 9–12 weeks of age. The development of neutralizing antibodies directly correlates with immune protection, and dogs with high neutralization titers are protected against clinical disease.

One of the most remarkable phenomena in veterinary practice has been the virtual disappearance of infectious canine hepatitis from regions where vaccination had been performed for many years. This may in part be a result of the shedding of vaccine virus by vaccinated dogs, thereby "seeding" the environment with attenuated virus, immunizing other dogs secondarily, and building up a high level of herd immunity.

CANINE ADENOVIRUS 2

Canine adenovirus 2 causes a localized respiratory disease in dogs and is a potential cause of the kennel cough syndrome (acute respiratory disease of canines). Respiratory disease in affected dogs is characterized principally by bronchitis and bronchiolitis. An essential difference between canine adenoviruses 1 and 2 is that, whereas canine adenovirus 1 causes systemic disease, canine adenovirus 2 infection results only in restricted respiratory disease. The molecular basis of this difference remains uncertain, but this property is exploited for vaccination of dogs: specifically, although the use of live-attenuated canine adenovirus 1 vaccines sometimes results in blue eye because of the ability of the vaccine virus to replicate systemically, canine adenovirus 2 vaccines do not replicate systemically. Canine adenovirus 2 vaccines, however, provide complete homologous and cross protection against disease induced by canine adenovirus 1.

EQUINE ADENOVIRUSES 1 AND 2

Two equine adenoviruses, equine adenoviruses 1 and 2, have been identified. Equine adenovirus 1 has been isolated worldwide from upper respiratory secretions of foals and horses with and without disease. Equine adenovirus 2 has been isolated from lymph nodes and feces of foals with upper respiratory disease and diarrhea. Most equine adenovirus infections are asymptomatic or present as mild upper or lower respiratory tract disease. The latter are marked by fever, nasal discharge, and cough. Secondary bacterial infections, which produce a mucopurulent nasal discharge and exacerbate the cough, are not uncommon.

Arabian foals that have genetically based (defective V(D)J recombination) primary severe combined immunodeficiency disease, an autosomal inherited defect in which there is a total absence of both T and B cells, are incapable of mounting an adaptive immune response to equine adenoviruses. As maternal antibody wanes, these foals become susceptible to adenovirus infection. Infection is progressive, and these foals invariably die within 3 months of age. Much research has been done on adenovirus infections in Arabian foals with primary severe combined immunodeficiency disease. Among all the potentially important opportunistic pathogens that may take advantage of the immune incompetence of these foals, the dominant role of equine adenovirus 1 in the overall pathogenesis of this syndrome is intriguing. In addition to causing bronchiolitis and pneumonia, the virus destroys cells in a wide range of other tissues in these foals, particularly the pancreas and salivary glands, but also renal, bladder, and gastrointestinal epithelium.

A diagnosis of adenovirus infection can, in most cases, be made by virus isolation, serology, or PCR detection and analysis of viral nucleic acid. Adenovirus antigen detection using enzyme immunoassay and virus-specific monoclonal antibodies may also be used. Virus isolation (from nasal swabs of suspect cases or tissues of foals with primary severe combined immunodeficiency disease) is performed in any of several cell lines of equine origin. Cytopathology typical of adenovirus infections (rounding and grape-like clustering of infected cells) occurs in most cases in 24–48 hours. Serologic diagnosis is usually made by hemagglutination-inhibition or neutralization tests. A variety of nucleic acid detection methods have been described, including DNA restriction endonuclease mapping (fingerprinting), Southern blot, dot-blot, *in-situ* hybridization and, most recently, PCR assay. Of these, the PCR assay is becoming the most widely used.

Like most other adenoviruses, equine viruses are probably transmitted by oral and nasopharyngeal routes. Nothing is done to prevent or control infections, given their self-limiting nature.

ADENOVIRUSES OF LABORATORY RODENTS AND LAGOMORPHS

Laboratory and wild mice (*Mus musculus*) are susceptible to two serologically distinct adenoviruses, known as mouse adenoviruses 1 and 2, and previously referred to as FL virus and K87 virus, respectively. Murine adenovirus 1 was isolated from the spleens of mice infected with Friend leukemia virus (thus the "FL" designation), and induces a multisystemic infection when inoculated into neonatal or immunodeficient mice. Naturally occurring disease appears to be non-existent, and the virus is very rare, if not extinct, in contemporary mouse colonies. A serologically related, but distinct adenovirus, murine adenovirus 2, is relatively more common, and may be associated with infant mouse runting and low mortality. Murine adenovirus 2 is enterotropic, producing adenoviral inclusions in enterocytes lining the villi of the small intestine. These inclusions are most apparent in infant mice, but may also be encountered in smaller numbers in adult mice. The serologic relatedness of these viruses involves a one-way cross-reactivity, with antibody against both murine adenoviruses 1 and 2 reacting with murine adenovirus 2 antigen, whereas antibody to murine adenovirus 2 does not react against murine adenovirus 1 antigen. Laboratory rats may also have intestinal adenoviral inclusions, and seroconvert to murine adenovirus 2, but the rat virus appears to be distinct from that of the mouse, as it is infectious only to rats. Syrian hamsters are also susceptible to an uncharacterized intestinal adenovirus, which is probably of rat origin.

Guinea pigs are susceptible to a respiratory adenovirus that causes pulmonary disease and inclusions in respiratory epithelium of young guinea pigs. Affected animals may be severely dyspneic, with high mortality, but morbidity within a population of guinea pigs is low. Disease cannot be reproduced by experimental inoculation of guinea pigs, so other susceptibility factors are suspected in natural disease. Enteritis with profuse diarrhea in young *Oryctolagus* rabbit kits has been described in Europe. Virus was isolated from several organs. There is evidence of seroconversion to adenovirus in North American rabbits, but no disease has been reported.

PRIMATE ADENOVIRUSES

There are numerous isolates of human adenovirus, which are now classified into six major species (human adenoviruses A–F). Adenoviruses of non-human primates are less well characterized, but are represented by at least 27 distinct serotypes that have been isolated from a wide variety of monkeys and apes, including macaques, vervet monkeys, baboons, gorillas, squirrel monkeys, tamarins, and chimpanzees. Most infections are subclinical, but respiratory disease, conjunctivitis, segmental ileitis, pancreatitis, and hepatitis, all with characteristic adenoviral inclusions, have been reported in various species. The non-human primate adenoviruses are genetically disparate from human adenoviruses, but serologically related.

MASTADENOVIRUSES OF CATTLE, SHEEP, GOATS, CAMELIDS, AND PIGS

The importance of mastadenoviruses in agriculturally important domestic animals is conjectural. Several serotypes of bovine adenoviruses have been isolated from calves with pneumonia, enteritis, conjunctivitis, keratoconjunctivitis, and weak calf syndrome. In sheep, adenoviruses are most often isolated from lambs and can be associated with respiratory and enteric infections/disease. Porcine adenoviruses have been associated with respiratory and/or enteric infection/disease or encephalitis; however, it is currently believed that porcine adenoviruses rarely cause severe disease. Protracted excretion of adenoviruses in feces has been described after experimental infections, including infections with those viruses that cause respiratory disease.

The classification of bovine adenoviruses is especially complicated because of the lack of genus-specific antigens. Therefore, some bovine adenoviruses (Subgroup I: bovine adenoviruses 1–3, 9, and 10) belong to the genus *Mastadenovirus*, whereas others (Subgroup II; bovine adenoviruses 4–8) are now classified in the genus *Atadenovirus*, which also includes ovine adenovirus 7 and caprine adenovirus 1. Ovine adenoviruses 1–5 are included in the genus *Mastadenovirus*, as is, tentatively, ovine adenovirus 6. Porcine adenoviruses 1–3 and, tentatively, caprine adenovirus 2 are also included in the genus *Mastadenovirus*. The sequence of adenoviruses isolated from camelids with enteric disease, pneumonia, and hepatitis place them in the genus *Mastadenovirus*, distinct from bovine and ovine isolates. These represent either camelid adenoviruses or spill-over viruses from some unidentified contact species. Clearly, additional epidemiological and experimental studies are needed to better define the virulence and pathogenesis of the adenoviral infections of livestock.

MEMBERS OF THE GENUS *AVIADENOVIRUS*

Aviadenoviruses infect only birds, and are serologically distinct from the adenoviruses in other genera. They are associated with a variety of important disease syndromes in birds. The role of most aviadenoviruses as pathogens is not well defined, with the notable exception of quail bronchitis and hydropericardium syndrome viruses. Aviadenoviruses were previously classified as Subgroup I avian adenoviruses, and include fowl adenoviruses 1–11, duck adenovirus 2, pigeon adenovirus, and turkey adenoviruses 1 and 2.

QUAIL BRONCHITIS VIRUS

Quail bronchitis is an important disease of wild and captive-bred bobwhite quail worldwide; in young birds it is seen as respiratory distress, open-mouth breathing, nasal discharge, coughing, sneezing, rales, lacrimation, and conjunctivitis.

In older birds there is also diarrhea. Mortality may be 100% in young birds, but falls to less than 25% in birds aged more than 4 weeks when infected. The disease is marked by tracheitis, air sacculitis, and gaseous, mucoid enteritis. The etiologic agent is avian adenovirus 1, which can be isolated readily from the respiratory tract of acutely affected birds and from the intestinal tract of mildly affected birds. The virus is highly contagious and spreads rapidly through flocks. Control is based on strict isolation, quarantine of introduced birds, and regular decontamination of premises and equipment. In some instances, recovered birds are retained as breeders, as there is no long-term shedding and immunity is long lasting.

HYDROPERICARDIUM SYNDROME (ANGARA DISEASE) VIRUS

Infectious hydropericardium syndrome first appeared in 1987 in broiler fowl in Pakistan, and has spread throughout the Middle East and parts of central and eastern Asia. A milder variant of the disease has been reported in Central and South America. The disease is typically associated with infection by fowl adenovirus type 4, but the most severe manifestations of the disease require co-infection with an immunosuppressive agent or exposure to immunosuppressive aflatoxins. The disease causes 20–80% mortality, usually beginning in birds aged 3 weeks of age, and peaking at 4–5 weeks in meat chickens. A milder disease can occur in older chickens such as breeders and layers. Affected birds exhibit pericardial effusion, pulmonary edema, and hepatomegaly, and have enlarged kidneys. A vaccine is available in some countries.

OTHER AVIADENOVIRUSES

Various disease syndromes have been associated with aviadenovirus infections, but experimental studies are lacking and, in some instances, experimental infections with these viruses have failed to reproduce the associated disease without secondary infections. Such syndromes include inclusion-body hepatitis, gizzard erosions, reduced egg production or growth rate, tenosynovitis, and respiratory disease in chickens. Similar infections by aviadenoviruses have been reported in turkeys, geese, ducks, pigeons, and ostriches. Pancreatitis has been associated with aviadenovirus infection in guinea fowl.

MEMBERS OF THE GENUS *ATADENOVIRUS*

Members of the genus *Atadenovirus* have a broad host range that includes reptiles, birds, and mammals.

REPTILIAN ADENOVIRUSES

Adenoviruses included in the genus *Atadenovirus* genus have been described in many reptile species, including several different species of snake, lizards (including emerald monitor, Mexican beaded lizard, bearded dragon, and Gila monster), chameleons, and crocodiles. Lesions in reptiles include hepatitis, esophagitis, enteritis, splenitis, and encephalopathy, often with characteristic adenoviral inclusions in affected tissues.

CERVINE ADENOVIRUS (ODOCOILEUS ADENOVIRUS 1)

In 1993, a novel adenovirus was determined to be the cause of an epizootic of severe systemic disease in mule deer (*Odocoileus hemionus*) in California. The causative virus, cervine adenovirus (odocoileus adenovirus 1) has tentatively been classified in the genus *Atadenovirus*. The disease caused by this virus also occurs amongst deer in Oregon, and in other regions of North America. Odocoileus adenovirus 1 has been isolated from naturally infected wild and/or captive white-tailed deer, mule deer, black-tailed deer, and moose, often in association with a fatal hemorrhagic disease syndrome. The disease is marked by pulmonary edema and erosions, ulcerations, hemorrhage, and abscesses of the intestinal tract (Figure 10.4A). Histologically, there is widespread vasculitis with endothelial intranuclear inclusions (Figure 10.4B). Laboratory diagnosis is based on the detection of viral antigen in tissues by immunofluorescence and by the detection of virions by electron microscopy or virus-specific PCR assay.

EGG DROP SYNDROME VIRUS

Egg drop syndrome, first reported in 1976, is characterized by the production of soft-shelled and shell-less eggs by apparently healthy chickens. The disease has been recognized in fowl, and in both wild and domestic ducks and geese worldwide, although the disease is not present in the United States. The virus originated in ducks and spread to chickens through a contaminated vaccine. Chickens are the major species affected by the disease. The virus grows to high titers in embryonating eggs of ducks or geese, or cell cultures derived from ducks, geese, or chickens—especially well in duck kidney, duck embryo liver, and duck embryo fibroblasts.

In chicken flocks without prior experience of these viruses, the first clinical signs of infection are loss of color in pigmented eggs and soft-shelled, thin-shelled, and shell-less eggs. Thin-shelled eggs may have a rough or even sandpaper-like surface. Because birds tend to eat the shell-less eggs, they may be missed, but egg production numbers decrease by a maximum of 40%. In flocks in which there is antibody, the disease is seen as a failure to achieve production targets. There is also an enzootic form of the disease, similar but more difficult to detect. Major lesions in infected birds are seen in the pouch shell gland and oviduct, where epithelial cells become necrotic and contain intranuclear inclusion bodies. There is associated inflammatory infiltration. These findings are virtually pathognomonic, but diagnosis may be confirmed by virus isolation or serology. Hemagglutination-inhibition or neutralization assays are specific for this virus and do not cross-react with antibodies from aviadenovirus infections.

The main route of transmission is through contaminated eggs. Droppings also contain virus, and contaminated fomites such as crates or trucks can spread virus. The virus is also transmitted by needles used for vaccinations. At one time these viruses were spread by the contamination of Marek's disease vaccine, which was produced in duck embryo fibroblasts. Breeding flocks were infected and the viruses were spread widely through fertile eggs. Because

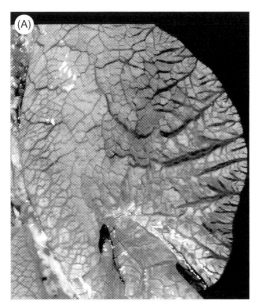 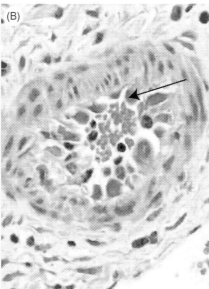

FIGURE 10.4 Cervine adenovirus infection. (A) Severe pulmonary edema in experimentally infected black-tailed deer (*Odocoileus hemionus*). (B) Intranuclear inclusions in endothelial cells (arrow) lining an affected arteriole. (*Courtesy of L. Woods, CA Animal Health and Food Safety Laboratory.*)

infection usually remained latent until birds reached sexual maturity and because the viruses are transmitted vertically in eggs, the detection of this source of contagion was very difficult. Sporadic outbreaks have also been traced to contact of chickens with domestic ducks or geese, and to water contaminated with wildfowl droppings.

This disease has been eradicated from primary breeder flocks in most countries. Its entry into layer flocks is further managed by: (1) preventing contact with other birds, especially waterfowl; (2) disinfecting all equipment regularly; (3) chlorination of water. Inactivated vaccines are available for use in chickens before they begin laying eggs, but they only reduce, rather than eliminate, virus transmission.

OTHER ATADENOVIRUSES

As described previously, the classification of ruminant adenoviruses is somewhat confusing, with some members being classified in the genus *Atadenovirus* (bovine adenoviruses 4–8, ovine adenovirus 7, goat adenovirus 1), whereas the majority are included in the genus *Mastadenovirus*. The pathogenic significance of many of these viruses awaits definitive characterization.

MEMBERS OF THE GENUS *SIADENOVIRUS*

The genus *Siadenovirus* includes viruses that infect amphibians, birds, and reptiles.

TURKEY ADENOVIRUS 3 (HEMORRHAGIC ENTERITIS OF TURKEYS, MARBLE SPLEEN DISEASE OF PHEASANTS, AND AVIAN ADENOVIRUS SPLENOMEGALY VIRUS)

Several important disease syndromes of different bird species are caused by siadenovirus (Subgroup II avian adenoviruses) infections. Hemorrhagic enteritis is a common acute infection of turkeys older than 4 weeks; it is characterized by splenomegaly and intestinal hemorrhage. Clinically, the disease is characterized by acute onset, depression, bloody droppings, and death. Infection causes both humoral- and cell-mediated immunosuppression, so opportunistic bacterial infections are often an intercurrent problem. Flock mortality may reach 60%, although the usual mortality is 1–3%.

A serologically indistinguishable virus causes marble spleen disease of pheasants and avian adenovirus splenomegaly in broiler chickens.

The lesions are pathognomonic: there is prominent reticuloendothelial hyperplasia and intranuclear inclusion bodies in the spleen, distended bloody intestines, and pseudomembranous (fibrinonecrotic) inflammation in the duodenum. Diagnosis of infection may be confirmed by serology using an immunoassay or agar gel immunodiffusion, or by virus isolation with identification of the isolates by immunohistochemistry, immunofluorescence or PCR assay.

The virus is transmitted readily by contact and fomites, and is very stable in contaminated droppings, litter, etc. Control of the disease in turkeys or pheasants is based on vaccination, using an attenuated virus produced either in turkey spleen cells or in turkey B lymphoblastoid cells. Vaccine is administered via drinking water. Because maternal antibody interferes with vaccination, the optimum age for vaccination (usually 4–5 weeks) may vary according to the level of antibody in the flock.

OTHER SIADENOVIRUSES

Frog adenovirus 1 is the prototype virus of the genus *Siadenovirus*. Genetically related viruses have been identified in the tissues of dead raptors (raptor adenovirus 1), and from budgerigars with fatal systemic disease. A siadenovirus also was recently isolated from Sulawesi tortoises (*Indotestudo forsteni*) that exhibited anorexia, lethargy, oral erosions, diarrhea, and nasal and ocular discharge. Virus was detected by PCR assay, and isolated from plasma and tissue samples.

OTHER ADENOVIRUSES

Although adenoviruses have been identified in the tissues of several species of fish, including cod, dab, Japanese eel, and bream, to date a virus has been isolated only from white sturgeon (*Acipenser transmontanus*). Genetic analyses indicate that this virus is distinct from those in the other four recognized genera within the *Adenoviridae*, thus it is proposed that this virus serve as the prototype of a new (fifth) genus, *Ichtoadenovirus*.

Chapter 11

Papillomaviridae and Polyomaviridae

Chapter Contents

Viruses in the families *Papillomaviridae* and *Polyomaviridae* are taxonomically and biologically distinct, but they share striking similarities in their genome organization, virion structure, and mechanisms of replication, cell cycle regulation, and tumor induction.

Papillomaviruses are the cause of papillomas (warts), which have been recognized in animals for centuries: a stable master for the Caliph of Baghdad described equine "warts" in the 9th century. That papillomas have a viral etiology was recognized as long ago as 1907, and in the 1970s it was determined that papillomas in cattle and in other species are caused by several different viruses. In 1935, Peyton Rous observed that benign rabbit papillomas occasionally progressed to carcinomas; this was one of the earliest associations of viruses with cancer. Cutaneous papillomas are common in cattle, and less so in other domestic species. Papillomas occur with some frequency in cervids (deer, moose, etc.). Young animals preferentially are affected, and in both dogs and goats there is breed predisposition to development of cutaneous papillomas.

Papillomaviruses cannot yet be grown in conventional cell cultures, but their genomes readily can be sequenced with molecular methods, without need for culture. The discovery in the 1980s that specific papillomaviruses are a primary cause of cervical and certain other carcinomas in humans prompted much research on the nature and mechanisms of papillomavirus-induced oncogenesis, which in turn has advanced understanding of papillomavirus infections in animals.

Polyomaviruses are ubiquitous, but individual viruses are highly host-species specific. Cell lines contaminated with simian polyomavirus [simian virus 40 (SV40)] were used to propagate some batches of the original human polio vaccine, which was disconcerting at the time because of the proven oncogenic potential of the SV40 virus in laboratory animals. However, it is now clear that polyomaviruses are ubiquitous in humans and animals but generally do not cause significant disease even though they often persist in a life-long subclinical state. They may cause rare neurological (progressive multifocal leukoencephalopathy) and renal diseases (polyomavirus nephropathy) in immunocompromised hosts, including humans and non-human primates, and may be associated with various types of neoplasia. Pathogenic polyomavirus infections occur with some frequency in psittacine birds.

MEMBERS OF THE FAMILY *PAPILLOMAVIRIDAE*

PROPERTIES OF PAPILLOMAVIRUSES

Classification

The family *Papillomaviridae*, like the family *Polyomaviridae*, includes viruses with circular double-stranded DNA genomes. The *Papillomaviridae* currently are divided into some 16 genera (*Alpha-*, *Beta-*, *Gamma-*, *Delta-*, *Epsilon-*, *Zeta-*, *Eta-*, *Theta-*, *Iota-*, *Kappa-*, *Lambda-*, *Mupa-*, *Nupa-*, *Xipa-*, *Omikron-* and *Pipapapillomavirus*), the member viruses of each being distinguished on the basis of host range, DNA sequence relatedness and genome organization, and their biological properties, including the disease that they cause. The distinction of individual virus types (species)

Fenner's Veterinary Virology. DOI: 10.1016/B978-0-12-375158-4.00011-0

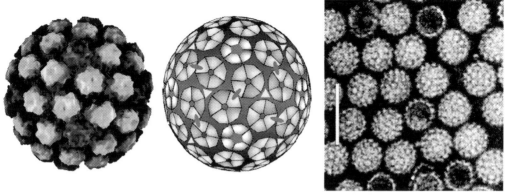

FIGURE 11.1 (Left) Atomic rendering of a papillomavirus capsid with combined image reconstructions from electron cryomicroscopy of bovine papillomavirus (BPV) at 9 A resolution with coordinates from the crystal structure of small virus-like particles of the human papillomavirus 16 (HPV-16) L1 protein (Modis, et al., 2002). (Center) Schematic diagram representing the 72 capsomers in a T = 7 arrangement of a papillomavirus capsid (the icosahedral structure includes 360 VP1 subunits arranged in 12 pentavalent and 60 hexavalent capsomers). (Right) Negative contrast electron micrograph of human papillomavirus 1 (HPV-1) virions. The bar represents 100 nm.) *[From* Virus Taxonomy: Eighth Report of the International Committee on Taxonomy of Viruses *(C. M. Fauquet, M. A. Mayo, J. Maniloff, U. Desselberger, L. A. Ball, eds.), p. 239. Copyright © Elsevier (2005), with permission.]*

TABLE 11.1 Diseases Caused by Papillomaviruses

Virus	Principal Species Affected	Disease
Bovine papillomaviruses 1–10	Cattle	Cutaneous fibropapilloma and papilloma, teat papilloma, and intestinal papilloma (type 4)
	Horses	Sarcoid (bovine papillomaviruses 1, 2)
Feline papillomavirus(es)	Cat	Cutaneous fibropapilloma (feline sarcoid), plaques and papillomas, squamous cell carcinoma
Ovine papillomavirus	Sheep	Cutaneous fibropapilloma
Equine papillomaviruses 1, 2	Horses	Cutaneous papilloma, aural plaques
Porcine genital papillomavirus	Swine	Cutaneous papilloma
Canine papillomaviruses 1–4	Dogs	Oral papilloma (type 1), endophytic papilloma (type 2), pigmented cutaneous plaques (types 3 and 4)
Deer papillomavirus	Deer	Fibropapilloma, papilloma, fibroma
Cottontail rabbit papillomavirus[a] and rabbit papillomavirus	Rabbits	Cutaneous papilloma (may become malignant)
Fringilla (finch) papillomavirus	Finches	Papilloma
Avian papillomavirus	Parrots	Papilloma

[a] *Also called Shope papillomavirus.*

is difficult and confusing, which has led to frequent misclassification. For example, current taxonomic criteria identify some 100 human papillomavirus types and 10 bovine papillomavirus types in at least three different genera, with additional types proposed. There also are several papillomaviruses of dogs (canine oral papillomavirus and several novel cutaneous canine papillomaviruses), cats, horses, rabbits (cottontail rabbit and rabbit oral papillomaviruses),

birds (chaffinch and psittacine papillomaviruses), and papillomaviruses have been described in cetaceans (*Phocoena spinipinnis* papillomavirus), deer (deer fibroma virus), elk and reindeer, non-human primates, elephant, opossum, and rodents (*Mastomys natalensis* papillomavirus), although many of these viruses have been only partially characterized (Table 11.1). There is little sequence homology between the genomes of papillomaviruses from different species.

The human papillomaviruses exhibit a remarkable genetic diversity. Of the animal papillomaviruses, bovine papillomaviruses are especially genetically divergent. Like the human papillomaviruses, the properties of individual strains of bovine papillomavirus differ, with some clearly being more capable of inducing neoplasms than others. In addition to cutaneous papillomas and fibropapillomas, bovine papillomaviruses also can induce papillomas of the mucosal lining of the upper gastrointestinal tract and, in concert with the chemical, quercetin, that is contained in bracken fern, these viruses can induce carcinomas in both the gastrointestinal and urinary tracts of cattle. Papillomaviruses also cause transmissible fibropapillomas of the genitalia of young cattle, with venereal spread analogous to that of human genital warts. In dogs, papillomaviruses are the cause of epithelial plaques and papillomas of the skin and mucosal lining of the oral cavity, conjunctiva, and external genitalia. In horses, they are the cause of papillomas, aural plaques, and sarcoids. Papillomaviruses are the cause of a similar spectrum of lesions in other animal species, although there is considerable variation in the lesions that are most common in each species.

Papillomaviruses can also be categorized according to their tissue tropism and the histologic character of the lesions they cause: for example, some bovine papillomaviruses (types 3, 4, 6, 9, and 10) and cottontail rabbit papillomavirus infect solely keratinocytes and induce squamous papillomas, whereas other bovine papillomaviruses (types 1, 2, and 5) infect both keratinocytes and underlying dermal fibroblasts to produce fibropapillomas, which consist of proliferative masses of both epithelium and fibrovascular (mesenchymal) tissue. Bovine papillomavirus type 4 can infect the epithelium of the mucosal lining of the upper gastrointestinal tract to produce purely epithelial papillomas. In contrast, other papillomaviruses such as deer papillomavirus infect mesenchymal cell to induce primarily fibromas, with minimal infection or proliferation of the overlying epidermis. Nevertheless, productive virus replication is restricted to the epithelial component of fibropapillomas and fibromas.

Virion Properties

Papillomavirus virions are non-enveloped, spherical, 55 nm in diameter, with icosahedral symmetry. Virions are composed of 72 hexavalent (six-sided) capsomers arranged in pentameric (five-sided) arrays (Figure 11.1). Both "empty" and "full" virus particles are seen by electron microscopy. The genome consists of a single molecule of circular double-stranded DNA, 6.8–8.4 kb in size. The DNA circle is covalently closed, supercoiled, associated with histones, and is infectious. The genome encodes some 8–10 proteins, two of which (L1 and L2) form the capsid (Figure 11.2). The remainder are non-structural proteins (designated E1–E8, depending on the individual virus) that exert important regulatory and replicative

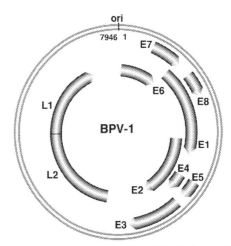

FIGURE 11.2 Diagram of the genome of the bovine papillomavirus (BPV 1). The viral dsDNA (size in bp—7946; origin of replication—ori). Inner arrows indicated the viral proteins encoded by each open reading frame, as well as the direction of transcription (L1, L2—capsid proteins; E1–E8—non-structural proteins). [*From* Virus Taxonomy: Eighth Report of the International Committee on Taxonomy of Viruses (C. M. Fauquet, M. A. Mayo, J. Maniloff, U. Desselberger, L. A. Ball, eds.), p. 240. Copyright © Elsevier (2005), with permission.]

functions. The genome organization differs between the individual genera of papillomaviruses, precise details of which are beyond the scope of this text (Figure 11.3).

Papillomaviruses are resistant to diverse environmental insults: infectivity survives lipid solvents and detergents, low pH, and high temperatures.

Virus Replication

Replication of papillomaviruses is linked intimately to the growth and differentiation of cells in stratified squamous epithelium of the skin and some mucous membranes, from their origin in basal layers to their shedding at the surface. Actively dividing basal cells in the stratum germinativum are infected initially, and maintain the virus in a proviral, possibly latent, state throughout cellular differentiation. Virus-induced hyperplasia, induced by early viral gene products produced during replication, leads to increased basal cell division and delayed maturation of cells in the stratum spinosum and stratum granulosum. These cells become massed into nascent papillomas. Late viral genes encoding capsid proteins are expressed first in cells of the stratum spinosum, and virions appear at this stage of cellular differentiation. The accumulation of large numbers of virions and associated cytopathology are most pronounced in the stratum granulosum. Virions are shed with exfoliated cells of the stratum corneum (keratinized layer) of the skin or non-keratinized cells of mucosal surfaces (Figure 11.4).

Virions attach to cellular receptors, enter via receptor-mediated endocytosis, and are transported to various locations, including the endoplasmic reticulum where they are

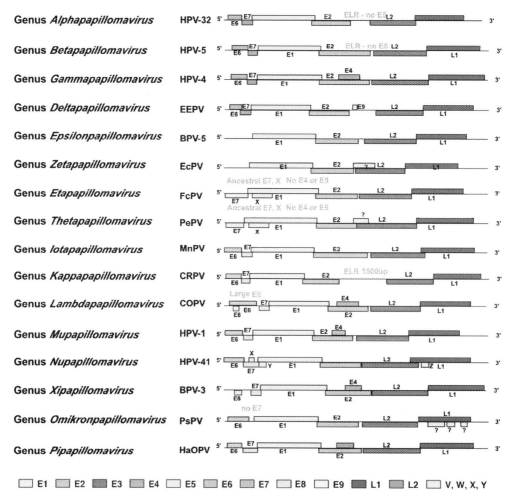

FIGURE 11.3 Comparison of the genome organization of the viruses corresponding to the type species of each genus in the family *Papillomaviridae*. The circular viral dsDNA genomes have been flattened for convenience and the origin of replication (ori) has been taken as the opening site. Similar open reading frames are indicated in similar colors for genes encoding structural (L1, L2) and non-structural proteins (E1–E9), and less well-characterized proteins described for individual viruses (V, W, X, Y). HPV, human papillomavirus; EEPV, European elk papillomavirus; BPV, bovine papillomavirus; EcPV, equine (*Equus caballus*) papillomavirus; FcPV, Fringilla coelebs papillomavirus; PePV, Psittacus erithacus timneh papillomavirus, MnPV, mastomys natalensis papillomavirus, CRPV, cottontail rabbit papillomavirus; COPC, canine oral papillomavirus; PsPV, Phocoena spinipinnis papillomavirus; HaOPV, hamster oral papillomavirus. [*From* Virus Taxonomy: Eighth Report of the International Committee on Taxonomy of Viruses (*C. M. Fauquet, M. A. Mayo, J. Maniloff, U. Desselberger, L. A. Ball, eds.), p. 241. Copyright © Elsevier (2005), with permission.*]

completely or partially disassembled. The genome and some viral proteins enter the nucleus, where they are replicated. The heparan sulfate proteoglycan, syndecan-3, can serve as a human papillomavirus receptor on dendritic cells, but receptors for other papillomaviruses remain to be thoroughly characterized. During productive infection, transcription of the viral genome is divided into early and late stages. Transcription of early and late coding regions is controlled by separate promoters and occurs on the same DNA strand. First, the half of the genome that contains the early genes is transcribed, forming messenger RNAs (mRNAs) that direct the synthesis of enzymes involved in virus replication and cell regulation. Late mRNAs that direct the synthesis of the structural proteins (L1, L2) that are involved in capsid assembly are transcribed from the

other half of the viral genome after DNA synthesis has begun. The regulated expression of the late (L1, L2) proteins of the papillomaviruses occurs only in differentiated epithelial cells, or in differentiating keratinocytes. Progeny DNA molecules serve as additional template, greatly amplifying the production of structural proteins. Several different translational strategies are utilized to enhance the limited coding capacity of the viral genomes.

DNA replication begins at a single unique origin of replication (ori) and proceeds bidirectionally, terminating about 180° away on the circular DNA (Figure 11.2). An initiation complex binds to the origin and unwinds a region (the replication bubble and fork); nascent DNA chains are formed, one strand being synthesized continuously in the direction of unwinding, the other synthesized discontinuously in the

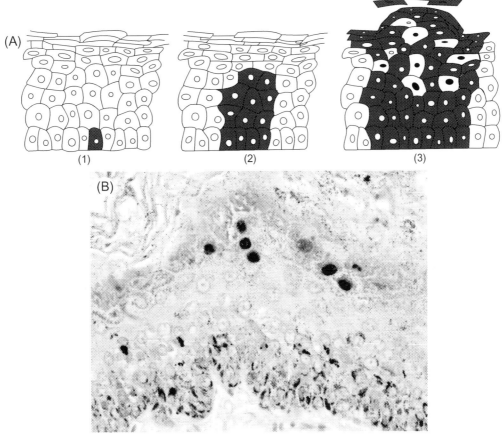

FIGURE 11.4   (A) Schematic representation of the events in papillomavirus infection of keratinocytes. (1) The primary infection occurs in a cell of the striatum germinativum, with the virus gaining entry via an abrasion, etc. (2) This results in a proliferating clone of infected cells that spreads laterally in association with virus-induced delay in the maturation of infected cells. (3) Cellular differentiation occurs eventually and large numbers of virions are produced in association with the formation of a papilloma. This is most pronounced in the stratum granulosum. Virions are shed with exfoliated cells of the stratum corneum. (B) Immunoperoxidase staining of papillomavirus antigen in a squamous plaque from a dog. Note intense, focally extensive nuclear staining (brown) of cells in a discrete region of the stratum spinosum (the granular cytoplasmic pigment in the other cell layers is melanin). *(A: Courtesy of H. zur Hausen. B: Courtesy of J. Luff, University of California, Davis.)*

opposite direction. As replication proceeds, the torsional strain created by the unwinding of the parental strands of DNA is released by the action of a specific viral helicase. Bidirectional replication proceeds around the full genomic DNA circle, at which point the progeny DNA circles separate.

Virions are assembled in the nucleus and are released on cell death, often simply as a consequence of cellular replacement in epithelia through obsolescence. Some cells exhibit a characteristic cytopathic effect, marked by cytoplasmic vacuolization. An infected cell may produce 10,000 to 100,000 virions.

Some papillomaviruses are able to transform cells through the activities of one or more of their non-structural proteins that corrupt normal cellular control signals. Specific strains of papillomavirus express proteins with particular affinity for cellular proteins such as Rb and p53, which are involved in the regulation of the cell cycle and/or apoptosis. For example, the E6 protein is a key component of the

transforming ability of some bovine papillomaviruses, whereas in other bovine papillomaviruses the E6 protein is absent but its oncogenic functions are expressed by other non-structural viral proteins. The E6 protein is a transcriptional activator, and interacts with and inhibits or degrades a variety of cellular proteins, including the transcription coactivator, CBP/p300, and p53 tumor suppressor. It also interacts with activating protein 1 in *trans*-Golgi processes, and it blocks the activity of the cellular molecule, paxillin, that contributes to focal adhesions between cells. Papillomavirus proteins also reduce the expression of major histocompatibility complex class I protein through a number of processes, compromising recognition of viral antigens and elimination of virus-infected cells by the immune system.

The host immune response to papillomavirus infection is directed against the virus, affording protective immunity to subsequent infection, and against the virus-induced tumor, resulting in regression of the papilloma or fibropapilloma. This dichotomous response involves separate antigenic targets, and was initially described by Richard Shope in early studies with rabbit papillomavirus-induced tumors, leading to the first descriptions of "T" (tumor) antigen and tumor-specific transplantation antigens. Antiviral immunity could be induced by vaccination with inactivated virus, but could be circumvented by inoculation of rabbits with infectious DNA (which lacks the viral antigen). However, once rabbits became immune to the tumor, neither virus nor DNA could induce papillomas. The tumor-directed immune response is cell mediated, and results in regression of tumors. Because of this dichotomous response, hosts may be immune to induction of new papillomas, but existing papillomas may continue to flourish, or regress, independent of immunity. These principles pertain to both papillomas and fibropapillomas of several species, in which regressing tumors typically contain infiltrates of T cells. Once an animal is immune to virus or has undergone tumor regression, it is strongly resistant to reinfection, but that immunity is virus-strain specific. Clinical approaches to papilloma therapy often continue erroneously to immunize against virus in an effort to induce tumor regression.

BOVINE PAPILLOMAVIRUS

Papillomas or warts occur more commonly in cattle than in any other domestic animal. All ages can be affected, but the incidence is highest in calves and yearlings. There currently are at least 10 recognized types of bovine papillomavirus, and additional types have been proposed. Bovine papillomavirus types 1 and 2 belong to the genus *Deltapapillomavirus* and exhibit a somewhat broader host range and tissue tropism than other types; they cause fibropapillomas in cattle and sarcoids in horses. Bovine papillomavirus types 3, 4, 6, 9, and 10 belong to the genus *Xipapillomavirus*; they are restricted to cattle and infect only epithelial cells to induce true papillomas. Bovine papillomavirus types 5 and 8 are members of the genus *Epsilonpapillomavirus* and appear to cause both fibropapillomas and true papillomas. Bovine papillomavirus type 7 is currently unclassified. The biological properties of many bovine papillomaviruses remain to be adequately defined, including those of many of the proposed additional types.

Clinical Features and Epidemiology

Bovine papillomavirus are probably transmitted between animals by fomites, including contaminated milking equipment, halters, nose leads, grooming and earmarking equipment, rubbing posts and wire fences, and other articles contaminated by contact with affected cattle. Sexual transmission of venereal warts in cattle is likely, as such lesions are rare in animals that are artificially inseminated. The disease is more common in housed cattle than in cattle on pasture. Natural bovine papillomavirus infection of horses may occur after exposure of the horses to cattle or to fomites contaminated from exposure to infected cattle.

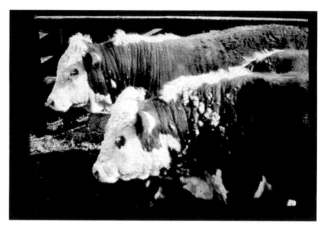

FIGURE 11.5 Cattle with papillomas.

Surveys for papillomavirus DNA in normal bovine skin and dermal tissues show that the viruses are widespread, most often without any obvious lesions. This apparently latent DNA may be reactivated at sites of injury, leading to papilloma formation. Where disease occurs, the various papillomaviruses in cattle are associated with distinct lesions, some in different anatomic locations. Many of the viruses are associated with teat and udder lesions, probably as a result of transmission during milking. Bovine papillomavirus types 1, 2, and 5 infect both mesenchymal and epithelial cells to cause "teat frond" warts, common cutaneous warts, and "rice grain" fibropapillomas. Papillomas have a fibrous core covered to a variable depth with stratified squamous epithelium, the outer layers of which are hyperkeratinized. The lesions vary from small firm nodules to large cauliflower-like growths; they are grayish to black in color and rough and spiny to the touch (Figure 11.5). Large masses are subject to abrasion and may bleed. Fibropapillomas are common on the udder and teats and on the head, neck, and shoulders; they may also occur in the omasum, vagina, vulva, penis, and anus.

In contrast, bovine papillomaviruses 3, 4, 6, 9, and 10 induce epithelial and cutaneous lesions without fibroblast proliferation. Lesions caused by bovine papillomavirus 3 have a tendency to persist, and are usually flat with a broad base, unlike the more usual fibropapillomas that protrude and are often pedunculated. In upland areas of Scotland and northern England, and in other parts of the world where bracken fern (*Pteridium aquilinum*) or closely related ferns are common, progressive papillomas caused by bovine papillomavirus 4 may occur in the alimentary tract, which can progress to squamous cells carcinomas. Although bovine papillomavirus 4 can cause transient papillomas in the alimentary tract, ingestion of the bracken fern is a major contributing factor, because the carcinogens, mutagens, and immunosuppressive chemicals that it contains are essential for the transition to invasive carcinoma of the alimentary tract. In cattle that eat bracken fern, papillomavirus types 1 and 2 may also contribute to the syndrome of "enzootic hematuria" that is characterized by hematuria and/or urinary bladder cancer; over half the bladder tumors include both (mixed) mesenchymal and epithelial components, and the remainder are exclusively of one or the other tissue type. Like fibromas, these tumors exhibit cellular transformation, but do not manifest virus replication.

Pathogenesis and Pathology

Papillomas develop after the introduction of virus through abrasions of the skin, or by activation of viruses already present. Infection of epithelial cells results in hyperplasia, with subsequent degeneration and hyperkeratinization. These changes begin usually 4–6 weeks after exposure. In general, papillomas persist for 1–6 months before spontaneous (immune-mediated) regression; multiple warts usually regress simultaneously. There is a sequential pattern of papilloma development: stage 1 papillomas appear as slightly raised plaques, starting—at about 4 weeks after exposure—with fibroplasia of the underlying dermis and early epithelial proliferation in association with nascent fibroma. Stage 2 fibropapillomas are characterized by virus-induced cytopathology, virus replication, and crystalline aggregates of virions in the keratinizing epithelium of lesions, starting at about 8 weeks. During this stage, the proliferating epidermis extends invasively into the underlying fibroma. Stage 3 fibropapillomas are characterized by fibrotic, pedunculated bases and rough, lobate, or fungiform surfaces, starting after about 12 weeks.

Diagnosis

The clinical appearance of papillomas is characteristic, and laboratory diagnosis is seldom necessary. Virions can be seen by electron microscopic examination but are restricted to the keratinizing epithelium. Polymerase chain reaction (PCR) tests can be readily used to detect papillomavirus DNA, and for typing the virus involved, but the common presence of papillomavirus DNA in samples from many clinically unaffected animals makes it important to interpret any positive results with care, and to associate the virus with the clinical disease. Immunohistochemical staining with appropriate antisera is very useful to confirm the presence of papillomavirus antigen within proliferative ("wart-like") lesions in the skin and mucosal surfaces.

Immunity, Prevention, and Control

Prevention and treatment of papillomas are difficult to evaluate, because the disease is self-limiting and its duration varies. Bovine interferon-α and photodynamic therapy have been used to treat affected cattle, but not widely. Inoculation with homogenized, autologous wart tissue, treated with formalin, has been used for many years, but its efficacy has always been evaluated anecdotally. Vaccination with viral capsid proteins produced by recombinant DNA technology has been encouraging for protection against viral infection, but vaccines must contain several virus types, because there is no cross protection between types. "Debulking" the overall tumor mass on an affected animal may stimulate general fibropapilloma regression, and the same appears to be true for papillomas in other species.

EQUINE PAPILLOMAVIRUS

Equine papillomaviruses are the cause of aural plaques and cutaneous papillomas. Papillomas are usually small, elevated, keratinized lesions that are most common around the lips and noses of young horses, but that also can occur on the ears, eyelids, genitalia, and limbs. They generally regress after 1–9 months. Warts that interfere with the bit, bridle, or other tack can be removed surgically. Congenital equine papillomas have been described.

Aural plaques are discrete, raised, smooth or hyperkeratotic depigmented plaques or nodules on the inner surface of the pinnae of the ear. They are neither pruritic nor painful and, unlike papillomas, they do not spontaneously regress. The presence of papillomavirus in these lesions can be confirmed by immunohistochemical staining, PCR assays, or by electron microscopy.

EQUINE SARCOID

Sarcoid is the most common skin tumor of horses, mules, and donkeys. Sarcoids are most common in horses less than 4 years of age, and may occur singly or in groups, with a predilection for the head, ventral abdomen, and limbs (Figure 11.6A). Although sarcoids are locally aggressive and frequently recur after surgical excision, they are not malignant, and they do not metastasize despite their histological resemblance to that of locally invasive fibrosarcomas. Specifically, the majority of the tumor consists of an irregular mass of proliferating, haphazardly arranged fibroblasts, accompanied by characteristic proliferation of the overlying epidermis with extensions into the dermal mass (Figure 11.6B). Superficial ulceration and secondary trauma are common. On the basis of their appearance, sarcoids have been classified into several types, including a verrucous (wart-like) type, a fibroblastic type, a mixed type, and a flat type.

It has been repeatedly confirmed that distinct variants of bovine papillomavirus types 1 or 2 are present in equine sarcoids, along with their E5 transforming protein that can modulate cellular regulatory signals. Interestingly, bovine papillomavirus DNA also can be detected in the unaffected skin of horses with sarcoids, and sometimes even in the skin of completely unaffected horses. However, transmission trials with sarcoid material are usually unsuccessful, and there is no strong evidence that productive replication of bovine papillomaviruses with production of infectious virions occurs in horses. Viral DNA persists episomally (not integrated into cellular genome) within the nucleus of infected fibroblasts and is not present within epithelial cells.

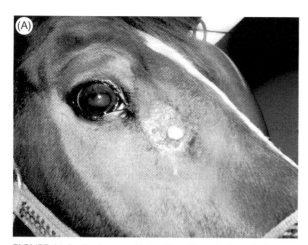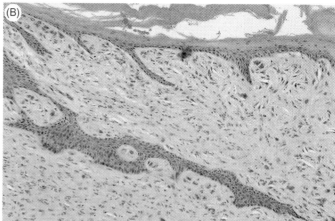

FIGURE 11.6   Equine sarcoid. (A) Sarcoid on the face of a horse. (B) Histological appearance, with proliferation of dermal fibroblasts and hyperplastic overlying epithelium. *(A: Courtesy of H. Hilton, University of California, Davis. B: Courtesy of V. Affolter, University of California, Davis.)*

Horses are susceptible to experimental infection with bovine papillomaviruses 1 and 2, and the tumors produced are morphologically similar to sarcoids. Bovine papillomavirus DNA sequences have been detected in high copy number by hybridization or quantitative PCR in both experimental and natural lesions. Also, bovine papillomaviruses have been shown to transform equine fibroblasts *in vitro*. These data, together with the observation that sarcoids can occur in epizootic form, indicate that certain bovine papillomaviruses cause equine sarcoids. However, unlike their natural counterparts, the induced tumors regress spontaneously, and horses infected experimentally develop antibodies against bovine papillomaviruses, which are absent in horses with naturally occurring sarcoids. Thus much remains to be determined regarding the precise mechanisms whereby specific strains of papillomavirus naturally induce equine sarcoids.

The variable success and hazards of attempted therapies (surgery, laser surgery, radiation, topical drugs) have led to an interest in immunotherapy. Stimulation of cell-mediated responses by the injection of immunopotentiators has met with limited success. Ocular sarcoids have regressed after the injection of viable bacille Calmette–Guérin (BCG) mycobacteria. Experimental vaccines containing mixtures of bovine papillomavirus type 1 virus-like particles and the E7 protein were associated with increased regression of sarcoids, suggesting that therapeutic or protective vaccines may be possible in the future.

CANINE PAPILLOMAVIRUS

Several genetically distinct canine papillomaviruses have been identified and sequenced, each associated with a specific clinical manifestation—specifically, canine oral papillomavirus from oral papillomas, canine papillomavirus 2 from endophytic papillomas, and canine papillomaviruses 3 and 4 associated with pigmented cutaneous plaques.

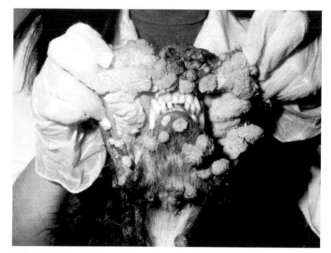

FIGURE 11.7   Oral papillomas in a dog. *(Courtesy of R. A. Rosychuk, Colorado State University, and S. White, University of California, Davis.)*

The most commonly encountered infection is canine oral papillomavirus (genus *Lamdapapillomavirus*), which is associated with, often multiple, exophytic lesions within the oral mucosa of young dogs. The warts usually begin on the lips, and can spread to the buccal mucosa, tongue, palate, and pharynx (Figure 11.7). They are characterized histologically by epithelial hyperplasia and cytoplasmic vacuolization (koilocytosis, which is a feature of all papillomas, regardless of species) with occasional intranuclear viral inclusion bodies. There is a 4–8-week incubation period, and lesions typically regress spontaneously after a further 4–8 weeks. The lesions occasionally become extensive and/or may not regress spontaneously, and progression to squamous cell carcinoma occurs very rarely.

Canine cutaneous exophytic and endophytic papillomas usually occur as single masses in older, often immunosuppressed, dogs. Exophytic papillomas are proliferative masses that exhibit acanthosis, koilocytosis, and occasional intranuclear viral inclusions, whereas endophytic papillomas are cup-shaped and occur below the level of surrounding normal skin. Progression of these lesions to highly invasive, metastatic squamous cell carcinoma has been described in a research colony of dogs with canine X-linked severe combined immunodeficiency.

Pigmented plaques are heavily pigmented cutaneous lesions that occur most frequently in pug dogs. The lesion is characterized by locally extensive epithelial hyperplasia often lacking distinct viral inclusions, with rare progression to squamous cell carcinoma.

FELINE PAPILLOMAVIRUS

Papillomavirus sequences can be amplified (using PCR) from the skin of apparently normal, healthy cats. However, viral sequences have been identified in characteristic proliferative cutaneous lesions in both domestic cats and various wild felids, including leopards, bobcats, and panthers. Some of these viral sequences have been designated as Felis domesticus papillomavirus type 1 (genus *Lambdapapillomavirus*), and these viruses are associated with dermal plaques and with squamous cell carcinomas. Viral sequences from other felid species are divergent, and suggest that these viruses may have co-evolved over time with their respective hosts, typically causing little or no disease.

In cats, individual papillomaviruses are variously associated with feline cutaneous fibropapillomas (feline sarcoids), viral plaques in immunosuppressed animals, cutaneous papillomas, and, recently, *in-situ* (early) squamous cell carcinomas. Feline cutaneous fibropapillomas are characterized by dermal fibroblastic proliferation and occur most often in young cats, on the head, neck, and digits. Partial sequence analysis of a papillomavirus present in these lesions suggests that it is a potentially novel virus most closely related to bovine papillomavirus 1. Feline hyperkeratotic viral plaques associated with feline papillomavirus 1 infection are most common in old, immunosuppressed cats. Feline *in-situ* carcinoma, also referred to as multicentric squamous cell carcinoma *in situ*, appears as multiple cutaneous, often pigmented, plaques that rarely invade the underlying dermis; genetically distinct strains of papillomavirus have been identified in these lesions. Recently, a portion of a human papillomavirus 9 was amplified from a feline cutaneous papilloma.

PAPILLOMAVIRUSES OF OTHER MAMMALIAN SPECIES

Classic studies on viral oncogenesis were carried out in the late 1930s with the Shope rabbit papillomavirus. Papillomas caused by this virus often progress to carcinomas both in their natural host, the cottontail rabbit (*Sylvilagus* spp.), and in laboratory rabbits infected experimentally. Virus replication, however, only occurs in the natural host.

Oral papillomatosis occurs naturally in domestic rabbits (*Oryctolagus cuniculus*); the tumors are small, gray-white, filiform or pedunculated nodules (5 mm in diameter) and are localized mostly on the underside of the tongue. The causative papillomavirus is distinct from the Shope rabbit papillomavirus (cottontail rabbit papillomavirus). Experimentally, oral papillomatosis has been reproduced in various rabbit species, and in nature it is widespread among domestic rabbits, particularly young animals. Virus spread in animal rooms seems not to occur, but transmission from the mother to offspring during the suckling period is common. Oral papillomas of rabbits show no tendency to malignancy, and may persist for many months.

Papillomaviruses are remarkably absent in rodents, despite concerted efforts to find murine variants to serve as models in the laboratory. Exceptions are the papillomaviruses in the "multimammate rat" or African soft-furred rat (*Mastomys natalensis*) and the European harvest mouse (*Micromys minutus*). Because of the strong species specificity of papillomaviruses, these cannot be transmitted to laboratory mice or rats.

PAPILLOMAVIRUSES OF BIRDS

The Fringilla (finch) papillomavirus causes papillomas in wild common chaffinch (*Fringilla coelebs*), brambling (*Fringilla montifringilla*) and Eurasian bullfinch (*Pyrrhula pyrrhula*). Infection with a second papillomavirus-like virus has been described in African grey parrot (*Psittacus erithacus*). Both viruses have been demonstrated in papillomatous lesions in their respective host species. In finches, papillomas occur exclusively on the toes and distal legs, and show stages of development from a slight node on a digit to heavy involvement of the foot and adjacent regions, with obscuring of the individual digits and resulting overgrowth and distortion of the claws. In severe cases the tumor may account for up to 5% of the bird's total body weight, but affected birds seem to remain in good condition otherwise. Cutaneous papillomas have been described in various psittacine birds, but many of these lesions are associated with herpesvirus infections and not papillomaviruses.

MEMBERS OF THE FAMILY *POLYOMAVIRIDAE*

Polyomaviruses have highly restricted host ranges, and these viruses typically cause life-long, inapparent infections in their respective hosts. The oncogenic potential of polyomaviruses is only evident when they are inoculated experimentally into heterologous hosts or their cells in culture. The family *Polyomaviridae* contains a single genus, *Polyomavirus*, which includes viruses identified in: humans; non-human primates (African green monkey, baboon, stump-tail and rhesus macaque); rodents, including mice (polyomavirus and K virus), hamsters (hamster

TABLE 11.2 Properties of *Papillomaviridae* and *Polyomaviridae*

Virions are non-enveloped, spherical in outline, with icosahedral symmetry. Virions are 55 nm (*Papillomaviridae*) or 45 nm (*Polyomaviridae*) in diameter

The genome consists of a single molecule of circular double-stranded DNA, 6.8–8.4 kbp (*Papillomaviridae*) or 5 kbp (*Polyomaviridae*) in size. The DNA has covalently closed ends, is circular and supercoiled, and is infectious

Members of both families replicate in nucleus; members of the *Polyomaviridae* grow in cultured cells; most members of the *Papillomaviridae* have not been grown in conventional cultured cells, but will transform cultured cells; infectious virions produced only in terminally differentiated epithelial cells

During replication, *Polyomaviridae* DNA is transcribed from both strands, whereas *Papillomaviridae* DNA is transcribed from one strand

Integrated (*Polyomaviridae*) or episomal (*Papillomaviridae*) DNA may be oncogenic

polyomavirus), and rats (rat polyomavirus); rabbits (rabbit kidney vacuolating agent); birds (avian polyomaviruses, including budgerigar fledgling disease polyomavirus); cattle (bovine polyomavirus); equine (equine polyomavirus). The avian polyomaviruses segregate independently of the mammalian ones on the basis of genome sequence analyses, indicating long-standing evolutionary divergence that may result in their being included in different genera in the future. Polyomaviruses of veterinary importance occur in laboratory animals and birds.

The genome organization, virion structure, and replication strategy of polyomaviruses is generally similar to that of papillomaviruses (Table 11.2). Virions (40–45 nm) and the genome (approximately 5 kb) of polyomaviruses are slightly smaller than those of papillomaviruses, and their replication is analogous to that of papillomaviruses, except that transcription of coding regions occurs on opposite DNA strands in the case of polyomaviruses and on the same strand with papillomaviruses. Like the papillomaviruses, polyomaviruses regulate the cell cycle and can transform infected cells through the activities of one or more of their nonstructural proteins (so-called T proteins). Transformation of infected cells occurs in some instances by specific inactivation of the cellular *p53* tumor suppressor gene that normally limits infection by inducing apoptosis of virus-infected cells.

Reactivation of persistent, latent polyomavirus infections can occur as a consequence of immunosuppression, regardless of the cause, potentially as a result of mutations in the transcriptional control region of the viral genome. Reactivation of virus in the kidney leads to shedding of virus in the urine of infected humans.

AVIAN POLYOMAVIRUSES, INCLUDING BUDGERIGAR FLEDGLING DISEASE POLYOMAVIRUS

Polyomaviruses have been identified in numerous species of birds, although most infections are not associated with clinical disease. The avian polyomaviruses are all related, but there is considerable genetic diversity amongst them. Disease syndromes associated with polyomavirus infections in birds include increased mortality in a variety of young captive psittacine birds [lovebirds (*Agapornis* spp.), macaws (*Ara* spp.), conures (*Aratinga* and *Pyrrhula* spp.), ring-necked parakeets (*Psittacula krameri*), caiques (*Pionites* spp.), Eclectus parrots (*Eclectus roratus*), occasionally nestlings of Amazon parrots (*Amazona* spp.) and cockatoos (*Cacatua* spp.)], and an acute generalized disease in fledgling budgerigars (*Melopsittacus undulatus*). So-called budgerigar fledgling disease polyomavirus may also be responsible for "French molt," a milder disease of budgerigars that results in chronic disorders of feather formation. Subclinical polyomavirus infection has been described in European raptors, zebra finches (*Poephila guttata*), Ross's turaco (*Musophaga rossae*) and a kookaburra (*Dacelo novaeguineae*). The only species shown to be infected in its natural setting is the sulfur-crested cockatoo (*Cacatua gallerita*) in Australia. A polyomavirus has been described in 3–16-week-old domestic geese with bloody diarrhea, subcutaneous hemorrhage, tremors, ataxia, and variable mortality. An avian polyomavirus of unknown significance has been isolated from wild buzzards (*Buteo buteo*) and Eurasian kestrel (*Falco tinnunculus*).

Avian polyomavirus-associated diseases have repeatedly been reported from captive populations. Infection and disease are widespread in budgerigars and lovebirds, with mortality rates ranging between 30 and 80% of infected nestlings. The virus can be shed in the feces for up to 6 months. Affected birds typically die suddenly with minimal clinical warning, but they briefly manifest weakness, pallor, subcutaneous hemorrhages, anorexia, dehydration, inappetence, and crop stasis. Two additional, but less frequent presentations are described. The first is an acute form of disease that results in birds that present with generalized edema and ascites, full crops, reddened skin, feather dystrophy, and acute death. Gross lesions in affected birds include hydropericardium, cardiomegaly (enlarged heart), hepatomegaly (enlarged liver), and scattered cutaneous hemorrhages. Histologic lesions include focal necrosis in several organs, including the liver, with characteristic clear-to-light basophilic intranuclear inclusions in cells adjacent to necrotic foci. Polyomavirus virions can be visualized by electron microscopy in the nuclei of epithelial cells—for example, in renal tubules. The second atypical form occurs mostly in cockatoo, which have reduced weight gains, and develop interstitial pneumonia and pulmonary edema.

POLYOMAVIRUSES OF PRIMATES AND LABORATORY ANIMALS

Progressive multifocal leukoencephalopathy caused by simian polyomaviruses (SV40) occurs in immunosuppressed non-human primates, typically rhesus macaques (*Macaca mulatta*) infected with simian immunodeficiency virus. The same disease occurs in some humans with acquired immunodeficiency syndrome, but is generally associated with a distinct human polyomavirus, JC virus.

Polyomavirus infections involve a number of common laboratory animal species, including mice, rats, hamsters, and rabbits. Polyomavirus of mice is the namesake virus for this family, but its previous status as the prototype virus for the family has been usurped by SV40 virus. Components of the T antigen genes of polyomavirus are often used in transgenic constructs in order to induce transformation. Polyomavirus biology is well understood in the mouse. Young mice are globally immunodeficient at birth and, when experimentally inoculated with polyomavirus as neonates, they develop multisystemic infections with cytolytic replication of the virus in several organs. If the mice survive, foci of transformed cells arise, resulting in the evolution of many (poly) types of tumor (oma), including tumors of mesenchyme as well as epithelium. Tumors of skin resemble papillomas, with virus replication in the keratinizing epithelium, but, otherwise, tumors do not contain replicating virus. Under natural conditions, neonatal mice in enzootically infected populations are protected from infection by maternal antibody, and acquire infection when maternal antibody is waning. Under these circumstances, infection is subclinical, without tumor induction, and may be persistent, with chronic shedding of virus in the urine. This feature of subclinical persistent urinary shedding is common among many species of polyomaviruses.

The mouse is host to another polyomavirus, known as K virus, or Kilham's virus, and more recently erroneously named as "murine pneumotropic virus." K virus is not truly pneumotropic, but rather may induce pulmonary edema and hemorrhage as a result of its tropism for, and cytolytic replication in, vascular epithelium. This only occurs when mice develop disseminated infections as immunodeficient neonates. Like polyomavirus of mice, K virus may be chronically shed in the urine, but, unlike polyomavirus of mice, it has no known oncogenic activity. Both polyomavirus and K virus are essentially non-existent as naturally occurring infections in contemporary mouse colonies. However, because polyomavirus continues to be studied experimentally, it has occasionally been the cause of iatrogenic contamination of laboratory mice. This is most significant in athymic nude (T-cell-deficient) mice, which have been found to develop neoplasia following natural exposure.

Both laboratory and pet Syrian hamsters (*Mesocricetus auratus*) and European hamsters (*Cricetus cricetus*) have been found to be infected with a hamster polyomavirus of unknown origin, which probably arose in Eastern Europe when wild European hamsters were mixed with laboratory Syrian hamsters. Hamster polyomavirus is biologically similar to most other polyomaviruses, with initial multisystemic cytolytic infection, tumor induction in immunodeficient animals, and chronic infection with shedding of virus in the urine. This cycle is enhanced in the hamster, because Syrian hamsters are highly inbred, with an undefined cellular immune deficiency which renders them susceptible to the virus and to tumor induction at all ages. When initially introduced to a naïve population of hamsters, hamster polyomavirus will induce massive epizootics of transmissible lymphomas among young hamsters, generally arising initially in the mesenteric lymph nodes, but involving several organs. These epizootics can be devastating, and have resulted in the loss of several valuable inbred lines of laboratory hamsters. When infection becomes enzootic within the population, the prevalence of lymphomas decreases, and animals often manifest multiple cutaneous epitheliomas. As in polyomavirus of mice, lymphomas represent transformed cells without virus replication, whereas virus replication occurs in the keratinizing epithelium of epitheliomas. This feature initially resulted in the erroneous classification of the hamster agent as a papillomavirus.

Other common laboratory animals may also incur polyomavirus infections. One of the earliest polyomaviruses to be discovered was the rabbit kidney vacuolating agent, which induced cytopathic change in cottontail rabbit kidney cultures. Thus the virus is indigenous to *Sylvilagus* spp., but polyomavirus-like intranuclear inclusion bodies may also be found in renal tubules of *Oryctolagus* spp. rabbits, suggesting the presence of a similar virus in this species. Polyomaviruses are clinically inconsequential in rabbits.

Finally, laboratory rats may be infected with an as yet to be characterized polyomavirus, which has been manifest clinically on several occasions in athymic nude rats with respiratory disease. These animals have robust intranuclear inclusion bodies in the respiratory epithelium and lungs, as well as salivary glands, but not involving the kidneys. This observation parallels the recent discovery of human polyomaviruses in children with respiratory disease (KI and WU viruses), and in adults with Merkel cell carcinomas (MC virus).

BOVINE POLYOMAVIRUS INFECTION

Bovine polyomavirus is frequently present in bovine sera, especially fetal and neonatal calf sera. Furthermore, cross-reacting antibodies have been detected in the serum of a high proportion of veterinarians in some regions. However, despite the ubiquitous presence of this virus in cattle, no disease has been associated with bovine polyomavirus infection, and its significance remains uncertain.

Parvoviridae

Chapter Contents

Parvoviruses infect many animal species and are the causative agents of several important animal diseases (Table 12.1). There probably are many more parvoviruses that cause only mild or subclinical infections, and infections with such viruses are increasingly diagnosed using molecular assays. Parvovirus-induced diseases such as that caused by feline panleukopenia virus have been recognized for more than 100 years, whereas others such as canine parvovirus disease have emerged more recently.

Despite their complex taxonomic organization, the parvoviruses are all related and probably derive from a common ancestor. They share common biological properties, including their resistance to desiccation in the environment and their requirement for cells that are passing through mitotic S phase in order to replicate their DNA. The relative availability of mitotically active cells in specific tissues during differentiation in early life confers an age-dependent susceptibility to several parvovirus-induced diseases. Thus certain parvovirus infections are most severe in fetuses (after transplacental infection) and neonates. This requirement for mitotically active cells also is reflected in the tropism of some parvoviruses for rapidly dividing hemopoietic precursors and lymphocytes, and progenitor cells of the intestinal mucosal lining.

PROPERTIES OF PARVOVIRUSES

Classification

The family *Parvoviridae* comprises two subfamilies: the subfamily *Parvovirinae*, which contains viruses of vertebrates, and the subfamily *Densovirinae*, which contains viruses of insects that will not be discussed further. There are five genera in the subfamily *Parvovirinae*. The taxonomic organization of parvoviruses can be confusing, as a single animal species may be host to more than one species of parvovirus, but the parvoviruses are taxonomically grouped into genera according to their molecular properties and not their species of origin. The genus *Parvovirus* includes: feline panleukopenia virus and the closely related canine parvovirus, mink enteritis virus, and raccoon parvovirus; parvoviruses of rodents and lagomorphs; porcine and chicken parvoviruses. The genus *Erythrovirus* includes human parvovirus B19 and related viruses of non-human primates and, tentatively, bovine parvovirus type 3 and chipmunk parvovirus. The genus *Dependovirus* includes the so-called adeno-associated viruses that are themselves replication defective and do not cause disease as they are unable to replicate except in the presence of a helper virus, usually an adenovirus. This

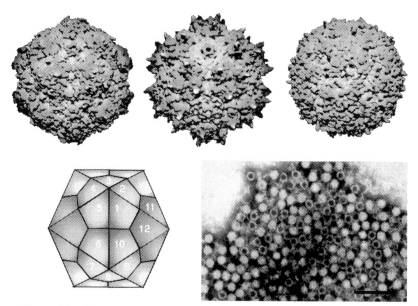

FIGURE 12.1 (Top) Space-filling models of the capsid structures of canine parvovirus (CPV) (left); adeno-associated virus - 2 (AAV-2) (center) and Galleria mellonella densovirus (GmDNV) (right). Each model is drawn to the same scale and is colored according to distance from the viral center. In each case, the view is down a twofold axis at the center of the virus, with threefold axes left and right of center, and fivefold axes above and below (Courtesy of M. Chapman). (Bottom left) Diagram representing a T = 1 capsid structure. (Bottom right) Negative contrast electron micrograph of CPV particles. The bar represents 100 nm. *[From Virus Taxonomy: Eighth Report of the International Committee on Taxonomy of Viruses (C. M. Fauquet, M. A. Mayo, J. Maniloff, U. Desselberger, L. A. Ball, eds.), p. 353. Copyright © Elsevier (2005), with permission.]*

TABLE 12.1 Manifestations of Parvovirus Diseases in Animals[a]

Virus	Disease
Feline panleukopenia virus	Generalized disease in kittens, with panleukopenia, enteritis; cerebellar hypoplasia
Canine parvovirus 1 (minute virus of canines)	Minimal
Canine parvovirus 2 (subtypes 2a, 2b, 2c)	Generalized disease in puppies; enteritis, myocarditis (rarely), lymphopenia
Porcine parvovirus	Stillbirth, abortion, fetal death, mummification, infertility.
Mink enteritis virus	Leukopenia, enteritis
Aleutian mink disease virus	Chronic immune complex disease, encephalopathy. Interstitial pneumonia in neonates
Mouse parvoviruses, minute virus of mice, rat parvoviruses, H-1 virus of rats	Subclinical or persistent infection; congenital fetal malformations; hemorrhagic syndrome in rats
Goose parvovirus	Hepatitis, myocarditis, myositis
Duck parvovirus	Hepatitis, myocarditis, myositis

[a] *Parvoviruses have also been detected in a variety of animal species, frequently in the absence of obvious clinical disease.*

genus also includes goose and duck parvoviruses and, provisionally, bovine parvovirus 2. Aleutian mink disease virus is the sole member of the genus *Amdovirus*. Bovine parvovirus and canine minute virus are included in the genus *Bocavirus*. Thus individual parvoviruses from dogs, birds, rodents, cattle, and mink are classified in several genera.

Virion Properties

Parvovirus virions are non-enveloped, 25 nm in diameter, and have icosahedral symmetry (Figure 12.1). The capsid displays a number of surface features that are associated with its functioning, include a hollow cylinder at each fivefold axis of symmetry that is surrounded by a circular depression, prominent protrusions around the threefold axis of symmetry, and, in most viruses, a depression at each twofold axis of symmetry. The receptor binding site of feline and canine parvoviruses, which determines their host and tissue tropism, is located on the surface of the spike, which is also the site of binding of most antibodies directed against the capsid.

The parvovirus capsid is composed of a total of 60 protein molecules, approximately 90% being VP2 and approximately 10% being the overlapping but larger VP1 protein. VP1 and VP2 are formed by alternative splicing of the same messenger RNA (mRNA), and the entire sequence of VP2 is encoded within the *VP1* gene. In some viruses a third structural protein, VP3, is formed (only in DNA-containing capsids) by cleavage of a peptide from the amino terminus of VP2. The parvovirus capsid proteins all contain a central eight-stranded, antiparallel β-barrel motif, and the strands of the β-barrel are linked by four extensive loops; these loops form most of the outer surface of the virus particle and are responsible for their receptor binding, their antigenic properties, and their environmental stability. Indeed, parvoviruses are extremely stable to environmental conditions, including extremes of heat and pH, and disinfection of contaminated premises using commercially available disinfectants is a major challenge.

The genome consists of a single molecule of linear single-stranded DNA, approximately 4.5–5.5 kb in size (Figure 12.2). Some parvoviruses encapsidate only the negative-sense DNA strand (e.g., canine parvovirus, minute virus of mice). Others encapsidate different proportions of both negative and positive strands, so that individual virions of these viruses may contain single-stranded DNA of either polarity. The genome contains two major open reading frames: an open reading frame in the 3′ half of the genome that encodes the non-structural proteins that are required for DNA transcription and replication, and another open reading frame towards the 5′ half encodes the structural proteins (variously designated as CAP, VP, or S) of the capsid. Both reading frames are present on the same DNA strand of members of the *Parvovirinae*. The genome has terminal palindromic sequences, enabling each end to form hairpin or other complex base-paired structures required for virus replication.

Virus Replication

Receptor binding at the plasma membrane initiates viral infection of susceptible cells, and virions are then taken up into the cell by endocytosis. Transferrin receptor is the receptor for canine parvovirus and feline panleukopenia virus, and it also directs the virus into the clathrin-mediated uptake pathway. Utilization of the transferrin receptor probably also facilitates replication of these viruses, as it is markedly upregulated on proliferating cells; parvovirus

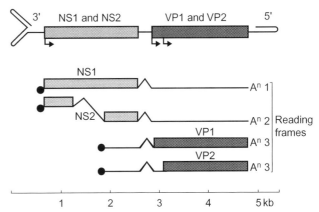

FIGURE 12.2 Genomic DNA of canine parvovirus and its transcription strategy. The genome has terminal palindromic sequences enabling each end to form hairpin structures; these structures serve as the origin of DNA replication and also facilitate encapsidation (packaging) of viral DNA within nascent virions. The 5′ ends of RNA transcripts are capped (black circles) and the 3′ ends are polyadenylated (A^n). VP1 and VP2, which are produced in very large amounts, are encoded in the same mRNA. They are formed by alternative initiation codons (arrowheads)—the entire sequence of VP2 is encoded within the *VP1* gene. The non-structural protein NS1, also produced in very large amounts, serves a number of functions: (1) it binds to DNA and is required for viral DNA replication; (2) it serves as a helicase; (3) it serves as an endonuclease; (4) it interferes with cellular DNA replication, causing the arrest of the cell division cycle in the S phase. NS2, which is encoded in two open reading frames and is formed by splicing, also regulates viral gene expression. Among the different parvoviruses, there is a remarkable diversity in transcription details (frameshifting, splicing, etc.) and products that cannot be shown using any one virus as a model. *(Courtesy of C. R. Parrish.)*

replication is intimately associated with cellular replication, because virus replication occurs only in cells that pass through mitotic S phase. Many parvoviruses also bind sialic acid residues, consistent with their ability to hemagglutinate erythrocytes of various species; sialic acid is an essential component of the cell receptor binding process utilized by some rodent parvoviruses. Other determinants of parvovirus tropism are not well understood. The known receptors for most animal parvoviruses do not appear to be sufficiently tissue specific to explain the tropism of the viruses, although it is likely that the binding affinity of specific virions to their receptors might influence the pathogenesis of infections with these viruses.

Once inside cells, virions traffic through the endosomal pathways within the cytoplasm, including the early and late endosomes and, in some cases, the recycling endosomes. Exactly how the particles exit from the endosomal system is unclear. However, the viral VP1 protein contains a phospholipase A2 enzyme activity in its N-terminal unique region that may be involved in modifying the endosomal membrane and facilitating capsid release. This unique region of VP1 is buried inside the newly made particle, and so exposure within the endosome requires a structural transformation of the capsid to release that activity. The particles that enter the cytoplasm are trafficked to the nuclear pore, and the more-or-less intact particle enters the nucleus, where replication occurs.

Viral DNA replication and capsid assembly take place in the nucleus and require host-cell functions of S phase of the cell division cycle. The requirement for cycling cells for virus replication is due to a viral requirement for host DNA replication machinery for replication of the viral DNA, as the virus does not encode or package such an enzyme. Instead, cellular DNA polymerases replicate the viral DNA to form a double-stranded DNA intermediate, which is then used as a template for transcription of viral mRNAs. Alternative splicing gives rise to several mRNA species that are translated into four major proteins, and additional small and less well-characterized proteins. The most abundant mRNA, which is encoded in the 5′ half of the genome, directs the synthesis of the structural proteins. The non-structural protein (NS1) that is encoded in the 3′ portion of the genome serves a number of functions: (1) it becomes attached to the 5′ end of the viral DNA during replication; (2) it serves as a helicase during replication and DNA packaging; (3) it serves as a site-specific nickase; (4) it mediates arrest of the cell in the G_1 phase of the cell cycle.

The mechanism of replication of the genome is described as a rolling-hairpin replication; it is complex, and some details still are not completely understood. The 3′-terminal hairpin on the negative-sense DNA genome serves as a self-primer for the initiation of synthesis of a double-stranded DNA replicative intermediate. The detection of a dimeric form of the replicative intermediate—that is, a head-to-head concatemer of two covalently linked double-stranded forms—has led to a model in which the growing DNA strand replicates back on itself to produce a tetrameric form from which two complete positive strands and two complete negative strands are generated by a complicated series of reopening of closed circular forms, reinitiation of replication at transiently formed hairpins, and single-strand endonuclease cleavages (Table 12.2).

A major determinant of the pathogenesis of parvoviruses is their requirement for cycling cells for virus replication. Parvovirus infections of the fetus (pig or cat) or newborn (dog or cat) at critical stages of organogenesis when there is considerable cell division may result in widespread infection and tissue destruction that cause developmental defects. Thus feline panleukopenia virus infection selectively destroys the developing cerebellum in feline fetuses or kittens infected in the perinatal period, whereas the developing heart (myocardium) may be affected in parvovirus-infected pups and goslings. Typically, replication of these same viruses is restricted in older animals with differentiated organs; however, continuously dividing cells such as hemopoietic precursors, lymphocytes, and progenitor cells of the intestinal mucosa are susceptible in animals of all ages. Selective parvovirus infection and destruction of these rapidly dividing cell types leads to tissue injury analogous to that induced by radiation—hence the designation of some

parvovirus infections as being "radio-mimetic." The tropism of Aleutian mink disease virus also changes with age; in neonates lacking maternal immunity there is infection and destruction of type II pneumocytes, leading to acute interstitial pneumonia, whereas older animals (or neonates in which antibodies are present) develop chronic infections with less infection of type II pneumocytes.

While many parvoviruses cause acute infections that last only a few days, others persist for long periods in the face of apparently robust host immune responses. The precise mechanisms of parvovirus persistence are not well understood, as most of the viruses appear to be susceptible to antibody-mediated neutralization. Aleutian mink disease virus persistently replicates to high levels in many mink, perhaps because of capsid-associated phospholipids that reduce antibody binding or neutralization. Disease develops in persistently infected mink as a result of the high levels of circulating antigen–antibody complexes that deposit in tissues and initiate a type III hypersensitivity reaction that results in tissue injury and destruction.

MEMBERS OF THE GENUS *PARVOVIRUS*

Virions of some members of the genus *Parvovirus* contain exclusively negative-sense DNA, whereas those of other viruses in the genus also include variable proportions of positive-sense DNA.

FELINE PANLEUKOPENIA VIRUS

All members of the family *Felidae* are probably susceptible to infection with feline panleukopenia virus, which occurs worldwide. Some members of the families *Viverridae*, *Procyonidae* and *Mustelidae* also are susceptible, including the raccoon, mink, and coatimundi. The associated

---

TABLE 12.2 Properties of Parvoviruses

Five genera: *Parvovirus, Erthrovirus, Dependovirus, Amdovirus, Bocavirus*

Virions are icosahedral, 25 nm in diameter, and composed of 60 protein subunits

The genome is a single molecule of single-stranded DNA, approximately 4–6 kb in size; some viruses encapsidate exclusively negative-sense DNA, whereas others encapsidate both positive- and negative-sense DNA

Replication occurs in the nucleus of dividing cells; infection leads to large intranuclear inclusion bodies

Viruses are very stable, resisting 60°C for 60 minutes and pH 3 to pH 9

Most viruses hemagglutinate red blood cells

disease, feline panleukopenia, can be very severe and cause substantial mortality in susceptible animals.

Clinical Features and Epidemiology

Feline panleukopenia virus is highly contagious. The virus may be acquired by direct contact with infected cats or via fomites (bedding, food dishes); fleas and humans may act as mechanical vectors. Virus is shed in the feces, vomitus, urine, and saliva, and is very stable in the environment.

Feline panleukopenia is most common in kittens infected around the time of weaning when maternal antibody wanes, but cats of all ages are susceptible. The incubation period is approximately 5 days (range 2–10 days). At the onset of clinical signs, there is a profound leukopenia and the severity of the disease and the mortality rate parallel the severity of the leukopenia; the prognosis is grave if the white blood cell count falls below 1000 cells per ml of blood. Clinical signs include fever (greater than 40°C), which can persist for 24 hours or more. Death occurs during this phase in the peracute form of the disease. In cats that survive, temperature returns to normal and increases again on the 3rd or 4th day of illness, at which time there is lassitude, inappetence, a rough coat, and often repeated vomiting. A profuse, persistent, and frequently bloody diarrhea may develop at approximately the 3rd or 4th day of illness. Dehydration from severe malabsorption diarrhea frequently is a major contributing factor to fatal infections.

Perinatal or *in-utero* infection of kittens can cause abnormal development of the cerebellum (cerebellar hypoplasia/atrophy syndrome). Affected kittens are noticeably ataxic when they become ambulatory around 3 weeks of age (so-called spastic or wobbly cat syndrome); they have a wide-based stance and move with exaggerated steps, tending to overshoot the mark and to pause and oscillate about an intended goal.

Pathogenesis and Pathology

After virus entry in the oropharynx, initial virus replication occurs in pharyngeal lymphoid tissue. From here the virus is distributed in a free and cell-associated viremia to other organs and tissues via the blood stream. Cells that have appropriate receptors and are in the S phase of the cell cycle are infected and killed or prevented from entering mitosis; there also may be "indirect" effects on uninfected cells through receptor binding, or resulting from the regulatory and cytotoxic effects of virus-induced cytokines such as tumor necrosis factor. The characteristic profound leukopenia involves all white blood cell elements, including lymphocytes, neutrophils, monocytes, and platelets. These cells are destroyed—both those present in the circulation and those in lymphoid organs, including the thymus, bone marrow, lymph nodes, spleen, and Peyer's patches. Resting peripheral leukocytes may be stimulated

to proliferate, thereby becoming permissive for virus replication. The presence of virus bound to the surface of cells may also render them targets for cytotoxic lysis.

Rapidly dividing epithelial cells lining the intestinal glands (crypts) are also highly susceptible to infection. These cells are progenitors of the entire intestinal mucosa, so their destruction results in mucosal collapse with contraction and fusion of the villi of the small intestine, and attenuation of the lining epithelium. The functional consequence is maldigestion and malabsorption, with resultant diarrhea. At necropsy, there may be segmental congestion of the mucosa and/or petechial hemorrhages on the bowel serosa, although gross lesions are often very subtle, even in severely affected cats. Histologically, in addition to marked contraction of the intestinal villi and attenuation of the lining epithelium, the crypts are dilated and distended with mucus and cell debris. Attenuation of the enterocyte lining of the intestinal mucosa in acute infections occurs as individual cells spread out, preventing exposure of the basement membrane to intestinal contents, but ulceration and breach of this important barrier is frequent. Rarely, intranuclear inclusions may be present in crypt enterocytes. Proliferation and expansion of crypt enterocytes are prominent in the recovery phase of infection as those cells attempt to repopulate the damaged mucosa. Maldigestion and malabsorption may occur during the repair phase because of immaturity of the intestinal mucosal lining. Lymph nodes may be enlarged and edematous; histologically, there is evidence of widespread destruction of lymphocytes.

In fetuses infected during the last 2 weeks of pregnancy and the first 2 weeks of life, dramatic lesions are present in the external granular layer of the cerebellum—this is the basis for the characteristic cerebellar hypoplasia/atrophy that occurs in cats infected at this stage of development (Figure 12.3). During this period, cells of the external granular layer of the cerebellum normally undergo rapid division and migrate to form the internal granular and Purkinje cell layers; this proliferation and migration is arrested, and affected kittens remain permanently ataxic.

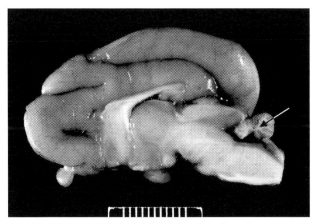

FIGURE 12.3 Cerebellar hypoplasia/atrophy (arrow) induced by feline panleukopenia virus in a young kitten. *(Courtesy of J. Peauroi and University of California, Davis.)*

Diagnosis

Clinical signs, hematological data, and postmortem findings are characteristic and sufficient for presumptive diagnosis of feline panleukopenia. The usual confirmatory tests include either antigen-capture enzyme immunoassay or immunofluorescence for the detection of antigen in tissues, or polymerase chain reaction (PCR) assay for the detection of viral DNA in feces or tissues. Virus isolation or hemagglutination assays also can be used. Serologic diagnosis is by hemagglutination-inhibition assays, enzyme immunoassay, or indirect immunofluorescence.

Immunity, Prevention, and Control

Following natural infection in previously healthy cats there is a rapid immune response. Neutralizing antibody can be detected within 3–5 days of infection and may increase to very high levels. The presence of high-titer antibody is correlated with protection against reinfection, and immunity after natural infection or vaccination with modified live vaccines is probably life-long. The titer of passively acquired antibody in kittens is related to the maternal antibody titer, and falls at a constant rate. Thus kittens are protected for varying periods related to their initial titer, and varying from a few weeks to as long as 16 weeks. Vaccination is widely practiced, with both inactivated and live-attenuated virus vaccines available. Although each vaccine type has its own inherent perceived advantages and disadvantages, attenuated live vaccines are safe and potentially better than inactivated vaccines for the control of disease.

The stability of the virus and the very high rates of virus excretion result in high levels of environmental contamination, hence it may be difficult to disinfect contaminated premises. The virus may be acquired from premises after the introduction of susceptible cats weeks or even months after previously affected cats have been removed. The virus may also be carried a considerable distance on fomites. In large catteries, strict hygiene and quarantine of incoming cats are essential if the virus is to be excluded; cats should be held in isolation for about 2 weeks before entry, sick cats should be removed and isolated, and vaccines should be used rigorously. For disinfection, 1% sodium hypochlorite applied to clean surfaces will destroy residual contaminating virus, but it is less effective in the presence of organic matter. Organic phenolic or iodine- or glutaraldehyde-based disinfectants, together with thorough cleaning with detergent-based cleansers, can also be used in these circumstances.

MINK ENTERITIS VIRUS

Mink enteritis is caused by a parvovirus that is related very closely to feline panleukopenia virus. In mink, the virus produces a syndrome similar to that caused by feline panleukopenia virus in cats, except that cerebellar hypoplasia/atrophy has not been recognized. The disease in mink appears to have resulted from the introduction of feline panleukopenia virus into commercial mink farms in Ontario, Canada, during the 1940s.

CANINE PARVOVIRUS 2

Canine parvovirus disease, caused by canine parvovirus 2, was first described as a new disease in 1978. After its initial recognition, the virus spread rapidly around the world, causing a "virgin-soil" panzootic that was marked by high incidence rates and high mortality rates. Sequence analyses and retrospective serologic studies indicate that the immediate ancestor of the virus began infecting dogs in Europe during the early or mid-1970s; this conclusion is based on the finding of virus-specific antibodies in sera from dogs in Greece, the Netherlands, and Belgium in 1974, 1976, and 1977, respectively. During 1978, antibodies were first found in dogs in Japan, Australia, New Zealand, and the United States, confirming that the virus spread around the world in less than 6 months. The stability of the virus, its efficient fecal–oral transmission, and the near-universal susceptibility of the dog population of the world probably explain the occurrence of this remarkable panzootic.

All members of the family *Canidae* (dogs, wolves, foxes, coyotes) are susceptible to natural infection with canine parvovirus 2. Infection by some virus strains has been described in members of the families *Mustelidae* and *Felidae*—specifically cats, mink, and ferrets. The virus continues to be a very important cause of infectious diarrhea in both wild and domestic canids.

Canine parvovirus 2 is distinct genetically from a previously described parvovirus of dogs, minute virus of canines, which is now called canine parvovirus 1. Since its emergence in the 1970s, continuing genetic variation has resulted in the appearance of novel strains of canine parvovirus 2, with three major variants (2a, 2b, and 2c) having now been recognized. Interestingly, some of the more recently emergent variant 2a and 2b viruses are more infectious to cats than the original strains of canine parvovirus 2 that first emerged in the 1970s.

Clinical Features and Epidemiology

The epidemiological features of canine parvovirus 2 infections are similar to those of feline panleukopenia. The virus is highly contagious and very stable in the environment, so most infections result from the exposure of susceptible dogs to virus-contaminated feces. Severe disease is most common in rapidly growing pups between 6 weeks and 6 months of age; however, many dogs that are naturally infected with canine parvovirus 2 exhibit only mild or subclinical disease.

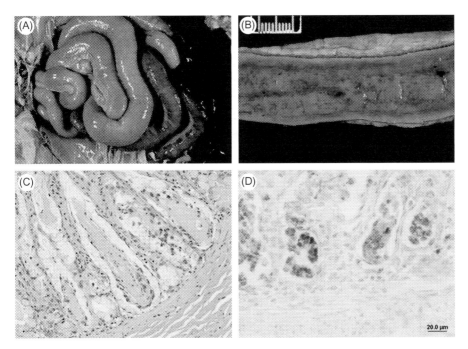

FIGURE 12.4 Canine-parvovirus-induced intestinal lesions. (A) Serosal hemorrhage. (B) Mucosal hemorrhage. (C) Crypt necrosis. (D) Immunohistochemical staining of parvovirus antigens in crypt epithelium. *(Courtesy of P. Pesavento, University of California, Davis.)*

Canine parvovirus 2 is the cause of an enteritis syndrome analogous to feline panleukopenia, although leukopenia is often less severe in dogs. Further, intestinal hemorrhage with severe bloody diarrhea is more characteristic of canine parvovirus disease than of feline panleukopenia. The incidence of the enteritis syndrome has fallen since the virus first emerged, thanks to widespread vaccination, but canine parvovirus 2 is still an important cause of infectious diarrhea in young dogs. Vomiting is often the initial sign and can be severe and protracted; there is accompanying anorexia, lethargy, and diarrhea that quickly can lead to severe dehydration. The feces are often streaked with blood or are frankly hemorrhagic and remain fluid until recovery or death. Death is uncommon except in young pups. Some genetic strains of canine parvovirus may be more virulent than others, and it appears that some dog breeds are more susceptible to severe disease than others.

A myocarditis syndrome that results from infection in the first week of life is usually manifest as acute heart failure and sudden death in pups, often without preceding clinical signs. Pups that survive acute myocardial injury may subsequently develop cardiomyopathy at 4–8 weeks of age. This syndrome was relatively common when the virus first emerged, but is now rare as a result of the widespread immunity in breeding bitches that protects most puppies during the susceptible period.

Pathogenesis and Pathology

The pathogenesis of canine parvovirus infection in the dog is similar to that of feline panleukopenia virus infection in the cat, but the absence of cerebellar hypoplasia/atrophy and the occurrence of myocarditis in pups distinguish the diseases. Parvovirus infection of the myocardium can occur because of the rapid proliferation of myocytes that occurs in the first week after birth. Infection leads to myocardial necrosis and inflammation in affected puppies, which in turn results in pulmonary edema and/or hepatic congestion from acute heart failure. Eccentric hypertrophy (dilated cardiomyopathy) occurs in pups that survive for some time, with associated lymphocytic myocarditis and myocardial fibrosis.

Parvovirus infection of dogs results in systemic infection following oropharyngeal entry of the virus (analogous to feline panleukopenia virus infection). Intestinal lesions in affected dogs result from infection and destruction of enterocytes populating the intestinal crypts, with subsequent mucosal collapse, maldigestion and malabsorption diarrhea (Figure 12.4). Mucosal and serosal hemorrhage can be severe, perhaps reflecting terminal disseminated intravascular coagulation in affected dogs. Hemorrhages may occur in other organs, and hemorrhage in the central nervous system can cause neurological signs, for example. Lymphoid tissues also are affected, with widespread destruction of lymphocytes, and the resultant immunosuppression can predispose to secondary infections.

Diagnosis

The sudden onset of foul-smelling, bloody diarrhea in young dogs is suggestive, but certainly not diagnostic, of canine parvovirus infection. Fecal enzyme immunoassays now facilitate rapid detection of the virus, although virus shedding is transient (between days 3 and 7 after infection). Laboratory diagnosis of canine parvovirus infection also can be made using hemagglutination of pig, cat, or rhesus monkey red blood cells (pH 6.5, 4°C) by virus present in fecal extracts, and the specificity of this hemagglutination is determined by titrating the sample in parallel in the presence of normal and immune dog serum. Fecal samples from dogs with acute enteritis may contain many thousands of hemagglutinating units of virus, reflecting very high titers of virus. Electron microscopy, virus isolation, and amplification of viral DNA using PCR assay on fecal samples are also used for laboratory confirmation of clinical diagnosis. Retrospective diagnosis can be done with serology, typically using the immunoglobulin IgM and/or IgG-capture enzyme-linked immunosorbent assay on paired sera.

Immunity, Prevention, and Control

Following natural infection there is a rapid immune response. Neutralizing antibodies can be detected within 3–5 days of infection and increase rapidly to very high titers. Immunity after natural infection appears to be life-long. Most maternal antibody is transferred with colostrum; and the titer of the antibody in pups parallels the maternal antibody titer and is therefore quite variable, providing protection for only a few weeks or for as long as 16 weeks. Cytotoxic T cells are also generated after both infection and vaccination.

Live-attenuated virus vaccines are available and widely used; however, vaccine failure in weanling pups may occur as a result of maternal antibody interference during immunization, and is the most common cause of failure. Pups receive about 10% of their maternal antibody via transplacental transfer and 90% through colostrum (the half-life of canine IgG is 7–8 days). It has been determined that an antibody titer of 80 or greater is protective (as measured by the hemagglutination-inhibition assay); thus pups born to bitches with low antibody titers may become susceptible to wild-type virus as early as 4–6 weeks after birth, whereas those born to bitches with high titers may be immune to infection for 12–18 weeks. Of course, pups born to seronegative bitches are susceptible at birth. The level of maternal antibody that is able to protect pups against infection by the wild-type virus is different than that which interferes with an attenuated vaccine virus. In addition to the difference in their intrinsic properties, the wild-type virus is introduced via the oronasal rather than the parenteral route. In effect, as maternally acquired immunity wanes, there is an approximately 1-week period when antibody titers have declined to levels where pups are susceptible to wild virus but are still refractory to immunization. The time of this gap may be estimated for each pup by serologic testing, but this is expensive and, in most instances, impractical. The usual approach is to administer pups a series of vaccinations at 2- to 3-week intervals, starting at 6–8 weeks of age and continuing through 16–20 weeks of age. Another approach has been to use very high-titer vaccine, thereby partially

overcoming immune interference. Yet another approach has been to use vaccine containing a lower passage, slightly more virulent virus, favoring more virus replication in the recipient and a better chance to overcome interference.

Problems in parvovirus disease prevention and control are encountered commonly in breeding colonies or facilities that house large numbers of puppies, such as shelters, breeding facilities, or kennels, and in veterinary clinics, where high viral loads can occur. Along with any vaccination strategy, in contaminated environments it may help to isolate pups to minimize their chances of becoming infected during their most vulnerable period. It is especially important in kennels to isolate pups from other dogs, beginning around 6 weeks of age and continuing until their vaccination series is complete. In household settings, if true isolation is not possible, pups should at least be kept from areas where puppies or infected dogs congregate.

PORCINE PARVOVIRUS

Porcine parvovirus disease is an infectious cause of reproductive failure in swine throughout the world. When the virus is introduced into a fully susceptible breeding herd, it can have devastating effects. Some manifestations of the disease are described by the acronym, SMEDI (stillbirth, mummification, embryonic death, infertility). Infection of older swine causes only a mild or subclinical disease, but the virus has also been associated more rarely with respiratory disease and vesicular disease, and systemic disease of neonates. Although there are genetic differences between some porcine parvovirus strains, only a single serotype is recognized.

Clinical Features and Epidemiology

Porcine parvovirus occurs worldwide and is enzootic in many herds, although the occurrence of disease has been dramatically diminished by vaccination. Because the virus is so stable, premises may remain infected for many months, even where hygiene appears satisfactory. Losses are most extreme if the virus is introduced into a seronegative herd at a time when many sows are pregnant. There is a possibility that some pigs infected *in utero* may survive as long-term immunotolerant carriers, but this is unproven. In most herds, a large proportion of gilts are infected naturally before they conceive, and hence are immune. Passively acquired maternal antibody can persist for up to 6 months or more, which interferes with active immunization following either natural infection or vaccination. Consequently, some gilts may conceive and then, when their residual maternal antibody levels decline to non-protective levels, their pregnancy is at very high risk. Boars play a significant role in the dissemination of virus, in that they may shed virus in semen for protracted periods.

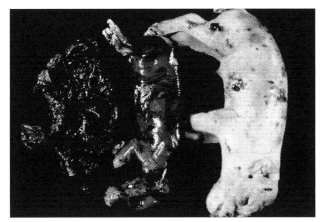

FIGURE 12.5 Porcine parvovirus infection. Infected fetuses in various stages of mummification, consistent with stillbirth, mummification, embryonic death and infertility (SMEDI) syndrome.

The major impact of porcine parvovirus results from infection of pregnant gilts or sows, and the stage of gestation at which infection occurs determines the particular clinical signs seen, and runs the full gamut of the SMEDI syndrome. The first sign of infection in a herd is frequently an increase in the number of gilts or sows returning to estrus 3–8 weeks after breeding. Some sows may remain "endocrinologically pregnant," not returning to estrus until after the expected time of farrowing. These clinical features are caused by fetal infection and resorption. Infection occurring later in gestation is evident at farrowing by smaller than normal litters and by mummified fetuses, due to only some of the fetuses becoming infected and the variable course of the disease in those fetuses that do become infected (Figure 12.5). In addition, some piglets at birth may be smaller than normal, or so weak that they do not survive. In young pigs, infection has been associated with a vesicular disease of the feet and mouth.

Pathogenesis and Pathology

It has been shown experimentally that it takes about 15 days after maternal infection for the virus to reach the fetus. When infection occurs less than 30 days after conception, the fetus dies and is resorbed; when infection occurs between 30 and 70 days after conception, the fetus often fails to develop an immune response and is usually affected severely and dies. Fetuses infected 70 or more days after conception, although frequently developing lesions, are affected less severely and mount an immune response (immunocompetence of swine fetuses starts at 55–70 days). The virus replicates in lymph nodes, tonsils, thymus, spleen, lungs, salivary glands, and other organs. It replicates well in blood lymphocytes, and both infection and the immune response stimulate cell proliferation, thereby increasing the viral load. Monocytes and macrophages also can become lytically infected. More so than with the other parvoviruses, swine parvovirus causes persistent infection, with chronic shedding.

Diagnosis

Infected fetuses may contain very large amounts of virus. Frozen-section immunofluorescence of fetal tissues using standardized reagents is rapid and reliable and the preferred diagnostic test. Hemagglutination of guinea pig red blood cells by virus contained in extracts of fetal tissues may also be used. PCR assay is very sensitive, but the interpretation of results is important, as the assay may detect viral DNA even when the virus is not the primary cause of the disease. Serologic tests are of limited value, because the virus is so widespread in swine, and vaccination may interfere. Diagnosis is difficult if infection occurs in the first few weeks of gestation; commonly, fetuses are resorbed completely and there may be no suspicion of the presence of the virus, and hence no specimens collected for laboratory diagnosis.

Immunity, Prevention, and Control

Vaccination is practiced widely as the only means of assuring that all gilts are protected. Inactivated and attenuated virus vaccines are used. There is often only a brief window of opportunity to immunize gilts that are bred before 7 months of age. The duration of immunity is uncertain, but there seems to be good immunological memory, and infection in vaccinated pigs rarely leads to fetal disease.

RODENT PARVOVIRUSES

More than 30 distinct parvoviruses in at least 13 serogroups have been isolated from laboratory rodents, thus they represent a broad genetic spectrum. Several of these viruses commonly cause enzootic infections in rodent colonies: parvoviruses of mice, including minute virus of mice, mouse parvovirus types 1, 2, and 3; parvoviruses of rats, including Kilham's rat virus, Toolan's H-1 virus, rat minute virus type 1 and rat parvovirus type 1; a hamster parvovirus, which is genetically identical to mouse parvovirus 3 and therefore represents cross-species transmission. There is also a high prevalence of mouse and rat parvoviruses in wild mice and rats, respectively. The major importance of these viruses is their confounding effect on research, especially immunology and cancer research. They may also contaminate cell lines and tumor virus stocks, sometimes causing little cytopathology, which can allow them to be introduced into clean colonies.

Rodent parvoviruses most commonly cause subclinical infection, but they may rarely cause fetal and neonatal abnormalities, with granuloprival cerebellar hypoplasia, as in feline panleukopenia. Rodent parvoviruses destroy dividing cells, but with a more limited spectrum compared with parvoviruses of other species. Most importantly, none of the rodent parvoviruses infects intestinal epithelium, but rather they tend to have primary tropism for hemopoietic and lymphoid tissues. The overwhelming majority of parvovirus infections in rodents are clinically silent, but often with significant effects upon immune response. In rats, clinical disease is most often associated with Kilham's rat virus, resulting in cerebellar injury, hemorrhagic encephalopathy and hepatitis in young rats, and outbreaks of peritesticular and intra-abdominal hemorrhage in older rats. The hemorrhagic lesions are probably a result of tropism of the virus for vascular endothelium, as well as tropism for megakaryocytes, resulting in thrombocytopenia. Periodontal and craniofacial deformities have been observed in hamsters naturally infected with hamster parvovirus (mouse parvovirus 3), and can be experimentally induced with several other rodent parvoviruses.

One consequence of rodent parvovirus infections, particularly mouse parvovirus, can be persistent virus carriage, even in the presence of high titers of neutralizing antibody. This is important, because some experimental manipulations, especially those that are immunosuppressive, may cause virus reactivation and recrudescent shedding. In turn, infection can be immunosuppressive (e.g., abrogating cytotoxic T lymphocyte responses and helper T cell dependent B cell responses), again affecting experiments in which infected animals are used unknowingly.

Diagnosis is primarily based on serology (hemagglutination-inhibition, indirect immunofluorescence, neutralization, or enzyme immunoassay) and virus isolation in rodent cell cultures. Reference reagents are used to identify particular virus strains, or viral DNA can be identified by PCR and the specific virus type determined by DNA sequencing. Both serologic and nucleic acid detection methods may be challenging with some mouse strains, such as C57BL/6 mice, which may be infected with undetectable levels of antibody or viral DNA. Thus direct-contact sentinel animals of a more susceptible genotype are needed to detect infection within such colonies.

In laboratory colonies, these viruses are transmitted horizontally by contact and fomites. Young animals born from infected dams are protected by maternal antibody for the first few weeks of life, but then are infected via the oronasal route. As with other parvoviruses, rodent viruses are extremely stable and resistant to desiccation, and may be carried between rodent colonies by fomites; the strictness of facility quarantine must be rigorous. When virus is detected, elimination is effected by depopulation, meticulous disinfection of the premises, and introduction of new founding stock that is screened and free of virus and/or antibody. Unlike the situation in rebuilding a colony after eliminating some other rodent viruses, colonies that have had parvovirus infections cannot always be repopulated by cesarean section and use of foster mothers. Under such circumstances, embryo transfer may be effective.

RABBIT PARVOVIRUSES

Serologic evidence indicates that lapine parvovirus is very common among domestic rabbits, but is clinically silent. Experimental infection of young kits has been shown to result in disseminated infection, mild enteritis, clinical signs of depression, and anorexia.

MEMBERS OF THE GENUS *ERYTHROVIRUS*

Populations of mature virions of viruses within the genus *Erythrovirus* contain equivalent proportions of positive- and negative-sense DNA. The genus includes parvoviruses of humans, non-human primates, and bovine parvovirus 3.

NON-HUMAN PRIMATE PARVOVIRUSES

Several parvoviruses have been identified in macaques, including simian parvovirus in cynomolgus monkeys (*Macaca fascicularis*), rhesus parvovirus in rhesus macaques (*M. mulatta*) and cynomolgus parvovirus in cynomolgus monkeys. Considering the large number of species and subspecies of macaques, it is likely that there are many other parvoviruses among non-human primates. Of the three characterized to date, they are genetically related to but distinct from each other, and are also related to B19 virus of humans. These viruses may be associated with clinical anemia and fetal abnormalities.

MEMBERS OF THE GENUS *AMDOVIRUS*

Virions of viruses in this genus include genomes exclusively of negative-sense DNA.

ALEUTIAN MINK DISEASE VIRUS

The Aleutian Mink Disease Virus naturally infects mink, skunks, and ferrets, generally causing a mild or subclinical disease. When clinical disease occurs in mink, it is characterized by chronic antigenic stimulation leading to expansion of plasma cells in multiple tissues (so-called plasmacytosis), hypergammaglobulinemia, splenomegaly, lymphadenopathy, arteritis, glomerulonephritis, hepatitis, anemia, and death. Lesions result from chronic infection in which there is a sustained production of virus and a failure to eliminate virus–antibody (immune) complexes. Despite extremely high levels of virus-specific antibody, the virus is not neutralized, and infectious virus can be recovered from circulating immune complexes. Immune stimulation and immune-complex-mediated disease follow. The disease occurs primarily in mink that are homozygous for the recessive gene for a commercially desirable pale ("Aleutian") coat color. This coat color gene is linked to a gene associated with a lysosomal abnormality of the Chediak–Higashi type that inhibits destruction of internalized immune complexes. The level of the hypergammaglobulinemia is cyclical, with death typically occurring during a peak response between 2 and 5 months after infection. Immunization of mink carrying the Aleutian gene with inactivated virus vaccine increases the severity of the disease. Conversely, immunosuppression diminishes the severity of the disease. As the virus appears to be only poorly transmissible, and mink are seasonal breeders, Aleutian disease can be controlled in a farmed mink population by serological testing and elimination of seropositive animals.

MEMBERS OF THE GENUS *DEPENDOVIRUS*

Populations of mature virions contain equimolar amounts of positive- and negative-sense DNA. The genus includes adeno-associated viruses from several animal species, as well as certain avian parvoviruses and bovine parvovirus 2.

GOOSE PARVOVIRUS

Goose parvovirus causes a lethal disease in goslings 8–30 days of age that is characterized by focal or diffuse hepatitis and widespread acute necrosis and degeneration of striated, smooth, and cardiac muscle. Inclusion bodies occur in the liver, spleen, myocardium, thymus, thyroid, and intestines. Control is achieved by the vaccination of laying geese with attenuated virus vaccine; maternal antibody persists in goslings for at least 4 weeks, the period of maximum vulnerability.

DUCK PARVOVIRUS

An apparently new disease of Muscovy ducklings was described in France in 1989. Although clearly a distinct virus type, it is most closely related to adeno-associated viruses and so is classified in the genus *Dependovirus*. Mortality has been high, and clinical and postmortem findings have resembled those found in geese infected with goose parvovirus. Ducks that survive are stunted and feathering is delayed. Effective vaccines are available, including one that consists of recombinant VP2 and VP3 viral proteins expressed in a baculovirus system.

MEMBERS OF THE GENUS *BOCAVIRUS*

In contrast to other parvoviruses, the bocaviruses contain an additional open reading frame that encodes a non-structural protein (NP1) of unknown function. Bocaviruses recently have been identified in humans, specifically in children with lower respiratory disease.

BOVINE PARVOVIRUS

A parvovirus has been isolated from cows, which is widespread but only rarely associated with clinical disease. In neonatal calves, the bovine parvovirus may cause mild watery to mucoid diarrhea. Infection of enterocytes occurs throughout the intestine, especially the small intestine. Disease lasts for 4–6 days, and virus may be shed for up to 11 days after infection.

CANINE MINUTE VIRUS (CANINE PARVOVIRUS 1)

A parvovirus isolated from a clinically normal dog in 1967 was originally named the minute virus of canines (also known as canine minute virus or canine parvovirus type 1). By serological testing, it appears that this virus is widespread in dogs, but that the vast majority of infections are very mild or subclinical. The most common clinical disease associated with canine minute virus is diarrhea or sudden death in neonatal puppies. Some cases were apparently associated with primary infection with the canine minute virus, but in other instances the affected dogs were also infected with another pathogen. Fetal infections have been reported, although these appear to be rare.

OTHER PARVOVIRUSES

Intestinal parvovirus infections recently were identified in chickens and turkeys. Novel parvoviruses related to human parvovirus 4 also were recently isolated from cattle and pigs. Human parvovirus 4 has been detected in human plasma and liver tissue, and these viruses all share a distinctive genome organization, so they probably constitute a new genus within the family *Parvoviridae*, subfamily *Parvovirinae*.

Circoviridae

Chapter Contents

The family *Circoviridae* includes viruses with circular single-stranded DNA genomes, and which share common physicochemical and genomic properties. Together with members of the family *Parvoviridae*, these are the smallest known DNA viruses of vertebrates, and have similarities to single-stranded DNA viruses of plants. The family *Circoviridae* includes important pathogens of birds and swine. Torque teno viruses are genetically heterogeneous single-stranded DNA viruses that are morphologically similar to circoviruses, but which are classified in a free-standing genus, *Anellovirus*, because of other distinctive characteristics (see Chapter 32).

PROPERTIES OF CIRCOVIRUSES

Classification

The member viruses of the family *Circoviridae* have somewhat similar virion and genome properties, but are ecologically, biologically, and antigenically quite distinct. The family currently contains two genera (*Circovirus*, *Gyrovirus*). Porcine circovirus 1 is the type species of the genus *Circovirus*, members of which use an ambisense genome strategy, with viral genes in different orientations. The genus *Circovirus* includes beak and feather disease virus, canary circovirus, goose circovirus, pigeon circovirus, and porcine circoviruses 1 and 2. Chicken anemia virus is the type (and only) member of the genus *Gyrovirus*, in which the viral genes are all in the same orientation.

Virion Properties

The properties of circovirus virions are summarized in Table 13.1. They are small (approximately 20–25 nm in diameter), non-enveloped, spherical in outline, with T = 1 icosahedral symmetry. Virions are made up of 60 capsid subunits that package the viral circular single-stranded DNA. Virions of individual circoviruses differ in surface structure, with chicken anemia virus having 12 trumpet-like structures that are less obvious in the other circoviruses (Figure 13.1). Mature virions often appear in infected cells and free

---

TABLE 13.1 Properties of Circoviruses

Virions are small (20–25 nm), non-enveloped, spherical in outline, with icosahedral symmetry

Mature virions can be seen in infected cells as well as in linear arrays in cell-free diagnostic specimens

The genome consists of a single molecule of circular (covalently closed ends) single-stranded ambisense (genus *Circovirus*) or positive-sense (genus *Gyrovirus*) DNA, 1.7–2.3 kb in size

Chicken anemia virus encodes a protein (VP3) that induces apoptosis in chicken lymphocytes (apoptin)

Replication takes place in the nucleus of cycling cells, producing large intranuclear inclusion bodies

Virions are very stable, resisting 60°C for 30 minutes and pH 3 to pH 9

Fenner's Veterinary Virology. DOI: 10.1016/B978-0-12-375158-4.00013-4

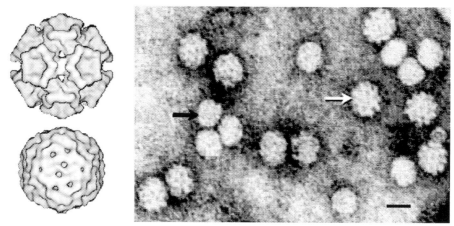

FIGURE 13.1 (Left upper) Cryo-electron microscopy image of a particle of an isolate of chicken anemia virus. A structural model comprising 60 subunits (T=1) arranged in 12 protruding pentagonal trumpet-shaped units pentameric rings has been proposed. (Left lower) Cryo-electron microscopy image of a particle of an isolate of porcine circovirus 2. A structural model comprising 60 subunits (T=1) arranged in 12 flat pentameric morphological units has been proposed. (Right) Negative contrast electron microscopy of particles of an isolate of chicken anemia virus (black arrow) and beak and feather disease virus (BFDV) (white arrow), stained with uranyl acetate. The bar represents 20nm. *[From* Virus Taxonomy: Eighth Report of the International Committee on Taxonomy of Viruses *(C. M. Fauquet, M. A. Mayo, J. Maniloff, U. Desselberger, L. A. Ball, eds.), p. 327. Copyright © Elsevier (2005), with permission.]*

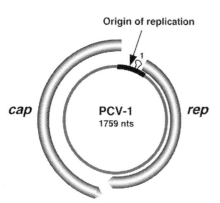

FIGURE 13.2 Genome organization of an isolate of porcine circovirus 1 (PCV-1). The origin of replication is located between the start sites of the two major, divergently-arranged ORFs, *cap* and *rep* (thick arrows). The *cap* gene, encoding the capsid protein (CP), is expressed from a spliced transcript, and the *rep* gene directs the synthesis of two distinct proteins, Rep and Rep', using differentially-spliced transcripts. *[From* Virus Taxonomy: Eighth Report of the International Committee on Taxonomy of Viruses *(C. M. Fauquet, M. A. Mayo, J. Maniloff, U. Desselberger, L. A. Ball, eds.), p. 329. Copyright © Elsevier (2005), with permission.]*

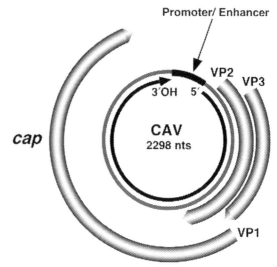

FIGURE 13.3 Genome organization of chicken anemia virus (CAV). The unspliced CAV transcript (5'-3') contains three partially overlapping ORFs, which are expressed in CAV-infected cells. The non-transcribed region possesses promoter-enhancer activity. Open reading frame (ORF) 1 (*cap* gene) encodes the capsid protein VP1; ORF2 encodes VP2, a protein phosphatase, and ORF3 encodes VP3 also known as apoptin. *[From* Virus Taxonomy: Eighth Report of the International Committee on Taxonomy of Viruses *(C. M. Fauquet, M. A. Mayo, J. Maniloff, U. Desselberger, L. A. Ball, eds.), p. 332. Copyright © Elsevier (2005), with permission.]*

in diagnostic specimens and in linear "strings of pearls" in cell-free diagnostic specimens. The genome consists of a single molecule of circular (covalently closed ends) single-stranded ambisense (genus *Circovirus*) or negative sense (genus *Gyrovirus*) DNA, approximately 1.7–2.3kb in size.

Beak and feather disease virus, porcine circoviruses 1 and 2, and the other members of the genus *Circovirus* utilize an ambisense transcription strategy—that is, some genes are encoded in the viral sense DNA and others in the complementary strand (Figure 13.2). Beak and feather disease virus has three open reading frames and porcine circovirus has four; in each case there is one major capsid

protein. In contrast, the genes of chicken anemia virus, genus *Gyrovirus*, are all encoded in the complementary positive-sense DNA strand that is transcribed to give a single polycistronic transcript (Figure 13.3); however, the existence of minor spliced transcripts was also recently described. Chicken anemia virus has three open reading frames, one of which encodes the major capsid protein (VP1) that is present in virions. Another virus-encoded protein (VP3), termed apoptin, induces apoptosis of

T lymphocytes and is probably important to the pathogenesis of infections in chickens.

These viruses are all very stable in the environment; they are not inactivated by heating at 60°C for 30 minutes, are resistant to many disinfectants, and may require long exposure to efficacious chemicals.

Virus Replication

The receptors responsible for cellular attachment of circoviruses are uncertain, but some circoviruses hemagglutinate erythrocytes and thus they are likely to bind to sialic acid on the cell surface. Virus particles are taken up by endocytosis, although the specific mechanisms also are not well understood. Viral DNA replication occurs in the nucleus and requires cellular proteins and other components produced during the S phase of the cell cycle. Replication of the genome is believed to occur via a rolling circle that originates at a stem-loop structure. Three distinct proteins are produced during replication of chicken anemia virus.

A major feature of the circoviruses that determines their pathogenesis is the requirement for dividing cells to facilitate their DNA replication, thus virus replication typically is maximized in actively dividing cells in the tissues of young animals. Similarly, replication of porcine circovirus 2 in swine is enhanced during periods of immune stimulation that result in proliferation of lymphocytes in which the virus can replicate. Circoviruses typically cause persistent infections of their respective hosts, although the mechanisms responsible are poorly characterized, as the viruses persist despite apparently robust host antiviral immune responses. In the case of chicken anemia virus, virus replication in the oviduct of chickens may be regulated by estrogen, and hence is differentially stimulated, particularly during egg laying, to allow more efficient vertical transmission. The apoptin protein of chicken anemia virus may itself cause destruction of infected lymphocytes, and hence promote a relative immune suppression that favors virus persistence.

BEAK AND FEATHER DISEASE VIRUS

It had long been known that many species of Australian parrots undergo permanent loss of feathers and develop beak and claw deformities when in captivity. In 1984, thin-section electron microscopic examination of affected tissues from such birds revealed large numbers of virions that resembled the previously described porcine circovirus 1. More recently, similar viruses have been identified in most species of parrots and related psittacine birds, and viruses of this type or their DNA have been detected in many other birds, including canaries, ostriches, pigeons, ducks, geese, finches, gulls, ravens, and starlings.

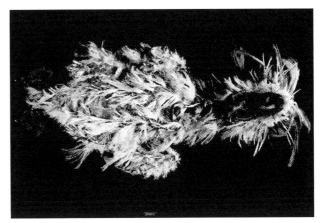

FIGURE 13.4 Beak and feather disease in a cockatoo. *(Courtesy of L. Lowenstine, University of California, Davis.)*

Clinical Features and Epidemiology

Many infections with these circoviruses are mild or subclinical. Where it occurs, beak and feather disease is a debilitating disease of cockatoos, parrots, and budgerigars, although is principally a disease of cockatoos. Natural infection occurs primarily in birds less than 5 years of age, most often in young birds during first feather formation. Typical findings include feather loss, abnormal pin feathers (constricted, clubbed, or stunted), abnormal mature feathers (retention of sheaths, blood in shaft, fracture of rachis), and various beak abnormalities (Figure 13.4). The beaks of affected birds are variously described as being shiny, overgrown, or broken, exhibiting delaminations, or with palatine necrosis. Birds may have feather lesions, beak lesions, or both. Severe leukopenia and non-regenerative anemia have been reported in some parrots, but usually without feather lesions.

Pathogenesis and Pathology

The disease can be reproduced experimentally by exposing psittacine birds to homogenates of feather follicles from affected birds. The virus replicates in the basal epithelial layer of the feather follicles, beak, and claw. Basophilic intracytoplasmic ("botryoid") inclusions occur in follicular epithelium, which by electron microscopy contain masses of virions. Inclusions also occur in macrophages and the epithelium of the cloacal bursa, but as a consequence of phagocytosis and not virus replication. Lymphoid depletion occurs, perhaps as a result of indirect effects of the infection. The disease is progressive; some birds die after the first appearance of malformed feathers or beak abnormalities, whereas, if cared for, others may live for months or years in a featherless state. Infection can result in persistent immunosuppression, so that affected birds are often also affected by other (secondary) viral, fungal, or bacterial infections.

Diagnosis

Diagnosis of beak and feather disease is made on the basis of clinical signs and signalment, and the presence of characteristic basophilic intracytoplasmic inclusion bodies as determined by histopathologic examination of biopsy specimens of affected feather follicles. The presence of virus can be confirmed using electron microscopy, immunohistochemical staining with virus-specific antisera, or demonstration of circovirus genome by polymerase chain reaction (PCR), which can detect viral DNA in feather tips, blood, biopsy samples, or swabs.

Immunity, Prevention, and Control

The contagious nature of beak and feather disease and its persistent, progressive course may lead to requests for euthanasia of infected birds. Beak and feather disease virus is highly prevalent as a consequence of subclinical infections in many birds and, as a result, eradication of the virus is difficult once it is present in a colony. Strict hygiene, screening protocols, and lengthy quarantines are used in cockatoo and other affected breeding colonies to prevent introduction of the virus. The virus persists and is shed by adult birds, and virus transmission can be via either vertical or horizontal routes. Antibodies are protective, but vaccines are not available because the virus has yet to be propagated in cell-culture systems. However, experimental vaccines have been developed that utilize either preparations of virus recovered directly from affected birds or capsid protein alone expressed from recombinant baculoviruses.

OTHER AVIAN CIRCOVIRUSES

Circovirus infections have been reported in a variety of wild and domestic avian species, including pigeons, canaries, geese, ducks, and ostriches, typically causing immunosuppression and developmental abnormalities. Most cases are in young birds. Infected pigeons may manifest poor performance, diarrhea and ill thrift, but feather lesions are rare in racing pigeons. In contrast, infected doves may exhibit feather loss. Atrophy of the cloacal bursa is common and results in immunosuppression. Mulard ducks have feather dystrophy, growth retardation, and mortality throughout rearing. Canaries have abdominal distension and failure to thrive. Circoviruses are implicated in, but not proven to cause, a fading chick syndrome in ostriches, characterized by listlessness, anorexia, and diarrhea.

PORCINE CIRCOVIRUSES

Porcine circovirus 1 was first isolated in Germany in 1974 from a pig kidney cell line (PK15) persistently infected

with this virus. Initial serologic studies suggested that the virus was widespread in all tested swine populations; however, at least some of this apparent seropositivity to porcine circovirus 1 may represent cross-reactive antibodies to the replicase protein, which is highly conserved between porcine circoviruses 1 and 2. More recent studies, using more specific serological tests, indicate that porcine circovirus 1 infection is not as highly prevalent in pigs as first thought. Of various animals tested, only domestic swine, mini-pigs, and wild boars have antibodies. Porcine circovirus 1 is considered to be apathogenic in swine; however, it has been isolated from stillborn piglets. Porcine circovirus 2 is an antigenically distinct virus that was first isolated in France in 1997. Subsequent studies have clearly shown the virus was present in pigs long before that time, as determined by the presence of porcine circovirus 2 capsid-specific antibodies and the virus itself in archival tissues and sera. The virus has been isolated in most regions of the world where swine are raised, including North America, Asia, Europe, and Oceania. Global isolates of porcine circovirus 2 are quite similar (96% identical), and they are distinct (<80% homology) from porcine circovirus 1, primarily on the basis of differences in the capsid proteins.

The potential pathogenic significance of porcine circovirus 2 was quickly recognized following its initial identification. Porcine circovirus 2 is associated with several disease syndromes, collectively designated *porcine-circovirus-associated disease*, which occur most commonly in weanling piglets at 7–15 weeks of age, but sometimes also in adults. Two genetically distinct subgroups of porcine circovirus 2 are recognized, each of which can be further subdivided into subgroups based on their DNA sequences, which may or may not be associated with disease expression. Although retrospective studies have clearly shown that porcine circovirus 2 infection has been present in swine populations for many years, for as yet undetermined reasons both the frequency and clinical severity of infections appear to have increased dramatically since 1997.

Clinical Features and Epidemiology

Porcine circovirus 2 strains are widespread in most pig populations, and it is clear that infections are often subclinical or very mild. Transmission occurs through direct contact and fomite transmission, with virus being shed in the feces, respiratory secretions, and urine. Vertical transmission occurs in swine, although maternal antibodies protect piglets against infection.

Porcine circovirus infections can be associated with substantial mortality (up to 50%) and disease occurrence in pig-rearing enterprises. Porcine circovirus 2 has been associated with a remarkable variety of disease syndromes, including postweaning multisystemic wasting syndrome, porcine dermatitis and nephropathy syndrome, porcine

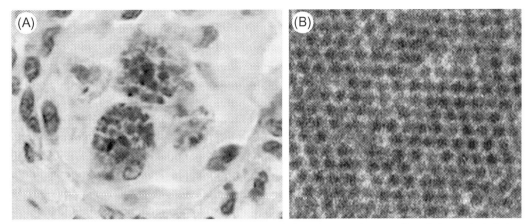

FIGURE 13.5   Porcine circovirus infection. (A) Macrophages with "botryoid" inclusions. (B) Paracrystalline viral array in inclusions. *(Courtesy of D. Imai, University of California, Davis.)*

respiratory disease complex, reproductive failure, granulomatous enteritis, exudative epidermitis, and necrotizing lymphadenitis. The precise role of porcine circovirus 2 infection in the pathogenesis of each of the porcine circovirus associated diseases remains to be clearly defined. The porcine respiratory disease complex, for instance, is typically manifest as bronchointerstitial pneumonia associated with combinations of pathogens, including *Mycoplasma hyopneumoniae* and other viral infections; however, abundant porcine circovirus 2 antigen can be detected in the lesions in some cases.

Pathogenesis and Pathology

The expression of clinical disease in pigs infected with porcine circovirus typically involves secondary microbial infections that may directly or indirectly influence the type of disease expressed. Infections that appear to enhance the replication and pathogenicity of porcine circovirus 2 include porcine parvovirus, swine influenza virus, porcine reproductive and respiratory syndrome virus, and *M. hyopneumoniae*, but other agents also might predispose. For example, torque teno viruses have recently been implicated as potentially contributing to the pathogenesis of porcine circovirus associated disease. It appears that the common feature of those infections is immune activation, which somehow enhances the replication of porcine circovirus 2 in a variety of target cells. Indeed, immune stimulation alone (without any associated infection) can promote the replication of porcine circovirus 2. However, immune suppression by corticosteroids may also result in increased expression of disease, thus the pathogenesis of porcine circovirus associated diseases is highly complex.

The porcine circovirus associated disease identified as postweaning multisystemic wasting syndrome is characterized by individual to coalescing foci of granulomatous inflammation in lymphoid tissues, lungs, liver, kidney, heart, and intestines, sometimes with prominent "botryoid" inclusion bodies

in virus-infected macrophages (Figure 13.5). Porcine dermatitis nephropathy syndrome has also been associated with porcine circovirus 2 infection, and is further characterized by infarctive (ischemic necrosis) skin lesions, particularly on the rear legs, and the kidneys of affected pigs exhibit vasculitis and glomerulonephritis; however, porcine circovirus 2 antigens or nucleic acid are rarely demonstrated in these lesions. The pathogenesis of the various porcine circovirus associated disease syndromes is not well characterized, including the role of co-infecting pathogens and immune-mediated mechanisms of tissue injury.

Diagnosis

Because porcine circovirus 2 is widespread in pig populations and often causes subclinical infections, diagnosis requires careful interpretation to determine the specific role of the virus in any diseases that occur. Assessment of the extent of infection in individual swine by quantitation of the number and distribution of virus-infected cells by immunohistochemistry, and/or viral load by quantitative PCR, is critical to interpretation.

Immunity, Prevention, and Control

Control of porcine circovirus associated diseases should involve several approaches, including general management practices to limit both circovirus infections and those caused by other, presumably "secondary," pathogens that can act as triggers for enhanced replication of porcine circovirus 2. Good nutrition and hygiene are critical, as is disinfection to prevent transmission of the virus between groups. Inactivated or baculovirus-expressed virus-like particles that include the capsid protein of the virus are available as vaccines, and new generation chimeric vaccines have been developed that utilize the non-pathogenic porcine circovirus 1 as a genetic backbone for expression of the immunogenic capsid protein of porcine circovirus 2. Vaccines can be effective in reducing viral load and subsequent shedding, and they can significantly reduce porcine circovirus 2 associated disease and mortality.

CHICKEN ANEMIA VIRUS

Chicken anemia virus associated disease was first recognized in Japan in 1979, although it is not a new virus and had probably been present in chickens for many years. Infection occurs worldwide and is a problem in all countries with industrial poultry industries. The virus is not known to infect birds other than chickens, and only a single serotype has been recognized, although low levels of variation have been reported among virus isolates both within and between countries.

Clinical Features and Epidemiology

Chicken anemia virus is transmitted horizontally by direct contact and contaminated fomites. The virus is also transmitted vertically through the egg. Horizontal transmission is through inhalation or oral exposure, and virus is shed in feces and feather dander. Breeder flocks may become infected before they begin to lay fertile eggs, and virus subsequently is transmitted vertically for as long as the hen is viremic. If hens are seropositive, maternal antibody generally protects chicks from disease, but not from infection. Many flocks of otherwise specific-pathogen-free chickens carry chicken anemia virus, and it is often difficult to eradicate the virus once it is present.

Chicken anemia virus causes an acute, immunosuppressive disease of young chickens, characterized by anorexia, lethargy, depression, anemia, atrophy or hypoplasia of lymphoid organs, cutaneous, subcutaneous, and intramuscular hemorrhages, and increased mortality. Disease occurs in chicks hatched to asymptomatically infected breeder hens that have been infected before egg laying. At 2–3 weeks of age the chicks become anorectic, lethargic, depressed, and pale. They are anemic, and develop bone marrow aplasia and atrophy of the thymus, cloacal bursa, and spleen. Disease is most severe in chicks that are co-infected with other viruses such as avian reoviruses, avian adenoviruses, reticuloendotheliosis virus, Marek's disease virus, or infectious bursal disease virus. There is usually no illness or loss of egg production when adult chickens are infected, but as the infected birds can become chronically or persistently infected, transmission can occur both horizontally and vertically.

Pathogenesis and Pathology

When 1-day-old susceptible chicks are inoculated with chicken anemia virus, viremia occurs within 24 hours and virus can be recovered from most organs and rectal contents for up to 35 days. The virus infects hemocytoblasts, causing pancytopenia evident as anemia, leukocytopenia, and thrombocytopenia. Packed cell volumes are low, and blood smears often reveal anemia and leukopenia. Blood may be watery and clot slowly as a consequence of thrombocytopenia. Mortality rates usually are low (10% or less), but may be higher than 50%. Histologically, there is depletion of lymphoid cells in all lymphoid organs and panmyelophthisis of bone marrow. Secondary bacterial infection is common. Age resistance to disease (but not infection) begins at about 1 week of age and is complete by 2 weeks after hatching. However, protective effects of maternal antibody and age resistance can be overcome where there is co-infection with other immunosuppressive viruses. Infection with chicken anemia virus also can suppress the immune system of chickens, and dual infections involving the virus and other avian pathogens are often more severe than would otherwise be expected.

Diagnosis

Diagnosis of chicken anemia virus infection in chickens is based on history, clinical signs, and gross and microscopic pathologic findings. Viral DNA is readily detected by PCR and virus isolation can be done in MDCC-MSB1 cells (a lymphoblastoid cell line derived from Marek's disease tumors), 1-day-old chicks, or chick embryos (which must be virus- and antibody-negative). Because the virus is noncytopathic when first isolated, immunologic methods must be used to identify its presence. Methods for serological identification of chicken anemia virus infection include enzyme-linked immunosorbent assay, indirect immunofluorescence, and virus neutralization.

Immunity, Prevention, and Control

Immunity to chicken anemia virus is complex. Neutralizing antibodies are protective against disease, but do not completely protect chickens against infection or result in virus clearance. The presence of antibodies in breeders greatly reduces vertical as well as horizontal transmission. Several commercial vaccines are available and are mainly used in broiler breeders. Maternal antibodies and controlled exposure are primary methods for control in broilers.

Young breeder hens may be infected deliberately with wild-type virus by adding crude homogenates of tissues from affected chickens to drinking water. This ensures infection and seroconversion before hens begin to lay eggs, but is not recommended because it can maintain high levels of virus in the population. Because severe disease results from co-infection with immunosuppressive viruses such as Marek's disease virus, control of these other pathogens also is important.

Retroviridae

Chapter Contents

Retroviruses infect a wide variety of animals, including humans, and have long been associated with important diseases in veterinary medicine. Depending on the particular retrovirus and respective host, they are the causative agents of certain types of cancer, immunosuppressive or immune-mediated diseases, or they may exist as stable components of the host genome. Retroviruses were so named in the mid-1970s after the discovery of a key enzyme, reverse

Fenner's Veterinary Virology. DOI: 10.1016/B978-0-12-375158-4.00014-6

transcriptase, by Drs Howard Temin and David Baltimore, but diseases associated with retrovirus infections were described much earlier. Equine infectious anemia, bovine leukosis, and Jaagsiekte (pulmonary adenomatosis) of sheep all were recognized in the mid-1800s. In 1904, Vallée and Carré demonstrated that equine "infectious" anemia was transmitted by a filtrate and the causative agent was subsequently confirmed as the first described retrovirus. Retroviruses in tissue filtrates from chickens with leukosis were investigated by veterinarians Ellerman and Bang in Denmark in 1908 and, subsequently, a medical pathologist, Rous, produced sarcomas by injecting filtrates in chickens as early as 1911. The two related viruses—avian leukosis and avian sarcoma viruses—are prototypic of the etiologic agents of similar infectious malignant tumors now recognized in many other animal species, including cattle, cats, mice, and primates.

The family *Retroviridae* is classified currently into two subfamilies (*Orthoretrovirinae* and *Spumaretrovirinae*) and seven genera (Table 14.1). The family includes many viruses of importance in veterinary and human medicine, and to biomedical science in general. The term *retro* (reverse, backward) reflects the property of retroviruses to use their RNA genome to produce DNA intermediates using reverse transcriptase (RT), an RNA-dependent DNA polymerase that is present within the virions of all members of the family. The study of the enzymes and proteins encoded by retroviruses has defined fundamental mechanisms of cell transformation and other important paradigms of cell biology. Since the 1980s, retroviruses have been demonstrated to cause a number of important human diseases, including lymphomas, leukemias, and acquired immunodeficiency disease syndrome (AIDS), which has further catalyzed intensive investigation of both human and animal retroviruses.

PROPERTIES OF RETROVIRUSES

Retroviruses are a diverse group of RNA viruses that all replicate utilizing reverse transcriptase, a virus-encoded enzyme

TABLE 14.1 Retrovirus Classification

Genus	Viruses and Examples of Diseases
Subfamily *Orthoretrovirinae*	
Alpharetrovirus	Avian leukosis, myeloblastosis and sarcoma viruses. Exogenous and endogenous viruses of birds, simple retroviruses with type C morphology. Some contain oncogenes. Avian leukosis and sarcoma viruses are classified into at least 10 subgroups (designated A–J) based on their tropism and cell receptors.
Betaretrovirus	Mouse mammary tumor virus, Jaagsiekte sheep retrovirus (ovine pulmonary adenocarcinoma virus), and various simian Type D retroviruses
Gammaretrovirus	Exogenous and endogenous viruses of rodents, carnivores, birds, and primates. Some further classified by host range and species distribution of receptors (e.g., ecotropic). Includes feline leukemia virus, feline sarcoma virus, porcine type C virus, murine leukemia and sarcoma viruses, guinea pig type C virus, viper type C virus and avian reticuloendotheliosis viruses
Deltaretrovirus	Complex exogenous viruses associated with B cell lymphoma and lymphocytosis of adult cattle (bovine leukemia virus), T cell lymphoma/leukemia, and other inflammatory disorders of humans (human T lymphotropic virus type 1), persistent infection with sporadic case reports of neurologic disease and lymphoproliferative disease (human T lymphotropic virus type 2), asymptomatic, persistent infections (human T lymphotropic viruses 3 and 4) and T cell lymphoma and persistent asymptomatic infections of non-human primates [simian T lymphotropic viruses (STLV) 1, 2, and 3]
Epsilonretrovirus	Walleye dermal sarcoma virus, walleye epidermal hyperplasia viruses types 1 and 2. These cause seasonal proliferative lesions on the skin of affected fish
Lentivirus	Complex exogenous viruses associated with immunologic and neurologic disease (some indirectly with cancer). Members in a variety of species, including: sheep [ovine lentiviruses (OvLV); *syn.* Visna-Maedi virus], goats [caprine arthritis encephalitis virus (CAEV)], equine [equine infectious anemia virus (EIA)], humans [human immunodeficiency viruses (HIV-1 and -2)], bovine [bovine immunodeficiency virus (BIV)], non-human primates, such as African green monkey, sooty mangabey, stump-tailed macaque, pig-tailed macaque, rhesus macaque, chimpanzee, and mandrill viruses [simian immunodeficiency virus (SIV)], and feline domestic and exotic species [feline immunodeficiency virus (FIV)]
Subfamily *Spumaretrovirinae*	
Spumavirus	"Foamy" viruses (named for cytopathic effects produced in cell culture). Complex retrovirus group with unique replication features that are distinct from those of other retrovirus genera, infect a variety of species, including bovine, feline, simian, and humans, but not yet associated with disease

that synthesizes a DNA copy from the RNA viral genome. All retroviruses contain reverse transcriptase and a diploid genome with two copies of single-stranded, positive-sense RNA. Virions are enveloped and typically form by budding from cell membranes. Retroviruses integrate into host cell genomes using another unique virus-encoded enzyme, integrase. This property allows them to acquire, but also alter, host genetic sequences. The ability of retroviruses to integrate into the host cell genome can result in activation or inactivation of specific host cell genes near integration sites. Integration has also been exploited in the construction of retrovirus vectors for intentional delivery of genes into DNA.

Classification

The family *Retroviridae* is subdivided into two subfamilies (*Orthoretrovirinae*, *Spumaretrovirinae*) and seven genera (*Alpharetrovirus*, *Betaretrovirus*, *Gammaretrovirus*, *Deltaretrovirus*, *Epsilonretrovirus*, *Lentivirus*, and *Spumavirus*), as illustrated in Table 14.1. Individual viruses within these genera infect nearly all species of importance to veterinary medicine, and many are associated with some form of chronic disease characterized by immunopathology or cancer. The spumaretroviruses are an obvious exception as, to date, they have not been associated with disease.

Initial classification of retroviruses was based on their respective host species of origin, virion morphology, and morphogenesis as determined by electron microscopy, and biological properties including their route of transmission (exogenous versus endogenous), host cell restrictions, and ability to resist cross-neutralization by specific antiserum. Morphologically, four different types of particles were recognized, designated A, B, C, and D (Figure 14.1). This classification terminology is still found in the scientific literature. For example, type C retrovirus morphogenesis involves the formation at the cell membrane of distinctive crescent-shaped nascent nucleocapsids (hence the name *type C retrovirus*). Oncogenic retroviruses include those with either type B (e.g., mouse mammary tumor virus) or type C (e.g., feline leukemia virus) particle morphology. Type A particles were described as intermediate forms of type B virions or were found in cell lines as unique "intracisternal" A particles.

Exogenous retroviruses are transmitted horizontally and are rarely transmitted via *in-utero* or germ-line infection. In contrast, endogenous retroviruses or retroviral elements are included in the genome of most, if not all animals. These endogenous viruses or elements (collectively known as *retro-elements*) are transmitted vertically as part of the genome of their host species and are passed from generation to generation as inherited genetic sequences. Retro-elements

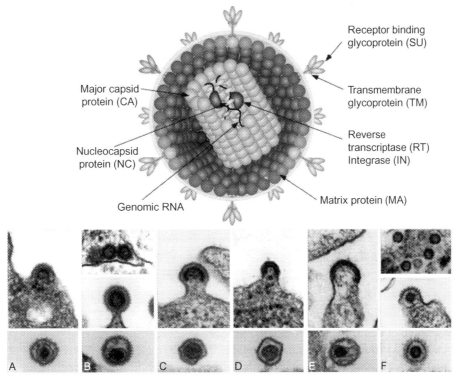

FIGURE 14.1 (Top) Schematic cartoon (not to scale) shows the inferred locations of the various structures and proteins of a retrovirus virion. (Bottom) In panel (A) *Alpharetrovirus*: Avian leukosis virus (ALV); type "C" morphology; panel (B) *Betaretrovirus*: Mouse mammary tumor virus (MMTV); type "B" morphology; panel (C) *Gammaretrovirus*: Murine leukemia virus (MLV); panel (D) *Deltaretrovirus*; Bovine leukemia virus (BLV); panel (E) *Lentivirus*: Human immunodeficiency virus 1 (HIV-1); panel (F) *Spumavirus*: Simian foamy virus (SFVcpz(hu)) (formerly called HFV). *(Courtesy of M. Gonda reproduced from "Retroviruses", CSH Press, with permission). [From* Virus Taxonomy: Eighth Report of the International Committee on Taxonomy of Viruses *(C. M. Fauquet, M. A. Mayo, J. Maniloff, U. Desselberger, L. A. Ball, eds.), p. 421. Copyright © Elsevier (2005), with permission.]*

can represent a large fraction of the total DNA in a mammalian genome, but sequences similar to those of exogenous retroviruses are typically only a small percentage of the total retro-element complement of most species. It has been estimated that up to 10% of animal genomes contain retro-elements (or related sequences), which presumably represent vestiges of retroviral DNA integration events throughout the course of evolution. The laboratory mouse is remarkable in this regard, as it is estimated that up to 37% of its genome represents retro-elements.

Nucleotide sequencing is the basis for current comparison of retroviral genomes, regardless of species of origin. The antigenic relationships among different retroviruses can be complex, as some envelope glycoprotein epitopes are retrovirus type-specific, whereas others are strain-specific. Host-derived antibodies that neutralize viral infectivity in cell culture typically are directed against surface envelope glycoproteins, but are not always predictive of protection from natural infections. Core protein epitopes specified by the *gag* gene are often common to the retroviruses of particular animal species—that is, they are group-specific antigens and referred to as "Gag." Some conserved epitopes (e.g., those of reverse transcriptases) are shared between retroviruses (interspecies antigens).

Virion Properties

Retrovirus virions are enveloped, 80–100 nm in diameter, and have a unique three-layered structure (Figure 14.1). Innermost is the genome–nucleoprotein complex, which includes about 30 molecules of reverse transcriptase, and has helical symmetry. This structure is enclosed within an icosahedral capsid, about 60 nm in diameter, which in turn is surrounded by an envelope derived from the host cell membrane, from which surface envelope glycoprotein spikes (peplomers) project (Table 14.2).

The genomes of retroviruses are diploid, meaning there are two RNA copies packaged in virions as an inverted dimer of two molecules of linear positive-sense, single-stranded RNA. Each RNA genome copy is between 7 and 11 kb (depending on the retrovirus) and has a 3′-polyadenylated tail and a 5′ cap; specific details of the organization of the genomes of the various viruses vary widely (Figure 14.2). Virions are enveloped, and so they are inactivated relatively easily by lipid solvents or detergents and by heating. However, they are more resistant than other viruses to ultraviolet and X-irradiation, in part because their dimeric (diploid) genomes can compensate for radiation-induced mutations during reverse transcription.

Retroviruses require reverse transcriptase for their replication. Among its many functions, reverse transcriptase serves as an RNA-dependent DNA polymerase, a DNA-dependent DNA polymerase, and an RNase, with each distinctive function being carried out by a different part of the

---

TABLE 14.2 Properties of Retroviruses

A diverse group of RNA viruses, which replicate via reverse transcription (synthesize a DNA copy of their RNA genome during their replicative cycle)

Infect a wide variety of animals, including humans, and are associated with certain types of cancer

Some retroviruses may induce immunosuppressive or immune-mediated diseases, or may exist as stable members of the host germ line (endogenously)

Virions are enveloped, 80–100 nm in diameter, and have a three-layered structure: an innermost genome–nucleoprotein complex with helical symmetry, surrounded by an icosahedral capsid, in turn surrounded by an envelope with glycoprotein spikes (surface and transmembrane components)

The genome is diploid, consisting of a dimer of two molecules of linear positive-sense, single-stranded RNA, each 7–11 kb in size. Genomic RNA has a 3′-polyadenylated tail and a 5′ cap

All non-defective retroviruses have *gag*, *pol*, and *env* genes; some acquire an oncogene and are usually defective in their own replication as a consequence. Complex retroviruses, such as lentiviruses, have a variety of auxiliary (non-structural) genes that encode proteins important in replication and virus spread in hosts

Viral reverse transcriptase transcribes DNA from virion RNA following the formation of long terminal repeats; linear and circular double-stranded DNA is formed and linear DNA forms integrate into cellular chromosomal DNA as a provirus, through the action of a virally encoded integrase enzyme and host-cell DNA repair mechanisms

In productive infections, virions assemble at and bud from the plasma membrane

Key biological features of retroviruses include: ability to acquire and alter host-derived genetic sequences; ability to integrate into host-cell genome; activation or inactivation of specific genes near integration site; ability to undergo mutation and recombination; can be used to generate vectors to deliver genes

---

protein molecule (Figure 14.3). Reverse transcriptase has been cloned and exploited as a laboratory reagent because of its remarkable properties, for example in reverse-transcriptase-mediated polymerase chain reaction (RT-PCR). Replication of retroviruses also is dependent on host-cell RNA polymerases for transcription of the integrated DNA copy of the viral genome. The genome of replication-competent (exogenous/non-defective) retroviruses contains three major genes, each encoding two or more proteins. The *gag* gene encodes the virion core proteins [capsid (CA); nucleocapsid (NC); and matrix (MA)], the *pol* gene encodes reverse transcriptase (RT) and integrase (IN), and the *env* gene encodes the virion envelope proteins [surface (SU) and transmembrane (TM)]. Genome termini have several distinctive components, each of which is functionally important. For example, the R (repeat) and U (5′ and

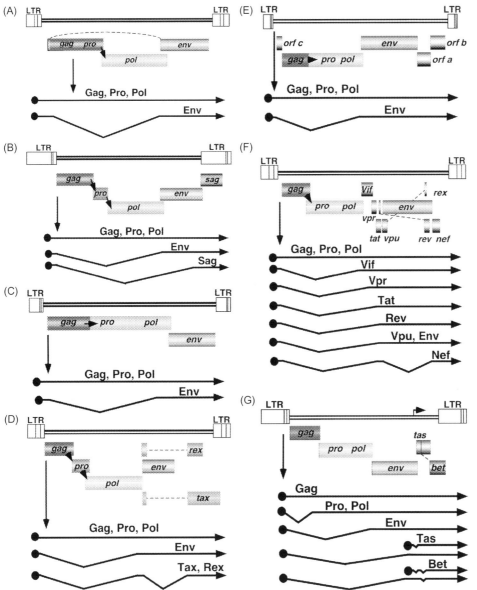

FIGURE 14.2 Genomic maps of the genera of the family *Retroviridae*. (A) *Alpharetrovirus*; (B) *Betaretrovirus*; (C) *Gammaretrovirus*; (D) *Deltaretrovirus*; (E) *Epsilonretrovirus*; (F) *Lentivirus*; (G) *Spumavirus*. Colored block lines, encoded genes in their relative reading frames; arrowheads, frameshifts or ribosomal read through sites; dotted lines, RNA splicing; solid line arrows, primary gene products. LTR, long terminal repeats; Gag (gag), internal virion proteins; Pro, protease; Pol (pol), replicase enzymes; Env (env), envelop protein. Refer to Table 14.3 for definitions of other genes and proteins. *[From Virus Taxonomy: Eighth Report of the International Committee on Taxonomy of Viruses (C. M. Fauquet, M. A. Mayo, J. Maniloff, U. Desselberger, L. A. Ball, eds.), pp. 425, 427, 429, 431, 432, 434, 437. Copyright © Elsevier (2005), with permission.]*

3' unique regions) are critical for reverse transcription, integration, and viral transcription after integration (Table 14.2).

Retroviruses are often classified as having acute transforming or chronic transforming biologic characteristics, based on the presence or absence of key transforming genes in the viral genome. Those viruses that are capable of acute cellular transformation have also been referred to as rapidly or strongly transforming, because these retroviruses typically contain viral oncogenes (v-*onc*) that, under direct control of a viral promoter, increase the probability of expression of v-*onc*. The presence of the v-*onc* gene, which was originally acquired from a host genome, is often associated with deletions elsewhere in the viral genome as a result of a "trade" of a viral gene for a host-cell

gene ("*onc*") during recombination. This trade of a viral gene for a cellular one reflects the packaging constraints imposed during replication and the viral *env* gene is usually exchanged. Thus most v-*onc*-containing viruses are unable to synthesize a complete envelope, are replication defective and must associate with non-defective viruses that are replication competent that act as helper viruses to accomplish replication and spread to other hosts. Rous sarcoma virus is an exception; its genome contains the viral oncogene, v-*src*, but it also contains complete *gag*, *pol*, and *env* genes and is therefore replication competent. Chronic, also referred to as slowly transforming, retroviruses induce neoplasia by insertional mutagenesis through random integration into regions of the host genome that influence cell division, activating host oncogenes.

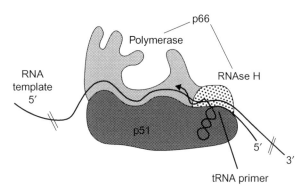

FIGURE 14.3 Schematic diagram of a reverse transcriptase molecule showing its multiple functional domains. The virion reverse transcriptase is coded for as a component of the Gag-Pol precursor and is processed by a virus-coded protease to yield a homodimer of p66 molecules; a portion of the C terminus is subsequently cleaved from one subunit to produce a heterodimer, composed of one molecule of p66 and one of p51. Because of its three-dimensional structure the molecule has been compared to a clenched right hand—specific domains are designated as the palm, thumb, and fingers. A short connection joins the reverse transcriptase domain to the RNase H domain. The viral RNA template and the transfer RNA (tRNA) primer are positioned within the palm. *[From J. M. Coffin. Retroviridae: the viruses and their replication. In: Field's Virology (B. N. Fields, D. M. Knipe, P. M. Howley, R. M. Chanock, J. L. Melnick, T. P. Monath, B. Roizman, S. E. Straus, eds.), 3rd ed., pp. 1767–1848. Copyright © 1996 Lippincott-Raven, Philadelphia, PA, with permission.]*

In addition to encoding *gag*, *pol*, and *env* genes, which are common to all retroviruses, complex retroviruses such as lentiviruses encode several other regulatory and "accessory" genes (Table 14.3). The key regulatory genes of human immunodeficiency virus type 1 (HIV-1), a prototype for the lentiviruses, include *tat*, which encodes a potent transactivator that enhances the efficiency of transcription by cellular RNA polymerase, mainly by preventing premature termination of transcription, and *rev*, which encodes a protein that facilitates the export of non-spliced or singly spliced viral RNA from the nucleus to the cytoplasm. The HIV-1 and simian immunodeficiency viruses (SIV) accessory gene, *nef*, is not required for virus replication in cell culture, but is essential for replication and disease expression *in vivo*. The Nef protein can downregulate expression of cell receptors such as CD4 and may alter the state of activation of target cells *in vivo*. The Vif protein (encoded by the *vif* gene) of human and simian immunodeficiency viruses accumulates in the cytosol of infected cells and is incorporated in virions to enhance virus replication in lymphocytes. Vif binds to and promotes the degradation of a cell-derived cytidine deaminase, APOBEC 3G, blocking APOBEC 3G from inhibiting retrovirus replication by promoting the incorporation of deoxyuridine in the first minus-strand complementary DNA produced during reverse transcription.

Other accessory proteins that occur in primate lentiviruses include the Vpr and Vpx virion-associated proteins

TABLE 14.3 Complex Retrovirus Genes and Protein Functions

Virus and Gene	Protein Function
Human T Cell Lymphotropic Virus (HTLV) and Bovine Leukosis Virus (BLV)	
tax = transactivating gene	Tax: transactivation of viral and cell promoters
rex = regulator of transcription gene	Rex: expression of full-length and env RNAs
pX accessory genes, e.g., *pX ORF 1*	Example: HTLV-1 p12, BLV G4: viral infectivity
hbz = Antisense gene	HBZ: viral infectivity/ regulates viral gene expression
Lentiviruses (e.g., Simian Immunodeficiency Virus)	
tat = transactivating gene	Tat: transactivation of viral promoter, i.e., LTR
rev = regulator of transcription gene	Rev: expression of full-length and env RNAs
nef = "negative factor"	Nef: degradation of CD4 receptor/cell signaling/ infectivity
vif = viral infectivity factor	Vif: counteracts cell restriction, e.g., ABOBEC
vpu = viral infectivity factor	Vpu: degradation of CD4 receptor/infectivity factor
vpx = viral infectivity factor	Vpx: infectivity factor
vpr = viral infectivity factor	Vpr: proviral DNA transport/ infectivity factor
Spumaviruses	
bel 1 = between env and LTR	Transactivation of virus transcription
sag = superantigen gene	Superantigen promotes cell proliferation and spread

that probably contribute to nuclear localization of preinitiation complexes, influence cell-cycle regulation, and alter cell signaling within infected cells. Vpu is an amphipathic membrane protein of primate lentiviruses that promotes efficient release of virions from cells during budding. The precise role of these "accessory" proteins in natural lentivirus infections awaits full clarification; however, it is clear that they can be important in the establishment and maintenance of retrovirus infections in their respective hosts.

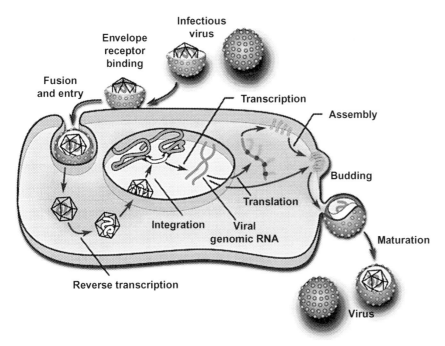

FIGURE 14.4 An overview of the replication cycle of retroviruses. Virions enter their host cells either by fusion or by receptor-mediated endocytosis (top, left), and mature by budding through the plasma membrane (right). *[After J. M. Coffin. Retroviridae: the viruses and their replication. In:* Field's Virology *(B. N. Fields, D. M. Knipe, P. M. Howley, R. M. Chanock, J. L. Melnick, T. P. Monath, B. Roizman, S. E. Straus, eds.), 3rd ed., pp. 1767–1848. Copyright © 1996 Lippincott-Raven, Philadelphia, PA, with permission.]*

Virus Replication

Cell Binding and Penetration

The process of retrovirus replication begins when virion envelope glycoproteins bind to cellular receptors (Figure 14.4 and Figure 2.9). The specific cellular receptors responsible for virus attachment are unique to each retrovirus genus, so many retroviruses are species restricted in their host range; for example, Moloney murine leukemia virus binds receptors that are present only on mouse cells. After attachment, the viral envelope and the cell membrane fuse, allowing the virion core to enter the cytoplasm; less commonly, entry involves receptor-mediated endocytosis. Cells infected with a particular retrovirus are often resistant to superinfection by another closely related retrovirus. Even within a particular species, inbred animals or lines exhibit susceptibility to retrovirus infections based on receptor expression; for example, strains of avian leukosis virus have distinct interference patterns that reflect their individual effects on receptor expression.

Reverse Transcription and Integration

Once present in the cytoplasm, a double-stranded DNA (dsDNA) copy of the retrovirus genomic single-stranded RNA is synthesized within the viral capsid by the virion-associated reverse transcriptase. The reverse transcriptase enzyme contains a domain for polymerase activity, as well as an RNase H that degrades the RNA moiety of RNA–DNA hybrids. Reverse transcription is dependent upon unique features of the reverse transcriptase enzyme such as its ability to "jump" between template strands.

In the process of reverse transcription during retrovirus replication, some 300 to 1300 base pairs are added to the ends of each genomic RNA molecule. These termini, called long-terminal repeats (LTRs), have a complex secondary structure and are central in the replication strategy of all retroviruses. Host-cell-derived transfer RNAs (tRNAs) unique to each genera of retroviruses bind viral 5′-LTR sequences and act to prime the reverse transcriptase. During the process of creating a DNA copy of its RNA genome, the RNase H portion of the reverse transcriptase molecule selectively degrades the RNA strand to create short single-strand DNA, which then hybridizes to the R region of the same (intramolecular) or different (intermolecular) genomic RNA molecule to complete synthesis of first-strand DNA. Eventually the digestion of all viral RNA occurs, except short regions used as second DNA strand primers. Second-strand DNA synthesis occurs by elongation to create the dsDNA intermediate and, ultimately, a linear dsDNA copy of the viral RNA genome that is then transported to the nucleus before integration into the host chromosomal DNA using the virus-encoded integrase enzyme.

Most retroviruses, except lentiviruses, must rely upon cell division for efficient passage into the nucleus and for integration to occur. Once these DNA forms are integrated into the host cell chromosome, the retroviral genomic copies are designated as "proviruses." Proviruses are templates for transcription, including the transcription of full-length genomic RNA and various spliced messenger RNAs (mRNAs). Transcription by cellular RNA polymerase, initiated in the 5′-LTR and ending in the 3′-LTR, generates new virion RNA. The essential features in the replication cycle of a non-defective retrovirus are shown in Figure 14.4.

Retrovirus genomic integration mediated by integrase does not specifically target particular host cell sequences. Local chromatin structure such as sites of DNA bending or so called "open" chromatin structures that are transcriptionally active are favored sites of integration. These cellular integration tendencies may, in part, explain mechanisms of carcinogenesis, as certain retroviruses tend to integrate near, and activate, cellular oncogenes.

Although the process of reverse transcription defines the retroviruses, hepadnaviruses such as hepatitis B virus, endogenous retroviral elements such as retrotransposons, and caulimoviruses of plants also use reverse transcription during their replication.

Transcription of Provirus

After the provirus is integrated, it may remain latent (transcriptionally muted) or, depending on the cellular environment, be transcriptionally active. The viral LTR promotes and initiates transcription of different RNA species that are processed similarly to host cell RNA. After transport to the cytoplasm, the mRNA forms two pools: one for full-length genomic RNA that is subsequently packaged in virions as genomic RNA, and another that includes mRNAs encoding various combinations of Gag, Pro, Env, and Pol species.

A major function of the LTR is to provide signals to initiate RNA synthesis and to control the rate of transcription, in concert with both viral and cellular factors. Thus the LTR may determine disease progression by controlling replication of the retrovirus in specific cell types. Because the LTR is repeated in the proviral forms of retroviruses, they must suppress the 3'-LTR from initiation of transcription. This is accomplished by adjacent *gag* signals that allow the 5'-LTR to be used for initiation at the 3'-LTR. All subgenomic RNAs have a splice start at the common 5' donor. Most simple retroviruses are "passive" and rely upon the cellular splicing mechanisms to obtain splice messages. Complex retroviruses like bovine leukemia virus produce a regulator protein (i.e., Rex) that promotes genomic RNA or single-splice RNA species to be selectively transported from the nucleus to the cytoplasm.

Mutation of Retroviruses

Replication of retroviruses is accompanied by a high mutation frequency that is principally due to the lack of a 3' to 5' exonuclease proofreading mechanism (e.g., editing) by reverse transcriptase. Whereas many loci can tolerate mutation, others in genes encoding either enzymes or structural proteins may not tolerate high mutation rates if they result in defects that block replication or virus assembly. Thus *gag* and *pol* genes are typically more conserved, as are certain critical portions of *env*, whereas other regions of *env*, particularly those regions encoding sites to which antibody binds, are highly variable. The ability for the portions of *env* to tolerate variation without adversely impacting virus

viability facilitates the evolution of new virus strains, including those that can escape immune control.

There is also a high frequency of recombination and gene rearrangements between retrovirus genomes in cells infected with more than one virus. Deletions, duplications, and inversions are relatively common (perhaps as high as 1 in every 25 proviral copies produced), but most are probably lethal for the virus. These events are postulated to occur during reverse transcription, during which there are a number of chances for the reverse transcriptase enzyme to jump templates, produce duplications, or lead to mispriming. Retroviruses also have a relatively high rate of recombination (ranging from <1% to 20% of a genome per replication cycle).

Translation

In infected cells, retroviral protein synthesis occurs in the cytoplasm and is regulated similarly to that of the host cell machinery. Spliced mRNAs are used for translation of envelope proteins and a variety of "accessory proteins" of complex retroviruses. Full-length, non-spliced RNA serves as genomic RNA (packaged in virion) or as mRNA for Gag-Pro-Pol proteins. Translation occurs by ribosomal scanning of mRNAs with frameshifts and read-through translation occurring to produce some proteins. The precursor protein transcribed from 35S mRNAs includes both structural and enzymatic proteins and is associated with free polyribosomes, whereas the 22–24S mRNAs encode the envelope proteins and are associated with membrane-bound ribosomes.

The Env protein is glycosylated as it is processed in the endoplasmic reticulum and Golgi complex before trafficking to the plasma membrane as a result of targeting modifications such as myristoylation. Together with viral RNA, Gag and Gag-Pol precursors begin to assemble nucleocapsids on the inner side of the plasma membrane. Budding proceeds with nucleocapsids binding to Env proteins already fixed as spikes in the plasma membrane. Virus particle assembly is initiated with interaction of the NC domain of Gag precursor protein with packaging signals in genomic RNA. An electron-dense core is formed at the surface of infected cells before virus budding. Proteolytic processing of structural precursor proteins is initiated during budding of virus particles, and continues in newly released virus particles when the virions are fully infectious. Recent studies indicate that key retroviral late-budding (L) domains in Gag are required for the efficient release of nascent virions in concert with cellular co-factors involved in protein trafficking and sorting.

With the notable exception of some lentiviruses, many retroviruses replicate predominantly in dividing cells, often without obvious cytopathology or dramatic alteration of the metabolism of the cells they infect; others, such as the lentiviruses, cause cell death in a number of ways, including syncytium formation (an inherently unstable event) and

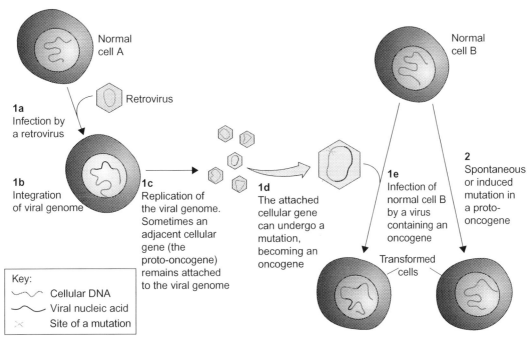

FIGURE 14.5   Mechanism of oncogene capture by retroviruses. Cellular oncogenes incorporated into virus genome often are mutated and lack normal control leading to transformation of infected cells. (*Courtesy of M. Lairmore and T. Vojt, the Ohio State University.*)

apoptosis. In some instances, infected cells may continue to divide while producing large numbers of virions.

Oncogenesis

Oncogenes were discovered through the study of retroviruses associated with animal cancers. Cellular "oncogenes" (c-*onc* or proto-oncogenes) are responsible for normal cell growth and differentiation. During retrovirus replication, viral oncogenes (v-*onc*) can be created from c-*onc* through processes such as read-through transcription (Figure 14.5). Viral oncogenes typically include features that result in the loss of cellular control of v-*onc* activity. Viral oncogenes generally affect cell growth control (dysregulation) by influencing or acting as growth factors, receptors, intracellular signal transducers, or intranuclear factors such as transcription factors.

Oncogene capture is a unique feature of retrovirus replication and is considered an "illegitimate" recombination event. Current models favor a non-homologous recombination event during reverse transcription. This occurs by two potential mechanisms each occurring when retroviruses integrate within or adjacent to a proto-oncogene; specifically, packaging of deleted and wild-type genomes can be followed by recombination, resulting in additional sequences "captured" by the virus. Alternatively, packaging of read-through transcripts can occur as RNA polymerases transcribe the provirus, and subsequent recombination results in the incorporation of additional sequences into the new viral genome. Many of these events may block replication, but those that lead to a transformation event may ultimately be expressed as cancer in the infected host.

MEMBERS OF THE SUBFAMILY *ORTHORETROVIRINAE*, GENUS *ALPHARETROVIRUS*

AVIAN LEUKOSIS AND SARCOMA VIRUSES

Retrovirus infections are responsible for a remarkable variety of disease syndromes in poultry, and much of our current understanding of the biology of oncogenic retroviruses derives from research on the viruses affecting birds. Retrovirus infections of chickens fall into two distinct groups: (1) the avian leukosis, myeloblastosis, and sarcoma viruses, which belong to the genus *Alpharetrovirus*; (2) the avian reticuloendotheliosis viruses, which belong to the genus *Gammaretrovirus* (Table 14.1). Each of these groups of viruses has numerous individual members (virus species).

Like other retroviruses, avian retroviruses come in various forms, including: (1) *endogenous*; (2) *exogenous replication competent*; (3) *exogenous replication defective*. Endogenous avian leukosis viruses occur in the genome of every chicken as DNA proviruses. These endogenous retroviruses are typically not expressed or pathogenic unless recombination events create viruses associated with rare tumors such as glioma. Exogenous avian leukosis viruses are replication competent and have a standard complement of *gag*, *pol*, and *env* genes. These exogenously transmitted avian retroviruses are generally non-pathogenic, but in the course of lifetime infection a small percentage of infected birds develop leukemia or lymphoma. Also, some exogenous viruses acquire an oncogene (v-*onc*) from a cellular *onc* (c-*onc*) gene and then can induce malignant tumors rapidly. The great majority of such rapidly

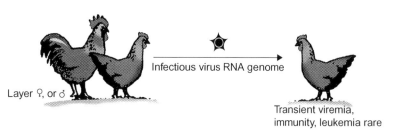

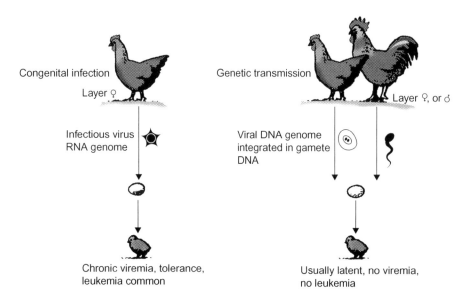

FIGURE 14.6 Horizontal and vertical transmission of avian leukosis viruses. *(Courtesy of R. A. Weiss.)*

transforming (oncogenic) viruses lose part of their genome when they acquire their oncogene, so that they become replication defective and dependent on the helper activity of a replication-competent virus. A few viruses, however, like Rous sarcoma virus, have a full complement of viral genes plus a v-*onc* gene—they are rapidly oncogenic while at the same time capable of replication without a helper virus. Oncogenic retroviruses may be transmitted from one chicken to another horizontally or vertically, and vertical transmission may occur through infectious virus (complete virions) or through provirus integrated into the DNA of the host germ cells (Figure 14.6). All routes of transmission occur, including germ cell (ova or sperm) transmission, which complicates efforts at disease prevention.

With most of the avian retroviruses, if chickens are infected horizontally when more than 5 or 6 days of age they are unlikely to develop leukemia; instead they develop a transient viremia and produce neutralizing antibody. If virus is transmitted congenitally via the egg or within the first few days of life, the chicken develops a viremia that persists for life because of the induction of immunological tolerance. Such birds may appear to grow normally, but they subsequently can develop leukemia and associated diseases and are a major source of exogenous virus that can be spread to contact birds.

Avian sarcoma and leukosis viruses are classified into at least 10 different subgroups (designated A–J) based primarily on the unique cellular receptors these viruses use to infect the host cell. Six subgroups occur in chickens (A, B, C, D, E, and J). The various subgroups are associated with distinct patterns of disease. In general, avian leukosis viruses are widespread in most commercial layer flocks of chickens, and most chickens in a flock will have been infected within a few months of hatching. Historically, if rapidly transforming viruses are not present, disease occurs sporadically in birds more than 14 weeks of age, with an overall incidence of about 1–2%, but sometimes the incidence of disease may be as high as 20%, as occurred in the 1990s with Leukosis J in broiler breeding birds. However, today the commercial layer and broiler breeding industries have nearly eradicated avian leukosis from primary breeding flocks, and the occurrence of avian leukosis in the field is generally from horizontal transmission of the virus amongst commercial layer birds. The variety of syndromes produced by avian leukosis/sarcoma viruses is shown in Table 14.4.

In chickens infected with exogenous non-defective viruses, tumors occur only when infection occurs congenitally and there is persistent viremia. Over the course of the life of the chicken, proviral DNA is integrated into many different kinds of cells—sometimes, by chance, in a location where the activity of a c-*onc* gene is disturbed

TABLE 14.4 Syndromes Produced in Chickens by Avian Retroviruses

Virus[a]	Syndrome	Rate of Tumor Development	Viral Oncogene	Cell First Affected	Type of Lesion
Replication-Competent (Avian Leukosis Viruses)					
	Lymphoid leukosis	Slow	–	Lymphoblast (B cell)	Lymphoid cell infiltrations of various organs
	Osteopetrosis	Slow	–	Osteoclast or osteoblast	Thickened long bones
	Renal tumors	Slow	–	Renal cells	Nephroblastoma, carcinoma
Replication-Defective (Avian Erythroblastosis, Avian Myeloblastosis, Avian Myelocytomatosis Viruses)					
	Erythroblastosis	Rapid	v-*erbB*	Erythroblast	Anemia
	Myeloblastosis	Rapid	v-*myb*	Myeloblast	Anemia, leukemia
	Myelocytomatosis	Rapid	v-*myc*	Myelocyte	Sarcoma
	Hemangioma	Rapid	?	Capillary endothelium	Hemangioma
	Sarcomas	Rapid	v-*fps*, v-*yes*	Various mesenchymal cells	Sarcoma
Replication-Competent Rapidly Transforming (Rous Sarcoma Virus)					
	Sarcoma	Very rapid	v-*src*	Various mesenchymal cells	Sarcomas

[a] *In addition to these exogenous viruses, all chickens carry endogenous retroviral DNA as part of their genome.*

in such a way as to initiate tumor production (*cis*-acting transformation).

A variety of neoplasms are generated by replication-defective leukemia viruses propagated by co-infection with a non-defective helper, which is usually an exogenous avian leukemia virus. These defective viruses, for the most part, arise as a rare event in each individual bird in which they are found; because they are defective in their own replication and are so rapidly fatal that they are seldom, if ever, transmitted horizontally or from generation to generation. The very different pathogenic potential of the various viruses is attributable to the different v-*onc* genes they carry, and is reflected in the different tumors that they induce (Table 14.4).

Diseases Caused by Replication-Competent Avian Retroviruses

Lymphoid leukosis

Lymphoid leukosis (synonymous with visceral lymphomatosis) is the most common form of avian leukosis and occurs in chickens approximately 14–30 weeks of age. Clinical signs are non-specific, but the comb may be pale, shriveled, and occasionally cyanotic, and affected birds may exhibit inappetence, emaciation, weakness, and abdominal swelling. Tumors may be present for some time before clinical illness is recognized, although the course may be rapid from the onset of disease. Often, tumor formation is only detected after slaughter at poultry processing plants, but results in condemnation of the carcass.

Hematological changes are variable in infected birds, with overt leukemia rarely observed. Tumors, usually as discrete, nodular lesions, occur first in the cloacal bursa (bursa of Fabricius), with subsequent metastasis to liver, spleen, and other internal organs. These multicentric tumors consist of aggregates of lymphoblasts that express B lymphocyte markers. These cells may secrete large amounts of immunoglobulin M (IgM), but their capacity to differentiate into IgG-, IgA- or IgE-producing cells is arrested. Bursectomy (removal of the cloacal bursa), even up to 5 months of age, abrogates the development of lymphoid leukosis. Tumor induction is typically caused by virus activation and overexpression of the *c-myc* oncogene, with contributions from B*lym*-1 and *c-bis*.

Osteopetrosis

Osteopetrosis (*syn.* "thick leg" syndrome) affects bones of chickens infected with certain strains of avian alpharetroviruses, resulting in uniform or irregular diaphyseal thickening that may progress to metaphyseal thickening of the affected bones. Lesions are usually most obvious in the long bones of the leg, but may also occur in the pelvis, shoulder girdle, and ribs, and are typically bilaterally symmetrical. Birds with osteopetrosis also frequently have secondary anemia and lesions of lymphoid leukosis.

Renal tumors

Renal tumors associated with alpharetrovirus infection are usually found coincidentally at slaughter of affected birds, but may lead to emaciation and weakness before death. Two forms occur: nephroblastomas, which originate from both epithelial and mesenchymal elements of nephrogenic blastema (embryonic nephrons and embryonal rests in the kidneys), and carcinomas, which originate only from the epithelium of the embryonal blastema.

Diseases Caused by Replication-Defective Avian Retroviruses

This group of diseases is characterized by cellular transformation by oncogenic viruses that have acquired an oncogene through the loss of an essential viral gene, thus they require the presence of a helper virus for their replication.

Erythroblastosis

The incubation period for erythroblastosis may be 21–100 days for chicks exposed at 1 day of age, but most clinical cases manifest with lesions at 3–6 months of age. Two patterns are recognized: a proliferative form characterized by the presence of many erythroblasts in the blood, and an anemic form in which there is anemia with few circulating erythroblasts. The primary target cells are progenitor erythroblasts, with viral infection activating the c-erb oncogene. Virus-infected erythroblasts have a normal appearance, except that retrovirus particles can be demonstrated either within cytoplasmic vacuoles or budding from their plasma membranes. In affected birds, the liver and kidney are diffusely swollen, cherry red to dark mahogany in color, soft, and friable.

Myeloblastosis

Myeloblastosis is uncommon, and usually seen in adult chickens. In this form of disease, clinical signs are similar to those of erythroblastosis and develop after an incubation period that may be as short as 10 days. The target cells are myeloblasts in the bone marrow. The v-myb oncogene of acute transforming defective retroviruses is responsible for neoplastic transformation of the myeloblasts. Leukemia is a major feature of myeloblastosis, with very high numbers of up to 10^9 per ml of circulating myeloblasts in the blood; indeed, leukocytes may actually outnumber erythrocytes. Bone marrow displacement (myelophthisis) may result in secondary anemia and

thrombocytopenia. The liver is enlarged, firm, and gray from the diffuse infiltration of neoplastic cells.

Fowl glioma (a central nervous system tumor) has been associated with recombinant viruses, with envelope regions most closely related to endogenous myeloblastosis-associated avian retroviruses, suggesting a causal role in this rare but lethal tumor.

Myelocytomatosis

Birds with myelocytomatosis can exhibit clinical signs similar to those in birds with erythroblastosis or myeloblastosis. The incubation period after infection is 3–11 weeks. Target cells are non-granulated myelocytes (morphologically distinct from myeloblasts) that proliferate following infection, to occupy and efface much of the bone marrow. The neoplastic cells may extend through the cortex and periosteum of affected bones. The tumors are distinctive and characteristically occur on the surface of bone, in association with the periosteum and near cartilage, although any organ or tissue may be affected. With avian leukemia virus J, in addition to involvement of bones, tumor cells also infiltrate and enlarge the spleen, liver, and other organs. Histologically, the tumors consist of compact masses of uniform, well-differentiated myelocytes packed with acidophilic cytoplasmic granules, similar to normal bone marrow myelocytes.

Myelocytochromatosis is caused by either replication defective or non-defective avian leukemia viruses. Acute transforming virus strains possess the v-myc oncogene, whereas the slow transforming virus strains activate the c-myc oncogene.

Hemangioma

Affected birds typically develop a single or multiple hemangioma(s) in the skin or on the surface of the viscera within 3 weeks of initial viral infection of vascular endothelial cells. The lesion takes the form of a "blood blister," which may rupture, causing death from acute hemorrhage. The obvious presence of these lesions in the skin also encourages cannibalism.

Connective Tissue Tumors

A variety of sporadic mesenchymal tumors in young and adult birds, including fibrosarcoma, fibroma, myxosarcoma, myxoma, histiocytic sarcoma, osteoma, osteogenic sarcoma, and chondrosarcoma, are caused by infections with avian retroviruses containing v-onc genes, either replication-defective viruses acting in concert with a helper virus, or replication-competent viruses that carry their own oncogene such as Rous sarcoma virus.

Diagnosis

History, clinical signs, and gross and histopathologic findings are usually sufficient to make a diagnosis of avian leukosis. The most important differential diagnosis for retrovirus-induced avian leukosis is Marek's disease (see Chapter 9), and distinction of these two entities is important because Marek's disease can be controlled by vaccination.

Rous sarcoma virus and other replication-competent, acutely transforming avian retroviruses can be directly quantitated using proliferative focus formation assays in chick embryo fibroblast cell cultures. Replication-defective rapidly transforming viruses, which carry v-*onc* genes, can also be assayed by focus formation, but virions can only be obtained in cells carrying a replication-competent leukosis virus; the yield always consists of a mixture. Replication-competent leukosis viruses do not transform cells *in vitro*; because they interfere with transformation by viruses that carry a v-*onc* gene, interference assays are used. Assays for the presence of leukosis viruses can also be carried out by serologic methods using enzyme immunoassay or radioimmunoassay. Sequence analyses can be used to identify new virus subgroups associated with unusual disease patterns. This information, combined with receptor usage assays, has provided novel insights into the pathogenesis of avian retroviruses.

Immunity, Prevention, and Control

Transmission of avian retroviruses may occur either horizontally or vertically (Figure 14.6). Only a few chicks are infected vertically, but this route of transmission allows the virus to persist from generation to generation. Congenital infection is usually a consequence of the presence of virus in the oviduct of viremic hens that results in high titers of virus in the albumin of eggs, with subsequent embryo infection commencing as early as the 8-cell blastocyst. The pancreas of infected embryos contains large amounts of virus, and these birds shed virus in their meconium and feces after hatching. Most chickens become infected horizontally by close contact with congenitally infected chicks, especially in the hatchery and in the first few weeks after hatching, but virus present in the saliva and feces of older chickens contributes to horizontal transmission and environmental contamination. Horizontal transmission of the virus also provides the source of virus for egg-borne vertical transmission. Transovarial infection is apparently unimportant. Individual infected hens may transmit virus either continuously (these are typically viremic, seronegative birds) or intermittently (these are typically viremic, seropositive birds). Transmission is less efficient in hens more than 18 months of age. Congenitally infected chickens may be immunologically tolerant and their blood may contain up to 10^9 infectious particles/ml. These birds excrete virus in saliva and feces, but are otherwise healthy, although some eventually develop leukosis. Congenital transmission is most prevalent in backyard and hobby flocks.

Most 1-day-old chicks have maternal antibody titers between 1 and 10% of those of their dams. Thus the efficiency of passive antibody transfer is low, and the titer declines, so that chicks are seronegative by 4–7 weeks of age. Then, if they have not been infected congenitally, they become infected by horizontal transmission and develop a transient viremia followed by high levels of antibody; virus is usually eliminated and the antibody persists for life. However, some birds remain persistently infected and act as a source of virus for both horizontal and vertical transmission. Roosters may be involved in the germ line transmission of endogenous (non-pathogenic) retroviruses, but they play no part in congenital infection because sperm cells are acytoplasmic.

Hygiene is important in minimizing the level of viral contamination, particularly in the immediate post-hatching period when the age, population density, and levels of virus are highly conducive to horizontal transmission. The "all-in–all-out" management system, with thorough cleaning and disinfection of incubators, hatcheries, brooding houses, and equipment, is standard practice. The risk of introducing additional strains of virus is minimized if stocks are obtained from a single source.

When intensive methods for broiler and egg production were introduced in the 1940s, there was an unwitting selection of genetically susceptible chicken lines. Today, most commercial flocks consist of genetically resistant lines and, accordingly, there has been a sharp reduction in the incidence of leukosis. Resistance correlates with the virus subgroup and with the absence of receptors for viral envelope glycoproteins; the genes encoding viral receptors are located on an autosomal chromosome, so it is possible to select for genetically resistant birds by challenging chorioallantoic membranes or chick embryo fibroblast cell cultures derived from leukosis-free birds with appropriate pseudotypes of Rous sarcoma virus. Failure to produce foci of cell transformation correlates with resistance, and lines of chickens can be bred that are homozygous for the resistance allele. Viral mutants able to bypass resistance emerge frequently, so that, in practice, genetic resistance as a basis for control requires a continuing selection program.

Eradication of horizontally transmitted virus has been accomplished in flocks of breeding and egg-laying birds, especially those used as a source of eggs for vaccine production. This is the case whether the eggs are for human, domestic mammal, or avian virus vaccines. Establishment and maintenance of leukosis-free flocks, which still carry endogenous avian retroviruses, are expensive, but can be a method of control. In addition to eliminating the occurrence of tumors, eradication has a number of other benefits, including reduced mortality from other causes, improved growth rate, and improved production, quality, fertility, and hatchability of eggs. Immunization with either inactivated or live-attenuated virus vaccines has not been commercially or experimentally successful.

MEMBERS OF THE SUBFAMILY *ORTHORETROVIRINAE,* GENUS *BETARETROVIRUS*

JAAGSIEKTE SHEEP RETROVIRUS (OVINE PULMONARY ADENOMATOSIS VIRUS)

Ovine pulmonary adenomatosis or ovine pulmonary carcinoma is a significant retrovirus-induced disease in sheep in certain regions of the world. In affected adult sheep, the disease leads to chronic wasting and severe respiratory distress. The causative virus is a type D retrovirus classified as a member of the genus *Betaretrovirus.* Significant progress in the understanding of the etiologic agent occurred after the virus was cloned, sequenced, and studied in cell culture and animal models. Originally described in South Africa, where it was called Jaagsiekte, the disease occurs worldwide, except in Australia and New Zealand, where it has not been documented, and Iceland, where it was eradicated in 1952. Ovine pulmonary adenomatosis occurs sporadically in the Americas and in some countries in Europe. In Peru, the virus may be responsible for perhaps a quarter of the annual mortality in adult sheep.

Clinical Features and Epidemiology

Jaagsiekte was recognized and described by sheep farmers in South Africa in the early 1800s. The word "Jaagsiekte" is an Afrikaans term that depicts the clinical outcomes of affected sheep—"chase" (Jaag) and "sickness" (sieckte), which accurately describes the respiratory disease. A retrovirus cause of the disease was identified much later when virus particles were observed in lung cells of affected sheep and subsequently confirmed experimentally by reproducing the disease using cell-free lung fluid filtrates and then using molecular clones of the Jaagsiekte virus in young lambs. The viral infection is naturally transmitted in aerosolized lung fluid between sheep that are housed in close contact. Following exposure, clinical disease may be prolonged and, generally, significant losses occur in adult sheep that are over 2 years of age.

Sheep with pulmonary adenomatosis exhibit progressive dyspnea, anorexia, and cachexia. Severely affected animals may die of respiratory failure from the massive amount of fluid that is secreted from proliferating Type II pneumocytes in neoplastic foci (nodules) that are disseminated throughout the lung. The incubation period varies from 1 to 3 years, but may be shorter when young lambs are infected. The onset of disease is insidious, with progressive respiratory distress, bouts of spasmodic coughing, and the production of large amounts of surfactant-containing viscous fluid by tumor cells, leading to blockage of small airways and death from anoxia, secondary bacterial pneumonia, or concurrent ovine lentivirus (visna-maedi) infection. In affected sheep, variably sized neoplastic nodules are scattered through the lungs. The disease is typically restricted to the lung, and metastases are extremely rare.

Pathogenesis and Pathology

The viral cause of ovine pulmonary adenomatosis is designated as JSRV (denoting Jaagsiekte sheep retrovirus) for the original disease description. JSRV uniquely induces transformation of differentiated lung epithelial cells such as type II pneumocytes in the alveoli (airspaces) and Clara cells in the bronchioles (terminal airways). Integrated viral DNA can also be detected in lymphoid tissues, alveolar macrophages, and peripheral blood mononuclear cells, which may allow virus spread within an infected sheep or between sheep from contaminated lung fluid. Recent evidence indicates that the JSRV envelope and LTR regions are key factors in both determining the cell tropism and the expression of JSRV. The viral surface glycoprotein interacts with a member of the hyaluronoglucosaminidase family, hyaluronidase 2, to gain cell entry. However, active replication of JSRV is restricted to bronchoalveolar epithelial cells, in part because of restriction of cellular transcription factors capable of binding the viral LTR and promoting virus expression. The JSRV envelope has also been demonstrated to be a major determinant for the cellular transformation via alteration of cellular signaling pathways that promote cellular proliferation.

Lesions associated with ovine pulmonary adenomatosis are often detected at slaughter of culled sheep. Characteristic nodules in affected lungs are confirmed by histological evaluation to include a bronchoalveolar pattern of epithelial proliferation that can resemble human bronchoalveolar carcinomas. Histologically, these lesions are classified as adenomas or adenocarcinomas; they represent neoplastic transformation of type II secretory epithelial cells and nonciliated bronchiolar epithelium. Less commonly, metastases to regional pulmonary lymph nodes may occur.

Diagnosis

JSRV infection elicits no specific circulating antibodies against the virus that can be detected in infected sheep using conventional methods; this lack of response may be due to immune tolerance caused by the presence of endogenous retroviruses closely related to JSRV. Unique JSRV proviral DNA sequences, however, are detectable by PCR assay of blood leukocytes in clinically affected and in a percentage of contact animals. Improved methods have been successfully used to screen flocks for the presence of JSRV, providing a tool for control programs in countries with enzootic ovine pulmonary adenomatosis.

Immunity, Prevention, and Control

There are no reports of effective immune responses against JSRV in individual animals, and vaccines against the viral infection have not been produced. Outbreaks occur when infected sheep are introduced into uninfected flocks, especially where sheep are confined. Infected animals shed virus in saliva, milk, colostrum, and respiratory secretions; natural infection is presumed to be acquired and maintained principally via the respiratory route.

Eradication in Iceland involved the near depopulation of the entire sheep population of the country; in the absence of a sensitive test to detect preclinical cases, eradication in other countries has proven unfeasible. Nevertheless, the incidence of the disease can be reduced greatly by strict isolation of flocks and removal of sick animals (ewes and their lambs) immediately upon the onset of clinical signs.

ENZOOTIC NASAL TUMOR VIRUS

Enzootic nasal tumor virus (ENTV) is related closely to JSRV retrovirus and the cause of nasal adenocarcinoma (also called enzootic nasal adenocarcinoma, enzootic nasal tumor, and infectious nasal adenopapillomatosis), which is a relatively rare and contagious tumor of sheep and goats (Figure 14.7). Although sheep may be co-infected with both viruses (JSRV and ENTV), associated disease is rare. Animals infected with ENTV are susceptible to development of nasal tumors, and sheep with these tumors characteristically exhibit copious nasal discharge, respiratory distress, exophthalmos, and bone lesions that can result in skull deformity. Both ENTV and JSRV utilize hyaluronidase 2 as a receptor for attachment; however, ENTV targets epithelial cells lining the upper airways, whereas JSRV infects lung epithelial cells. *In-vitro* studies suggest that JSRV requires a lower pH for cell membrane fusion than does ENTV. Interestingly, the envelope protein of ENTV itself appears capable of transforming epithelial cells, an apparently unique mechanism amongst retroviruses of oncogenesis.

Etiologic confirmation of ENTV in nasal carcinomas of sheep requires amplification of a portion of the

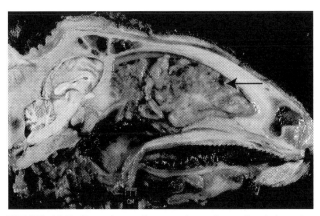

FIGURE 14.7 Enzootic nasal tumor in a sheep. Saggital section showing expansive tumor (arrow) in the nasal passages. *(Courtesy of B. Murphy and University of California, Davis.)*

viral genome by PCR. Other routine diagnostic tests are not available. Virus-specific immune responses are not detected in infected sheep.

ENDOGENOUS RETROVIRUSES OF SHEEP

The sheep genome contains at least 27 copies of endogenous retroviruses. An extensive family of endogenous retroviruses, designated enJSRV (for endogenous JSRV) because they are closely related to JSRV, occurs in domestic and wild sheep and goats. These endogenous retroviruses are transmitted as stable genes of sheep of unknown biological significance. Interestingly, these endogenous retroviruses are expressed in the placenta and genital tract of many mammals, including sheep and humans. Whether this expression is advantageous to placenta formation or function remains unclear, but recent studies indicate that enJSRVs are required for normal reproductive function in sheep, and it has been further suggested that they mediate protection against exogenous retrovirus infections. Thus there is considerable research currently to establish the contribution of enJSRV to the normal physiology and various diseases of sheep.

Endogenous retroviruses have been used recently as genetic markers to study the domestication of sheep, which parallels human migration patterns. The endogenous retrovirus sequences of "primitive" sheep breeds are distinct from those of modern breeds of sheep, and mirror the influx of human populations in Europe and Asia, who were dependent upon them for food and fiber.

TYPE D SIMIAN RETROVIRUSES

The first type D retrovirus described was Mason-Pfizer monkey virus; it was isolated in 1983 from a rhesus macaque and is now recognized, along with other simian retroviruses (SRV), as the cause of a severe, often fatal, immunosuppressive disease, in addition to being associated with a distinctive syndrome of retroperitoneal fibrosis that is actually caused by rhesus monkey rhadinovirus (a herpesvirus that is closely related to the human Kaposi-sarcoma-associated herpesvirus). The macaque immunosuppressive disease syndrome was the first to be called simian-acquired immunodeficiency syndrome (SAIDS), but the term has become too vague to be useful because simian immunodeficiency viruses (lentiviruses) also cause a similar syndrome.

Exogenous type D simian retroviruses are naturally indigenous to various species of the genus *Macaca* (subfamily *Cercopithecinae*). These viruses have been divided into five (and possibly seven) major neutralizing serotypes—known as SRV-1, SRV-2, SRV-3, etc.—with considerable variability within each serotype. The Mason-Pfizer virus is SRV-3. In addition, nearly all Old World non-human primates (excepting apes), as well as squirrel monkeys (*Saimiri sciureus*) and langurs (*Presbytis obscurus*) possess endogenous retroviruses in their genomes that have not been associated with disease. The macaque exogenous viruses, particularly SRV-1 and SRV-2, are of significance in their association with immunodeficiency syndrome in captive *Macaca* species.

Clinical Features and Epidemiology

Simian type D retrovirus infections are important problems among macaques in primate centers and research colonies, where they are frequently associated with disease but can be difficult to detect. Some infected macaques can be viremic and spread the virus, but without detectable antibody production. Thus considerable effort has been placed on the breeding of specific-pathogen-free animals that are antibody and virus-specific PCR assay negative for simian retroviruses and other common infections. Animals that are positive for simian retroviruses may remain so throughout their lifetime and, in severe forms, may develop immunodeficiency and suffer from a variety of opportunistic infections and neoplastic and inflammatory diseases that render them unsuitable for experimental studies.

Pathogenesis and Pathology

There are a variety of potential pathogenic outcomes associated with simian retrovirus infections in various species of macaques, with cynomolgus macaques (*Macaca fascicularis*) being relatively resistant to disease. In severe forms of disease, macaques may develop devastating immune deficiency and become susceptible to a variety of opportunistic infections by ubiquitous agents in addition to inflammatory, proliferative, or even neoplastic diseases such as lymphoma. A typical presentation in virus-positive animals is weight loss, diarrhea, lymphocytopenia, and anemia. At necropsy, there may be inflammatory lesions in several organs, including lymph nodes, salivary gland, spleen, thymus, and brain. Retroviruses are indigenous to wild macaques, but their potential as pathogens in this species is greatest among captive animals exposed as infants, which develop ineffective immune responses to the virus. When infected as juveniles, rhesus macaques (*Macaca mulatta*) may die within 1 year.

Diagnosis

Diagnosis of simian retrovirus infections may require repeated serologic tests for detection of virus-specific antibodies using enzyme-linked immunosorbent assay (ELISA) and western blot assays, as some animals may be infected but fail to mount a detectable antibody response. Typically, PCR assays in combination with nucleotide sequencing are required to confirm infection and/or to differentiate virus

subtypes in valuable animals. Using carefully managed test and removal methods, primate colonies can be established that exclude these viruses; this approach has dramatically reduced the incidence of simian type D retrovirus-associated diseases.

Immunity, Prevention, and Control

Animals that have high titer viremia and RNA levels in their peripheral blood are more likely to spread these viruses. Transmission requires close contact, with virus being present in saliva and blood and spread occurring via biting, grooming, and fighting. Effective inactivated virus vaccines have been produced against three of the viruses, but their use has been limited in favor of strict isolation of primate colonies, and intensive diagnostic screening with removal of infected animals. Because retroviruses are present in many tissues and most bodily fluids from infected animals, control can be complicated. Furthermore, although many animals are antibody positive and viremic, some animals may be seronegative and not be considered positive unless tested repeatedly or by alternative methods such as PCR assays for detection of viral nucleic acid. The shedding of virus from infected animals may be quite variable, and thus transmission may also be intermittent. A strong antibody response against the virus, especially against surface envelope glycoprotein (gp70) typically suppresses viral loads and thus reduces transmission. However, animals with strong antibody responses may intermittently shed virus and females may spread virus to their offspring even in the presence of a substantial antibody titer. Naïve animals (not previously exposed to simian retroviruses) typically form a detectable antibody and cell-mediated immune response against the viral infection within 6–8 weeks after exposure. These animals, however, can still shed virus and serve as a source of infection, especially if they are stressed or exhibit immune suppression.

Cross-reactive antibodies between simian retrovirus strains have been reported and are usually directed to the conserved major capsid, p27, or transmembrane, gp20, proteins. Information on the virus strain responsible for infection of a group of animals can be used to design more specific antibody-binding assays. A serious concern in the control of simian retrovirus infections are animals that have low or undetectable antibody responses and are viremic and transmit virus. The mechanism of how these animals remain virus positive, but antibody negative, may be related to immunotolerance, as these animals are often juvenile or infants born to antibody-positive mothers.

Also potentially complicating control programs is the occurrence of multiple strains of simian retroviruses, which may require the use of strain-specific primers for detection of these viruses in PCR assays. These assays also must distinguish exogenous simian retroviruses from closely related endogenous retroviral sequences that are present in monkeys, and which may lead to false-positive results. Thus positive PCR tests should be confirmed by nucleotide sequencing of the amplified product to confirm the presence of exogenous virus.

MURINE MAMMARY TUMOR VIRUSES

Mouse mammary tumor viruses are structurally similar to murine leukemia viruses, but they encode a protein known as a superantigen (Sag) that is important to the pathobiology of the virus in their murine hosts. All inbred strains of mice contain one or more (in some strains more than 50) endogenous mammary tumor virus loci in their genome, and the genomic distribution of these loci is unique to each inbred strain of mouse. In contrast, some wild mouse populations do not contain these loci. In inbred mice, most mammary tumor virus loci do not encode infectious virus or are transcriptionally inactive, but those mouse strains (DBA, C3H, GRS) that possess the loci known as *Mtv1* and *Mtv2* encode infectious virus. In addition to these endogenous mammary tumor viruses, mice are susceptible to exogenous mammary tumor viruses, although these exogenous viruses have been eliminated from contemporary mouse colonies (unless purposely maintained for experimental purposes). Both endogenous and exogenous viruses are transmissible to pups in the milk from virus-positive dams, where the virus initially replicates in gut-associated lymphoid tissue. Although mouse mammary tumor viruses are named for their tropism and disease potential in mammary tissue, they are highly B lymphocytotrophic. The Sag proteins encoded by the LTR of mouse mammary tumor viruses are presented in the context of major histocompatibility complex (MHC) class II molecules on dendritic and B cells, and are thereby recognized by T cells, which results in T cell reactivity. Reactive T cells stimulate massive B cell proliferation, which in turn fosters virus integration and replication. Blood-borne B lymphocytes with replicating virus home to and infect the mammary gland, where virus replicates to extremely high titer in mammary tissue, and may induce mammary cancer through insertional mutagenesis. Various inbred strains of mice have several means to subvert this cycle of susceptibility, thereby contributing to mouse-strain-related differences in susceptibility to mammary cancer. Mammary tumor viruses may also cause lymphomas in some strains of mice. In addition to its role in Sag expression, the LTR region of mouse mammary tumor virus confers an important determinant for mammary tissue tropism, and has been used in transgenic constructs that possess specificity to mammary tissue expression.

Other species of animals, including humans, contain sequences related to mouse mammary tumor virus in their genomes, but the mouse appears to be the only known species that encodes replication-competent virus.

MEMBERS OF THE SUBFAMILY *ORTHORETROVIRINAE*, GENUS *GAMMARETROVIRUS*

The gammaretroviruses are a diverse group of avian and mammalian retroviruses that cause infections in their respective hosts characterized by prolonged clinical latency that may or may not result in induction of disease. Moloney murine leukemia and feline leukemia viruses are prototypes of this group of retroviruses. Despite their names, leukemia viruses are often not oncogenic, or may induce systemic, non-leukemic forms of disease. Depending upon host species, they may be either exogenous or endogenous viruses.

FELINE LEUKEMIA AND SARCOMA VIRUSES

Clinical Features and Epidemiology

Feline leukemia and sarcoma viruses are responsible for a variety of disease syndromes, some neoplastic and others relating to effects on cells of the hemopoietic and immune systems. Three major types of neoplasia are caused by these viruses: lymphosarcoma (*syn.* malignant lymphoma or lymphoma), myeloproliferative disease, and fibrosarcoma. In addition, infection is associated with several types of non-neoplastic diseases such as anemia, immune-mediated inflammatory diseases, and immunodeficiency disease with opportunistic infections. Neoplastic and non-neoplastic diseases caused by feline leukemia virus occur worldwide and remain a common non-accidental cause of death in cats; however, the prevalence of feline leukemia virus infection in countries such as the United States has plummeted in recent years with the advent of testing and control measures.

Feline leukemia virus is a naturally occurring exogenous gammaretrovirus that is enzootic in domestic cats, but cats also possess endogenous retroviruses within their genomes. Feline leukemia virus infection, apparently of domestic cat origin, has been documented in wild North American pumas, and in captive South American and African felids, including leopards and cheetahs. Infection is typically lifelong and associated with a number of clinical presentations, but disease outcomes within individual virus-positive animals may be variable. The natural infection among cats with feline leukemia virus was discovered in 1964 by its association with immunodeficiency diseases (and associated increased occurrence of opportunistic infections and anemia) and malignant or proliferative diseases such as lymphosarcomas and leukemias of lymphoid, myeloid, or erythroid origin. Knowledge about naturally occurring infections and associated diseases provided important foundations for researchers who later investigated human retroviruses and their association with immunodeficiency and neoplastic diseases.

Like feline immunodeficiency virus (a lentivirus) infection in cats, feline leukemia virus infection in healthy cats is usually low in prevalence (<2%), but can be increased as much as 30% in cats that are presented with certain illnesses or that are at a high risk of infection, for instance in cats from high-density populations. Common risk factors that increase the likelihood of infection include having free access to the outdoors, age (older cats are more likely to be positive), and male gender (because of fighting). In cats infected with feline leukemia virus, a prolonged clinical latency before exhibiting disease complicates control of the infection. Effective methods to identify and prevent the spread of the infection to naïve cats remain a key to controlling the infection in susceptible populations.

Feline leukemia virus is commonly transmitted horizontally by bite wounds and grooming, or from infected queens to kittens by transplacental transmission or from nursing. Kittens are more susceptible to infection than are older cats. The presence of viral antigens in serum and blood generally correlates with viremia and is used diagnostically. Some cats are infected but do not exhibit detectable antigen in their blood. Infected cats shed virus from most body fluids, including saliva and milk.

Pathogenesis and Pathology

Feline leukemia virus infection typically commences in the oral or pharyngeal lymphoid-associated tissues, and virus is then spread via monocytes and lymphocytes to peripheral tissues. It appears that most cats that are infected with feline leukemia virus will remain so for life, but a proportion of infected cats can have periods of time in which they are negative for viral antigen in blood as well as virus culture. The presence of provirus in blood leukocytes from these cats can be detected with sensitive PCR assays, confirming that they are indeed persistently infected. These "regressively" infected cats must develop immune responses that temporarily control virus replication and so limit their ability to shed virus and spread infection. These cats also do not usually succumb to feline leukemia virus-associated diseases. In contrast, cats that undergo "progressive" infection (e.g., those that are viral antigen positive) have pronounced virus replication in lymphoid tissues, bone marrow, and mucosal and glandular epithelial tissues. At mucosal sites the virus is shed in body fluids such as saliva. These cats do not appear to have sufficient immunity to control virus replication, and typically suffer from virus-associated diseases. Rarely, cats may be exposed to the virus but not become infected.

Feline leukemia virus infection is characterized by mixed infections of several genetically distinct, but related, virus strains. This variability is related to both changes within the infecting virus and its recombination with endogenous feline retroviruses in the infected cat. The viral determinants of feline leukemia virus pathogenicity are located within both the LTR (e.g., promoter regions of the provirus) and the SU (surface glycoprotein) of the virus. Thus unique strains may be more likely to be associated with particular disease outcomes (e.g., multicentric lymphosarcoma versus anemia). Genetic changes associated with pathogenic strains may result in a replication advantage for these strains and predict a more virulent outcome following natural infection of cats.

The SU protein is a major pathogenic determinant of feline leukemia virus. Subtle changes in SU can dramatically alter receptor use and disease outcomes. This protein has a receptor binding domain that controls virus entry into cells. On the basis of receptor usage and sequence variation in the *env* gene (encoding the SU protein), strains of feline leukemia virus have been subclassified in four subgroups: FeLV-A, -B, -C, and -T. In addition, FeLV-B and FeLV-C subgroups can arise from recombination of FeLV-A *env* gene with closely related endogenous FeLV elements in the cat genome, resulting in changes in receptor usage and disease outcomes. Without undergoing recombination or mutations in *env* genetic sequences, FeLV-A subgroups are minimally pathogenic; however, molecular clones of FeLV-A with particular *env* gene mutations can cause severe immunodeficiency. Strains of FeLV-C have been associated with severe aplastic anemia, and FeLV-B isolates have been linked to a number of disease outcomes. The most common clinical form of FeLV-B-associated disease is the thymic form of lymphosarcoma, but non-regenerative anemia and other lymphoid tumors and myeloid leukemia can also occur.

Feline leukemia virus associated lymphosarcoma has been linked to at least six conserved cellular integration sites. These sites are associated with dysregulation of cellular oncogenes controlling cell proliferation or represent v-*onc* transduced by feline leukemia virus infection. The first and most extensively studied is c-*myc* and, in some circumstances, v-*myc* (virus associated), in transformed lymphocytes. Insertion of feline leukemia provirus in the *flvi-2* locus, which encodes *bmi-1* and *pim-1* related genes, is also associated with c-*myc* dysregulation. Other integration sites include *flvi-1* in non-T-cell lymphomas, *flit-1* in thymic lymphomas, and *fit-1* in T-cell lymphomas (linked with c-*myb* control). Overexpression of a cell-surface receptor from the transforming growth factor-beta superfamily has also been associated with provirus insertion in *flit-1*.

Feline Lymphosarcoma (Lymphoma)

Feline lymphosarcoma is perhaps the most common naturally occurring lymphoid malignancy of mammals, and in some surveys accounts for up to 30% of all tumors in cats. There are both retrovirus-associated and non-viral forms of feline lymphosarcoma. The incidence of feline leukemia virus associated lymphomas has declined markedly in the United States since the advent of testing and control measures, whereas as many as 70% of feline lymphosarcomas by the presence of large numbers of neoplastic cells in the bone marrow, a non-regenerative anemia, and immunosuppression. Transformation of erythropoietic cells may produce erythroblastosis, erythroblastopenia, other cytopenias, or pancytopenia, all of which are associated with anemia.

Immunopathologic Disease Associated with Feline Leukemia Virus Infection

This group of conditions includes both immune-complex-mediated and immunodeficiency diseases. Persistently high levels of feline leukemia virus antigens are sometimes produced during infection, which, when bound in immune complexes, produce glomerulonephritis after the immune complexes are deposited within glomerular capillaries. In other cases, lymphocytes are depleted in part by antibody-dependent cytotoxicity, with feline oncovirus membrane-associated antigens (FOCMA) being the target. This leads to a variety of opportunistic infections in which the cat fails to thrive and can suffer from any one of several inflammatory diseases, including chronic stomatitis, gingivitis, non-healing skin lesions, subcutaneous abscesses, chronic respiratory disease, and a higher incidence of feline infectious peritonitis. In addition, toxoplasmosis and infection with *Mycoplasma haemofelis* are more common in cats infected with feline leukemia virus than in normal cats. Poor reproductive performance, including infertility, fetal deaths, and abortions, is also more likely to occur in feline leukemia virus infected cats.

Feline Fibrosarcoma

Fibrosarcomas usually manifest as solitary tumors in older cats. In young kittens infected with feline leukemia virus, feline sarcoma virus may, on rare occasions, induce a multifocal subcutaneous fibrosarcoma—a highly anaplastic form that grows rapidly with frequent metastasis. There is no evidence that feline sarcoma virus is transmitted horizontally, because it is replication defective; the tumors and the virus (feline sarcoma virus) arise after feline leukemia virus infection as a result of recombination and v-*onc* acquisition.

Rarely, cats will develop feline sarcoma after receiving vaccines or medications that are administered subcutaneously or intramuscularly and components of which persist at the site of injection for extended periods of time. These are very rare; however, they remain a concern for owners, but there is no evidence of an infectious etiology of these tumors.

Diagnosis

Commercially available test kits are used routinely for diagnostic screening for the p27 antigen of feline leukemia virus. This antigen is commonly found in the blood of

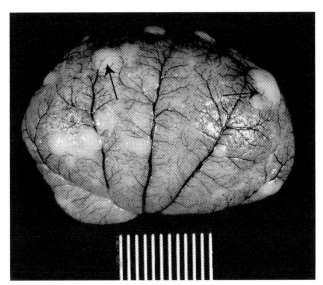

FIGURE 14.8 Lymphosarcoma in a cat. Variably sized neoplastic nodules (arrows) protrude from the cortex of the kidney. *(Courtesy of M. Lairmore and the Ohio State University.)*

were previously attributed to feline leukemia virus infection (before the 1980s). Four major forms of lymphosarcoma are recognized in cats, based on the location of the primary tumor: (1) *multicentric lymphosarcoma*, in which tumors occur in various lymphoid and non-lymphoid tissues; (2) *thymic lymphosarcoma*, occurring particularly in kittens; (3) *alimentary lymphosarcoma*, usually occurring in older cats in which lymphoid tissues of the gastrointestinal tract and/or mesenteric lymph nodes are affected; (4) *unclassified lymphosarcomas*, an uncommon finding in which tumors occur in non-lymphoid tissues such as the skin, eyes, and central nervous system. Of these various different types of lymphosarcoma, feline leukemia virus-induced tumors are typically of T cell lineage and are either multicentric, thymic, or affect the eyes or central nervous system. The appearance of lymphosarcoma is characteristic, regardless of location: lesions consist of variably sized accumulations of firm, homogeneous pale tissue composed of neoplastic lymphocytes (Figure 14.8).

Feline Myeloproliferative Diseases and Anemia

In this group of diseases, transformation of one or a combination of bone marrow cell types is induced by feline leukemia virus. Four types are recognized: (1) *erythremic myelosis*, in which the target is an erythroid progenitor cell; (2) *granulocytic leukemia*, in which a granulocytic myeloid progenitor cell, often of the neutrophil lineage, is targeted; (3) *erythroleukemia*, in which both erythroid and granulocytic myeloid precursors become neoplastic; (4) *myelofibrosis*, a proliferation of fibroblasts and cancellous bone resulting in medullary osteosclerosis and myelofibrosis. These diseases, which are similar to those produced by the acutely transforming avian retroviruses, are characterized progressively infected cats within 1 month of exposure. Within individual cats, particularly kittens, the test may need to be repeated, as variability occurs as to when antigenemia is first detectable. In low-risk or asymptomatic cases or when discordant test results occur, virus-specific PCR assay can be used to increase the sensitivity of detection or to confirm an antigen-positive test. Less commonly, immunofluorescence tests have been used as a confirmatory test to detect feline leukemia virus antigens, but this assay is prone to false-positive results and requires experienced operators. Virus culture in reference laboratories is possible, but not typically used in clinical practice. Discordant test results (e.g., antigen-positive and immunofluorescence assay-negative) occur, often as a result of variability in the cat's response to infection, timing of exposure, and laboratory errors. In such cases repeat testing is recommended. Vaccination does not typically interfere with feline leukemia virus antigen tests unless blood is sampled immediately after vaccination.

Immunity, Prevention, and Control

Feline leukemia virus infection is controlled through testing and prevention of virus spread among susceptible cats. Transmission via direct contact such as biting or grooming is common; thus identification and removal of infected cats from susceptible populations is central to effective control. Additional potential sources of contact such as nursing of infected queens and sharing of food, water, and litter pans must be considered in any control plan. A number of commercially available vaccines have been produced against feline leukemia virus, and these can be incorporated into control plans for susceptible animals and populations. Vaccine efficacy may vary, and does not eliminate the need for diagnostic testing before or as part of a postvaccination control program. In addition, the duration of immunity after vaccination may be variable. Vaccination of cats that already are positive for feline leukemia virus is of little value and not recommended. Although vaccines can protect against progressive infection and disease, they may not prevent infections after exposure to the virus.

Feline leukemia virions are unstable in the environment because of their lipid envelope, and can be inactivated with most commercial detergents or disinfectants. Thus cleaning procedures are important to an effective control plan against indirect infections, as debris such as dried blood may protect virions and prolong viability. Infected animals must be housed away from susceptible cats to prevent further spread, and immunosuppressed cats must be protected from cats with other infectious agents. Additional control measures include practices to limit spread from animal handling and instruments or equipment that may come in contact with infected cats. Animals housed indoors are less likely to be infected or pose a threat to infection control procedures.

In situations in which large numbers of cats are co-mingled, such as catteries or for outdoor cats, testing and removal combined with a vaccination program are recommended. Prior testing for infection is recommended for cats used for breeding or in situations in which new cats are brought into a group setting. Good management practices for cat shelters require testing and appropriate control procedures to reduce the risk of infections. Because virus-infected but asymptomatic cats, or symptomatic cats with proper veterinary care may live for months to years, decisions to euthanatize infected cats should be based on individual circumstances and the risk for further spread of the infection to susceptible cats. Virus-positive cats should be confined to prevent spread to virus-free cats, should undergo frequent health checks by a veterinarian, and should be neutered. Because infected cats may be immunosuppressed or prone to immune suppression, corticosteroids and other types of immune-suppressive drugs should be used with caution.

MURINE LEUKEMIA AND SARCOMA VIRUSES

Murine leukemia viruses were identified originally in the 1920s and 1930s; several viruses were isolated and passaged in mice, each somewhat different, and each given the name of the person identifying it, such as Gross, Friend, Moloney, Rauscher, and many other murine leukemia viruses. Gross murine leukemia virus was originally a mixture of non-oncogenic endogenous leukemia viruses (which recombined to become the oncogenic Gross murine leukemia virus), and the Friend, Moloney and Rauscher group of viruses appear to be most closely related to exogenous viruses that are no longer enzootic in laboratory mice, but are still used experimentally. These differently named viruses induce distinct tumors: Gross and Moloney viruses induce T cell lymphomas, whereas Friend and Rauscher viruses induce erythroleukemia. Some viruses are immunosuppressive, leading to the designation "murine acquired immunodeficiency syndrome (MAIDS)."

All mice carry endogenous murine leukemia virus sequences in their genome. The most recognized endogenous retroviruses of the mouse are the C-type murine leukemia viruses and the B-type murine mammary tumor viruses. These endogenous retroviruses both have closely related exogenous counterparts, which are transmitted primarily through the milk rather than as genetic determinants. The replication-competent endogenous retroviruses are therefore considered to be evolutionarily young introductions to the genome, whereas there are far greater numbers of replication-defective and more distantly related retrovirus-like sequences, including IAPs, VL30, Etns, and others, collectively known as retro-elements. These elements have been truncated, mutated, methylated, etc., to become non-infectious. However, these non-infectious elements are far from insignificant, in that they continue to re-integrate into the genome during cell division, resulting in many randomly distributed copies throughout the genome. These integrations have been responsible for mouse genetic drift, spontaneous mutations, and important mouse phenotypes, such as the nude allele, the hairless allele, rodless retina, and others.

Various inbred strains of mice were selectively bred for different patterns of lymphoma, mammary cancer, etc. This inbreeding resulted in selection of homozygous genomes containing unique combinations of endogenous retroviruses, presence or absence of cell receptors for those viruses, and cellular susceptibility factors for virus replication. These events are unique to the inbred nature of the laboratory mouse. The evolution of lymphomas has been extensively studied, revealing expression of non-oncogenic endogenous retroviruses at different ages and in different tissues, with sequential recombination of multiple endogenous retroviral genomes, resulting in evolution of infectious oncogenic viruses. Within any given inbred strain, endogenous viruses may be capable of infecting other mouse cells (ecotropic viruses) or may be incapable of infecting mouse cells but infectious to cells of other species (xenotropic viruses), or may be capable of infecting cells of mice in addition to other species (polytropic viruses). As mice age, endogenous retroviruses, the parental viruses of which were xenotropic and incapable of infecting other cells in the mouse, may acquire polytropic characteristics through recombination of multiple endogenous retroviruses, and thereby infect and transform cells in the host mouse. It took decades to unravel these complex events in lymphoma-susceptible inbred mice, such as AKR mice. Murine leukemia viruses are considered to be chronic transforming viruses, and induce tumors with latencies ranging from 2 to 18 months, depending on the strain of virus and strain of mouse. Acute transforming viruses, which have usurped cellular oncogenes such as v-*onc* genes, are largely experimental phenomena, but are used extensively for research. The Abelson murine leukemia virus serves as one such example and, because of its additional v-*onc*, is replication defective, requiring a replication-competent helper virus to replicate (the Moloney murine leukemia virus is often used for this purpose). Murine leukemia viruses are widely distributed in laboratory and wild mice. The wild mouse viruses have been important because they have shown new receptor specificities and distinct lesion patterns. Infections of laboratory mice with these viruses have been the cause over the years of many compromised experiments, especially long-term experiments and experiments that required mouse strains that express high levels of endogenous virus (e.g., AKR, C58, PL, HRS, CWD). The effect on experiments of the immunosuppression caused by some murine leukemia/sarcoma viruses has also not been well appreciated. Unlike the situation with other important murine viruses, there

is no way to eliminate murine leukemia/sarcoma viruses from a colony; nevertheless, in some circumstances, testing is warranted to assess viral load.

Friend virus isolates contain at least two viral components: a replication-competent Friend murine leukemia virus (F-MuLV) and a replication-defective spleen focus forming virus (SFFV). This pair of Friend viruses has been a useful model of retrovirus-induced leukemias. The murine leukemia virus component compensates for the replication-defective functions to the replication defective SFFV, whereas SFFV is the pathogenic component responsible for cell transformation leading to acute erythroleukemias. The molecular events of SFFV infection have provided evidence that the envelope of SFFV (gp55) interacts with the receptor for erythropoietin. This receptor is highly expressed on bone marrow precursor cells and, following binding of gp55, results in proliferation and differentiation of erythroid progenitor cells. This model has revealed that the leukemic progression depends on the cooperation of at least two oncogenic events, one interfering with differentiation and one conferring a proliferative advantage for the virus, similar to that proposed for the development of human acute myeloid leukemia.

RETROVIRUSES OF OTHER LABORATORY RODENTS

Endogenous retroviruses have been documented in laboratory rats, hamsters (both European and Syrian), and guinea pigs. Virus expression occurs in tumors and cell lines derived from these species, but viruses have not proven to be oncogenic when experimentally inoculated into any of these species. Rat endogenous retrovirus sequences have contributed to the development of murine sarcoma viruses, such as the Harvey murine sarcoma virus and the Kirsten sarcoma virus, which evolved from rats inoculated with mouse Moloney murine leukemia virus and mouse Kirsten erythroblastosis virus, respectively. These sarcoma viruses are defective, acute-transforming viruses that produce solid tumors of fibroblast origin, or transform fibroblasts *in vitro*.

PORCINE ENDOGENOUS RETROVIRUSES

All pigs, both domestic and wild, have multiple copies of endogenous gammaretroviruses called porcine endogenous retroviruses (PERV). The concern for potential transmission of these viruses during xenotransplantation (pig tissue to humans) has stimulated research on them. They are classified—in a manner analogous to the feline leukemia virus strains—as classes A (PERV-A), B (PERV-B), or C (PERV-C), on the basis of a combination of envelope sequence variation, receptor interference patterns, and cell-line tropism. PERV-A and -B can infect both pig and human cells in culture, whereas PERV-C infects only cells of porcine origin. The transmission of porcine endogenous retroviruses to humans following xenotransplantation has not been reported to date, but concerns persist because putatively human-tropic viruses have been reported after recombination from cell culture experiments. Furthermore, transmission of porcine endogenous retroviruses to mice has been reported following pig islet xenotransplantation. Porcine endogenous retroviruses also have host cell integration preferences near transcription start sites, similar to those of the murine leukemia viruses, which raises concerns for the use of these viruses as vectors for gene therapy.

AVIAN RETICULOENDOTHELIOSIS VIRUS

Reticuloendotheliosis viruses are pathogenic avian retroviruses that are antigenically and genetically unrelated to the avian leukosis/sarcoma retroviruses, but have a wider avian host range. Replication-competent avian reticuloendotheliosis viruses are considered simple retroviruses. Reticuloendotheliosis viruses are responsible for three syndromes: (1) runting disease syndrome; (2) neoplasia of lymphoid and other tissues; (3) acute reticulum cell neoplasia, which is not a spontaneous disease in the field. The runting syndrome has been associated primarily with use of contaminated vaccine in chickens, which has been corrected by improved quality-assurance testing of avian vaccines. Lymphomas induced by avian reticuloendotheliosis virus are rare in commercial poultry, but occur after a prolonged latency similar to that associated with lymphoid leukosis caused by avian leukosis virus. These reticuloendotheliosis-virus-induced tumors are B cell lymphomas that arise in the cloaca after transformation of IgM-bearing B cells, thus the name "reticuloendotheliosis" is inappropriate. These tumors have been linked to *cis*-activation of the cellular oncogene, *c-myc*. Five viruses have been recognized. The prototype of the group, reticuloendotheliosis virus-T, was isolated from an adult turkey with visceral reticuloendotheliosis and nerve lesions. Reticuloendotheliosis virus-T is replication defective and carries a v-*onc* gene, v-*rel*. The other avian reticuloendotheliosis viruses are non-defective strain T (reticuloendotheliosis virus A), duck infectious anemia virus, duck spleen necrosis virus, and chick syncytial virus. These viruses are all replication competent.

When inoculated into 1-day-old chicks, reticuloendotheliosis virus-T produces severe hepatosplenomegaly, with either marked necrosis or lymphoproliferative lesions. Major outbreaks of disease involving the deaths of large numbers of chickens have occurred as a consequence of contamination of turkey herpesvirus Marek's disease vaccine with reticuloendotheliosis virus-T. There is some evidence that the virus may also be transmitted mechanically by mosquitoes.

Epidemiologic studies using antibody screening methods indicate that reticuloendotheliosis virus infections are relatively common in commercial layer, broiler, and turkey flocks in the United States, but these infections cause minimal disease and so are of minor economic impact. The infection is naturally transmitted by direct contact among infected birds or vertically from infected birds to their offspring. Specific control procedures are not commonly practiced because of the low incidence of disease among commercial flocks.

MEMBERS OF THE SUBFAMILY *ORTHORETROVIRINAE*, GENUS *DELTARETROVIRUS*

BOVINE LEUKEMIA VIRUS

Bovine leukemia (*syn.* enzootic bovine leukosis) was first described in 1871, but attracted significant attention early in the 20th century in several European countries, notably Denmark and Germany, where clusters of herds with a high incidence of a similar disease suggested a viral etiology. However, the viral etiology of this disease was not described until 1969. Bovine leukemia virus is classified in the genus *Deltaretrovirus*, which also includes the related viruses human T lymphotropic virus type 1 (HTLV-1) and simian T lymphotropic viruses (STLV-1, -2, and -3). Bovine leukemia virus infection occurs worldwide, but varies in prevalence depending on the country and type of cattle herd, with dairy cattle often having a high rate of infection. Successful eradication programs recently have been implemented in some countries, notably those of the European Union.

Two patterns of disease associated with bovine leukemia virus are recognized. In addition to the sporadic and lethal form of the disease, bovine leukemia virus infection is also associated with persistent lymphocytosis caused by a sustained increase in numbers of circulating B lymphocytes. The majority of infected cattle remain asymptomatic throughout their lives, but a significant proportion (approximately 1–5%) of adult cattle infected with this virus will develop multicentric lymphosarcoma.

Clinical Features and Epidemiology

Bovine leukemia virus is horizontally transmitted between cattle through the transfer of infected cells via direct contact, through milk, and possibly mechanically from insect bites. Importantly for veterinarians and owners, the virus can be spread via routine procedures involving blood from infected animals if proper decontamination practices are not followed. Despite the low incidence of diseases associated with bovine leukemia virus, the infection does cause significant economic losses for some countries, such as the United States, from culling of high-producing dairy cattle and restrictions on exportation of cattle. The virus and disease have been eradicated from many countries in Europe and Scandinavia using control programs, and the European Commission recently announced Austria, Belgium, Cyprus, Czech Republic, Denmark, Finland, France, Germany, Iceland, Ireland, Luxembourg, Netherlands, Norway, Slovenia, Sweden, the Slovak Republic, and the United Kingdom to be free, in addition to extensive portions of Italy and Poland.

The natural host for bovine leukemia virus is domestic cattle, and some studies suggest that water buffaloes are also naturally infected. The infection can be experimentally transmitted to several species, including rabbits, rats, chickens, pigs, goats, and sheep. Sheep develop an accelerated course of leukemia and lymphoma from experimental infection, and have been used as a model of the disease. There is no evidence that bovine leukemia virus infects humans, and extensive epidemiological studies have failed to show any connection between milk consumption and leukemia in people drinking raw milk from infected cattle.

Pathogenesis and Pathology

Most bovine leukemia virus infections are asymptomatic and are recognized only by serological testing. Among infected cattle, about 30% develop persistent lymphocytosis, but this is not associated with any clinical signs. In those few animals that do develop disease, clinical signs are seen in adults typically between 4 and 8 years of age. These animals develop multicentric lymphoid tumors (i.e., lymphosarcomas) in lymph nodes, abomasum, heart, spleen, kidneys, uterus, spinal meninges, retrobulbar region, and brain (Figure 14.9), but not any consistent

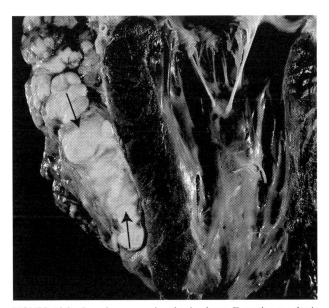

FIGURE 14.9 Lymphosarcoma in a bovine heart. Extensive neoplastic involvement (arrows) of the epicardial surface. *(Courtesy of M. Lairmore and the Ohio State University.)*

presence of large numbers of malignant cells in the blood as suggested by the name of the disease and the virus.

The primary target cells of bovine leukemia virus are B lymphocytes that express IgM, but the virus also infects monocytes and macrophages. Following infection, a polyclonal expansion of lymphocytes occurs that is probably driven by the virus to promote virus spread and establish sufficient integrated proviruses to maintain the infection. Infection of cattle is typically life-long, and the animals harbor lymphocytes that will divide and maintain the virus by clonal expansion of infected cells. Virus replication during early dissemination of the virus is dependent upon viral proteins that either are required for transactivation of viral promoters or are involved in cell activation or survival. A key determinant is the transactivating protein, Tax, which acts to enhance transcription of the viral promoter (LTR), but key cellular genes that promote lymphocytes to proliferate are also important.

After a prolonged clinical latency, a certain percentage of cell clones dominate and survive following somatic mutation and immune evasion. Within this population, those clones that develop a growth advantage continue to proliferate as transformed lymphocytes. Transformation of lymphocytes is not the result of insertion of provirus into particular cellular sequences (c-oncogenes) or the insertion of viral oncogene. Instead, bovine leukemia virus produces the oncoprotein, Tax, that promotes cell survival and proliferation, leading ultimately to the emergence of transformed cells. Additionally, bovine leukemia virus probably escapes immune elimination by tightly controlling viral gene expression *in vivo* by a self-attenuating process that allows the virus to maintain low levels of virus transcription while promoting cell survival by inhibiting apoptosis. In fact, some tumors, particularly those from terminal cases, do not contain the complete viral genome and fail to express viral antigens unless they are placed in culture and stimulated.

Diagnosis

The presence of bovine leukemia virus infection in cattle herds is indicated by an abnormally high prevalence of multicentric lymphosarcoma in adult animals. Enzyme immunoassay, agar gel diffusion, and syncytium-inhibition assays are used for serological diagnosis of bovine leukemia virus infection. Test and removal programs have been adopted by numerous European countries, and these countries require that imported cattle be serologically negative using standardized tests. In other countries, including the United States and Canada, individual owners have undertaken test and removal programs on a voluntary basis, but national programs are not in place. Virus-specific PCR assays have been developed.

Immunity, Prevention, and Control

Following infection, virus-specific antibodies can be detected within a few weeks by most assays and persist throughout the life of the infected animal. Antibodies are directed at most structural components, but are particularly strong against viral envelope (gp51) and capsid (p24) proteins; however, antibodies can be directed at regulatory proteins such as Tax. These antibodies have been demonstrated to mediate antibody-dependent cell lysis. Concurrently, cytotoxic T lymphocytes (CTLs) are produced and appear to be directed at either viral envelope or Tax. In cattle, γ/δ T lymphocytes make up a significant portion of the CTL response. Although robust, the immune response of bovine leukemia virus infected cattle does not eliminate the infection. These responses persist throughout the lifetime of the infected animal, but the cytotoxic and helper T cell responses may diminish over time, leaving these animals more susceptible to infection by opportunistic pathogens.

The transmission of bovine leukemia virus is highly cell dependent, thus natural or iatrogenic routes of transmission invariably are the result of transfer of infected cells. Transmission of the virus has been associated with trauma, restraint devices, gloves used for rectal examination, re-use of needles and surgical instruments, and, rarely, by insects acting as mechanical vectors. Some infected cattle have lymphocytes with very high virus copy numbers per cell whereas others have low copy numbers, thus making some animals more at risk for transmission of the virus. Fewer than 10% of calves born to infected dams are infected at birth. Although definitive data are lacking, it has been proposed that calves nursing infected mothers may become infected from lymphocytes in the colostrum or milk.

Virus may be eliminated from a herd if all cattle are tested serologically at 2–3-month intervals and positive animals removed immediately. The length of time required to obtain a virus-free herd varies, depending on the initial prevalence of infection. If the prevalence of infection is too high to permit removal of all serologically positive animals, segregation of seropositive and seronegative animals may be attempted. Calves from infected dams should be isolated, tested, and allowed to enter the seronegative cohort only if seronegative at 6 months of age. Vaccination is not used for control of the infection, although an experimental inactivated vaccine has been shown to prevent disease following virus challenge.

MEMBERS OF THE SUBFAMILY *ORTHORETROVIRINAE*, GENUS EPSILONRETROVIRUS

RETROVIRUSES OF FISH (WALLEYE DERMAL SARCOMA VIRUS)

A number of proliferative lesions of fish are attributed to retrovirus infection, including those associated with walleye dermal sarcoma virus, discrete epidermal hyperplasia virus types 1 and 2, and Atlantic salmon swim bladder sarcoma virus. In some cases these lesions occur in a seasonal pattern—that is, they develop and regress annually. One of the best characterized members of this group is the walleye dermal sarcoma virus that is associated with a multicentric skin tumor of the walleye (*Sander vitreus*), an important North American sport fish. Tumor prevalence ranges from 27% of adult walleyes in densely populated lakes such as Oneida Lake, New York, to 1% in less populated waters. Phylogenetic analysis of virus isolates from different regions of North America indicates that there are distinct genotypic clusters, suggesting that the various viral genotypes have a long association with fish in various lakes. Two other retroviruses have been isolated from walleyes—walleye epidermal hyperplasia viruses 1 and 2—and other retroviruses have been isolated from snakeheads, sea bass, and salmon. The sea bass virus has been associated with an erythrocytic disease and the salmon virus with leukemia.

The molecular and cellular events leading to the seasonal induction and regression of walleye dermal sarcoma are not completely understood, but are likely to include complex interactions of viral and host factors—for example, hormonally regulated changes in viral gene expression, and variations in the immune response of fish at different water temperatures. The genomic structures of these retroviruses of fish include genes that encode unique proteins that regulate cell survival and may contribute to lesion development and regression. For example, there are two non-overlapping open frames, *orf-A* and *orf-B*, distal to *env* in the walleye dermal sarcoma virus and, importantly, *orf-A* encodes a retroviral cyclin (rv-cyclin) that is distantly related to cellular cyclins that control the cell cycle.

The epsilonretroviruses do not appear to reinfect feral walleyes or cause tumors or proliferative lesions in subsequent years. In addition, experimentally, walleye fingerlings with lesions induced by walleye dermal sarcoma virus are more resistant to new tumor production than are fingerlings that have experienced no previous virus challenge. The immune system, however, does not appear to play a major role in the regression of established lesions.

MEMBERS OF THE SUBFAMILY *ORTHORETROVIRINAE*, GENUS *LENTIVIRUS*

Lentivirus-associated diseases have long been recognized and described in veterinary medicine; however, the discovery in 1983 that human AIDS is also caused by a lentivirus (HIV) rapidly accelerated the study of this genera of retroviruses. There has been remarkable progress in defining the basic properties of these viruses and the pathogenesis of the diseases they cause. Human AIDS now serves as a paradigm for the better understanding of the lentivirus diseases of veterinary importance, and the lentivirus diseases of animals are used as models for the study of the human disease. This "cross-fertilization" even involves the surrogate testing of drugs and vaccines in the equivalent AIDS-like primate, equine, and feline disease models, with the aim of developing preventive and therapeutic regimens for animals as well as humans. In this regard, all the animal lentiviruses and the diseases they cause are of interest, each providing particular lessons and particular experimental advantages.

VISNA-MAEDI (OVINE PROGRESSIVE PNEUMONIA) VIRUS

In 1933, 20 Karakul sheep were imported into Iceland from Germany, and within 2 years two diseases, respectively called *maedi* (dyspnea) and *visna* (wasting), emerged, which in the following years were responsible for the deaths of 105,000 sheep. These same Karakul sheep reportedly were also the source of pulmonary adenomatosis virus infection in Icelandic sheep. A further 600,000 sheep were slaughtered in 1965, when the diseases were declared eradicated. These diseases have an incubation period of more than 2 years, an insidious onset, and a protracted clinical course, lasting 6 months to several years, unless terminated by concurrent disease. Björn Sigurdsson, a physician, performed pioneering work to demonstrate that both Icelandic diseases were transmissible with cell-free filtrates, described the diseases as "slow virus infections," and introduced this concept into the field of virology.

It is now clear that maedi and visna are caused by the same or very closely related lentiviruses that have more recently been designated as small ruminant lentiviruses, a grouping that includes ovine lentivirus (*syn.* visna-maedi virus) and closely related caprine arthritis-encephalitis virus. Ovine lentivirus infection occurs in all sheep-producing countries except Australia and New Zealand, and associated respiratory disease (maedi) has been described in several countries in Europe (where in the Netherlands it is called "Zwoegerziekte" and in France "la bouhite"), in South Africa (where it is called "Graaf Reinet disease"), and in the North America (where it is called "ovine progressive pneumonia").

Comparative studies of the *gag-pol* or *pol* regions have led to grouping of small ruminant lentiviruses into four related groups, designated A–D. Group A viruses are further divided into at least seven subtypes, A1–A7, where the subtype A1 is identified by the genetically and geographically heterogeneous visna-maedi viruses and group B refers to the caprine arthritis-encephalitis virus and comprises only two distinct subtypes, B1 and B2. Groups C and D are represented by just a few virus isolates or recognized only by *pol* sequences. Direct evidence for natural sheep-to-goat and goat-to-sheep transmissions of particular subtypes has been reported.

Clinical Features and Epidemiology

The onset of clinical signs of maedi (ovine progressive pneumonia) is insidious and is seldom detected in sheep less than 3 years of age. Incubation periods of up to 8 years have been recorded. There is progressive weight loss; dyspnea, initially detectable only after exercise, becomes progressively more apparent over time. Affected sheep lag behind when the flock is driven. The head may jerk rhythmically with each inspiration, nostrils are flared, and there may be a slight nasal discharge and a concurrent cough. Severely dyspneic sheep spend much time lying down. The clinical course may last 3–8 months; it may be prolonged by careful nursing or shortened by pregnancy, stress such as occasioned by inclement weather or poor nutrition, or concurrent disease, particularly bacterial pneumonia. Pregnant ewes may abort or deliver weak lambs.

The incubation period of visna varies from a few months to as long as 9 years. The onset of clinical signs is insidious and usually begins with slight weakness of the hind legs. Affected sheep may not be able to keep up with the flock and may stumble and fall for no apparent reason. There is progressive weight loss and trembling of facial muscles and lips. The paresis eventually leads to paraplegia. There is no fever, appetite is maintained, and sheep remain alert. The clinical course may last several years, with periods of remission. The cerebrospinal fluid contains increased numbers of mononuclear cells.

The prevalence of ovine lentivirus infections varies in enzootic regions, depending on husbandry conditions and management practices. The virus is transmitted from infected ewe to nursing lambs through colostrum or milk and, where animals are housed together, direct transmission from nasal secretions and sexual transmission can occur. Seroprevalence of approximately 10–40% has been documented amongst sheep in North America.

Pathogenesis and Pathology

Before 1933, Icelandic sheep were genetically isolated for approximately 1000 years and it has been suggested, but not proven, that there may be a genetic predisposition to lentivirus disease, especially visna. The virus is probably acquired most commonly by droplet infection via the respiratory tract, followed by a monocyte-associated viremia. It appears that the cell and tissue tropism varies amongst virus strains, perhaps reflecting variation in the long terminal repeat (LTR) region of the genome.

Apart from neurogenic muscle atrophy, there are no characteristic gross lesions of visna, and histological lesions are usually confined to the central nervous system, although lesions also may be present in the lungs. The characteristic lesion in the central nervous system is a demyelinating leukoencephalomyelitis. The meninges and subependymal spaces are infiltrated with mononuclear cells, mainly lymphocytes, with some plasma cells and macrophages. There is perivascular cuffing, neuronal necrosis, malacia, and demyelination scattered patchily throughout the central nervous system.

Gross findings in maedi (ovine progressive pneumonia) are restricted to the lungs and associated lymph nodes. The lungs are extensively consolidated, and do not collapse and show rib impressions when the thoracic cavity is opened. The parenchyma is pale with a few small gray foci and has a uniformly rubbery texture. Bronchial and mediastinal lymph nodes are enlarged greatly. Histologically, there is hyperplasia of the fibrous tissue and muscle of the alveolar septa and a mononuclear cell inflammatory infiltration. Interstitial pneumonia is accompanied by lymphoid nodules surrounding vessels and airways.

The lesions of visna in particular appear to be immunologically mediated, as lesions are minimal in sheep subjected to immune suppression before infection. Similarly, it is proposed that cellular immune responses to persistently infected cells in the respiratory system are responsible for the lesions of maedi.

In addition to chronic pneumonia and weight loss, ovine lentivirus infection can be associated with indurative mastitis with agalactia and, more rarely, arthritis. With mastitis, the affected udder is diffusely firmer than normal, and histologically there is diffuse interstitial lymphocytic infiltration and formation of lymphoid nodules that are often periductal with extension and protrusion into the duct lumen.

Diagnosis

A presumptive diagnosis of ovine lentivirus infection can be made on the basis of clinical signs, although only a small proportion of animals are typically affected. Histologic lesions are characteristic, and useful to correlate with serologic results; however, these changes are not pathognomonic. The most common method to diagnose ovine lentivirus infection is to test for the presence of antibodies. A number of serologic tests are available including: agar gel immunodiffusion (AGID), ELISA, radioimmunoprecipitation (RIPA), and western blotting. The specific method used may depend on resources available and number of samples to be tested. The most widely used diagnostic tests for the detection of virus-specific antibody are enzyme immunoassays in which either or both core and surface viral antigens are present. Western blots are more sensitive and are used frequently to confirm a diagnosis. Virus can be detected in blood, although viral loads are often low. Viral DNA may be detected in tissues by virus-specific PCR assays or by *in-situ* hybridization. Virus can be isolated by co-cultivation of gradient-purified peripheral blood leukocytes with mitogen-stimulated purified sheep peripheral blood leukocytes in the presence of interleukin 2.

Immunity, Prevention, and Control

Lentiviruses are refractory to clearance by host immune responses, including the production of neutralizing antibodies in addition to cell-mediated immune responses; neither virus nor infected cells are eliminated. In fact, immune suppression can delay the progress of degenerative changes associated with lesions induced by ovine lentivirus, suggesting an immunopathologic element in lesion development. In infected sheep, antigenic variation in the envelope antigens of the virus occurs over time, which may be an important mechanism for circumventing virus elimination and a key in the pathogenesis of the disease.

Prevention of ovine lentivirus transmission is difficult in enzootic situations, as these viruses are shed in a variety of body fluids, including blood, semen, bronchial secretions, tears, saliva, and milk. Droplet transmission is facilitated by housing and close confinement, and was important in Iceland, where sheep are housed for 6 months of the year. Natural transmission occurs from infected ewes to their lambs via colostrum and milk, thus removal of lambs prior to colostrum ingestion can be used as a means to generate a virus-free lock. Evidence for transplacental infection is conflicting, but virus may be shed in semen of rams with a high viral load. Contaminated surgical equipment or needles can readily transmit virus mechanically from viremic sheep if correct decontamination procedures are not followed.

Visna-maedi was eradicated from Iceland by a drastic slaughter policy, before the availability of any diagnostic test. Test and removal programs are used elsewhere.

CAPRINE ARTHRITIS-ENCEPHALITIS VIRUS

First recognized in the United States in 1974 by Dr Linda Cork and co-workers, caprine arthritis-encephalitis is now known to occur worldwide. In the United States, the disease is an economically important disease of goats, with infection rates as high as 80% in some herds. The causative virus is most closely related to North American isolates of visna-maedi virus. Two syndromes are recognized: encephalomyelitis in kids 2–4 months of age and, more commonly, arthritis in goats from about 12 months of age onward. The virus is not known to be transmitted naturally to other animal species, although experimentally the virus infects sheep and causes arthritis. Despite the high incidence of caprine arthritis-encephalitis virus infection in goats in Australia and New Zealand, infection of sheep has not been reported in these countries.

Clinical Features and Epidemiology

The central nervous system disease, now a rare outcome of infection, is a progressive leukoencephalomyelitis associated with ascending paralysis. Affected goats also show

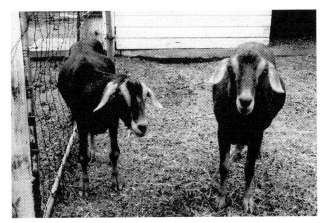

FIGURE 14.10 Caprine arthritis encephalitis. Swollen joints in affected goats. *(Courtesy of M. Lairmore and the Ohio State University.)*

progressive wasting and trembling and the hair coat is dull, but they remain afebrile, alert, and usually maintain good appetite and sight. Terminally there is paralysis, deviation of the head and neck, and paddling. The onset of arthritis is usually insidious and progresses slowly over months to years, but in some cases disease may appear suddenly and remain static. The joints are swollen and painful (Figure 14.10), particularly the carpal joints, but also hock, stifle, shoulder, fetlock, and vertebral joints. Cold weather exacerbates the signs. Bursae—particularly the atlanto-occipital—and tendon sheaths are thickened and distended with fluid. Progressive thickening of the capsules and lining of affected joints can result in restricted movement and flexion contracture. Infected goats may also exhibit lymphocytic mastitis and interstitial pneumonia similar to those observed in sheep infected with visna-maedi virus.

Pathogenesis and Pathology

At necropsy, central nervous system lesions may be visible as focal malacia in predominantly white matter, but are identified more reliably microscopically as foci of mononuclear cell inflammation and demyelination. The characteristic lesion in affected joints is a proliferative synovitis; tendon sheaths and bursae are characterized by villus hypertrophy, synovial cell hyperplasia, and infiltration with lymphocytes, plasma cells, and macrophages. Progression is accompanied by degenerative changes, including fibrosis, necrosis, mineralization of synovial membranes, and osteoporosis. A lymphocytic mastitis with accumulation of lymphoid nodules can occur in affected animals, as can mild interstitial pneumonia with hyperplasia of pulmonary lymphoid tissue. A very florid and severe interstitial pneumonia occurs rarely.

Diagnosis

Caprine arthritis encephalitis virus-specific antibodies can be detected by agar gel diffusion, indirect immunofluorescence, or ELISA, and form the basis of voluntary control programs that are based on test and removal. As with visna-maedi of sheep, the presence of proviral DNA in seropositive animals can be confirmed using virus-specific PCR assay.

Immunity, Prevention, and Control

Infection of goats with caprine arthritis encephalitis virus is acquired during the neonatal period, via colostrum or milk. The rate of infection of newborn goats can be reduced by more than 90% by removing kids from infected does as they are born, providing them with colostrum that has been heated to 56°C for 1 hour, feeding them pasteurized goat's or cow's milk, and raising them in isolation from infected goats. Serological tests such as the AGID test can be used to monitor herd status.

EQUINE INFECTIOUS ANEMIA VIRUS

Equine infectious anemia (EIA) was first described in France in 1843 and was subsequently associated with infection by a "filterable agent" in 1904, becoming one of the first animal diseases to be assigned a viral etiology. Equine infectious anemia is an important disease of horses that occurs worldwide, and which may manifest as an acute syndrome that ends fatally within a month of onset or as a chronic relapsing disease. It may also remain silent for the life of the infected horse.

Clinical Features and Epidemiology

After primary infection, most horses develop fever after an incubation period of 7–21 days. The disease is recognized as four interchanging, overlapping syndromes: In *acute* equine infectious anemia there is a marked fever, weakness, severe anemia, jaundice, tachypnea, and petechial hemorrhages of the mucosae. Many acute cases are fatal, whereas others pass into the *subacute* form, in which continuing moderate fever is followed by recovery. Recovery from either the acute or the subacute disease is followed by *life-long persistent infection*. Recovered viremic horses may appear and perform well, but some experience recurrent episodes of disease, whereas others develop *chronic disease* that varies from mild signs of illness and failure to thrive to episodic or persistent fever, cachexia, anemia, and ventral edema.

Tabanid flies and stable flies (*Stomoxys* spp.) can serve as mechanical vectors for equine infectious anemia virus. Transmission occurs particularly in the summer months in low-lying, humid, swamps. Prevalence can be very high on farms where infection has been enzootic for many years. Iatrogenic transmission by the use of non-sterile equipment has been responsible for some major outbreaks. Transplacental infection has been recognized; colostrum and milk, saliva, urine, and semen are other unproved but possible modes of transmission.

Pathogenesis and Pathology

Equine infectious anemia virus initially infects macrophages, and life-long, cell-associated viremia develops in all infected horses. The precise mechanism of the anemia and thrombocytopenia that occur in some infected horses remains uncertain, although complement is implicated in the lysis of red cells. The vasculitis and glomerulonephritis that occur in some animals result from deposition of immune complexes of viral antigen and specific antibody. Hemorrhages may be a consequence of thrombocytopenia.

Envelope gene variation that occurs during virus-replication-induced mutations leads to the emergence of virus variants during the course of persistent infection; these novel variants possess new neutralization-sensitive epitopes within the gp90, and recurrent episodes of disease are associated with the emergence of these antigenic variants of the gp90 envelope protein. Neutralization assays confirm that serum collected during early febrile episodes can neutralize isolates associated with establishment of infection, but fail to neutralize viruses isolated from subsequent febrile episodes.

Diagnosis

Clinical diagnosis can be confirmed by either enzyme immunoassay or the immunodiffusion test (the so-called Coggins test, named after its inventor, Dr Leroy Coggins). Foals nursing infected dams test positive temporarily, and recently infected horses may test negative. As with other retrovirus infections, a positive serological result can be confirmed by western immunoblot analysis and the presence of proviral DNA in peripheral blood leukocytes confirmed by virus-specific PCR assay.

Immunity, Prevention, and Control

Initial equine infectious anemia virus infection causes a high-titer, infectious plasma viremia within 3 weeks of exposure. Both humoral and cellular virus-specific responses are required to terminate the initial viremia, via the action of virus-specific cytotoxic T cells and non-neutralizing virus-specific antibodies. Infected horses develop strong responses against both the surface (gp90) and transmembrane (gp45) proteins of the virus. However, low levels of viral infection and virus replication occur in tissue macrophages of asymptomatically infected carrier horses, with associated presence of virus in plasma. The critical importance of immune control has been demonstrated in experimental settings, in which immune suppression is associated with reactivation of the virus and occurrence of disease symptoms long after the initial infection.

Cytotoxic T lymphocytes (CTLs) that are generated in infected horses recognize and lyse cells expressing epitopes of either Gag or Env. CTLs directed to Rev epitopes have been found in subclinically infected horses, suggesting that responses against this key regulatory protein may control disease outcome. Virus-specific neutralizing antibodies that are able to block the infecting strain usually emerge only after 2 or 3 months following infection, suggesting that they are not responsible for the termination of the acute episode. The level of neutralizing antibodies does not correlate with the course of the disease, as titers of neutralizing antibodies fluctuate significantly during the course of infection and their role in controlling virus replication remains unclear.

Virus transmission in enzootic areas may be reduced by stabling of horses in insect-secure facilities during those times of the year (summer) and that time of the day (dusk) when biting insects are most active. Iatrogenic transmission is avoided by careful hygiene. Equine infectious anemia virus infection now is controlled in many countries by rigorous testing to identify infected horses, an approach that was made feasible with the advent of highly sensitive and specific serological tests such as the Coggins test. Seropositive horses are either euthanized or kept in quarantine for the remainder of their lives.

FELINE IMMUNODEFICIENCY VIRUS

Since its first isolation by Dr Niels Pedersen and co-workers in 1987, feline immunodeficiency virus infection in the domestic cat has been recognized as a significant cause of immune suppression in infected cats and as a useful model of HIV–AIDS. Feline immunodeficiency virus is associated with progressive immune suppression leading to an increased susceptibility to opportunistic infections.

Clinical Features and Epidemiology

Feline immunodeficiency virus infection occurs in domestic cats worldwide, and in a variety of wild feline species. The seroprevalence in random surveys in asymptomatic domestic cats is typically low ($\approx 1\%$), but increases to 30% in sick domestic cats. The incidence of infection is also much higher in certain regions. Feline immunodeficiency virus associated disease occurs in three stages: an acute stage marked by lymphadenopathy and fever, a long subclinical stage, and a terminal stage marked by progressive loss of immune function, opportunistic infections, and, sometimes, neoplasia. Common presenting clinical signs are similar to those of cats infected with feline leukemia virus, and include an insidious onset of recurrent fever of undetermined origin, lymphadenopathy, leukopenia, anemia, weight loss, and non-specific behavioral changes.

In the terminal stage, opportunistic bacterial and fungal infections are especially common in the mouth, periodontal tissue, cheeks, and tongue. About 25% of cats have chronic respiratory disease, and a lesser number have chronic enteritis, urinary tract infection, dermatitis, and neurologic signs. The terminal disease may resemble advanced human AIDS.

Pathogenesis and Pathology

The incubation period of feline immunodeficiency virus infection may last for several years; progression of the disease that follows parallels the decline in CD4$^+$ T lymphocytes. Infected cats have a higher than expected incidence of feline leukemia virus-negative lymphomas, usually of the B cell type, and myeloproliferative disorders (neoplasias and dysplasias). Cats infected with particular virus strains can develop inflammatory lesions in the brain, particularly affecting the cerebral cortex and basal ganglia. Cats remain infected for life; the presence of serum antibodies is correlated directly with the ability to isolate virus from blood cells and saliva.

The major mode of virus transmission is via bite wounds and, less commonly, from infected queens to their kittens. Sexual transmission appears to be uncommon, although semen of infected males contains virus. The initial infection is often not recognized by owners and is associated with transient fever, lymphadenopathy, and leukopenia. Following exposure, virus can be detected in blood by virus isolation methods or virus-specific PCR assay. Within the first few weeks of feline immunodeficiency virus infection, lymphopenia precedes an active immune response that is marked by the production of virus-specific antibodies, suppression of circulating viral load, and a rebound and persistent increase in numbers of CD8$^+$ T lymphocytes and inversion of CD4$^+$:CD8$^+$ T lymphocyte ratios. Eventually, both subsets of lymphocytes decline and immune suppression occurs, making infected cats susceptible to opportunistic pathogens.

Cats may remain asymptomatic for prolonged periods after the initial infection, despite a decline in CD4$^+$ T lymphocyte counts. Eventually, infected cats suffer from chronic inflammatory conditions, and in some cases neoplasia. Within 2 weeks of infection, antibodies against viral structural antigens are detected that typically persist throughout the course of infection, except during terminal immune-system exhaustion.

Diagnosis

Cats infected with feline immunodeficiency virus typically maintain detectable serum antibodies, which is useful for routine diagnostic screening, but will not differentiate the response of naturally infected cats from that of vaccinated animals. Commercial test kits can detect antibodies to several antigens, including the viral p24 capsid protein. The development of detectable antibodies may be delayed in some cats, and re-testing is necessary in some circumstances such as suspected recent exposures. Confirmatory testing is recommended for animals at low risk and in asymptomatic but exposed cats. Western immunoblot and immunofluorescence assays can detect antibodies against a range of viral antigens, but may be less sensitive and specific. Vaccinated cats produce antibodies that cannot be distinguished by any current commercially available antibody test and may persist for more than 4 years.

Positive antibody tests in kittens younger than 6 months must be carefully interpreted because of the presence of maternal antibodies. Because kittens do not commonly become infected with the virus, most that test positive for feline immunodeficiency virus antibodies are not truly infected and will test negative when re-evaluated. Although infection of kittens is uncommon, it does occasionally occur, and kittens older than 6 months that have virus-specific antibodies are considered to be infected.

Virus culture is considered a gold standard for identification of feline immunodeficiency virus infection, but is not routinely available. Confirmation of infection using PCR assays has been described; however, the sensitivities and specificities of individual assays appear to be variable.

Immunity, Prevention, and Control

The presence of virus-specific neutralizing antibodies does not correlate with virus clearance or disease progression in cats infected with feline immunodeficiency virus. In contrast, increases in CD8$^+$ T cell counts are associated with declining viremia, probably through both cytotoxic and non-cytotoxic mechanisms. CD8$^+$ cytotoxic activity appears to be antigen specific and MHC class I restricted, and is persistent in most cats. In virus-infected cats, a population of antigen-non-specific, non-cytotoxic, antiviral CD8$^+$ cells has also been described that suppresses virus replication.

Despite a vigorous immune response, feline immunodeficiency virus infected cats remain viremic and eventually suffer from progressive immune dysfunction and opportunistic infections, even before declines in CD4$^+$ T cells numbers are measurable. Several mechanisms appear to be responsible for this immune dysfunction, including cytokine dysregulation, immunologic anergy, and inappropriate activation of immune regulatory cells. Virus-infected cats have altered cytokine levels, including decreased interleukin (IL)-2 and increased IL-6 and tumor necrosis factor-α production by blood leukocytes in response to immune stimulation. Recent studies also suggest impairments in innate immune responses in the feline immunodeficiency virus infected cats. Overall, the infection appears to produce a shift from T-helper 1 (Th-1) to T-helper 2 (Th-2) cells, cytokine dysregulation, and suppressed innate and cellular immune responses, which ultimately cause anergy and apoptosis of lymphocytes in primary lymphoid tissues.

Following experimental feline immunodeficiency virus infection, a significant increase in the percentage of CD4$^+$ and CD8$^+$ T cells that express B7.1 and B7.2 molecules has been demonstrated in infected cats as compared with uninfected cats. The percentage of B7- and CTLA4-positive

CD4$^+$ and CD8$^+$ T cells appears to increase with disease progression. This dysregulation may explain the progressive loss of T cell immune function and increase in lymph node T cell apoptosis that is characteristic of persistent infection. Several studies have reported an activated T-regulatory (Treg) cell population in infected cats, which may contribute to suppression of T cell immune responses. It has been postulated that viral antigen presentation leads to activation of T and B cells, which in turn results in activation of Treg cells to dampen the immune response. This dampened immune response may permit continued virus replication, which, in turn, continues to activate T cells. This chronic activation of T cells would maintain Treg cell activation, resulting in a global immune suppression and the inability to respond to secondary infections.

Feline immunodeficiency virus is shed mainly in the saliva, and the principal mode of transmission is through bites. Because of this, free-roaming (feral and pet), male, and aged cats are at the greatest risk of infection. Feline immunodeficiency virus infection is uncommon in closed purebred catteries. Neither sexual contact nor maternal grooming appears to be a significant mode of transmission, although virus may be shed in semen. However, the virus is transmitted to kittens from acutely infected queens, through colostrum and milk.

Vaccines against feline immunodeficiency virus are available but of variable efficacy, in part because of poor induction of cross-protective immunity against the variety of virus strains that circulate among susceptible populations of cats. Thus feline immunodeficiency virus vaccines are typically considered discretionary (non-essential), although they may be considered for cats with lifestyles that put them at high risk of infection, such as outdoor cats or cats living with infected cats.

Appropriate test and removal programs and certification at the point of sale can be applied to control the infection. No human public health risks have been identified in association with the infection in cats.

SIMIAN IMMUNODEFICIENCY VIRUS

At least 40 species of African non-human primates are naturally infected with unique strains of simian immunodeficiency virus (SIV), suggesting that these viruses have evolved with adaption in each host species. For example, a high proportion of African green monkeys (*Cercopithecus aethiops*) in the wild in Africa (as well as in colonies in other areas) are infected. In most cases these viruses do not cause overt disease in their natural hosts; however, when some of these viruses gain entry into other species of monkeys, they can cause severe, even fatal, disease. For example, when virus from African green monkeys (SIV$_{agm}$) infects rhesus macaques (*Macaca mulatta*), it causes a disease similar to human AIDS. Antibodies against SIV have

been detected in workers exposed to virus-infected non-human primates. HIV probably evolved through infection of humans with a simian immunodeficiency retrovirus of chimpanzee (*Pan troglodytes*; HIV-1) or sooty mangabey (*Cercocebus atys*; HIV-2) origin.

Simian immunodeficiency virus macaque strain (SIV$_{mac}$) has not been identified in rhesus monkeys in the wild in Asia, but it is transmitted among animals in colonies, where it causes an AIDS-like disease. Months after exposure, the first signs of infection are an inguinal rash and lymphadenopathy. This progresses to a wasting syndrome, chronic enteritis, and the onset of opportunistic infections caused by organisms such as *Toxoplasma gondii*, *Pneumocystis carinii*, *Cryptosporidium* spp., *Salmonella* spp., in addition to adenoviruses, polyomaviruses, and cytomegaloviruses. There is often an encephalopathy with neural lesions similar to those seen in humans with AIDS dementia. The rhesus macaque model serves as an important model of HIV and AIDS to examine virus–host interactions, potential vaccines or therapeutics, and viral determinants of disease. Macaque monkeys, when experimentally infected with simian immunodeficiency virus, exhibit progressive lymphoid depletion in primary and secondary lymphoid organs as a result of increased apoptosis of several lymphocyte subsets. Concurrently, increases in the percentages of CD8$^+$ T cells are observed, altering the CD4$^+$: CD8$^+$ T lymphocyte ratio. In contrast, most African non-human primates are relatively resistant and generally do not develop a true AIDS syndrome. However, experimental infections of at least three African non-human primate species—the black mangabey (*Lophocebus aterricus*), the chimpanzee (*Pan troglodytes*) and the baboon (genus *Papio*)—with heterologous simian immunodeficiency viruses have all been reported to cause AIDS-like disease.

Natural SIV infections in African non-human primate species appear to lack the severe immunodeficiency patterns that characterize similar infections of Asian macaques; however, less is known of the clinical course of infection in wild African species. Infections in sooty mangabeys and African green monkeys are both characterized by high viral loads, low amounts of immune activation, a reduced longevity of virus-infected cells, and a modified adaptive immune response to the infection. These animals also have reduced expression of chemokine receptors on CD4$^+$ T cells. Interestingly, the level of mucosal CD4$^+$ T cells remains stable in sooty mangabeys, but progressively declines in SIV-infected rhesus macaques and in untreated human AIDS patients. Thus it has been postulated that, in natural SIV infection, the preserved mucosal lymphoid system is a key to avoiding microbial or microbial toxin effects. These animals appear to avoid a robust systemic immune activation phase and progressive loss of CD4$^+$ T cells in blood and lymph nodes. This, coupled with the low level of chemokine receptor expression on

CD4$^+$ T cells, may help protect the African species. The low level expression of this key viral receptor may protect these cells from cytotoxic virus replication or reduce the homing of activated CD4$^+$ T cells to inflamed tissues. Naturally infected African non-human primate species are also uniquely protected from vertical transmission of the infection. Overall, it appears that the primate lentiviruses and their natural hosts have co-evolved to allow virus replication, but not at the cost of killing the host.

The macaque model has been used extensively in efforts to develop a vaccine against HIV and AIDS. Although many vaccines have been produced, including live-attenuated virus vaccines, there has been no clearly efficacious vaccine produced to date that has directly resulted in the comparable vaccine against HIV-1 infection.

BOVINE IMMUNODEFICIENCY VIRUS

Bovine immunodeficiency virus was first isolated in 1972 from a dairy cow with progressive weakness, persistent lymphocytosis, lymphoid hyperplasia, and central nervous system lesions. Serologic studies indicate that the virus is present throughout the world and, in some cases, correlated with a decreased milk production in dairy cattle. However, unequivocal epidemiologic evidence is lacking to correlate bovine immunodeficiency virus infection with clinical immune deficiency and an increase in susceptibility to opportunistic infections in infected cattle. The virus has parallels with other lentiviruses in genomic organization and replication mechanisms. In addition to the structural *gag, pol* and *env* genes that are common to all retroviruses, bovine immunodeficiency virus encodes six putative non-structural/accessory genes. The genome is the most complex of the non-primate lentiviruses, in that, in addition to *tat, rev,* and *vif,* there are three other accessory genes, designated *vpy, vpw,* and *tmx.* Genetic variability is common among virus strains, in particular in viral envelope sequences.

Bovine immunodeficiency virus can be grown in monolayer cell cultures from a variety of bovine embryonic tissues, producing a cytopathic effect characterized by syncytium formation. When transmitted to calves by intravenous inoculation, it causes an immediate leukopenia followed, within 15–20 days, by lymphocytosis that persists. The virus infects a wide spectrum of cells; proviral DNA has been detected in CD3$^+$, CD4$^+$, and CD8$^+$ cells, in addition to γ/δ and B lymphocytes, null cells, and monocytes. Virus persists in naturally infected cows for at least 12 months.

The true economic impact of bovine immunodeficiency virus infection remains conjectural, although several reports have suggested infected cattle may be at increased risk for reproductive problems, abscesses, peritonitis, and arthritis. Experimentally, calves infected with bovine immunodeficiency virus reportedly exhibited lymphadenopathy, ataxia, meningoencephalitis, and a paraplegic syndrome. However, despite these reports, a direct role of bovine immunodeficiency virus in clinical disease in animals infected under natural conditions has not been clearly demonstrated.

JEMBRANA DISEASE VIRUS

In contrast to the relatively benign nature of bovine immunodeficiency virus infection in European cattle, a related virus has been established as the cause of a peracute disease of Bali cattle (*Bos javanicus*) in Indonesia. The disease, called Jembrana disease for the district, was recognized in 1964. Within 12 months, 26,000 of 300,000 cattle in the area died. The disease remains enzootic on Bali and has spread to Sumatra, Java, and Kalimantan. The origin of the virus has not been established. Disease is characterized by high morbidity and high mortality rates. After a very short incubation period of 5–12 days there is fever, lethargy, anorexia, and pronounced swelling of lymph nodes and panleukopenia. Jembrana disease virus infection results in high levels of virus replication—up to 10^{12} RNA genomes/ml plasma—during a prolonged febrile response which may last more than a week. Following recovery, viral loads are reduced but may persist for up to 2 years. Approximately 17% of acutely ill cattle die. Necropsy findings include widespread hemorrhages, lymphadenopathy, and splenomegaly. Histologically, the lymphoid tissues are populated by many lymphoblastoid cells.

The genome of Jembrana disease virus has been sequenced completely and is similar to, but distinguishable from, other isolates of bovine immunodeficiency virus. The Jembrana disease virus genome has an organization similar to that of bovine immunodeficiency virus, including accessory (*tat, rev*) and regulatory (*vif, tmx*) genes.

MEMBERS OF THE SUBFAMILY *SPUMARETROVIRINAE*

The subfamily *Spumaretrovirinae* includes only a single genus, *Spumavirus* (Table 14.1). The spumaviruses are also referred to as foamy viruses, because of the cytopathic effects they elicit in cell cultures. These viruses infect a broad range of species, including non-human primates, cats, cows, and horses, as well as humans. Human infections have been associated with cross-species transmission from non-human primates. Spumavirus infections, like those of other retroviruses, are life-long, although they have not been linked to disease.

Spumaviruses replicate in cell cultures and are common contaminants of primary cell cultures from non-human primates, where they cause characteristic cytopathic effects. These viruses were first described in 1954 as foamy viruses because they caused large multinucleated syncytia with a highly vacuolized appearance in cell cultures from non-human primates. These viruses have unique immature appearance to their virions on electron microscopy. Their proviral genome contains typical retrovirus elements, including LTRs as well as the *gag*, *pol*, and *env* genes. In addition, the spumaviruses encode two unique non-structural proteins, Tas (transcriptional activator of spumavirus) and Bet (a cytoplasmic protein of uncertain but possibly regulatory function). Spumaviruses, like orthoretroviruses, use reverse transcription to convert their RNA genomes into DNA that then becomes integrated into the host genome as proviruses. However, the reverse transcription step occurs during budding and assembly, so that the genome is actually DNA, similar to hepadnaviruses. Spumaviruses also differ by encoding separate Gag and Pol proteins from separate mRNA.

There have been no reports clearly linking spumaviruses to disease in their natural hosts, infected humans, or from experimental infections. The discrepancy between the dramatic cytopathic effects these viruses induce in cell cultures and their apparent lack of disease-producing capability has been the subject of investigation, but is not clearly understood. The prevalence of infection is high among captive non-human primates. The majority of animals seroconvert as juveniles, suggesting a non-sexual route of transmission; biting or licking has been hypothesized as a primary mode of transmission. Cross-species transmission to humans has been documented when people such as veterinarians, animal caretakers, bushmeat hunters, and zookeepers are in close contact with non-human primates. Spumavirus infections are often associated with a severe bite, which suggests that saliva is the means of transmission. No human-to-human transmission has been documented, suggesting that humans are dead-end hosts. A viral receptor has not been identified, but extensive studies from primate tissue cultures indicate that, *in-vitro*, these infections are not restricted to a particular species or cell type.

MISCELLANEOUS RETROVIRUS-ASSOCIATED DISEASES

A variety of diseases have been associated with retrovirus infection, but lack unambiguous proof of a cause-and-effect relationship. These are typically neoplastic or proliferative disorders in which a retrovirus has been detected using electron microscopy or indirect measurements of the presence of retroviruses such as reverse transcriptase assays. For example, investigations of endogenous retrovirus infections related to murine leukemia virus have described nucleotide sequences in amphibians, reptiles, birds, and mammals, and complete genomic sequences have been obtained from endogenous retroviruses from reptiles and amphibians. Some of these retroviral genomes have novel organizational structure as compared with retroviruses of mammals and birds. The endogenous amphibian retrovirus, Xen1, for instance, clusters with the epsilon retroviruses walleye dermal sarcoma virus and walleye epidermal hyperplasia (types 1 and 2) viruses.

INCLUSION BODY DISEASE OF SNAKES

Retroviruses have been reported in snakes, often associated with neoplasms. Retroviruses also have been incriminated as a cause of inclusion body disease of snakes, which affects primarily boas and pythons of the family *Boidae*. This disorder is characterized by the presence of widespread eosinophilic intracytoplasmic inclusions in several organs. The disease is contagious and typically fatal. Snakes with the disease exhibit intermittent regurgitation and are anorexic. The disease progresses to affect the central nervous system, with snakes showing head tremors, opisthotonos, ataxia, and behavioral changes. These nervous system signs may progress to complete paresis and result in the inability of the snake to capture prey. Other clinical signs include ulcerative stomatitis, pneumonia, and increased incident of cutaneous tumors such as sarcomas. An underlying immune suppression in affected snakes has been suggested, but not thoroughly investigated. Diagnosis is confirmed from histologic examination of typical inclusions from biopsies or tissues of affected organs at necropsy. Inclusions are variable in size, electron-dense, and may contain type C virus-like particles. The snake mite *Ophionyssus natricis* has been implicated, but not proven, as a vector for the disease.

Reoviridae

Chapter Contents

The family *Reoviridae* is one of the most complex in all of virology, currently comprising 12 recognized and three proposed genera of viruses with genomes composed of several (10–12) segments of double-stranded RNA (dsRNA) (Figure 15.1). Individual viruses within the family infect a remarkable variety of hosts, including mammals, birds, reptiles, amphibians, fish, mollusks, crustaceans, insects, plants, and fungi. Viruses in the different genera can be distinguished on the basis of several different features, including their capsid structure, number and size of genome segments, host range and associated diseases, serological properties, and, increasingly, by the nucleotide sequence of their genomes. The root term "reo" is an acronym for "respiratory enteric orphan," which was coined because the first members of the family were identified in the respiratory and the enteric tracts of animals and humans as "orphans"—that is, not associated with any disease. These viruses are now members of the genus *Orthoreovirus*. The later inclusion in the family of the genera *Orbivirus*, *Coltivirus*, *Rotavirus*, *Seadornavirus*, and *Aquareovirus* added important pathogens of humans and a variety of animal species, including aquatic animals (Table 15.1).

The distribution of the member viruses of the genus *Orthoreovirus* is ubiquitous, including viruses from cattle, sheep, swine, humans, non-human primates, bats, and birds; however, most of these infections are not associated with any significant clinical disease. Only reovirus infections of poultry, and perhaps primates, are of major pathogenic significance. The aquareoviruses resemble orthoreoviruses and have been isolated from fish and mollusks in both fresh and sea water, but their significance as primary pathogens remains conjectural.

Viruses of the genus *Orbivirus* are transmitted to animals primarily by arthropod vectors, which, depending on the individual virus, can be certain species of *Culicoides* midges, mosquitoes, black flies, sandflies, or ticks. The global and seasonal distribution of individual viruses, therefore, coincides with that of their specific biological vector and appropriate climatic conditions. Bluetongue and African horse sickness viruses economically are the most important members of this genus, although several others are potentially important, either regionally or globally. Although, historically, bluetongue virus infection has been restricted to relatively defined areas of the world that include much

Fenner's Veterinary Virology. DOI: 10.1016/B978-0-12-375158-4.00015-8

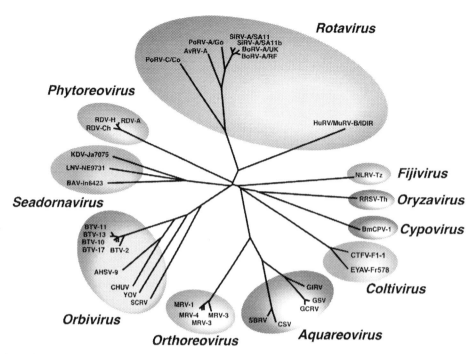

FIGURE 15.1   Phylogenetic map (neighbor joining tree) of the family *Reoviridae* based on the amino acid sequence of the RNA-dependent RNA polymerase (RdRP). AHSV, African horse sickness virus 9; AvRV, avian rotavirus A; BAV-In6423, Banna virus, Indonesian isolate 6423; BmCPV, *Bombyx mori* cypovirus; BoRv, bovine rotavirus; BTV, bluetongue virus; CHUV, Chuzan virus; CSV, chum salmon reovirus; CTFV-F1, Colorado tick fever virus serotype F1; EYAV-Fr578, Eyach virus (France-578); GCRV, grass carp reovirus; GIRV, golden ide reovirus; GSV, golden shiner aquareovirus; HuRV/MuRV-IDIR, human/murine rotavirus-IDIR; KDV-Ja7075, Kadipiro virus, Java isolate 7075; LNV-NE9731, Liao ning virus, isolate NE9731; MRV, mammalian orthoreovirus; NLRV-Tz, *Nilaparvata lugens* reovirus, Tanzanian isolate; PoRV, porcine rotavirus; RDV, rice dwarf phytoreovirus; RRSV-Th, Rice ragged stunt virus, Thai strain; SBRV, striped bass reovirus; SCRV, St Croix River virus; SIRV, simian rotavirus; YOV, Yunnan orbivirus. *[From* Virus Taxonomy: Eighth Report of the International Committee on Taxonomy of Viruses *(C. M. Fauquet, M. A. Mayo, J. Maniloff, U. Desselberger, L. A. Ball, eds.), p. 453. Copyright © Elsevier (2005), with permission.]*

of the tropical and temperate regions, several different viral serotypes have recently emerged throughout extensive portions of Europe, perhaps in part as a consequence of climate change in the region. There is concern that African horse sickness or other pathogenic orbiviruses might follow.

Rotaviruses are also widespread; essentially, every species of domestic animal and bird has been found to harbor at least one indigenous rotavirus that typically is responsible for causing diarrhea ("scours") in newborn animals. Rotavirus causes perhaps 600,000 childhood deaths yearly, mostly in developing countries. They also cause considerable economic losses to livestock industries worldwide.

Viruses included in the genera *Coltivirus* and *Seadornavirus* are, respectively, transmitted to humans and animals by ticks and mosquitoes. Viruses in these genera are the cause of serious but sporadic human diseases. Genetic analyses suggest an evolutionary link between coltiviruses and aquareoviruses, and between rotaviruses and seadornaviruses.

PROPERTIES OF REOVIRUSES

Classification

All animal viruses with multi-segmented dsRNA genomes are included in the family *Reoviridae*, with the notable exception of the birnaviruses and picobirnaviruses. Consequently, the family is complex, with substantial

differences among viruses in the different genera (Table 15.2; Figure 15.2). Because of their segmented RNA genomes, reassortment of genome segments among different strains of these viruses is common within the same virus species, as is a high rate of RNA mutations in individual genes. The resulting genetic shift and drift leads to a remarkable diversity of viruses, which is reflected by the numerous serotypes and myriads of strains of individual viruses within each genera.

The genus *Orthoreovirus* comprises at least five different virus species: species I includes four serotypes of mammalian reoviruses (designated 1–4); species II includes several serotypes of avian reoviruses that have been isolated from chickens, Muscovy and other species of duck, turkeys, and geese; species III includes relatives of a virus that was isolated from a fruit bat; species IV is represented by baboon reovirus; species V includes a group of reptilian reoviruses.

The genus *Aquareovirus* contains at least seven type species, designated A–G, that include a large number of viruses isolated from anadromous and marine fish (various species of Atlantic and Pacific salmon, smelt, turbot), freshwater fish (bass, catfish, carp), oysters, and clams. The pathogenic and economic significance of many of these viruses remains uncertain. Several diseases of crustaceans (e.g., shrimp and crabs) have been attributed to reoviruses; these probably represent a new genus of aquatic reoviruses,

TABLE 15.1 Characteristics of Reovirus Infections

Virus / Hosts / Serotypes	Disease / Symptoms	Transmission / Diagnostic Specimen	Prevention / Control
Orthoreovirus			
Reoviruses in mammals Serotypes 1–4	Asymptomatic infection experimental disease	Fecal–oral route; systemic infection	For mouse colonies good sanitation, regular testing, and preventive quarantine
Reoviruses in poultry Reoviruses in many bird species, multiple serotypes	Tenosynovitis/arthritis Respiratory disease, enteritis, with weight loss, stunted growth; often subclinical	Fecal–oral route; systemic infection Feces, serum, multiple target tissues	Good sanitation, regular testing, and preventive quarantine Attenuated and inactivated virus vaccines available
Orbivirus			
Bluetongue virus Sheep, cattle, goats, deer Serotypes 1–25	Bluetongue Fever, hyperemia, cyanosis, edema, oral, cavity erosions, nasal discharge, lameness	Vector transmission: *Culicoides* spp. Blood—virus detection; serum—antibody testing; spleen, lung, lymph nodes	Attenuated and inactivated virus vaccines available Prevent contact with *Culicoides* spp.
African horse sickness virus Horses; donkeys, mules, zebras (subclinical) Serotypes 1–9	Respiratory or cardiovascular failure Fever, edema	Vector transmission: *Culicoides* spp. Blood—virus detection; serum—antibody testing, spleen, lung, lymph nodes	Attenuated and inactivated virus vaccines available Prevent contact with *Culicoides* spp.
Equine encephalosis viruses Horses; donkeys, mules, zebras (subclinical) Serotypes 1–7	Subclinical often Fever, African horse sickness-like disease	Vector transmission: *Culicoides* spp. Blood—virus detection; serum—antibody testing, spleen, lung, lymph nodes	No vaccines Prevent contact with *Culicoides* spp.
Epizootic hemorrhagic disease of deer viruses Deer, cattle, sheep Serotypes 1–10 Ibaraki virus (EHDV setorype 2)	Hemorrhagic disease Fever, hyperemia, cyanosis, edema	Vector transmission: *Culicoides* spp. Blood—virus detection; serum—antibody testing, spleen, lung, lymph nodes	No vaccines Prevent contact with *Culicoides* spp.
Palyam virus Cattle, serotypes 1–13	Reproductive, central nervous system disease; Abortion, congenital abnormalities; hydranencephaly	Vector transmission: *Culicoides* spp.	No vaccines
Peruvian horse sickness Horses in South America and Australia	Neurological disease	Vector transmission: likely mosquitoes	No vaccines
Rotavirus			
Rotaviruses Virtually all species	Gastroenteritis/diarrhea	Fecal–oral route Feces	Dam innoculation with attenuated or inactivated virus Oral attenuated vaccines for neonates
Coltivirus			
Colorado tick fever virus Small animals, humans—zoonosis	Tick fever/Saddle-back fever Retro-orbital pain, myalgia, leukopenia	Trans-stadial vector transmission: wood tick (*Dermacentor andersonie*) Blood and serum	No vaccines or treatments Prevent contact with ticks
Eyach virus Small animals, humans—zoonosis	Antibodies found in patients with meningoencephalitis and polyneuritis	European *Ixodidae* ticks Blood and serum	No vaccines or treatments Prevent contact with ticks
Aquareoviruses			
Fish, shellfish	Uncertain	Uncertain	No vaccines or treatments

TABLE 15.2 Properties of Reoviruses

Virions are non-enveloped, spherical in outline, 55–80 nm in diameter

Virions are composed of three concentric capsid layers, all with icosahedral symmetry; the outer capsid differs in appearance in the various genera

Genome is composed of double-stranded RNA, divided into 10–12 segments, total size 18–27 kbp: genus *Orthoreovirus*, 10 segments, 23 kbp; genus *Orbivirus*, 10 segments, 18 kbp; genus *Rotavirus*, 11 segments, 16–21 kbp; genus *Coltivirus*, 12 segments, 27 kbp; genus *Aquareovirus*, 11 segments, 15 kbp

Cytoplasmic replication

Genetic reassortment occurs between viruses within each genus or serogroup

as they possess genomes of 12 segments of dsRNA, in contrast to other aquareoviruses that have 11 gene segments.

The genus *Orbivirus* is divided into at least 21 virus subgroups, which represent distinct virus species. Several of these include viruses that cause disease in domestic animals. Separate virus species encompass 24 (very likely 25) serotypes of bluetongue virus; 9 serotypes of African horse sickness virus; 10 serotypes of epizootic hemorrhagic disease virus, including Ibaraki virus (a variant of epizootic hemorrhagic disease virus serotype 2); 7 serotypes of equine encephalosis virus; 1 serotype of Peruvian horse sickness virus; 13 serotypes of Palyam virus, including Chuzan virus; certain other viruses affecting different animal species. These orbivirus species have been defined both serologically and genotypically, and viruses within each subgroup share a common antigen demonstrable by serologic tests. Genetic

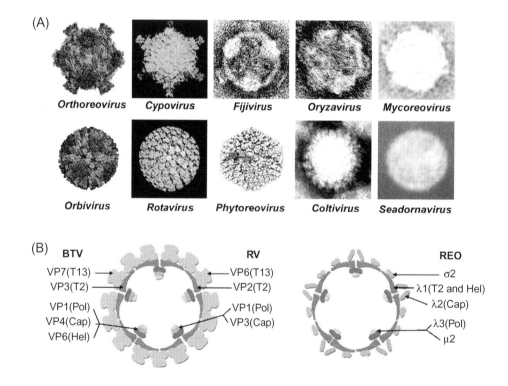

FIGURE 15.2 (Top and Center) A comparison of two distinct core particle morphologies (spiked and unspiked) present amongst members of different genera of the family *Reoviridae*. *Orbivirus*: a 3D model from x-ray crystallography of the core particle of an isolate of bluetongue virus serotype 1 (BTV 1). *Orthoreovirus*: a 3D model from x-ray crystallography studies of a core particle of an isolate of revirus 3. *Cypovirus*: a 3D cryo-EM reconstruction of a particle of an isolate of cypovirus 5, at 25 Å resolution. *Rotavirus*: a 3D cryo-EM reconstruction of a double shelled particle of an isolate of rotavirus A (SiRV-A/SA11), at 25 Å resolution. *Fijivirus*: an electron micrograph of a core particle of an isolate of maize rough dwarf virus. *Phytoreovirus*: a 3D cryo-EM reconstruction of the double-shelled particle of an isolate of rice dwarf virus, at 25-Å resolution (highlighted in colour are a contiguous "group of 5 trimers" found in each asymmetric unit). *Coltivirus*: an electron micrograph of a negatively stained double-shelled particle of an isolate of Colorado tick fever virus. *Oryzavirus*: an electron micrograph of a negatively stained core particle of an isolate of rice ragged stunt virus. *Mycoreovirus*: an electron micrograph of a negatively stained core particle of mycoreovirus 1 (Rosallinia necatrix mycoreovirus-1). *Seadornavirus*: an electron micrograph of a negatively stained core particle of an isolate of Banna virus. The reconstructions and electron micrographs are not shown to exactly the same scale. The outer capsid morphologies of members of the different genera of the family *Reoviridae* are more variable and may appear smooth, or with surface projections, or may even be absent. (Bottom) shows a diagrammatic representations (on the left) of the core particles of an orbivirus (BTV), or rotavirus (RV), which have a well defined capsomeric structure but lack large surface projections at the 5 fold icosahedral axes, as compared to the 'turreted' (spiked) core particle of an orthoreovirus (Reo). (Courtesy of J. Diprose). [*From* Virus Taxonomy: Eighth Report of the International Committee on Taxonomy of Viruses *(C. M. Fauquet, M. A. Mayo, J. Maniloff, U. Desselberger, L. A. Ball, eds.), p. 447. Copyright © Elsevier (2005), with permission.*]

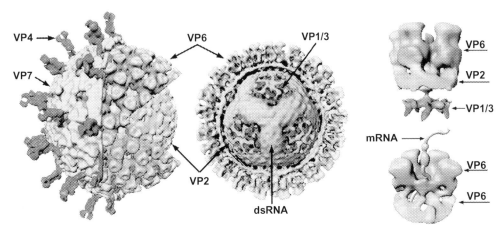

FIGURE 15.3 (Left) Cutaway view of the mature particle of simian rotavirus A/SA11 (SiRV-A/SA11), illustrating the triple-layered capsid structure taken from cryo-EM data and following image reconstruction at 24Å resolution. (Center) Cutaway view of the transcriptionally-competent double layered particle at 19Å. (Top right) Transcription enzyme complex composed of VP1 and VP3, shown anchored to the inner surface of VP2 at the icosahedral vertex. This figure has been computationally isolated from the 22Å reconstruction of a VP1/3/2/6-VLP (virus-like particle). (Bottom right) Proposed pathway of mRNA translocation through the double-layered capsid during genome transcription. The mass of density at the extremity of the mRNA represents the structurally discernible portion of nascent mRNA visible in the 25Å structure of the actively transcribing particle (Courtesy of B.V.V. Prasad). *[From Virus Taxonomy: Eighth Report of the International Committee on Taxonomy of Viruses (C. M. Fauquet, M. A. Mayo, J. Maniloff, U. Desselberger, L. A. Ball, eds), p. 485. Copyright © Elsevier (2005), with permission.]*

differences and relationships among the various viruses can be clearly identified by sequence analyses.

The classification of the member viruses of the genus *Rotavirus* is based on genotypic and serologic analyses. Variation in the group-specific capsid antigen on VP6 is used to define major groups or subgroups for group A rotaviruses (Figure 15.3). Rotavirus group A includes important pathogens of humans, cattle, swine, horses, gallinaceous poultry, laboratory mice, and other animals; group B includes pathogens of humans, cattle, sheep, ferrets, swine, and rats; group C includes only pathogens of humans, swine, and cattle; group E includes only viruses from swine; groups D and F include only pathogens of birds. Differentiation into serotypes is based on neutralization tests. Because both outer capsid proteins (VP4 and VP7) carry type-specific epitopes recognized by neutralizing antibodies, a binary system of classification of serotypes has been developed, akin to that used for influenza viruses. For example, in group A rotaviruses, 15 [G] genotypes (14 G serotypes) have been defined on the basis of differences in VP7, and 27 [P] genotypes (14 P serotypes), based on differences in VP4. Monoclonal antibodies, gel electrophoresis of viral RNA segments, RNA hybridization, and partial or complete sequencing of each RNA segment are used to make any further distinctions as may be necessary in molecular epidemiological studies to identify reassortants and potential inter-species transmission events.

There are only a few members of the genus *Coltivirus*. Colorado tick fever virus is the prototype virus, and Eyach virus is the European counterpart. A few other coltiviruses have been isolated from other areas of the western United States. The genus *Seadornavirus* includes mosquito-borne viruses that infect humans and animals in Asia, including

Banna, Kadipiro, and Liao ning viruses. These viruses initially were included in the genus *Coltivirus*.

Virion Properties

Orthoreoviruses and rotaviruses are resistant to lipid solvents and are stable over a wide range of pH, but orbiviruses and coltiviruses have a narrower zone of pH stability (pH 6–8) and lose some, but not all, infectivity on exposure to lipid solvents. Proteolytic enzymes increase the infectivity of orthoreoviruses and rotaviruses (e.g., chymotrypsin in the small intestine cleaves an outer capsid VP4 protein of rotavirus, thereby enhancing infectivity). Proteolytic cleavage of the outer capsid protein VP2 of bluetongue virus (genus *Orbivirus*) also increases its infectivity for cells of its insect vector (*Culicoides* species) but not for mammalian cells. Orbiviruses and rotaviruses are remarkably stable. Bluetongue viruses are relatively stable in the presence of protein, and have been re-isolated from blood stored for years at room temperature. Likewise, group A rotaviruses are stable for months, even when maintained at room temperature, or for years when stored frozen. Viral infectivity is inactivated by phenols, formalin, 95% ethanol, and β-propriolactone.

Reovirus particles are non-enveloped, spherical, and have a diameter of approximately 85 nm. Virions consist of a multilayered capsid, each with icosahedral symmetry (Table 15.2). The precise virion morphology varies with the genus (Figure 15.2). The genome consists of linear dsRNA divided into 10 (genus *Orthoreovirus* and *Orbivirus*), 11 (genus *Rotavirus* and *Aquareovirus*), or 12 (genus *Coltivirus, Seadornavirus,* and some currently designated members of genus *Aquareovirus*) segments. The overall genome size is approximately 23 kbp (genus *Orthoreovirus*), 19 kbp (genus *Orbivirus*), 16–21 kbp (genus *Rotavirus*), 29 kbp (genus *Coltivirus*), 21 kbp (genus *Seadornavirus*), or 24 kbp (genus *Aquareovirus*). The positive strands of each double-stranded segment have 5′-terminal caps (type 1 structure). The 3′ termini of both strands lack 3′-poly(A) tails. Each RNA segment is present in equimolar proportion in virions. Further detail requires separate mention of each genus.

Genus Orthoreovirus

The outer capsid forms a nearly spherical icosahedron, consisting predominantly of complexes of the proteins σ3 and μ1C (Figure 15.2). In addition to intact virions, there are two stable subviral particles. The first of these is missing only its outer capsid (i.e., it is lacking σ3 and contains cleaved forms of μ1 protein); this particle is called the *infectious subviral particle* (ISVP). The second subviral particle is missing both its outer and its middle capsids and is called the *core particle*. The protein by which virions attach to host cells, σ1, forms spikes that project through the outer capsid at each of the 12 vertices of the virion. Most importantly, when the outer capsid layer is removed, σ1 protein molecules remain attached to the infectious subviral particle and form extended fibers containing the cellular attachment domain at their tips. The core contains the viral RNA polymerase (transcriptase) and consists of three major proteins (λ1, λ2, and σ2) and two minor proteins (λ3 and μ2). The 10 genome segments of the orthoreoviruses fall into three size classes: large, medium, and small. Each segment encodes a single protein, except for one that is cleaved co-translationally to form two proteins. Each genome segment can be differentiated by size using gel electrophoresis, and these electropherotype patterns are used to type isolates of mammalian and avian viruses.

Genus Aquareovirus

Virions resemble those of the orthoreoviruses, although the genome consists of 11 or, in some viruses, 12 segments.

Genus Orbivirus

The outer capsid consists of a diffuse layer formed by two proteins, VP2 and VP5. This outer capsid is dissociated readily from the core particle, which has a surface composed of 260 VP7 trimers arranged in ring-like structures for which the genus is named. Both VP2 and VP5 are attached to VP7, which in turn is associated with a subcore shell composed of 120 copies of VP3 surrounding the transcriptase complex (VP1, VP4, and VP6), and the genomic RNA segments. Surface projections are observed only on virions that have been stabilized (e.g., frozen for cryo-electron microscopy). Otherwise, the surface of virions appears smooth and unstructured. The 10 genome segments of the orbiviruses are all monocistronic, except the smallest

gene segment (number 10), which includes a single open reading frame, but with two functional initiation codons near the 5′ end of the positive-sense strand. As with the orthoreoviruses, the gene segments form distinct size patterns during electrophoresis that can be used to identify the different orbivirus species. Variation can be detected between the RNAs of closely related viruses with this method, which can be used to distinguish strains within a single viral serotype. The 10 genome segments encode seven structural proteins (VP1–7) and four non-structural proteins (NS1–NS3, NS3A).

Genus Rotavirus

The outer capsid forms a nearly spherical icosahedron; it consists of the glycoprotein VP7, from which dimers of VP4 extend (Figure 15.3). The outer VP7 capsid and the middle capsid, which is composed of VP6 (the structural equivalent of VP7 of orbiviruses), are dissociated readily from the core, which is composed of three proteins: VP1, VP2, and VP3. The 11 genome segments of the rotaviruses are monocistronic, except gene 11, which encodes two proteins. In addition to the six structural proteins (VP1–4, VP6, VP7), the rotavirus genome also encodes six non-structural proteins (NS1–6). The genome segments can be differentiated by size using gel electrophoresis, and these electropherotype patterns are used to type isolates.

Genera Coltivirus and Seadornavirus

The virions of these viruses are approximately spherical, with concentric, multi-layered capsid shells. Coltivirus particles have a relatively smooth surface, whereas those of seadornaviruses have well-developed capsomeric structures. The double-layered core particle includes the 12 segments of the viral genome.

Virus Replication

The σ1 protein of orthoreoviruses mediates attachment to target cells. Virions or infectious subviral particles enter susceptible cells by receptor-mediated endocytosis. Junctional adhesion molecule A is a serotype-independent receptor for orthoreovirus, and sialylated glycoproteins can serve as a co-receptor for some strains. Variations in the σ1 protein, a filamentous trimer that projects as a spike from the virion, determine the cell and tissue tropism of each virus. Once internalized into the cytoplasm of infected cells, virions are degraded to core particles, within which virion-associated RNA polymerase (transcriptase) and capping enzymes repetitively transcribe 5′-capped mRNAs that are extruded into the cytoplasm through channels at core particle vertices. RNA polymerase (transcriptase) utilizes the negative strands of each of the dsRNA segments as templates; only certain genes are transcribed initially, four mRNAs appearing before the other six. The proportion of the various mRNAs found in infected cells varies, and the efficiency of the translation of each also varies (over a 100-fold range). How this regulation is mediated is not known.

After early mRNA synthesis, genomic RNA replication takes place within nascent progeny subviral particles in the cytoplasm of infected cells. The mechanism of genomic RNA replication is complex and not fully understood. Newly synthesized, dsRNA in turn serves as a template for the transcription of more mRNAs, which this time are uncapped. These mRNAs are translated preferentially to yield a large pool of viral structural proteins that self-assemble to form virions. The mechanism that ensures that one copy of each dsRNA segment is encapsidated into nascent virions is not known.

Shortly after virus entry, host-cell protein synthesis decreases abruptly; one proposed mechanism is that the cap-dependent host-cell mRNAs are less efficient in driving protein translation than uncapped viral mRNAs. Structures, termed viroplasms or virus factories, form in localized areas of the cytoplasm—these intracytoplasmic inclusion bodies can be dramatic in size and the number of associated virions (Figure 15.4, Figure 2.2A). Inclusion bodies have a granular and moderately electron-dense appearance in thin-section electron microscopy. Progeny virions tend to remain cell associated, but are eventually released by cell lysis.

Replication of orbiviruses and rotaviruses is generally similar to that of orthoreoviruses. Rotavirus infectivity requires triple-layered virus particles containing the outer capsid proteins, VP4 and VP7, for attachment. Proteolytic cleavage of VP4 (i.e., by chymotrypsin in the small intestine), is important for virus entry into the cells and increased infectivity. Some rotavirus strains bind to sialic acid residues

on the cell surface, but the cellular receptor has not been otherwise identified, and there are suggestions that rotavirus can enter cells either by receptor-dependent endocytosis or by direct penetration. Regardless, the process of cell entry removes the outer shell of the virion to generate the transcriptionally active double-layered particle that mediates transcription. Rotavirus progenitor particles acquire a temporary lipid envelope as they bud into cisternae of the endoplasmic reticulum of infected cells, which then breaks down, leaving VP7 as the major outer capsid protein.

Bluetongue virus—and presumably other orbiviruses—enter cells through clathrin-dependent, receptor-mediated endocytosis (Figure 15.5). Outer capsid (VP2 and VP5) and core (VP7) proteins have all been implicated in cell attachment and penetration. Indeed, bluetongue virus core particles (that lack the outer capsid proteins, VP2 and VP5) have infectivity comparable to that of fully intact virus particles for cells of the insect (*Culicoides*) vector, whereas core particles are less infectious for mammalian cells. Cell membrane glycoproteins can function as receptors, but these interactions are otherwise poorly characterized. Virus entry results in removal of the outer capsid, which activates the core-particle-associated transcriptase and capping enzyme. Transcription occurs within core particles associated with viral inclusion bodies. Distinctive tubules composed of the viral NS1 protein are characteristically present in the cytoplasm of infected cells, although their precise function remains uncertain. Before release of newly formed virus particles by lysis of the infected cell, particles can bud through the cell membrane in a process mediated by the NS3 protein.

MEMBERS OF THE GENUS *ORTHOREOVIRUS*

ORTHOREOVIRUS INFECTIONS OF MAMMALS AND BIRDS

The host range of reoviruses includes cattle, sheep, swine, humans, non-human primates, dogs, rodents, lagomorphs, bats, chickens, turkeys, Muscovy and other domestic and wild duck species, pigeons, woodcock, psittacine species, Bobwhite quail, crows, and geese. Only infections in primates, chickens, and turkeys are of major importance, but respiratory or enteric infections in other species, especially laboratory animals, may complicate diagnostic interpretation.

Clinical Features and Epidemiology

Orthoreoviruses, especially reovirus 3, cause an experimental disease syndrome in neonatal laboratory mice that is characterized by jaundice, diarrhea, runting, oily hair, and neurologic signs (e.g., ataxia). Natural infections in laboratory mice are invariably subclinical. Laboratory mice, rats, hamsters, guinea pigs and rabbits, and many other mammals as well, may be infected with any of the serotypes

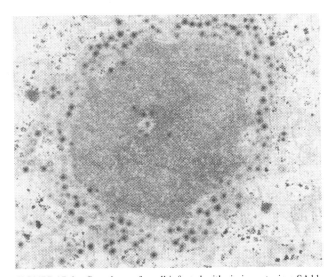

FIGURE 15.4 Cytoplasm of a cell infected with simian rotavirus SA11, showing a granular intracytoplasmic inclusion body (viroplasm or virus factory) with a large number of virions self-assembling at its margin. In many cases these inclusions can be dramatic in size and number of associated virions. Virions are largely cell associated and are released by cell lysis. Thin-section electron microscopy. Magnification: ×25,000.

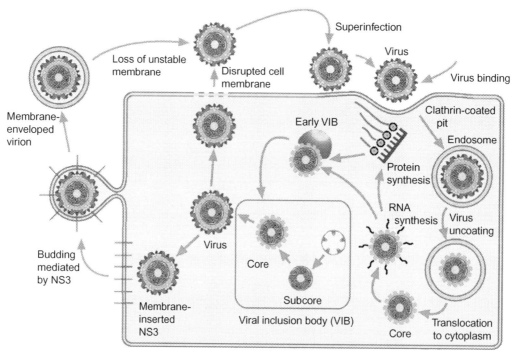

FIGURE 15.5 Schematic diagram of the reovirus (orbivirus) replication cycle. NS3, non-structural protein 3. *[From* Virus Taxonomy: Eighth Report of the International Committee on Taxonomy of Viruses *(C. M. Fauquet, M. A. Mayo, J. Maniloff, U. Desselberger, L. A. Ball, eds.), p. 450. Copyright © Elsevier (2005), with permission.]*

of reovirus. The greatest significance of reoviruses in laboratory animals is the cost of surveillance and prevention, which are questionable endeavors. These viruses have also been implicated as causes of respiratory and enteric disease in horses, cattle, sheep, swine, and dogs; however, as with mice, their true pathogenic significance is highly conjectural. Infection of primates has been associated with both hepatitis and meningitis.

The outcome of avian orthoreovirus infection in birds ranges from inapparent to fatal. Infection in some chicken, turkey, and goose flocks may be subclinical. The most frequent associated disease syndrome is tenosynovitis and arthritis in chickens, but other syndromes have been described after field or experimental infection, including respiratory disease, gastroenteritis, malabsorption syndrome, hepatic necrosis, hepatitis, myocarditis, hydropericardium, weight loss, runting/stunting, and increased mortality. Tenosynovitis and arthritis usually occur in meat-producing birds more than 5 weeks of age. Morbidity is often 100%, and mortality is usually less than 2%. In some turkey flocks, infection may be indicated only by enteritis.

Pathogenesis and Pathology

The pathogenesis of orthoreovirus infections in mice has been studied extensively as an experimental model system that requires infection of neonates for induction of disease. Virus is acquired via a fecal–oral transmission cycle and

infection is systemic, but lesions are rather nondescript, often appearing as focal necrosis and inflammatory infiltrations into the parenchyma of several organs.

Avian orthoreovirus infections most frequently cause necrosis, hemorrhage, and inflammation within tendons and tendon sheaths, and around joints. Necrosis in the liver, kidney, and spleen has been reported most often in Muscovy ducks, but occasionally in chickens. Historically, necrosis within the cloacal bursa and other lymphoreticular tissues, inclusion body hepatitis, and necrosis in the pancreas have all been attributed to reovirus infections, but subsequent studies have identified other agents as the cause of these conditions, and reoviruses were either incidental or, at most, mild co-pathogens. Reovirus has also been found in dead crows tested as part of the West Nile virus monitoring programs in the United States. Pathology associated with these cases was a severe enteritis.

Diagnosis

Orthoreovirus infections in laboratory rodents and lagomorphs are diagnosed serologically, usually by enzyme immunoassay using reovirus 3 antigen, which detects seroconversion to all major reovirus serotypes. Such assays are included in the battery of tests done regularly as part of the surveillance programs used to assure that animals used in research are free of intercurrent infections. Similar assays as well as immunofluorescence are used for the serological diagnosis of avian orthoreovirus infections; in addition, virus isolation using avian cell cultures is used when serology proves inadequate. Reoviruses produce vacuoles and syncytia in infected cell cultures, and are typed by neutralization assay.

Immunity, Prevention, and Control

The practices used in laboratory rodent colonies to maintain specific pathogen-free status are adequate to prevent the introduction of orthoreoviruses—the key is good sanitation, regular serologic testing, quarantine and testing before the introduction of new stock, and rodent control to prevent contact with wild mice. In chicken and turkey flocks, prevention of tenosynovitis and arthritis is principally through vaccination, in addition to biosecurity and good management practices. Vaccination is primarily through administration of live-attenuated or inactivated vaccine to breeder hens, which provides passive immunity to progeny via the yolk. Alternatively, live vaccines can be administered to chicks at 1 day of age, by coarse spray or subcutaneous inoculation, if field exposure is high and clinical disease a recurring problem. Such vaccination can, however, interfere with immunity to Marek's disease if given at the same time as turkey herpesvirus vaccine. Vaccination is ineffective in preventing enteric and stunting disease.

MEMBERS OF THE GENUS *ORBIVIRUS*

BLUETONGUE VIRUS

Bluetongue was first described in the Cape Colony of southern Africa, soon after the introduction of European sheep to the region. Epizootics of bluetongue subsequently were reported in the middle of the 20th century in countries of the Mediterranean basin, the United States, the Middle East, and Asia, and bluetongue virus infection was recognized in Australia during the 1970s. Infection has now been described on all continents except Antarctica, and the virus is present in most, if not all, countries in the tropics and subtropics. Since 1998, at least five different serotypes of bluetongue virus (serotypes 1, 2, 4, 9, and 16) have spread throughout formerly free areas of the Mediterranean basin, affecting ruminants in North Africa, the Iberian peninsula, the Mediterranean islands (Balearic Islands, Sardinia, Corsica, Cyprus), Italy, the Balkan countries, and Greece. Of these five serotypes, only serotype 1 has spread into northern Europe from the Mediterranean basin. Independently, another viral serotype (serotype 8) appeared in northern Europe in 2006 and this virus has rapidly spread to involve many countries, including the Scandinavian countries that are located farther north than bluetongue virus ever has previously been documented. The strain of bluetongue virus serotype 8 that spread throughout Europe is highly virulent to numerous animal species,

and has precipitated the most economically devastating outbreak of bluetongue in recorded history. In 2008, two additional bluetongue virus serotypes (6 and 11) also appeared in northern Europe, and a putative 25th serotype of bluetongue virus, designated Toggenberg virus, was isolated from goats in Switzerland.

Elsewhere in the world, bluetongue is of greatest economic importance to sheep production, although the severity of disease varies markedly depending on the virus strain, breed of sheep, and environmental stresses. Indeed, subclinical infection is characteristic of bluetongue virus infection in many regions of the world, including much of the Americas, and the major impact is through the imposition of non-tariff trade barriers that restrict the movement of live ruminants and germ plasm between bluetongue-virus-free and enzootic regions.

Clinical Features and Epidemiology

Bluetongue is most commonly a disease of certain breeds of sheep and certain wild ruminants. In sheep, it is characterized by fever that may last several days before onset of hyperemia of the mucous membranes of the oral cavity, excess salivation, and frothing at the mouth; a nasal discharge, initially serous but later mucopurulent, is common. Rarely, and in severe cases, the tongue may become cyanotic through vascular compromise, hence the name "bluetongue." There is a marked loss of condition and affected sheep may die, typically with increasing respiratory distress from pulmonary edema and, sometimes, acute secondary bacterial bronchopneumonia. The coronary bands of the feet exhibit hyperemia and may be so painful that affected animals become recumbent and are reluctant to move. Similarly, painful ulceration of the oral cavity makes affected sheep reluctant to eat. Edema of the head and neck is characteristic (Figure 15.6). Hyperemia of the skin may occur, leading to "wool break" some weeks later in animals that survive the acute infection. Muscle degeneration often is severe, with pronounced torticollis (wry neck) in some sheep. Convalescence frequently is protracted. Morbidity and mortality are highly variable, depending on the virus strain, environmental stressors, and the susceptibility of infected sheep. Bluetongue virus infection of white-tailed deer (*Odocoileus virginianus*) and pronghorn antelope (*Antilocapra americana*) can cause a peracute, fatal hemorrhagic disease. Bluetongue virus infection occurs in carnivores; specifically, infection and mortality occurred in Eurasian lynx fed meat that contained bluetongue virus serotype 8. Bluetongue virus specific antibodies also are common amongst free-ranging lion, leopard, and certain other large African carnivores. Bluetongue virus infection has been described in dogs, with associated high mortality in pregnant bitches that received a bluetongue virus-contaminated canine vaccine.

Bluetongue virus infection in cattle, goats, and the majority of wild ruminant species is typically subclinical

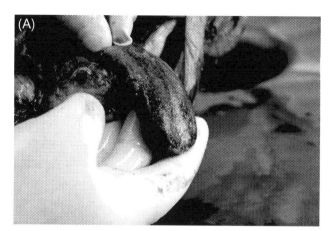
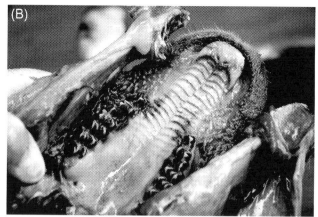

FIGURE 15.6 (A) Cyanosis and focally extensive mucosal necrosis and ulceration of the tongue in a sheep with bluetongue. (B) Acute hemorrhage, necrosis, and ulceration of the oral cavity in a sheep with bluetongue. [From N. J. MacLachlan, J. E. Crafford, W. Vernau, I. A. Gardner, A. Goddard, A. J. Guthrie, E. H. Venter. Experimental reproduction of severe bluetongue in sheep. Veterinary Pathology 45, 310–315 (2008), with permission.]

or asymptomatic; however, disease similar to that in sheep sometimes occurs in cattle, South American camelids and other non-African ungulates infected with bluetongue virus. Expression of the disease in cattle appears to result from infection with specific strains of the virus; notably, the strain of bluetongue virus serotype 8 that recently invaded northern Europe is highly pathogenic for cattle and other ungulates.

There is considerable confusion regarding the reproductive effects of bluetongue. Pregnant ewes that abort during outbreaks of bluetongue can do so in the absence of transplacental transmission of virus. Indeed, the majority of field strains of bluetongue virus rarely cross the placenta, whereas some laboratory-adapted viruses (such as live-attenuated vaccine strains, especially those propagated in embryonated eggs) readily cross the placenta to cause fetal infections and either fetal death or developmental anomalies (congenital hydranencephaly or porencephaly). Similarly, the few previously documented instances of fetal infection and virus-induced cerebral malformations in cattle occurred in areas where live-attenuated vaccines are used, suggesting perhaps that natural circulation of these vaccine viruses, or reassortant viruses that include specific genes of vaccine viruses, is responsible for these sporadic events. However, the field strain of bluetongue virus serotype 8 that recently spread throughout northern Europe does readily cross the ruminant placenta to cause fetal infection, causing considerable reproductive losses and a high incidence of fetal malformation (hydranencephaly).

Bluetongue viruses are almost exclusively transmitted by biting insects. Different serotypes of the virus are transmitted by different species of *Culicoides* (no-see-ums, midges) in different regions of the world. The epidemiology and natural history of the infection depend on interactions of vector, host, climate, and virus. Disease is most common amongst ruminants at the upper and lower limits of the global range of the

virus. Infection in these areas is seasonal, and disease occurs most commonly in late summer and early autumn. *Culicoides* insects are biological vectors of bluetongue virus, but, of the more than 1000 species, only a handful are proven vectors of the virus. Even amongst those species proven to be vectors, there are remarkable differences in their ecology and behaviour. Female *Culicoides* transmit bluetongue virus, but individual insects only become capable of transmitting the virus after an extrinsic incubation period of 7–10 days after feeding on a virus-infected animal. Thereafter, virus is shed in saliva at every subsequent blood meal.

Much remains to be determined regarding the mechanisms that allow bluetongue virus to persist between seasons in temperate zones. There is no concrete evidence of transovarial viral transmission in arthropods or of a true carrier state in ruminants. The virus also can be transmitted orally to newborn ruminants via ingestion of virus-contaminated colostrum; however, the epidemiological significance of this mechanism remains uncertain. The virus probably persists in tropical regions through a continuous, year-round cycle of infection between insect and vertebrate hosts, and available evidence suggests a similar phenomenon also occurs in temperate regions, but with a very low level of transmission in the colder months. There is clear evidence that the virus can be spread over very long distances by the wind-borne dispersal of infected *Culicoides*, introducing or reintroducing the virus to distant areas.

Pathogenesis and Pathology

After subcutaneous inoculation, bluetongue virus first replicates in the draining regional lymph node, from where it spreads to other organs, including the lungs, lymph nodes, and spleen, where virus replication occurs principally in macrophages, dendritic cells, and vascular endothelium. Virus then is released into the blood, where it promiscuously associates with all blood cell types, in titers reflective of the abundance of each cell type. Thus most virus is associated with platelets and red blood cells. Because of the abundance and extended lifespan of red blood cells—some 90–150 days in ruminants—bluetongue virus is almost exclusively associated with these cells late in the course of viremia. Association of bluetongue virus with red blood cells facilitates both prolonged viremia and infection of the hematophagous insect vector. Viremia very rarely exceeds 60 days in infected ruminants, and usually is considerably shorter.

Bluetongue virus infection causes vascular injury in susceptible species infected with virulent virus strains. Virus-mediated vascular injury results in thrombosis and tissue infarction. In white-tailed deer, extensive vascular injury results in disseminated intravascular coagulation and widespread hemorrhage, whereas widespread edema, especially pulmonary edema, is characteristic of fulminant bluetongue in sheep (Figure 15.6). It is not yet clear whether the vascular leakage that characterizes severe bluetongue in sheep is a consequence of direct virus-mediated vascular injury, or the result of vasoactive mediators released from virus-infected cells, or a combination of these two different mechanisms.

Sheep with bluetongue typically have extensive ulceration and hemorrhage in the mucosal lining of the oral cavity, esophagus, and forestomachs. Hemorrhage may also be present in the intestinal mucosa. The lungs are wet and heavy, and the airways filled with frothy fluid. There can be extensive pericardial and pleural effusion. Edema fluid is typically present in the subcutaneous tissues of the head and neck, and in the musculature of the neck and the abdominal wall. Subintimal and adventitial hemorrhages are characteristically present in the pulmonary artery, as are multifocal areas of necrosis in the myocardium of the left ventricle, as well as the skeletal musculature of the neck, limbs, and abdominal wall.

Diagnosis

The clinical presentation and lesions of bluetongue are very characteristic, as is the seasonal nature of the disease in temperate regions. Bluetongue viruses are often difficult to isolate in the laboratory, and washed blood cells, lung, or spleen are preferred. Virus isolation is carried out in embryonated eggs or in cell cultures of BHK21, Vero, or insect cells (usually by blind passage), but both systems can be quite insensitive. Reverse-transcriptase polymerase chain reaction (RT-PCR) assays, especially quantitative PCR assays, now are the standard for virus detection; however, ruminants remain positive by this assay months after infectious virus has been cleared from the blood.

Serologic techniques, most notably competitive enzyme immunoassays, based on the detection of antibodies to the VP7 group antigen, are used extensively for regulatory purposes involving the international livestock trade.

Immunity, Prevention, and Control

Animals infected with one serotype of bluetongue virus develop long-term immunity to reinfection with that serotype; however, immunity is serotype specific and dependent on the presence of virus neutralizing antibodies. Cellular immune responses are probably important in eliminating virus during primary infections, but these responses have been only partially characterized.

Control of bluetongue virus infection is almost exclusively by vaccination, as elimination of vector insects is generally impractical. Inactivated and live-attenuated bluetongue virus vaccines are available in different areas of the world. Live-attenuated vaccines to most viral serotypes were developed long ago in South Africa and the United States. These vaccines generally provide strong, serotype-specific protective immunity after a single inoculation, and they prevent clinical disease; however, attenuated virus vaccines also have inherent potential disadvantages: (1) some live-attenuated vaccines, especially those propagated in embryonated eggs, were associated with fetal death and cerebral abnormalities in sheep; (2) under-attenuated vaccine viruses can induce clinical reactions in vaccinated animals; (3) vaccine viruses can be acquired by vector insects, so their use may lead to the emergence of genetic reassortants. Inactivated vaccines are safe, but they are limited to a few serotypes and revaccinations are necessary. Recombinant bluetongue virus vaccines recently have been developed, but they are not yet commercially available.

It is clear that bluetongue virus can be translocated over long distances by either wind-borne midges or viremic animals. Thus only virus-free animals should be moved from infected to uninfected areas.

AFRICAN HORSE SICKNESS VIRUS

African horse sickness is a devastating disease of horses, with up to 95% mortality after infection of susceptible horses with some virus strains. Mules and donkeys are susceptible to infection, but typically develop a more mild disease. African horse sickness virus was first described in the Middle East in the 14th century, and epizootics have occurred in South Africa at regular intervals for some 300 years. An outbreak in 1855, for example, killed some 70,000 horses in the Cape of Good Hope region, representing more than 40% of the entire horse population at the time. More recently, major epizootics have occurred in the Middle East, the Indian subcontinent, North Africa, Spain, and Portugal. The virus is enzootic in sub-Saharan Africa, and periodically invades adjacent regions. African horse sickness has never been recognized in the Western Hemisphere, eastern Asia, or Australasia. Nine serotypes of African horse sickness viruses are described.

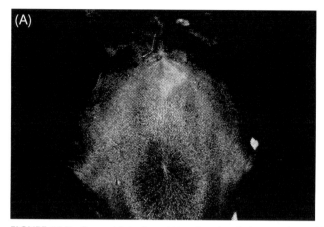 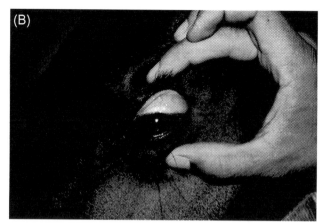

FIGURE 15.7　Supraorbital edema (A) and conjunctival congestion and hemorrhage (B) in a horse with acute African horse sickness. *(Courtesy of A. Guthrie, University of Pretoria.)*

Clinical Features and Epidemiology

The severity of clinical disease in susceptible horses, donkeys, and mules varies with the virulence of the specific strain of virus. There are several different forms of the disease, although these are somewhat artificial distinctions:

The *pulmonary form* ("Dunkop" or central form) is characterized by severe and progressive respiratory distress and death. After an incubation period of 3–5 days, horses develop fever for 1–2 days, the respiration rate then increases rapidly, and affected animals may stand with their forelegs apart, head extended, and nostrils dilated. Spasmodic coughing may occur terminally, accompanied by profuse sweating and a discharge of frothy fluid from the nostrils. This pulmonary form is most common in completely susceptible horses infected with a highly virulent virus.

The *cardiac form* ("Dikkop" or peripheral form) can be more protracted and somewhat milder. Fever lasts for 3–6 days, and, as the temperature falls, characteristic edema appears, involving the supraorbital fossae and eyelids, sometimes with accompanying congestion and hemorrhage in the conjunctiva (Figure 15.7). Subsequently, the edema extends to affect the lips, tongue, intermandibular space, and laryngeal region. Subcutaneous edema may also track down the neck toward the chest. Mortality rates for such cases may be as high as 50%; death occurs within 4–8 days of onset of fever.

Disease of intermediate severity (*mixed form*) is seen in some animals. Mortality is approximately 70%.

Horse sickness fever is manifest in animals that are partially immune or resistant to expression of disease, such as donkeys and zebra. Horses that are partially immune as a result of vaccination also may express this form, which is characterized by transient fever, inappetence, increased respiratory rate, and very low mortality.

The epidemiology of African horse sickness is similar to that of bluetongue, and *Culicoides imicola* and

Culicoides bolitinos are proven vectors of the virus in South Africa. However, *Culicoides* species from other regions of the world can be infected experimentally with African horse sickness virus. Infection and disease are highly seasonal, typically occurring in the late summer on swampy low-lying farms.

Pathogenesis and Pathology

The pathogenesis of African horse sickness has much in common with that of bluetongue. After the bite of an infected insect, the virus replicates in the local lymph node before spreading to other tissues and organs. As with bluetongue, the precise mechanisms by which the viruses cause the devastating vascular injury that characterizes fatal horse sickness are unknown, but it seems increasingly likely that pro-inflammatory and vasoactive mediators released from virus-infected cells (dendritic cells, macrophages, and endothelial cells) are important.

At necropsy, striking pulmonary edema is characteristic of infection of horses with the most virulent viruses. The lungs are distended and heavy, and frothy fluid may fill the trachea, bronchi, and bronchioles. This frothy exudate may ooze from the nostrils. There also may be pleural and pericardial effusion, along with pericardial hemorrhage. Thoracic lymph nodes may be edematous, and the gastric fundus congested. Gelatinous yellow fluid is present in the subcutis of horses infected with less virulent viruses and having a longer clinical course, especially in the tissues surrounding the jugular veins and ligamentum nuchae. The pulmonary form is occasionally seen in dogs that consume virus-contaminated meat.

Diagnosis

African horse sickness is an exotic disease outside sub-Saharan Africa. Clinical diagnosis of the pulmonary and cardiac forms is not difficult, because of the spectacularly severe nature of the disease and characteristic edema of the supraorbital fossae. Similarly, the severe pulmonary edema, and pericardial and pleural effusion at necropsy provide a further reason to suspect the disease, especially in enzootic areas and in the appropriate season. African horse sickness virus can be isolated in cell culture or by intracerebral inoculation of 2- to 6-day-old mice with blood or a spleen suspension from the suspect animal, using washed cell fractions to remove any early virus-neutralizing antibody. Identification of the particular virus (e.g., African horse sickness viruses 1–9) is achieved by neutralization assays, although RT-PCR assays increasingly now are available for rapid diagnosis of the infection.

Immunity, Prevention, and Control

Like bluetongue, horses that recover from natural African horse sickness virus infection develop life-long immunity against the homologous serotype and, in some instances, partial immunity against heterologous serotypes. Foals of immune dams acquire passive colostral immunity lasting for 3–6 months. Attenuated virus vaccines have been used in South Africa for many years. The current polyvalent vaccine consists of trivalent and quadrivalent preparations that are administered sequentially. Several courses of vaccination may be required to achieve complete immunity, and annual boosting is recommended. Serious disease can occur in a small percentage of well-vaccinated horses. Inactivated virus vaccines have been developed when required for some serotypes, but there is a clear need for safe and effective new-generation vaccines should African horse sickness emerge from its historic distribution range. Indeed, recent experiences with emergence of bluetongue throughout Europe provide a sobering reminder of the devastating impact of these *Culicoides*-transmitted diseases, and the inability of regulatory authorities to prevent their spread.

Human Disease

Very rarely, African horse sickness can be zoonotic. The first evidence of this came when laboratory workers, exposed to the virus during vaccine manufacture, developed encephalitis, chorioretinitis, and disseminated intravascular coagulation.

EQUINE ENCEPHALOSIS VIRUS

Sir Arnold Theiler first described a disease of horses he termed "ephemeral fever" at the beginning of the 20th century. Theiler recognized that the disease shared many similarities with African horse sickness, but that it constituted a distinct entity. What very likely is the same disease was "rediscovered" some 60 years later when it was given the unfortunate name of equine encephalosis, on the basis of rather nebulous signs and the lack of characteristic or severe gross or histological lesions in affected horses. Equine encephalosis virus infection is transmitted by *Culicoides* insects, thus its epidemiology is similar to that of African horse sickness virus. Most infections are subclinical; however, sporadic fatal infections—preceded by alternating periods of hyperexcitement and depression—occur in horses. Equine encephalosis virus can be isolated from affected horses or demonstrated by RT-PCR. There are at least seven different serotypes of equine encephalosis virus, and many strains. These viruses have been demonstrated to date only in South Africa and Israel, but they probably have a wider distribution. In addition to sporadic mortality in horses, the importance of equine encephalosis is that that infection can, on rare occasions, mimic African horse sickness.

EPIZOOTIC HEMORRHAGIC DISEASE VIRUS AND IBARAKI VIRUS

Epizootic hemorrhagic disease of deer was first shown to have a viral etiology in 1955 in the United States and in 1964 in Canada. The viruses are transmitted by *Culicoides* insects and have been isolated from wild and domestic ruminants and arthropods in North America, Asia, Africa and Australia, often without any associated clinical disease. With the notable exception of Ibaraki virus, which is a pathogenic variant of epizootic hemorrhagic disease virus serotype 2, most epizootic hemorrhagic disease virus infections of ruminants are mild or subclinical. However, disease occurs in some infected animals, and white-tailed deer are especially susceptible. Infected white-tailed deer develop disseminated intravascular coagulation and a generalized hemorrhagic disease (diathesis) that is indistinguishable from that caused by bluetongue virus infection. Similarly, cattle infected with certain strains of epizootic hemorrhagic disease virus develop oral lesions similar to those of bluetongue. Recent epizootics of apparent epizootic hemorrhagic disease have occurred amongst cattle in both North Africa and the Middle East.

Ibaraki disease was first recorded as an acute, febrile disease of cattle in Japan in 1959; the virus is now known to be present in many parts of Southeast Asia, although infection frequently is subclinical. Ibaraki disease is characterized by ulcerative stomatitis and dysphagia in affected cattle. Abortion and stillbirth are common in some outbreaks.

PALYAM VIRUS

Abortions and congenital malformations in cattle caused by Palyam virus infection have been described amongst cattle in both southern Africa and Japan. The Japanese virus is named Chuzan virus. Hydranencephaly and cerebellar hypoplasia were the characteristic congenital malformations that occurred in calves infected with these viruses in early gestation. Similar viruses, including D'Aguilar and CSIRO village viruses, have been isolated in Australia.

OTHER ORBIVIRUSES

Several additional and potentially important pathogenic orbivirus infections of animals have been identified and partially characterized. These include Peruvian horse sickness virus, which is the putative cause of regionally extensive outbreaks of fatal meningoencephalitis of horses in South America. A similar virus, designated Elsey virus, was isolated from horses with a similar disease syndrome in the Northern Territory of Australia. Yunnan and closely related viruses such as Rioja virus have been isolated from mosquitoes and cattle, sheep, equids, and dogs in Asia and South America, including animals with meningoencephalitis.

MEMBERS OF THE GENUS *ROTAVIRUS*

ROTAVIRUS INFECTIONS OF MAMMALS AND BIRDS

Rotaviruses have been recovered from diarrheal feces of a multitude of animal species, including cattle, sheep, goats, horses, dogs, cats, rabbits, mice, rats, non-human primates, and birds. Rotaviruses are a major cause of diarrhea in intensively reared farm animals throughout the world. The clinical signs, diagnosis, and epidemiology of disease are similar in all species; the severity of disease ranges from subclinical, through enteritis of varying severity, to death. Disease is usually seen only in young animals, 1–8 weeks of age, but more rarely during the first week of life. Based on sequence and phylogenetic analysis, rotavirus strains closely related to animal rotaviruses have been detected from humans. Recent sequencing of the complete 11 genome segments of several human rotaviruses has also revealed lineages closely related to porcine, bovine, or feline strains, suggesting their earlier zoonotic derivation from inter-species transmission events.

Clinical Features and Epidemiology

Rotavirus diarrhea in calves, piglets, foals, and lambs is often referred to as "white scours" or "milk scours." The incubation period is brief, only 1–24 hours. Some affected animals are only moderately depressed, and often continue to suckle or drink milk. The feces are voluminous, soft to liquid, and often contain large amounts of mucus. Ingestion of a large volume of milk is a contributory factor to the severity of the diarrhea, as the reduced production of lactase caused by rotavirus infection exacerbates osmotic dysregulation. Other factors, particularly reduced colostrum intake, but also infections with other enteric pathogens such as

Escherichia coli, poor hygiene, chilling, and overcrowding, may contribute to the severity of disease. Young animals may die as a result of dehydration or secondary bacterial infection, but most recover within 3–4 days. Outbreaks are particularly severe in intensive production systems.

Rotavirus infection of neonates in naïve mouse colonies results in a syndrome known as "epizootic diarrhea of infant mice" (EDIM). Mouse pups suffer from abdominal bloating, malabsorption, and pasting of unformed feces around the anus, which can result in obstruction. Pups continue to suckle, but are runted; mortality is usually low. Once infection becomes enzootic within a mouse breeding population, clinical signs of disease disappear, because pups are protected by maternal antibody during their period of age-related susceptibility. A similar syndrome has been reported in infant laboratory rats infected with a group B rotavirus. This syndrome has been named "infectious diarrhea of infant rats" (IDIR). The virus is no longer common in laboratory rat colonies, and appears to have arisen as an anthropozoonosis derived from humans.

Rotavirus infection can also be clinically significant in young rabbits, and can contribute to the multifactorial enteritis complex of this species. Rotavirus is an important and common disease agent in commercial rabbitries. During epizootic infections, rabbit kits may experience very high mortality. During enzootic infections, kits receive maternal antibody transplacentally, and experience low mortality but high morbidity. Rotavirus infections are common among both Old World and New World primates, according to seroprevalence studies, but clinical disease is equivocal. Mouse, rabbit, and simian rotaviruses are all used as experimental models for investigation of rotavirus pathogenesis and immunity.

Avian rotavirus infections that result in clinical disease are most frequent in young turkeys, but are also common in chickens, pheasants, guinea fowl, partridges, quail, and ratites. Sporadic infections have been described in pigeons and ducks. Initial signs are diarrhea and wet litter, which may be accompanied by litter eating, dehydration, poor weight gains, restlessness, huddling, stunting, and mortality.

Rotaviruses are excreted in the feces of infected animals in high titer (up to 10^{11} viral particles per gram); maximum shedding occurs on the 3rd and 4th days postinfection. Rotaviruses survive in feces for several months, so gross contamination of rearing pens can occur, which explains why intensively reared animals are commonly affected. Some rotaviruses are highly resistant to chlorination, and can survive for long periods in water, so that water-borne transmission is also a risk.

Pathogenesis and Pathology

Rotavirus infections cause intestinal malabsorption and maldigestion by destruction of the terminally differentiated

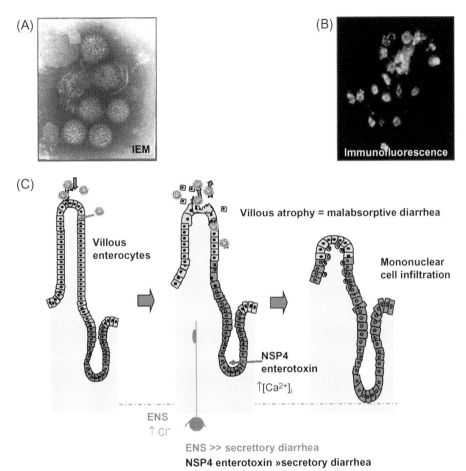

(A)

IEM

(B)

Immunofluorescence

(C)

Villous
enterocytes

Villous atrophy = malabsorptive diarrhea

Mononuclear
cell infiltration

NSP4
enterotoxin

$\uparrow[Ca^{2+}]_i$

ENS
$\uparrow$ Cl⁻

ENS >> secrettory diarrhea
NSP4 enterotoxin »secretory diarrhea

FIGURE 15.8 The pathogenesis of rotavirus-induced diarrhea, including the role of the enteric nervous system (ENS) and the rotaviral non-structural protein, NSP4. (A) Immunoelectron microscopic (IEM) of rotavirus particles. (B) Detection of rotavirus infection by immunofluorescence staining; note staining of rotavirus-infected cells lining the intestinal villi. (C) Mechanisms of rotavirus-induced diarrhea including destruction of enterocytes lining intestinal villi leading to maldigestion/malabsorption as well as NSP4 mediated secretory diarrhea. IEM, immuno-electron microscopy. *(Courtesy of L. Saif, the Ohio State University.)*

enterocytes lining the tips of the intestinal villi (Figure 15.8). The neonatal bowel is particularly susceptible to rotavirus infection and disease, because of the slow epithelial turnover rate and the high proportion of terminally differentiated epithelium. This is exemplified in globally immunodeficient mice, in which neonates are susceptible to disease, whereas adults are subclinically affected. Damaged villi become shortened and covered with immature, less differentiated epithelial cells that migrate from the crypts. These cells secrete reduced levels of disaccharidases such as lactase, and are less able to carry out glucose-coupled sodium transport. Undigested lactose in the milk promotes bacterial growth and exerts a further osmotic effect; both mechanisms contribute to the diarrhea.

Additional mechanisms of rotavirus diarrhea have been proposed, based on studies of mice. These include effects induced by the first viral enterotoxin reported, NSP4, and rotavirus stimulation of neurotransmitters, both of which activate secretory pathways. NSP4 triggers a signal transduction pathway that increases intracellular calcium concentrations and chloride secretion from crypt enterocytes that produces secretory diarrhea in neonatal mice, with resultant rapid loss of water and electrolytes (Figure 15.8C).

Diagnosis

Rotavirus infections are suspected in outbreaks of white scours, EDIM, and other enteritis syndromes among young animals. Rotaviruses were discovered by electron microscopy, and this remains a satisfactory approach to rapid diagnosis; virus particles are plentiful in the feces of affected animals, and have a highly distinctive appearance (wheel-like, hence the name "rotavirus"). The main disadvantage of this approach is that a high concentration of virions is required (at least 10^5 per gram of feces), but this can be offset somewhat by using immuno-electron microscopy (Figure 15.8A). Immuno-electron microscopy using rotavirus serogroup-specific antiserum has the advantage of being able to differentiate group A rotavirus from other rotavirus groups, and also to detect multiple viruses in a fecal specimen, as commonly seen in weaned pigs and calves. However, enzyme immunoassay is a more practicable and more sensitive method for the detection of rotaviruses in feces in most laboratories. The specificity of enzyme immunoassays can be manipulated by selecting either group- or serotype-specific or broadly cross-reactive antibodies as capture and/or indicator antibodies in an antigen-capture assay.

Recently, attention has turned to improving the sensitivity of diagnostic tests by identifying the viral genome in RNA extracted directly from feces. For example, polyacrylamide gel electrophoresis can distinguish rotavirus groups A, B, and C by RNA electropherotype pattern alone. Finally, the RT-PCR assay can be used to amplify viral RNA extracted from feces. The RNA is purified and then used as a template for reverse transcription and PCR amplification, using primer pairs appropriate for the degree of specificity desired (rotavirus groups based on VP6, or G and P genotypes based on VP7 and VP4, respectively). The rate of success of any diagnostic test for rotavirus is significantly affected by the time of sample collection; samples collected beyond 48 hours after onset of diarrhea are of limited value.

Rotaviruses are difficult to isolate in cell culture. The initial key to success was incorporation of trypsin or chymotrypsin in medium (serum-free) to cleave the relevant outer capsid protein (VP4), thus facilitating entry and uncoating of the virus. Immunofluorescence or immunohistochemistry is used to identify rotavirus antigen in infected cells (Figure 15.8B). Most bovine, porcine, and avian rotaviruses are not cytopathic initially, but can be passaged serially if grown in epithelial cells of intestinal or kidney origin (most commonly used are MA104 monkey kidney cells) in media containing trypsin/chymotrypsin. Neutralization tests using appropriate polyclonal antisera or monoclonal antibodies can be used to determine the serotype of isolates. Serum antibodies can be measured by enzyme immunoassay or neutralization tests.

Immunity, Prevention, and Control

Although the management of intensive rearing units for farm animals can be improved to reduce the incidence of disease, there is little likelihood that improved hygiene alone can completely control rotavirus infections. Local immunity in the small intestine is more important than systemic immunity in providing resistance to infection. In domestic mammals, rotavirus antibodies present in immune colostrum and milk are particularly important in protecting neonatal animals. Although much of the colostral antibody enters the circulation, serum antibody levels are not as critical for protection, except possibly in calves, in which passively acquired serum antibodies are transudated back into the intestine. Far more important for many species is the continued presence of antibody in the gut lumen. Ingestion of large volumes of colostrum for a short period gives protection for only about 48 hours after suckling ceases, whereas continuous feeding of smaller amounts of colostrum can provide protection for as long as it is available. Inoculation of the dam with inactivated or attenuated rotavirus vaccines promotes higher levels of antibody in the colostrum and milk, and a longer period of antibody secretion

in milk, with a corresponding decrease in the incidence of disease in neonates. Vaccines are not available for birds.

Recovery in severely affected calves or foals can be aided by administering oral electrolyte solutions containing glucose, to offset dehydration, shortly after the onset of diarrhea.

Because EDIM is a clinically significant disease syndrome in laboratory mice, considerable effort is expended toward serological surveillance and prevention. Laboratory mice can be protected from exposure through utilization of cage-level barriers, such as filter tops or ventilated rack systems.

MEMBERS OF THE GENUS *COLTIVIRUS*

COLORADO TICK FEVER VIRUS

Colorado tick fever is a zoonotic disease that occurs in forest habitats at 1000–3000 meters elevation in the Rocky Mountain region of North America. The vector is the wood tick, *Dermacentor andersoni*; virus is transmitted trans-stadially and overwinters in hibernating nymphs and adults. Some rodent species have prolonged viremia (more than 5 months), which may also facilitate virus persistence. Nymphal ticks feed on small mammals such as squirrels and other rodents, which serve as the reservoir for the virus. Adult ticks feed on larger mammals, including humans, during the spring and early summer. Eyach virus fills the same niche in Europe: it is widespread in ticks, and antibodies have been reported in patients with meningoencephalitis and polyneuritis, as well as a syndrome resembling that caused by Colorado tick fever virus.

The disease in humans is characterized by an incubation period of 3–6 days, followed by a sudden onset of illness. There is "saddle-back" fever, headache, retro-orbital pain, severe myalgia in the back and legs, and leukopenia; convalescence can be protracted, particularly in adults. More serious forms of the disease, notably meningoencephalitis and hemorrhagic fever, occur in perhaps 5% of cases, mainly in children. Virus can be isolated from red blood cells or detected inside them by immunofluorescence, even several weeks after symptoms have disappeared. This is a remarkable situation, as erythrocytes have no ribosomes and cannot support virus replication; however, the virus replicates in erythrocyte precursors in bone marrow, then persists in mature erythrocytes throughout their lifespan, protected from antibody during a viremia that can be as long as 100 days. The related Eyach virus, which is spread by Ixodid ticks, has been incrimintaed as a sporadic cause of human neurological disease in Europe.

MEMBERS OF THE GENUS *AQUAREOVIRUS*

Aquareoviruses are amenable to isolation in several established fish cell lines and are thus often encountered during routine examinations of healthy fish and mollusk populations. However, aquareoviruses also have frequently been incriminated as the cause of serious diseases among fish and mollusks (oyster and clams), although experimental studies have been ambiguous in confirming the pathogenic potential of individual virus strains. The aquareovirus from grass carp has received the most attention as the putative cause of widespread and significant mortality among fingerling and yearling grass and black carp in Asia. Affected fish exhibit numerous hemorrhages on the body surface, the base of the fins, and the eye, and mortality may reach 80%. However, the potential role of concomitant bacterial infections in many outbreaks has confused the role of grass carp aquareovirus in disease epizootics. Furthermore, experimental infections with grass carp reovirus and its close relative, golden shiner reovirus, have not caused obvious disease or mortality among several carp species or golden shiners.

Aquareoviruses have been isolated from marine mollusks (e.g., American oysters and hard clams) but their pathogenic role is unclear. It has been proposed that reoviruses identified among crustaceans (shrimp and crabs) be included as additional members of the genus *Aquareovirus*; however, their different genomes (12 vs. 11 segments) suggest they may be more closely related to insect reoviruses, or that they may constitute a new and distinct genus. These crustacean viruses are often associated with neurological diseases characterized by signs such as trembling and paralysis before death, but further characterization of these syndromes is needed.

OTHER REOVIRUSES

Viruses in the genus *Seadornavirus* circulate continuously in Asia and Southeast Asia, where they are transmitted by mosquitoes to humans and animals. Human infections are associated with influenza-like illness and neurological disease. These viruses have been isolated from naturally infected swine and cattle in China, and fatal disease has been described after experimental infection of adult mice.

Birnaviridae

Chapter Contents

The family *Birnaviridae* includes viruses with two segments of double-stranded RNA. Two members of the family, the agents of infectious bursal disease of chickens and infectious pancreatic necrosis of fish are economically significant pathogens.

Infectious bursal disease was first recognized in 1962 in an outbreak in Gumboro, Delaware; further outbreaks were subsequently referred to as "Gumboro disease." The most prominent lesion of this disease is located in the cloacal bursa (bursa of Fabricius), hence the present name of the disease. Large numbers of virions were observed by electron microscopy in the bursa of infected birds during early investigations of the disease, but these virus particles were initially misidentified as picornaviruses, adenoviruses, or reoviruses. Infectious pancreatic necrosis was first described in 1941 among rainbow trout (*Oncorhynchus mykiss*) in North America, although the viral etiology was not established until the 1950s. Infectious pancreatic necrosis virus and closely related viruses now occur worldwide and are responsible for considerable economic losses to salmonid aquaculture.

Birnavirus-like virions also have been observed in the feces of humans and animals with and without diarrhea, including rats, guinea pigs, cattle, swine, and a variety of zoo species. Some of these agents vary from true birnaviruses in characteristics such as their virion size and the number and length of genome segments, thus the designation "picobirnaviruses" has been proposed. These agents are potential but largely unproven causes of diarrhea in both humans and animals.

PROPERTIES OF BIRNAVIRUSES

Classification

The family *Birnaviridae* comprises three genera: *Avibirnavirus*, *Aquabirnavirus*, and *Entomobirnavirus*. Infectious bursal disease virus is the sole member of the genus *Avibirnavirus*. Members of the genus *Aquabirnavirus* include infectious pancreatic necrosis virus of salmonid fish and related viruses of mollusks and crustaceans. Members of the genus *Entomobirnavirus* infect only insects. The classification of the "picobirnaviruses"—that is, viruses that resemble birnaviruses but are smaller (30–40 nm diameter compared with 60 nm for the birnaviruses, and bi- or tri-segmented genomes), has not been resolved.

Virion Properties

Birnavirus virions are non-enveloped, approximately 60 nm in diameter, and hexagonal with a single shell having icosahedral symmetry (Figure 16.1). The genome is approximately 6 kbp and consists of two molecules of linear double-stranded RNA, designated A and B (Figure 16.2). Segment A ranges from >2.9 to <3.4 kbp in size and contains two open reading frames, the largest of which encodes a polyprotein that is processed to form two structural proteins, VP2 and VP3, and a viral protease (designated as VP4 or NS, depending on the virus) that autocatalytically cleaves the polyprotein. The major capsid protein, VP2, contains the principal antigenic site responsible for eliciting neutralizing antibodies, and is responsible for cellular

Fenner's Veterinary Virology. DOI: 10.1016/B978-0-12-375158-4.00016-X

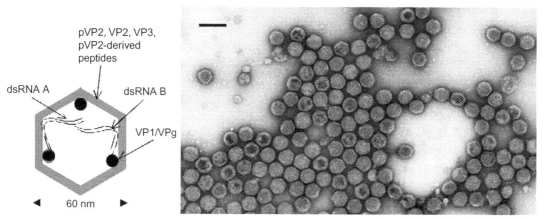

FIGURE 16.1 (Left) Diagram of a particle of infectious bursal disease virus (IBDV); (Right) negative contrast electron micrograph of IBDV virions. The bar represents 100 nm (Courtesy of J. Lepault). dsRNA, double-stranded RNA; VP2, VP3, capsid proteins; pVP2, precursor to VP2; VP1, RNA polymerase; VPg, genome-linked VP1. *[From* Virus Taxonomy: Eighth Report of the International Committee on Taxonomy of Viruses *(C. M. Fauquet, M. A. Mayo, J. Maniloff, U. Desselberger, L. A. Ball, eds.), p. 561. Copyright © Elsevier (2005), with permission.]*

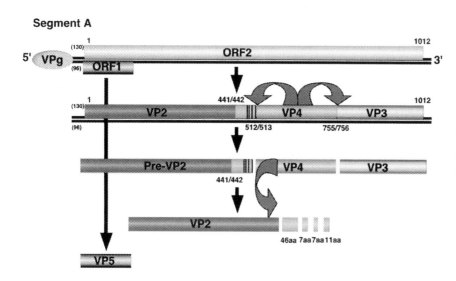

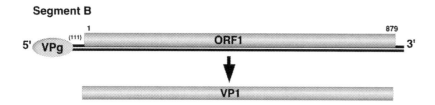

FIGURE 16.2 Schematic representation of the genome of infectious bursal disease virus (IBDV) and of the processing of the encoded proteins. ORF, opening reading frame; VP2 and VP3, capsid proteins; pre-VP2, precursor to VP2; VP1, RNA polymerase; VPg, genome linked VP1; VP4 protease; VP5 non structural protein; curved arrows indicate protease cleavage sites; numbers represent amino acid positions. *[From* Virus Taxonomy: Eighth Report of the International Committee on Taxonomy of Viruses *(C. M. Fauquet, M. A. Mayo, J. Maniloff, U. Desselberger, L. A. Ball, eds.), p. 564. Copyright © Elsevier (2005), with permission.]*

tropism and binding. The inner capsid protein, VP3, contains group-specific antigenic determinants and a minor neutralizing site. Segment B is approximately 2.7–2.9 kbp in size and encodes VP1, which is the RNA polymerase. VP1 exists as a genome-linked protein (VPg) that circularizes segments A and B by tightly binding to their ends. Termini of the genome segments resemble those of other segmented RNA viruses such as reoviruses and influenza viruses, in which both the 5′ and 3′ ends are homologous between the segments. At both ends of both segments, there are direct terminal and inverted repeats that are predicted to form stem and loop secondary structures and probably contain important signals for replication, transcription, and encapsidation.

Virions are relatively heat stable, and their infectivity is resistant to exposure at pH 3 and to ether and chloroform.

TABLE 16.1 Properties of Birnaviruses

Virions are non-enveloped, hexagonal in outline, approximately 60 nm in diameter, with a single shell having icosahedral symmetry; picobirnaviruses are smaller (30–40 nm) viruses with similar properties

Genome consists of two molecules of linear double-stranded RNA, designated A and B, approximately 6 kbp in overall size

Four structural proteins, and one or more non-structural proteins [RNA polymerase (transcriptase)]

Cytoplasmic replication

Survives at 60°C for 60 minutes; stable at pH 3 to pH 9

Member viruses occur in chickens (infectious bursal disease virus), fish (infectious pancreatic necrosis virus); picobirnaviruses have been detected in feces of humans and several species of animals, sometimes in association with diarrhea

Virus Replication

Infectious bursal disease virus replicates in both chicken and mammalian cells; however, highly pathogenic strains may be difficult to cultivate. Infectious pancreatic necrosis virus replicates in fish cell lines incubated below 24°C. Both avibirnaviruses and aquabirnaviruses can enter susceptible cells by the endocytic pathway, and heat-shock protein 90 is a component of the putative cellular receptor complex for infectious bursal disease virus. Many early events in the infection cycle, however, remain to be characterized.

Birnaviruses replicate in the cytoplasm without greatly depressing cellular RNA or protein synthesis. The viral mRNA is transcribed by a virion-associated RNA-dependent RNA polymerase (transcriptase-VP1). RNA replication is believed to be initiated independently at the ends of the segments and to proceed by strand displacement, with the inverted terminal repeats at the ends of each segment playing a part in replication (Table 16.1).

INFECTIOUS BURSAL DISEASE VIRUS

Infectious bursal disease occurs worldwide in chickens, and few commercial flocks are free of the causative virus. Infectious bursal disease is of great economic importance, principally as a result of the severe and prolonged immunosuppression that occurs during convalescence in infected birds. The disease also is of considerable scientific interest because of the distinctive tropism of infectious bursal disease virus for dividing pre-B lymphocytes within the cloacal bursa, which in turn leads to acquired B lymphocyte deficiency in affected birds.

There are two serotypes (1 and 2) of infectious bursal disease virus, but only serotype 1 is pathogenic, and only in chickens. Serotype 1 has three antigenic subgroups, all of which vary markedly in their virulence: (1) classic or standard viruses; (2) variant viruses; (3) very virulent viruses. Variant viruses produce no mortality, whereas classic (standard) or very virulent viruses can cause 10–50% and 50–100% mortality in young antibody-free chickens, respectively. Serotype 1 and 2 viruses exhibit minimal cross protection, and cross protection between serotype 1 viruses is variable. Very virulent strains of infectious bursal disease virus occur only in Europe, Africa, Asia, and South America, whereas classic and variant strains are distributed worldwide. Asymptomatic serotype 2 infections have been reported frequently in chickens and turkeys. Rarely, anti-infectious bursal disease virus antibodies have been reported in asymptomatic birds of other species, but such infections are insignificant to the ecology and epidemiology of the virus. There is no known public health significance from infectious bursal disease virus.

Clinical Features and Epidemiology

Infectious bursal disease virus is excreted in the feces of infected birds for 2–14 days; it is highly contagious, and transmission occurs directly through contact and oral uptake. The disease is most severe when the virus is introduced into an uninfected flock. If the disease then becomes enzootic or vaccination is practiced, its course is much milder and its spread is slower.

Infectious bursal disease is most severe in chicks 3–6 weeks of age, which is when the target organ, the cloacal bursa, reaches its maximal stage of development. Chicks less than 3 weeks of age may have subclinical infections because of their limited numbers of pre-B lymphocytes or from the presence of protective maternal antibodies. Birds older than 6 weeks rarely develop signs of disease, although they produce antibodies to the virus. After an incubation period of 2–3 days, chicks show distress, depression, ruffled feathers, anorexia, diarrhea, trembling, and dehydration; mortality is typically substantial. The clinical disease lasts for 3–4 days, after which surviving birds recover rapidly, although immunosuppression may persist, increasing susceptibility to other viral agents or bacteria.

Pathogenesis and Pathology

The most striking feature of the pathogenesis and pathology of infectious bursal disease is the selective replication of virus in the cloacal bursa, which, early in infection (3–4 days after exposure) becomes enlarged up to five times its normal size, with edema, hyperemia, and prominent longitudinal striations (Figure 16.3). Lymphoid follicles of the bursa collapse as a consequence of lymphocyte destruction through both necrosis and apoptosis, and in surviving birds the organ can be almost devoid of lymphocytes. Very virulent virus strains also produce depletion of cells in the thymus, spleen, and bone marrow. Hemorrhages occur beneath the serosa, and there are necrotic foci throughout the bursal parenchyma. At the time of death, the bursa may be atrophic, and the kidneys enlarged from accumulation of urate secondary to dehydration.

Following oral infection, the virus replicates first in gut-associated macrophages and lymphocytes in the ceca and small intestine (by 4–5 hours), from which it enters the portal circulation, leading to primary viremia. Within 11 hours of infection, virus is present in the lymphocytes of the cloacal bursa, with production and release of large amounts of virus, resulting in a secondary viremia and localization in other tissues, including other lymphoid tissues. The cloacal bursa plays a central role in pathogenesis, because bursectomized birds survive otherwise lethal infection without developing clinical signs or disease. However, the stage of differentiation of B lymphocytes in the cloacal bursa is crucial in supporting maximum virus replication, as only non-immunoglobulin-bearing B lymphoblasts or IgM-bearing B lymphocytes support virus replication, whereas stem cells and peripheral B cells do not. Interestingly, when lymphoid cells from the bursa are maintained in culture, only a fraction can be infected, but when the bursa is examined directly (by frozen section immunofluorescence or electron microscopy), nearly every cell is found to be infected productively. This phenomenon has been interpreted as indicating that the microenvironment of the bursa is important in maintaining the optimal level of differentiation of B lymphocytes to support virus replication. It is this exquisite virus tropism for only lymphocytes at a certain stage of differentiation that accounts for the age-dependent clinical disease in chickens.

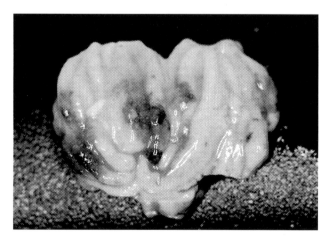

FIGURE 16.3 Infectious bursal disease. Swollen, edematous and hemorrhagic cloacal bursa from an infected chicken, with superficial hemorrhage. (*Courtesy of D. E. Swayne, University of Georgia.*)

The predilection of the virus for bursal lymphocytes leads to an important immunopathological manifestation in birds that recover from the infection. What has been called "viral bursectomy" results in a diminished antibody response and increased susceptibility to a wide range of opportunistic infectious agents, including *Salmonella* spp. and *Escherichia coli*. In addition, the immunosuppression leads to diminished antibody production after vaccination, so that outbreaks of other viral diseases may occur. These effects are most obvious in the weeks immediately following apparent recovery from infection with the virus. There is a correlation between the variety and severity of opportunistic infections and the age of the bird at the time of the viral infection: younger birds are affected more severely. Paradoxically, recovered birds develop high levels of antibody to the virus itself, because their mature peripheral B lymphocytes are still functional.

Diagnosis

Immunofluorescence staining of impression smears or sections of bursal tissue, gel diffusion tests with infected bursal tissue as the antigen, electron microscopy of bursal specimens, and virus isolation in embryonated eggs or specific chicken cell cultures such as lymphoblastoid cells are all useful in confirming the clinical diagnosis. The presence of virus or viral antigen can be detected in bursal tissue by immunofluorescence for 3–4 days after infection, for 5–6 days by immunodiffusion, and for up to 14 days by virus isolation. Detection of the infectious bursal disease virus genome by reverse transcriptase-polymerase chain reaction (RT-PCR) assay is increasingly common. Virus neutralization assays, agar gel precipitin testing, and enzyme immunoassays are reliable methods for serodiagnosis.

Immunity, Prevention, and Control

Infectious bursal disease virus is extremely stable and persists for more than 120 days in the farm environment and for more than 50 days in feed, feces, and water. The virus is resistant to inactivation by heat, cleaning, and disinfectants unless used at the correct concentration, temperature, and with sufficient contact time. Inactivation has been demonstrated with phenolic-based compounds, iodine complexes, formalin, and chloramine compounds. Improper cleaning and disinfection can lead to maintenance of the virus on contaminated premises and, hence, continued indirect transmission via contaminated feed, water, dust, litter, and clothing, or mechanical spread through insects. The virus is not vertically transmitted through the egg and birds are not persistently infected.

Vaccination is the primary method of control, although some breeds of chicken exhibit natural partial resistance to the disease. Protection against infection is primarily mediated by humoral immunity, but cell-mediated immunity has an additive effect. Because of the complexity of raising poultry, there is no one single vaccination program that fits all production systems and types of chickens. However, the basic premise is that breeding stock are vaccinated to produce immunity of progeny through maternal antibodies that are passively transferred via the egg yolk. Newly hatched chicks are protected for 1–3 weeks, but, with high serum titers in breeders, protection can extend up to 4–5 weeks after hatching. Vaccination programs vary with breeder companies, but a typical program would include oral live-virus vaccination of breeding stock after they have reached the age of about 18 weeks, with an injection of inactivated vaccine in oil adjuvant just before laying. The inactivated vaccine may be re-administered a year later, to ensure that high levels of neutralizing antibody are present throughout the laying life of the hens. In situations in which chicks have low or inconsistent levels of maternal antibodies, vaccination is carried out with an attenuated virus vaccine, beginning as early as 1–2 weeks of age. Broiler (meat-type) chickens can be vaccinated *in ovo* at 18 days of incubation with live-attenuated or virus–immune complex vaccines, to elicit an active immune response earlier in the chick's life.

Experimentally, the VP2 protein alone produces a protective immune response and has been expressed as an immunogen in yeast, baculovirus, and with various virus vectors such as recombinant fowl poxvirus or herpesvirus of turkeys. These potential vaccine products can induce high titers of neutralizing antibody, but they have not yet displaced conventional attenuated or inactivated vaccines, and only the herpesvirus of turkeys product is commercially available. A major challenge is to continue to modify vaccines so that they are effective against novel antigenic variants as those emerge in the field.

INFECTIOUS PANCREATIC NECROSIS VIRUS

Infectious pancreatic necrosis is a highly contagious and lethal disease of several salmonid fish species, but most often rainbow and brook trout in freshwater hatcheries. First feeding fry are the most apt to show clinical signs of disease, whereas virus exposures of fish older than 4 months often result in subclinical infections. Disease also occurs among young farmed Atlantic salmon (*Salmo salar*) in freshwater, but may also occur among smolts (juveniles) 6–8 weeks after transfer to sea water cages. Subclinical infectious pancreatic necrosis virus infection has been described in an ever increasing number of freshwater and marine fish species, which may in some cases be related to their proximity to farmed salmonid populations

that experience outbreaks of the disease. The potential spread of the virus from origins in North American salmonid fish to those in many other countries is probably related to historic and unrestricted movements of salmonid eggs and live fish. There are two distinct serogroups of infectious pancreatic necrosis virus, each with several serotypes, several of which contain viruses that are pathogenic.

Clinical Features and Epidemiology

Disease is usually observed in trout fingerlings shortly after they commence to feed in freshwater, and among Atlantic salmon smolts following transfer to sea water cages. With increasing age of the fish, the infection becomes subclinical. Subclinical infections are common and may persist for the lifetime of the fish, with periodic shedding of virus in the urine, feces, and reproductive fluids at spawning. Affected fish are dark in color, with a swollen abdomen, mild to moderate bilateral exophthalmos, and often pale gills. Cutaneous hemorrhages on the ventral body surface and at the base of the fins, and trailing fecal casts may also be present. A frantic corkscrew swimming followed by periods of rest is commonly observed before death. Mortality can range from 10 to 90%.

Pathogenesis and Pathology

In small fish, visceral organs, including the heart, liver, kidney, and spleen, are pale and the stomach and small intestine contain ropey mucus (Figure 16.4). Multiple petechiae may be present in visceral fat between intestinal ceca, especially in larger fish. Microscopic lesions are characterized by small to larger foci of necrosis in acinar cells of the pancreas, and may also be present in hemopoietic tissues of the kidney, liver, and intestinal mucosa.

Diagnosis

The diagnosis of infectious pancreatic necrosis in fish with typical gross or microscopic lesions is confirmed by virus isolation in standard fish cell cultures. Kidney is the tissue of choice for sampling, as high concentrations of virus are present in the kidneys of fish with either clinical or subclinical infections. Virus can be titrated in fish cells by plaque assay. Immunofluorescence (frozen sections or tissue smears) with virus-specific monoclonal or polyclonal antibodies may be used for direct detection of viral antigens in internal organs and as confirmation of virus identity from cell cultures. The identity of infectious pancreatic necrosis virus also can be determined by neutralization, enzyme-linked immunosorbent assay or RT-PCR assays. Antiviral

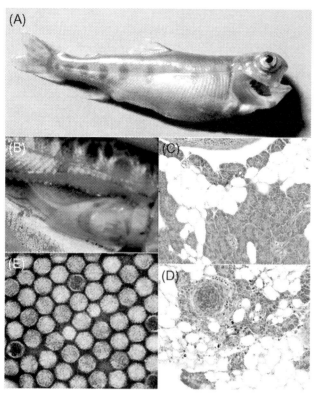

FIGURE 16.4 Infectious pancreatic necrosis. (A) Abdominal distention and pale gills in an infected brook trout. (B) Hemorrhages in the
mesentery adjacent to the intestines and ceca. (C) Normal acinar cells
of the exocrine pancreas. (D) Necrosis of acinar cells in proximity to an
islet. (E) Gradient-purified virions. *(A, B: Courtesy of K. Wolf, Cornell
University. C, D: Courtesy of R. Hedrick, University of California.)*

antibodies are present in fish with subclinical infections, but
serology is not routinely used as a diagnostic approach.

Immunity, Prevention, and Control

Virus shedding from persistently infected carrier fish contributes to transmission of the virus to fish that cohabit the
same waters. The presence of the virus in eggs may result
in vertical transmission to progeny, even when eggs are
subjected to standard disinfection procedures. The virus is
highly stable under various environmental conditions, surviving for months in fresh or sea water and retaining infectivity after passage through the gut of fish-eating birds.
Control strategies are based on hygiene, utilization of water
sources free of fish (e.g., well water), disinfection of equipment with iodophores, culling of infected breeder fish, and
depopulation and sanitization if an outbreak occurs.

It is now a common practice, before Atlantic salmon are
transferred to sea water, to immunize them with a multivalent vaccine containing both bacterial antigens and recombinant VP2 from infectious pancreatic necrosis virus. Recent
controlled-challenge studies confirmed that vaccination is a
cost-effective control measure against this disease.

The World Organization for Animal Health (OIE) lists
infectious pancreatic necrosis as one of several important
diseases that require control in the international commerce
of live fish and eggs. Procedures for the screening of fish to
demonstrate freedom from the virus are detailed in the OIE
Manual for Diagnostic Tests for Aquatic Animals (http://
www.oie.int/eng/normes/fmanual/A_summary.htm?e1d11).

Paramyxoviridae

Chapter Contents

The family *Paramyxoviridae* is included in the order *Mononegavirales*, along with the families *Rhabdoviridae*, *Filoviridae*, and *Bornaviridae*. This order was established to bring together viruses with distant, ancient phylogenetic relationships (Figure 17.1) that are also reflected in similarities in their gene order and strategies of gene expression and replication. All these viruses are enveloped and, other than bornaviruses, have prominent envelope glycoprotein

Fenner's Veterinary Virology. DOI: 10.1016/B978-0-12-375158-4.00017-1

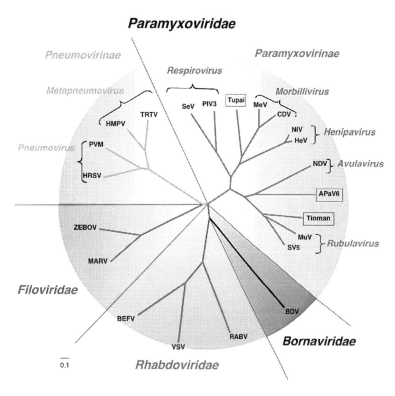

FIGURE 17.1 Phylogenetic tree of members of the order *Mononegavirales*. The tree was constructed using the sequences of the conserved domain III of the RNA polymerase. aPaV6, avian parainfluenza virus type 6; BDV, Borna disease virus; BEFV, bovine ephemeral fever virus; CDV, canine distemper virus; HeV, Hendra virus; HMPV, human metapneumovirus; HRSV, human respiratory syncytial virus; MARV, Lake Victoria marburgvirus; MeV, measles virus; MuV, mumps virus; NDV, Newcastle disease virus; NiV, Nipah virus; PIV3, parainfluenza virus 3; PVM, pneumonia virus of mice; RABV, rabies virus; SeV, Sendai virus; SV5, simian virus 5; TRTV, turkey rhinotracheitis virus; VSV, vesicular stomatitis virus; ZEBOV, Zaire ebolavirus. *[From* Virus Taxonomy: Eighth Report of the International Committee on Taxonomy of Viruses *(C. M. Fauquet, M. A. Mayo, J. Maniloff, U. Desselberger, L. A. Ball, eds.), p. 613. Copyright © Elsevier (2005), with permission.]*

TABLE 17.1 Distinguishing Characteristics of Four Families of the Order *Mononegavirales*

Characteristic	Family *Paramyxoviridae*	Family *Rhabdoviridae*[a]	Family *Filoviridae*	Family *Bornaviridae*
Genome size (kb)	15–19	11–15	19	9
Virion morphology	Pleomorphic	Bullet-shaped	Filamentous	Spherical
Site of replication	Cytoplasm	Cytoplasm	Cytoplasm	Nucleus
Mode of transcription	Polar with non-overlapping signals (except pneumoviruses) and stepwise attenuation	Polar with non-overlapping signals and stepwise attenuation	Polar with non-overlapping signals and stepwise attenuation	Complex with mRNA splicing and overlapping start/stop signals
Host range	Vertebrates	Vertebrates	Humans, non-human primates and bats	Horses, sheep, cats, birds, (humans?) shrews and possibly other small mammals
Pathogenic potential	Mainly respiratory disease	Mild febrile to fatal neurological disease	Hemorrhagic fever	Immune-mediated neurological disease Proventricular dilation syndrome in birds

[a]*Vertebrate virus members.*

spikes. All viruses included in the order have genomes consisting of a single molecule of negative-sense, single-stranded RNA. The features that differentiate the individual families of the order include genome size, nucleocapsid structure, site of genome replication and transcription, manner and extent of messenger RNA (mRNA) processing, virion size and morphology, tissue specificity,

host range, and pathogenic potential in their respective hosts (Table 17.1).

Several of the most devastating diseases of animals and humans are caused by members of the family *Paramyxoviridae*. In particular, the viruses causing rinderpest, canine distemper, Newcastle disease, measles, and mumps have arguably caused more morbidity and mortality than any other single group of related viruses in history. The impact of these diseases has been dramatically reduced through the use of vaccines in both humans and animals, in combination with depopulation and restrictions on animal movements for diseases such as rinderpest and Newcastle disease. Other viruses in this family also cause disease in a wide variety of mammals, birds, and reptiles—including, amongst many examples: respiratory syncytial viruses in cattle, sheep, goats, and wildlife; Sendai virus (murine parainfluenza virus 1) in mice; avian rhinotracheitis virus (metapneumovirus) in turkeys and chickens; phocine morbillivirus in seals; ophidian paramyxoviruses, including Fer-de-Lance virus in snakes. Of recent concern and interest are the paramyxoviruses of the genus *Henipavirus* that naturally infect various species of bats, but cause high mortality rates in infected humans and animals. As wildlife species come more in contact with humans and domesticated animals through changes in habitat, the opportunities increase for cross-species infections by these and additional, as yet unidentified, paramyxoviruses.

The history of the paramyxoviruses is replete with incorrect reports that complicate their taxonomic classification, and confuses assessment of their true ability to cause interspecies infections. Specifically, interpretation of the results of previous sero-surveys is frequently complicated by the considerable cross-reactivity that occurred as a result of inapparent contamination of the test antigens, as well as the stimulation of heterotypic antibodies after infection of animals with individual viruses. Failure to recognize these limitations led to erroneous conclusions, such as a putative link between parainfluenza virus 3 infection and abortion in cattle and respiratory disease in horses.

PROPERTIES OF PARAMYXOVIRUSES

Classification

The family *Paramyxoviridae* is subdivided into the subfamilies *Paramyxovirinae* and *Pneumovirinae*, the former containing the genera *Respirovirus, Avulavirus, Henipavirus, Rubulavirus*, and *Morbillivirus*, and the latter containing the genera *Pneumovirus* and *Metapneumovirus* (Table 17.2; Figure 17.2). The family continues to expand rapidly as new viruses are discovered in wild animal populations, with a growing list of relatively uncharacterized viruses from wild or feral rodents (J paramyxovirus, Nariva virus, and Mossman virus), tree shrews (Tupaia virus), and bats (Menangle virus and Mapuera virus). Several other members of the family have not yet been assigned to the existing genera, including: Fer-de-Lance and a variety of related ophidian paramyxoviruses of reptiles, Salem virus of equines, several viruses of penguins that are distinct from avian paramyxoviruses 1–9, and Atlantic salmon paramyxovirus. The list of members of the family *Paramyxoviridae* is certain to grow as more wildlife species are analyzed for their respective viruses. Indeed, the family *Paramyxoviridae* probably will

continue to expand, not just with new viruses, but also with new genera.

The nomenclature of viruses within the family *Paramyxoviridae* is confusing and fraught with inconsistencies, as individual viruses have variously been named according to their species of origin (e.g., porcine rubulavirus, avian paramyxoviruses 2–9), geographic sites of discovery (e.g., Sendai, Hendra, and Newcastle disease viruses), antigenic relationships (e.g., human parainfluenza viruses 1–4), or given names related to the diseases that they produce in affected animals or humans (e.g., canine distemper, rinderpest, measles, and mumps viruses). Indeed, it appears that many members of this family represent related lineages of viruses that are enzootic within one principal host species but periodically cross over to another species (species-jumping), underscoring the continuing potential for cross-species emergence of these viruses as pathogens.

VIRION PROPERTIES

Paramyxovirus virions are pleomorphic (spherical as well as filamentous forms occur), 150–350 nm in diameter (Figure 17.3). Virions are enveloped, covered with large glycoprotein spikes (8–14 nm in length), and contain a "herringbone-shaped" helically symmetrical nucleocapsid, approximately 1 μm in length and 18 nm (*Paramyxovirinae*) or 13–14 nm (*Pneumovirinae*) in diameter. The genome consists of a single linear molecule of negative-sense, single-stranded RNA, 13–19 kb in size. The RNA does not contain a 5′ cap and is not polyadenylated at the 3′ end, but does have functional 5′ and 3′ non-coding elements. With the exception of members of the *Pneumovirinae*, the genomic size follows the "rule of six"—that is, the number of nucleotides is a multiple of six, which appears to be a function of the binding properties of the N protein to the RNA molecule. There are 6–10 genes separated by conserved non-coding sequences that contain termination, polyadenylation, and initiation signals for the transcribed mRNAs; viruses in the genera *Respirovirus, Avulavirus, Henipavirus*, and *Morbillivirus* have 6 genes, those in the genus *Rubulavirus* have 7, the genus *Metapneumovirus* has 8, and the genus *Pneumovirus* has 10 (Figure 17.4). The genomes of viruses in the subfamily *Paramyxovirinae* encode 9–12 proteins through the presence of overlapping reading frames within the phosphoprotein (P) locus, whereas those in the subfamily *Pneumovirinae* encode only 8–10 proteins. Most of the gene products are present in virions either associated with the lipid envelope or complexed with the virion RNA. The virion proteins include three nucleocapsid proteins [an RNA-binding protein (N), a phosphoprotein (P), and a large polymerase protein (L)] and three membrane proteins [an unglycosylated matrix protein (M), and two glycosylated envelope proteins— a fusion protein (F) and an attachment protein, the latter being a hemagglutinin (H), a hemagglutinin–neuraminidase (HN),

TABLE 17.2 Paramyxoviruses and the Diseases they Cause

Subfamily/Genus Virus	Animal Species Affected	Disease
Paramyxovirinae/Respirovirus		
Bovine parainfluenza virus 3	Cattle, sheep, other mammals	Respiratory disease in cattle and sheep
Murine parainfluenza virus 1 (Sendai virus)	Mice, rats, rabbits	Severe respiratory disease in mice (sometimes rats and other laboratory animals)
Human parainfluenza viruses 1 and 3	Humans	Respiratory disease
Paramyxovirinae/Rubulavirus		
Avian paramyxovirus 1 (Newcastle disease virus-virulent isolates)	Domestic and wild fowl	Severe generalized disease with central nervous system signs
Avian paramyxoviruses 2–9	Fowl	Respiratory disease
Canine parainfluenza virus 5 (SV5)	Dogs	Respiratory disease
Porcine rubulavirus (La-Piedad-Michoacan-Mexico virus)	Swine	Encephalitis, reproductive failure, corneal opacities
Mumps virus	Humans	Parotitis
Human parainfluenza viruses 2, 4a, and 4b	Humans	Respiratory disease
Paramyxovirinae/Morbillivirus		
Rinderpest virus	Cattle, wild ruminants	Severe generalized disease
Peste des petits ruminants virus	Sheep, goats	Severe generalized disease like rinderpest
Canine distemper virus	Dogs and members of families *Procyonidae, Mustelidae, Felidae*	Severe generalized disease with central nervous system signs
Phocine distemper virus	Seals and sea lions	Severe generalized disease with respiratory system signs
Dolphin distemper virus	Dolphins	Severe generalized disease with respiratory system signs
Porpoise distemper virus	Porpoises	Severe generalized disease with respiratory system signs
Bovine morbillivirus (MV-K1)	Cattle	Poorly characterized—significance unknown
Measles virus	Humans	Measles, severe systemic disease with respiratory and central nervous system signs
Paramyxovirinae/Henipavirus		
Hendra virus	Horses and humans	Acute respiratory distress syndrome in horses and humans
Nipah virus	Swine and humans	Acute respiratory distress syndrome in swine and humans
Pneumovirinae/Pneumovirus		
Bovine respiratory syncytial virus	Cattle, sheep, goats	Respiratory disease
Pneumonia virus of mice	Mice and dogs	Respiratory disease
Human respiratory syncytial virus	Humans	Respiratory disease
Pneumovirinae/Metapneumovirus		
Turkey rhinotracheitis virus	Turkeys, chickens	Severe respiratory disease in turkeys, swollen head syndrome of chickens

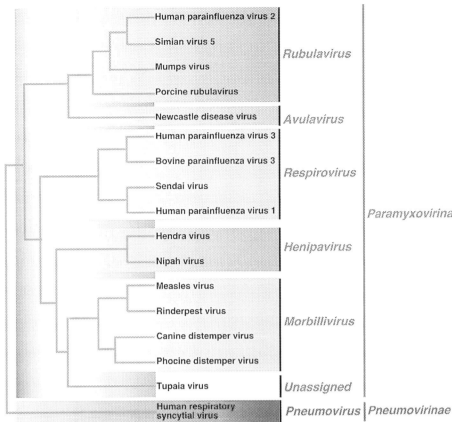

FIGURE 17.2 Phylogenetic relationships among the L protein sequences of member viruses of the family *Paramyxoviridae* [*From* Virus Taxonomy: Eighth Report of the International Committee on Taxonomy of Viruses (*C. M. Fauquet, M. A. Mayo, J. Maniloff, U. Desselberger, L. A. Ball, eds.), p. 667. Copyright © Elsevier (2005), with permission.*]

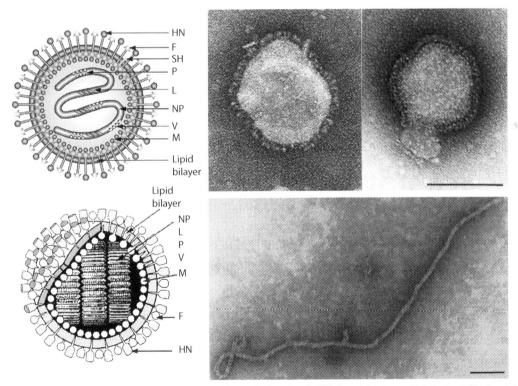

FIGURE 17.3   (Right) Negative contrast electron micrographs of intact simian virus-5 (SV-5) particles (genus *Rubulavirus*) (Top) and the SV-5 nucleocapsid after detergent lysis of virions (Bottom)(Courtesy of G.P. Leser and R.A. Lamb). The bars represent 100 nm. (Left top and bottom) Schematic diagrams of SV-5 particles in cross section (N) (formerly NP): nucleocapsid, P: phosphoprotein, L: large polymerase protein, V: cysteine rich protein that shares its N-terminus with P sequence and for SV-5 is found in virions, M: matrix or membrane protein, F: fusion protein, NH: hemagglutinin-neuraminidase, SH: small hydrophobic protein). Adapted from Kingsbury, D.W. (1990). *Paramyxoviridae*: the viruses and their replication. In: *Virology*, 2nd Edn (B.N. Fields and D.M. Knipe, eds). Raven Press, New York, and from Scheid, H. (1987). Animal Virus Structure, (M.V. Nermut, and A.C. Steven, eds). Elsevier, Amsterdam. With permission). [*From* Virus Taxonomy: Eighth Report of the International Committee on Taxonomy of Viruses (*C. M. Fauquet, M. A. Mayo, J. Maniloff, U. Desselberger, L. A. Ball, eds.), p. 655. Copyright © Elsevier (2005), with permission.*]

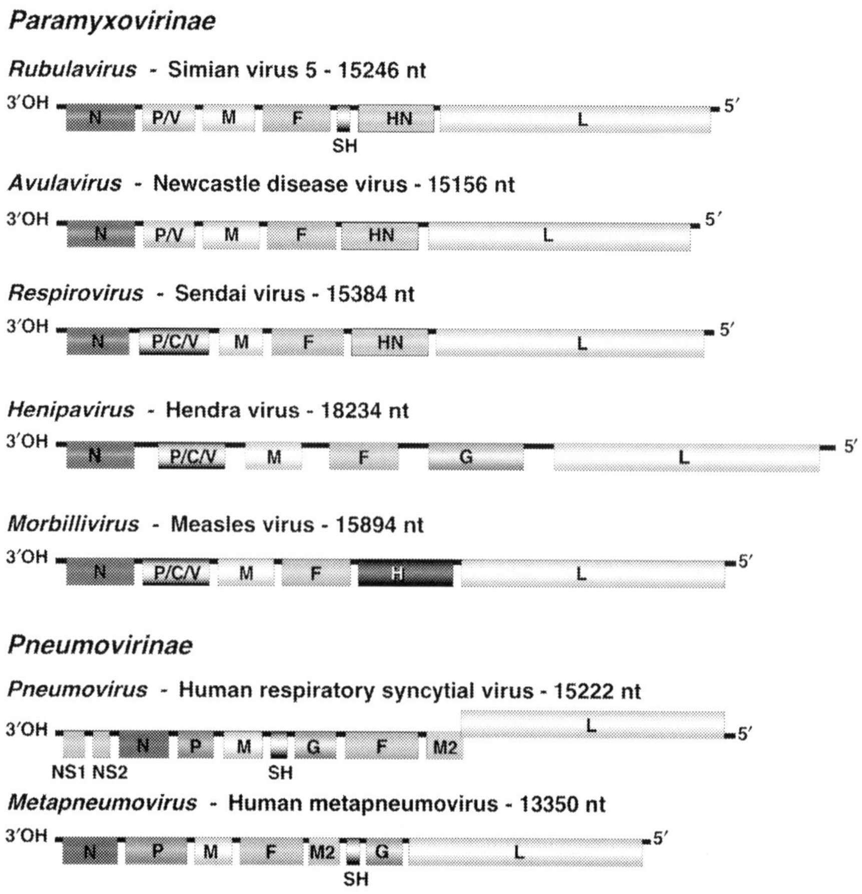

Paramyxovirinae

Rubulavirus - Simian virus 5 - 15246 nt

Avulavirus - Newcastle disease virus - 15156 nt

Respirovirus - Sendai virus - 15384 nt

Henipavirus - Hendra virus - 18234 nt

Morbillivirus - Measles virus - 15894 nt

Pneumovirinae

Pneumovirus - Human respiratory syncytial virus - 15222 nt

Metapneumovirus - Human metapneumovirus - 13350 nt

FIGURE 17.4 Maps of genomic RNAs (3' to 5') of viruses belonging to the seven genera of the family *Paramyxoviridae*. Each box represents a separately encoded mRNA; multiple distinct ORFs within a single mRNA are indicated by slashes. Numbers indicate nucleotide length of the genomic RNA. Protein letter codes are as in Figure 17.3. [*From* Virus Taxonomy: Eighth Report of the International Committee on Taxonomy of Viruses (*C. M. Fauquet, M. A. Mayo, J. Maniloff, U. Desselberger, L. A. Ball, eds.*), p. 657. Copyright © Elsevier (2005), with permission.]

TABLE 17.3 Functions and Terminology of Virion Proteins in the Family *Paramyxoviridae*

Function	Virion Protein		
	Genera *Respirovirus* and *Rubulavirus*	Genus *Morbillivirus*	Genus *Pneumovirus*
Attachment protein: hemagglutinin, induction of productive immunity	HN	H	G$^{\alpha}$
Neuraminidase: virion release, destruction of mucin inhibitors	HN	None	None
Fusion protein: cell fusion, virus penetration, cell–cell spread, contribution to induction of protective immunity	F	F	F
Nucleoprotein: protection of genome RNA	N	N	N
Transcriptase: RNA genome transcription	L and P/C/V	L and P/C/V	L and P
Matrix protein: virion stability	M	M	M
Other	(SH)	–	SH, M2

$^{\alpha}$No hemagglutinating activity.

or a glycoprotein G that has neither hemagglutinating nor neuraminidase activities]. Variably conserved proteins include non-structural proteins (C, NS1, NS2), a cysteine-rich protein (V) that binds zinc, a small integral membrane protein (SH), and transcription factors M2-1 and M2-2.

The envelope spikes of paramyxoviruses are composed of two glycoproteins: the fusion protein (F) and HN (*Respirovirus, Avulavirus, Rubulavirus*), H (*Morbillivirus*), or G (*Henipavirus, Pneumovirus, Metapneumovirus*) (Table 17.3). Both envelope proteins have key roles in the pathogenesis of all paramyxovirus infections. One glyco-protein (HN, H, or G) is responsible for cell attachment, whereas the other (F) mediates the fusion of the viral envelope with the plasma membrane of the host cell. Unlike entry of viruses through the endosomal pathway, membrane fusion initiated by the paramyxovirus F protein is not dependent upon a low pH environment. Neutralizing antibodies specific for the attachment glycoprotein (HN, H, or G) inhibit adsorption of virus to cellular receptors, but antibodies specific to F can also neutralize viral infectivity.

The fusion protein is synthesized as an inactive precursor (F0) that must be activated by proteolytic cleavage by cellular proteases. The cleaved peptides remain in close proximity by virtue of linking disulfide bonds. The specific nature of the cleavage process and the characteristics of the F0 protein differ among viruses in the different genera. However, the paramyxoviruses can be crudely divided into two groups: those with a single basic amino acid at the cleavage site and those with multiple basic amino acids at the cleavage site. The cleavage of F0 is essential for infectivity, and is a key determinant of pathogenicity; for example, virulent strains of avian paramyxovirus 1 (Newcastle disease virus) have multiple basic residues at the cleavage site, which means that the F protein can be cleaved intracellularly by furin, an endopeptidase in the *trans*-Golgi network (Table 17.4). The ubiquitous presence of this enzyme in cells facilitates the production of infectious virus in all cells capable of being infected by Newcastle disease virus. Avirulent forms of the virus have a single basic residue at the cleavage site, and the F0 protein is present in mature virions; these viruses are only activated by extracellular proteases with appropriate substrate specificity or trypsin-like enzymes in epithelial cells of, principally, the respiratory and gastrointestinal tracts. This limited "cleavability" restricts infectivity of the virus to fewer species of birds and significantly reduces the pathogenic potential of these viruses. After cleavage, the newly generated amino-terminal sequence of the F1 protein has a hydrophobic domain, and it is postulated that this is involved directly in fusion, in concert with the attachment protein.

The M or matrix protein is the most abundant protein in the virion. As with other viruses with similar proteins, M interacts with the lipid envelope, the cytoplasmic "tails" of the F- and HN-like proteins, and the ribonucleoprotein. These interactions are consistent with M having a central role in the assembly of mature virions, by providing the structural link between the envelope glycoproteins and the ribonucleoprotein. M proteins are also implicated in controlling the levels of RNA synthesis.

Virus Replication

Paramyxoviruses usually cause lytic infection in cell cultures, but adaptation of the virus (selection for mutants more

TABLE 17.4 Amino Acid Sequences at the F0 Cleavage Site of Strains of Avian Paramyxovirus 1

Virus Strain	Virulence for Chickens	Cleavage Site Amino Acids 111 to 117
Herts 33	High	-G-**R**-**R**-Q-**R**-**R***F-
Essex '70	High	-G-**R**-**R**-Q-**K**-**R***F-
135/93	High	-V-**R**-**R**-**K**-**K**-**R***F-
617/83	High	-G-G-**R**-Q-**K**-**R***F-
34/90	High	-G-**K**-**R**-Q-**K**-**R***F-
Beaudette C	High	-G-**R**-**R**-Q-**K**-**R***F-
La Sota	Low	-G-G-**R**-Q-G-**R***L-
D26	Low	-G-G-**K**-Q-G-**R***L-
MC110	Low	-G-E-**R**-Q-E-**R***L-
1154/98	Low	-G-**R**-**R**-Q-G-**R***L-
Australian isolates		
Peats Ridge	Low	-G-**R**-**R**-Q-G-**R***L-
NSW 12/86	Low	-G-**K**-**R**-Q-G-**R***L-
Dean Park	High	-G-**R**-**R**-Q-**R**-**R***F-
Somersby 98	Low	-G-**R**-**R**-Q-**R**-**R***L-
PR-32	?	-G-**R**-**R**-Q-G-**R***F-
MP-2000	Low	-G-**R**-**R**-Q-**K**-**R***L-

*Cleavage point. Basic amino acids are shown in **bold**. Note that all virulent viruses have phenylalanine (F) at position 117, the F1 N-terminus. [From Diseases of Poultry (Y. M. Saif, H. J. Barnes, J. R. Glisson, A. M. Fadly, L. R. McDougald, D. E. Swayne, eds.), 11th ed., p. 69. Copyright © 2003 Wiley-Blackwell, with permission.]

readily able to replicate in the *in-vitro* system) is usually necessary to achieve high-titer yields of virus. Formation of syncytia is a characteristic feature of many paramyxovirus infections in non-polarized cell cultures, but less so in polarized cell culture systems; similarly, syncytia are characteristic of some, but certainly not all, paramyxovirus infections in animals (Figure 2.2B). Acidophilic cytoplasmic inclusions composed of ribonucleoprotein structures are characteristic of paramyxovirus infections and, although their replication is entirely cytoplasmic, morbilliviruses also produce characteristic acidophilic intranuclear inclusions that are complexes of nuclear elements and N protein. Hemadsorption is a distinctive feature of paramyxoviruses that encode an HN protein (Figure 2.1D), and of some morbilliviruses, but not of pneumoviruses.

Paramyxoviruses replicate in the cytoplasm of infected cells; virus replication continues in the presence of actinomycin D and in enucleated cells, confirming that there is no requirement for nuclear functions. The virus attachment proteins (HN, H, G), recognize compatible ligands on the surface of host cells. For the rubulaviruses, respiroviruses, and avulaviruses, HN binds to surface molecules containing sialic acid residues—either glycolipids or glycoproteins. The neuraminidase activity of this protein is assumed, by analogy with influenza virus, to assist the virus in release from infected cells by removing the sialic acid residues that could bind virus to an already infected cell. For morbilliviruses, the cell receptor on lymphocytes, macrophages, and dendritic cells is the equivalent to the human CD150 [signaling lymphocyte activation molecule (SLAM)] glycoprotein, which explains the strong tropism of these viruses for these cell types. The receptors for henipaviruses (Hendra and Nipah viruses) are ephrin B2 and B3 cell-surface proteins, with single amino acid differences in the attachment glycoprotein G apparently determining which receptor is preferentially used. The distribution of these receptors may explain in part the pathogenesis of the systemic infections caused by henipaviruses, as these receptors are variably expressed on the surface of endothelial cells and brain stem neurons. The attachment molecules for respiratory syncytial virus (genus *Pneumovirus*) are ill defined, but may include heparan sulfate.

Following attachment, the processed F protein mediates fusion of the viral envelope with the plasma membrane at physiologic pH. The liberated nucleocapsid must remain intact, with all three of its associated proteins (N, P, and L) being necessary for initial transcription of the genomic viral RNA by the RNA-dependent RNA polymerase [transcriptase (L)]; mRNA synthesis is initiated in the absence of protein synthesis. The polymerase complex initiates RNA synthesis at a single site on the 3′ end of the genomic RNA, and the genome is transcribed progressively into 6–10 discrete mRNAs by a sequential interrupted-synthesis mechanism. This termination–reinitiation process controls the synthesis of mRNA such that the quantity of the individual mRNAs decreases with increasing distance from the 3′ end of the genome. The mRNAs are capped and polyadenylated.

When the concentration of the N protein reaches a critical level, a promoter sequence at the 3′ end of the genomic RNA is transcribed and N protein binds to the nascent RNA chain. This alters the polymerase to ignore the message-termination signals, and a complete positive-sense antigenome strand is made. This antigenome strand complexed with N protein then serves as a template for the production of negative-sense genomic RNA. A second phase of mRNA synthesis then begins from the newly made genomic RNA, thus amplifying dramatically the synthesis of viral proteins.

Whereas most genes encode a single protein, the *P* gene of the member viruses of the subfamily *Paramyxovirinae* encodes three to seven P/V/C proteins (Figure 17.4; Table 17.3). Remarkably different strategies for maximizing the coding potential of this gene complex have evolved in the different genera of the subfamily. For example, the gene complex of the member viruses of the genera *Morbillivirus*, *Henipavirus*, and *Respirovirus* encodes 4–7 proteins, the production of which utilizes two distinct transcription mechanisms: (1) internal initiation of translation from different start codons; (2) insertion of non-templated G residues into mRNA to shift the reading frame to that of an otherwise inaccessible open reading frame. Whereas the P protein itself is translated from a faithful mRNA copy of the complete gene, the smaller C protein is read in a different reading frame following initiation of translation from an internal initiation codon. Quite separately, the transcription of the *V* gene involves the insertion of an extra G nucleotide into its mRNA by polymerase site-specific stuttering ("editing"), which results in the production of a protein that displays N-terminal homology with the P protein, but with a different amino acid sequence downstream of the G insertion. Because the reading frame used to transcribe the *V* gene is also distinct, all three reading frames are utilized in the transcription of the *P/C/V* gene complex. In the case of parainfluenza virus 3, a fourth protein, D, is translated by insertion of two non-templated G residues. In the genus *Rubulavirus* there are additional variations in the transcription of the *P/C/V* gene complex and the products formed, but in the genus *Pneumovirus* each of the 10 genes encodes just a single protein, with none of the genomic coding economy and strategies utilized by viruses in the other genera.

The *P* gene is essential for virus replication but the function(s) of the proteins produced by the alternative transcription/translation of the gene are yet to be clearly defined. The C-terminal of the protein binds to the L protein and the N protein : RNA complex to form a unit that is essential for mRNA transcription. The N-terminal portion of the P protein is also proposed to bind to the newly synthesized N protein to permit synthesis of genomic RNA from the plus-strand template. Protein products of the "*P* gene" of several paramyxoviruses, including the henipaviruses and morbilliviruses, disrupt innate host defenses (Figure 17.5); specifically, mutations affecting these accessory proteins generally do not affect growth of the viruses in cell culture, but, *in vivo*, the mutants are attenuated. Available data suggest that products of the *P* gene compromise the interferon response network, possibly through inhibition of the signal transducers and activator of transcription (STAT) proteins, interferon regulatory factor 3 (IRF3), and other interferon response genes. Other activities ascribed to the accessory proteins involve regulation of levels of viral RNA synthesis.

Virion maturation involves: (1) the incorporation of viral glycoproteins into patches on the host-cell plasma membrane; (2) the association of matrix protein (M) and other non-glycosylated proteins with this altered host-cell membrane; (3) the alignment of nucleocapsid beneath the M protein; (4) the formation and release via budding of mature virions (Table 17.5).

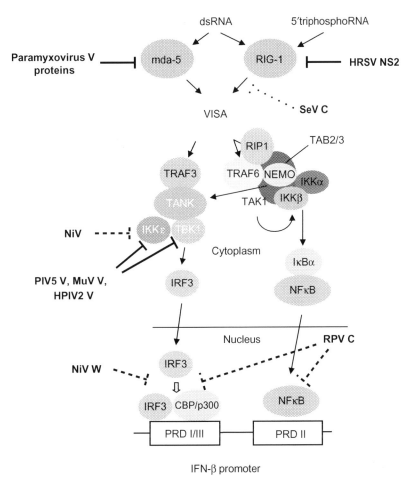

FIGURE 17.5   Paramyxovirus accessory proteins target the intracellular viral pattern recognition receptors (PRR). The signaling pathways leading from the RNA helicases mda-5 and RIG-1 to induction of interferon-β (IFN-β) are shown. Paramyxovirus V proteins interact with mda-5 and prevent its activation. Sendai virus (SeV) C protein targets RIG-1, although a specific molecular interaction has yet to be shown, The NS2 (non-structural) protein of human respiratory syncytial virus (HRSV) directly binds to RIG-1 and inhibits its activity. The V proteins of human parainfluenza virus 2 (HPIV2), simian virus 5 (PIV5, formerly SV5), and mumps virus (MuV) interact with and inhibit TBK1 and IKK , and the V protein of Nipah virus (NiV) inhibits IKK (although not TBK1). The C protein of rinderpest virus (RPV) and the W protein of NiV have uncharacterized nuclear targets that act downstream of transcription factors. CBP; IKK, inhibitory protein kappa B (IκB) kinase; IRF3, IFN regulatory factor 3; NEMO, NFκB essential modulator; NFκB, nuclear factor κB; PRD; RIP1, receptor-interacting protein 1; TAB2/3; TAK1, transforming growth factor-β-activated kinase 1; TANK, TRAF family member-associated NFκB activator; TBK1, TANK binding kinase-1; TRAF, tumor necrosis factor receptor-associated factor, VISA, *[From S. Goodbourn, R. E. Randall. The regulation of type I interferon production by paramyxoviruses. J. Interferon Cytokine Res. 29, 539–548 (2009), with permission.]*

TABLE 17.5 Properties of Members of the Family *Paramyxoviridae*

Two subfamilies: *Paramyxovirinae*, containing the genera *Respirovirus*, *Rubulavirus*, *Henipavirus*, and *Morbillivirus*, and *Pneumovirinae*, containing the genera *Pneumovirus* and *Metapneumovirus*

Virions are enveloped, pleomorphic (spherical and filamentous forms occur), and 150 300 nm in diameter. They are covered with large spikes (8–14 nm in length)

Virions contain a "herringbone-shaped" helically symmetrical nucleocapsid, 600–800 nm in length, and 18 nm (genera *Respirovirus*, *Rubulavirus*, *Morbillivirus*) or 13 nm (genera *Pneumovirus* and *Metapneumovirus*) in diameter

Virion envelope contains two viral glycoproteins and one or two non-glycosylated proteins

Genome consists of a single linear molecule of negative sense, single-stranded RNA, 13–19 kb in size, with seven to eight open reading frames encoding 10 to 12 proteins, including NP (or N), P, M, F, L, and HN (or H or G), which are common to all genera

Cytoplasmic replication, budding from the plasma membrane

Syncytium formation, intracytoplasmic and intranuclear inclusion bodies (genus *Morbillivirus*)

MEMBERS OF THE SUBFAMILY *PARAMYXOVIRINAE*, GENUS *RESPIROVIRUS*

The genus *Respirovirus* includes human parainfluenza viruses 1 and 3, bovine parainfluenza virus 3, and Sendai viruses. Counter-intuitively, human parainfluenza viruses 2 and 4 are included in the genus *Rubulavirus*, despite their antigenic cross-reactivity with the other human parainfluenza viruses. Segregation of these viruses is based on sequence analysis of specific genes (e.g., N protein) and distinctive properties of the viruses in each group. Although species designations are frequently used to identify individual parainfluenza viruses, these viruses do not necessarily respect host species boundaries.

BOVINE PARAINFLUENZA VIRUS 3

Bovine parainfluenza virus 3, although antigenically and genetically related to human parainfluenza virus 3, occupies a distinct branch of the parainfluenza virus 3 group. There is long-standing controversy as to whether bovine parainfluenza virus 3 infection alone causes disease in cattle and other ruminants, independently of its putative role of predisposing to secondary bacterial infections of the respiratory tract. It is the potential role of the virus in initiating so-called shipping fever of cattle, or bovine respiratory disease complex, which has prompted most attention and controversy. Shipping fever occurs in cattle subsequent to transportation or other stressful situations; the term refers to an ill-defined disease syndrome caused by a variety of agents acting in concert or sequentially, culminating in severe bacterial bronchopneumonia that is most commonly caused by *Mannheimia haemolytica*. The syndrome remains an economically important problem, particularly in feedlots.

Clinical Features and Epidemiology

Bovine parainfluenza virus 3 has a worldwide distribution and can infect many species of ungulates, including cattle, sheep, goats, and wild ruminants, as well as humans and non-human primates. In contrast to human parainfluenza virus 3, bovine parainfluenza virus 3 is both non-pathogenic and poorly transmitted between humans. The most important routes of transmission of bovine parainfluenza virus 3 in susceptible animals are by aerosol and fomites contaminated with nasal discharges, because this virus is exclusively a respiratory tract pathogen that rarely, if ever, becomes systemic. In calves, lambs, and goat kids, infection is generally subclinical, but sometimes may manifest as fever, lacrimation, serous nasal discharge, depression, dyspnea, and coughing. Some animals may develop bronchointerstitial pneumonia that selectively affects the anteroventral portions of the lungs. The uncomplicated respiratory infection caused by bovine parainfluenza virus 3 runs a brief clinical course of 3–4 days that is usually followed by complete and uneventful recovery. However, in stressful circumstances, cattle and sheep may subsequently develop severe bacterial bronchopneumonia—that is, shipping fever. In this case the infection, alone or in concert with other viral infections (e.g., bovine adenovirus, bovine coronavirus, bovine viral diarrhea virus, infectious bovine rhinotracheitis virus, bovine respiratory syncytial virus), predisposes to secondary bacterial infection, especially *Mannheimia haemolytica* infection. This syndrome is characterized by purulent nasal discharge, cough, rapid respiration, anorexia, fever, general malaise, and substantial mortality from acute fibrinous bronchopneumonia. Poor hygiene, crowding, transport, harsh climatic conditions, and other causes of stress typically initiate this important disease syndrome.

Pathogenesis and Pathology

Under farm conditions, clinical signs of bovine parainfluenza virus 3 infection are often obscured by concurrent infections with other agents. Upon intranasal or intratracheal inoculation of bovine parainfluenza virus 3 alone, calves show only mild fever and serous nasal discharge. Infection results in necrosis and inflammation in small airways in the lungs—specifically bronchiolitis and bronchitis—with accumulation of cellular exudate in the lumen of affected airways. Epithelial cells of the respiratory tract are the primary target cells for bovine parainfluenza virus 3, but type II pneumocytes and alveolar macrophages also are infected, sometimes with the presence of acidophilic intracytoplasmic and/or intranuclear inclusion bodies. Infection of alveolar macrophages and interference with the normal protective mucociliary clearance mechanisms of the lung predispose to bacterial invasion and pneumonia.

Diagnosis

The diagnosis of bovine parainfluenza virus 3 infection is most frequently made by virus isolation or by serology to demonstrate increasing antibody titers. Available serological assays include hemagglutination-inhibition and virus neutralization. The virus is easily isolated in a variety of cells, and virus isolation also provides a mechanism for screening for the other viruses associated with bovine respiratory disease. Nasal swabs or tracheal wash fluids are the samples of choice for virus detection, and the virus can be recovered from the nasal discharges for 7–9 days after infection, by cultivation in bovine cell cultures. The virus also may be identified in nasal discharges or respiratory tissues by immunofluorescence staining, reverse transcriptase-polymerase chain reaction (RT-PCR) tests, or immunohistochemistry. However, because of the extensive variety of agents associated with bovine respiratory disease and the high incidence of subclinical parainfluenza virus 3 infection, mere detection of the virus is not proof of any disease causality. Interpretation of results requires an assessment of the overall clinical condition in the individual animal and the herd.

Immunity, Prevention, and Control

Convalescent animals develop a strong immune response, indicated by the presence of virus-specific antibodies that mediate hemagglutination-inhibition, neuraminidase inhibition, and virus neutralization. These antibodies are predominantly directed against the hemagglutinin–neuraminidase protein. The role of the cellular response in protective immunity has not been thoroughly investigated. Sterile immunity is short lived, as it is with many respiratory pathogens, and animals become susceptible to reinfection after several months. Colostral antibodies prevent clinical disease. Inactivated and live-attenuated virus vaccines for intranasal and parenteral use are available that induce protective antibodies. Typically, combined vaccines are formulated to include various combinations of protective antigens of bovine herpesvirus 1 (infectious bovine rhinotracheitis virus), bovine respiratory syncytial virus, bovine viral diarrhea virus, and *Mannheimia haemolytica*. These vaccines are readily used to control disease problems associated with bovine parainfluenza virus 3 infection in dairy cattle, but the different management issues confronted in beef production complicate control of multifactorial disease syndromes such as the respiratory disease complex in feedlot cattle. Bovine parainfluenza virus 3 vaccines also have been used for protective immunization of sheep.

SENDAI VIRUS (MURINE PARAINFLUENZA VIRUS 1)

Sendai virus was discovered in 1952, after inoculation of lung material from pneumonic human infants into laboratory mice during attempts to isolate human respiratory viruses. These original studies occurred in Sendai, Japan, thus the designation as Sendai virus. It was subsequently shown that laboratory and feral rodents, rabbits, pigs, and non-human primates also may be infected with Sendai virus, which is closely related to human parainfluenza virus 1. This relationship has fuelled debate as to whether Sendai virus originated from humans or mice. However, although Sendai virus can replicate to an equivalent degree in a variety of animal species, including non-human primates, human parainfluenza virus 1 infects animals with markedly less efficiency.

Clinical Features and Epidemiology

Sendai virus infection of wild and laboratory rodents occurs worldwide. Although previously common in laboratory rodents, the virus has been curiously absent in recent decades. Sendai virus was a scourge of laboratory rodent colonies during the 1950s to 1980s, when it had a somewhat mysterious pattern of seasonal outbreaks in widely separated locations, suggesting exposure to human populations.

Sendai virus is among a very few naturally occurring viruses that can cause severe respiratory disease with high mortality in adult mice and, to a much lesser extent, in rats and other laboratory animals.

Sendai virus is highly contagious among rodents. Affected mice exhibit a roughened hair coat, crusting of the eyes, dyspnea, mortality in adult and post-weanling-aged mice, weight loss, and fetal resorption in pregnant animals. There is a remarkable genetic basis of susceptibility to clinical Sendai viral pneumonia among inbred strains of mice, some strains manifesting high mortality, whereas others are subclinically infected. T-cell-deficient animals such as athymic nude and severe combined immunodeficiency mice develop chronic wasting disease, with progressive weight loss and dyspnea. Immunocompetent mice that survive clinical infection recover with no persistence of the virus. Infection of other laboratory rodents and rabbits is generally subclinical or mild.

Pathogenesis and Pathology

The strict respiratory tropism of Sendai virus is related to the processing of the viral fusion (F) protein. A single basic amino acid at the cleavage site of the F protein precludes intracellular processing; rather, an endopeptidase similar to clotting factor Xa that is secreted by Clara cells within the bronchiolar epithelium of rats and mice is responsible for cleavage of the F protein, thereby allowing the virus to replicate and amplify within the respiratory tract. The pathogenesis of Sendai virus infection has been studied extensively, and provides insight into the pathogenesis of other parainfluenza virus infections. Sendai virus is largely non-cytolytic, and selectively infects respiratory epithelium in the nose, trachea, and bronchioles, as well as type II pneumocytes. Disease characterized by necrotizing rhinitis, tracheitis, bronchiolitis, and interstitial pneumonia arises during the "immune" phase of infection, wherein cytotoxic T cells destroy virus-infected cells. Thus clinical disease occurs in fully immunocompetent mice, with variable morbidity and mortality depending on the strain, immunocompetence, and age of the mice. A critical determinant of survival is the extent of immune-mediated destruction of infected type II pneumocytes, as extensive injury to these progenitor stem cells prevents repair. Older and genetically resistant strains of mice tend to develop less severe disease, because virus fails to reach the distal airways before the advent of the immune response. Likewise, when infection is enzootic within a population, young mice with waning maternal antibody are partially resistant. Animals devoid of cellular immunity, such as nude mice, do not develop the pathognomonic immune-mediated necrotizing bronchiolitis, but rather develop a chronic progressive interstitial pneumonia. Laboratory rats, other rodents, and lagomorphs usually develop very mild or subclinical infections.

Diagnosis

Enzyme immunoassays and immunofluorescence assays are most commonly used for the serological diagnosis of Sendai virus infections in laboratory rodent colonies. Antibodies are detected by approximately 7 days after infection, and their presence characteristically coincides with the advent of immune-mediated clinical signs of necrotizing bronchiolitis and pneumonia. The use of sentinel animals is a standard method for surveillance of infection in mouse colonies. The virus can be isolated in numerous cell culture systems (monkey kidney, Vero, and BHK-21 cells with trypsin in the culture medium) and embryonated eggs, and the presence of virus is confirmed by immunofluorescence or immunohistochemical staining of infected monolayers. RT-PCR testing now is standard for rapid testing and confirmation of isolates.

Immunity, Prevention, and Control

Sendai virus does not persist in immunocompetent animals that recover from infection, and antibodies remain detectable throughout life. When infections have been diagnosed, depopulation, disinfection of the premises, and screening of incoming animals are required for control. Infected colonies can be re-established by cesarean re-derivation and foster nursing, by embryo transfer, or by isolating seropositive (recovered) immunocompetent breeding mice, which will subsequently give birth to uninfected (but transiently seropositive) pups. Cesarean or embryo transfer derivation is useful for immunodeficient mice, because virus is restricted to the respiratory tract. Nevertheless, all progeny must be carefully screened to assure successful re-derivation before initiating breeding or reintroduction of animals into uninfected populations.

PARAINFLUENZA VIRUS 3 IN LABORATORY RODENTS

Guinea pigs are commonly infected asymptomatically with a parainfluenza virus 3 that is closely related to human parainfluenza virus 3. Parainfluenza virus 3 also causes natural infection and transient pulmonary lesions in laboratory rats. Parainfluenza virus 3 infections of laboratory rodents are generally discovered during sero-surveillance for Sendai virus infection, because antibodies to Sendai virus and human parainfluenza virus 3 are cross-reactive.

MEMBERS OF THE SUBFAMILY *PARAMYXOVIRINAE*, GENUS *RUBULAVIRUS*

The genus *Rubulavirus* includes mumps virus, human parainfluenza viruses 2 and 4, and simian viruses 5 (synonymous with canine parainfluenza virus 5), and 41 that are closely related to human parainfluenza virus 2, but distinguished on the basis of sequence analysis of specific genes (e.g., N protein) and their host range.

CANINE PARAINFLUENZA VIRUS 5 (SIMIAN VIRUS 5)

Canine parainfluenza virus 5 and simian virus 5 are essentially the same virus. Simian virus 5 was the first virus to be isolated from monkey cell cultures, but it is generally now believed that the dog is the natural primary host of this virus. There are unproven reports that canine parainfluenza virus 5 is zoonotic, but this debate is complicated by the antigenic cross-reactivity between human parainfluenza virus 2 and canine parainfluenza virus 5. Although the two viruses are genetically distinct, their close relationship is further reflected by the fact that the canine virus historically was referred to as parainfluenza virus 2, and it now is proposed that the virus be classified as type 5 parainfluenza virus, specifically canine parainfluenza virus 5. It also has been claimed that other species are naturally infected with this virus, but the validity of these claims is dubious, as they probably reflect either contamination or confusion with infection with closely related viruses such as human parainfluenza virus 3 infection in guinea pigs.

Canine parainfluenza virus 5 causes inapparent infection or mild respiratory disease in dogs, and the virus has been incriminated as an uncommon cause of congenital hydrocephalus also. Serological studies indicate that the infection of dogs occurs worldwide. Canine parainfluenza virus 5 is implicated in the pathogenesis of the acute respiratory disease of canines (kennel cough syndrome), and more serious, chronic respiratory disease may develop when additional microbial or viral agents, poor hygiene, or stress complicate infections. There is an incubation period of 3–10 days after infection, followed by disease that is characterized by the sudden onset of a serous nasal exudate, paroxysmal coughing episodes, and fever, lasting 3–14 days. Virus is shed for 6–8 days after infection and is spread by fomites or short-distance aerosols. Disease is most frequently seen in kennels, animal shelters, or day-care settings, and is more prevalent in younger dogs. The virus causes destruction of the ciliated epithelial cells of the respiratory tract, which predisposes infected dogs to secondary bacterial infections. Coughing can continue long after the virus has been cleared. In severe cases (mostly in malnourished or young dogs) there is also conjunctivitis, tonsillitis, anorexia, and lethargy. Because a number of other infectious agents (canine distemper virus, canine pneumovirus, canine influenza virus, canine adenovirus 2, canine herpesvirus) can induce similar clinical signs, definitive diagnosis depends on virus isolation or nucleic acid detection by RT-PCR from nasal or throat swabs. Serology can also be used to define the presence of canine parainfluenza virus 5. Vaccines are available and are usually used in various combination formulations containing antigens of other canine viral and microbial pathogens. Vaccination can complicate the interpretation of diagnostic test results, specifically RT-PCR and serology.

PORCINE RUBULAVIRUS (LA-PIEDAD-MICHOACAN-MEXICO VIRUS) AND MAPUERA VIRUS

A series of outbreaks of neurological disease, conjunctivitis, and corneal opacity, with moderate to high mortality, occurred among young pigs in commercial pig farms in central Mexico, beginning in 1980. Corneal opacity was the only manifestation of the disease in older non-pregnant animals, hence the common name for the disease, "blue eye." In pregnant sows there was an increase in abortions, stillbirths, and mummified fetuses. Characteristic histological changes in the brain were non-suppurative encephalomyelitis with perivascular cuffing, neuronal necrosis, and meningitis. A paramyxovirus was isolated from affected pigs and the disease syndrome was reproduced by inoculation of pigs with this virus. Sequence analysis resulted in designation of the causative virus as porcine rubulavirus, because of its similarities to human mumps virus. It is speculated that the virus spread to pigs from a wildlife reservoir, as porcine rubulavirus is genetically similar to a virus (Mapuera virus) that was isolated from a fruit bat in Brazil in 1979. A seropositive bat was detected in the affected region of Mexico, further supporting the speculation on the origin of porcine rubulavirus.

MENANGLE AND TIOMAN VIRUSES

In 1997, an apparently new paramyxovirus was isolated from mummified and deformed stillborn piglets in Australia. Abnormalities present in the stillborn piglets included arthrogryposis, spinal and craniofacial deformities, and central nervous system malformation. Disease was not evident in postnatal animals. There was a high seroprevalence amongst swine on the affected farm, and on several adjacent ones. Two humans on the property who had experienced undiagnosed febrile illnesses coincidentally with the recognition of the disease in the pigs had serum antibody to the new virus, named Menangle virus. As this outbreak occurred just 3 years after the initial identification of Hendra virus, it was quickly determined that fruit bats were the source of Menangle virus. Another related paramyxovirus (Tioman virus) was isolated in 2001 from pteropodid bats on Tioman Island, Malaysia. This virus can also infect pigs, although it caused only very mild disease. Both of these viruses are genetically distinct from other paramyxoviruses, and they have been tentatively placed in the genus *Rubulavirus*.

MEMBERS OF THE SUBFAMILY *PARAMYXOVIRINAE*, GENUS *AVULAVIRUS*

All viruses in the genus *Avulavirus* exhibit both hemagglutinin and neuraminidase activity. These viruses are most related to those in the genus *Rubulavirus*, but there are essential differences in the coding assignments of their respective genomes. The genus includes significant pathogens of birds, in particular Newcastle disease virus.

NEWCASTLE DISEASE AND OTHER AVIAN PARAMYXOVIRUS TYPE 1 VIRUSES

Newcastle disease has become one of the most important diseases of poultry worldwide, negatively affecting trade and poultry production in both developing and developed countries. The disease was first observed in Java, Indonesia, in 1926, and in the same year it spread to England, where it was first recognized in Newcastle-upon-Tyne, hence the name. The disease is one of the most contagious of all viral diseases, spreading rapidly among susceptible birds. Newcastle disease virus is by definition a virulent virus, classified in the genus *Avulavirus* in the avian paramyxovirus serotype 1 group, but some virus strains in this group are not Newcastle disease virus, as they are either avirulent or of low virulence. The genus *Avulavirus* also contains other species of low-virulent avian paramyxoviruses, designated as avian paramyxoviruses 2–9. Natural and experimental avian paramyxovirus serotype 1 group virus infections have been described in more than 240 bird species from 27 of the 50 orders of birds, but this virus group has the potential to infect most, if not all, bird species. The signs of the infection vary greatly depending on the species of bird and the strain of virus.

Because of the severe economic consequences of an outbreak of virulent Newcastle disease in commercial poultry, the disease is reportable to the World Organization for Animal Health (Office International des Epizooties: OIE). However, in view of the wide variation in disease caused by avian paramyxovirus serotype 1 strains, very specific criteria were established for defining an outbreak as Newcastle disease. The disease is defined as an infection of birds caused by an avian paramyxovirus serotype 1 virus that meets one of the following criteria for virulence: (1) the virus has an intracerebral pathogenicity index in day-old chickens (*Gallus gallus domesticus*) of 0.7 or greater, or (2) multiple basic amino acids have been demonstrated in the virus (either directly or deduced) at the C-terminus of the F2 protein and phenylalanine at residue 117, which is the N-terminus of the F1 protein (Table 17.4). The term "multiple basic amino acids" refers to at least three arginine or lysine residues between residues 113 and 116. Failure to demonstrate the characteristic pattern of amino acid residues as described above would require characterization of the isolated virus by an intracerebral pathogenicity index test.

As a corollary, Newcastle disease can only be caused by a virulent strain of avian paramyxovirus serotype 1 virus.

Clinical Features and Epidemiology

Chickens, turkeys (*Meleagridis gallapavo*), pheasants (*Phasianus colchicus*), guinea fowl (*Numida meleagris*), Muscovy (*Cairina moschata*) and domestic (*Anas platyrhynchos*) ducks, geese (*Anser anser*), pigeons (*Columba livia*), and a wide range of captive and free-ranging semi-domestic and free-living birds, including migratory waterfowl, are susceptible to avian paramyxovirus serotype 1 infections, including virulent strains—that is, Newcastle disease virus. Most low-virulent or avirulent avian paramyxovirus serotype 1 strains are maintained in migratory waterfowl and other feral birds, whereas others are maintained in domestic poultry. Newcastle disease virus strains are primarily maintained in and spread between domestic poultry, but cormorants (*Phalacrocorax auritus*) have been identified as reservoir hosts in North America that were implicated in the spread of the virus to domestic turkeys. Introduction of the Newcastle disease virus into a country has been documented through the smuggling of exotic birds and illegal trade in poultry and poultry products. Recent outbreaks of Newcastle disease in Australia and United Kingdom were the result of specific mutations within the fusion gene, changing an enzootic, avirulent avian paramyxovirus serotype 1 virus to a virulent Newcastle disease virus.

The clinical signs associated with avian paramyxovirus serotype 1 viral infections in chickens are highly variable and dependent on the virus strain, thus virus strains have been grouped into five pathotypes: (1) viscerotropic velogenic; (2) neurotropic velogenic; (3) mesogenic; (4) lentogenic; (5) asymptomatic enteric. The viscerotropic, neurotropic, and mesogenic strains are those that produce moderate to high mortality rates and are associated with officially designated Newcastle disease. Whereas velogenic strains kill virtually 100% of infected fowl, naturally avirulent strains of avian paramyxovirus serotype 1 virus (lentogenic and enteric strains) have even been used as vaccines against Newcastle disease because they induce cross-protective antibodies.

Virus is shed for up to 4 weeks in all secretions and excretions of birds that survive the infection. Transmission occurs by direct contact between birds via inhalation of aerosols and dust particles, or via ingestion of contaminated feed and water, because respiratory secretions and feces contain high concentrations of virus. Mechanical spread between flocks is facilitated by the relative stability of the virus and its wide host range. On rare occasions, vertical transmission has been documented for lentogenic virus strains, and virus-infected chicks have hatched from virus-containing eggs. It remains uncertain as to whether there is vertical transmission of more pathogenic viruses, although, in one experimental study, very low doses of virulent Newcastle disease virus inoculated into eggs resulted in isolation of the virus from a few hatched chicks. Vertical transmission is unclear, or a rare occurrence at best.

Legal trade of caged and aviary birds and poultry and their products has played a key role in the spread of Newcastle disease virus from infected to non-infected countries, but with implementation of stringent quarantine and testing procedures such introductions are now uncommon. However, smuggling of birds and products remains a high risk for spread of virulent Newcastle disease virus, especially with fighting cocks as occurred in Southern California in 2002–2003, and with psittacine birds as occurred in parts of the United States in 1991. Some psittacine species may become persistently infected with virulent Newcastle disease virus and excrete virus intermittently for more than 1 year without showing clinical signs. Virus may also be disseminated by frozen chickens, uncooked kitchen refuse, foodstuffs, bedding, manure, and transport containers. The greatest risk for spread is via human activity, through mechanical transfer of infective material on equipment, supplies, clothing, shoes, and other fomites. Wind-borne transmission and movement by wild birds are much less common modes of transfer.

Respiratory, circulatory, gastrointestinal, and nervous signs are all characteristic of avian paramyxovirus serotype 1 viral infections in chickens; the particular set of clinical manifestations depends on the age and immune status of the host and on the virulence and tropism of the infecting virus strain. The incubation period ranges from 2 to 15 days, with an average of 5–6 days. The velogenic strains may cause high mortality—close to 100%—without clinical signs. Other velogenic strains may cause increased respiration rate, loss of appetite, listlessness, occasionally edema around eyes and head, and typically ending in a few hours with prostration and death. Respiratory signs may be absent to severe, depending on virus strain. Some birds will have neurological signs including muscle tremors, torticollis, paralysis of legs and wings, and opisthotonos. Neurotropic strains produce severe respiratory disease followed, in 1–2 days, by neurological signs and near cessation of egg production. The infection produces 100% morbidity, but only 50% mortality, in adult chickens; mortality is higher in young birds. Mesogenic strains produce respiratory disease, reduced egg production and, uncommonly, neurological signs, and low mortality. Lentogenic strains usually cause no disease unless accompanied by secondary bacterial infections that result in respiratory signs.

The disease in turkeys is similar but usually less severe than that in chickens; there are signs of respiratory and nervous system involvement. Airsacculitis, rather than tracheitis, is the most common lesion. In ducks and geese most infections are inapparent, although a few cases of severe disease have been reported in domestic ducks. Game birds of most species have experienced outbreaks of Newcastle disease. In pigeons, avian paramyxovirus serotype 1 viral infections cause diarrhea and neurological signs, and the pigeon virus produces signs similar to velogenic or neurotropic virus strains in chickens.

Pathogenesis and Pathology

Strains of avian paramyxovirus serotype 1 virus differ widely in virulence, depending on the cleavability and activation of the fusion (F) glycoprotein. The importance of this feature of the viruses is reflected in the criteria set by the OIE for defining a virulent virus. Low-virulent or avirulent virus strains produce precursor F proteins that are cleaved only by a trypsin-like protease that has a restricted tissue distribution, and which is usually present extracellularly or in epithelial cells of only the respiratory and digestive systems. In contrast, in virulent virus strains these precursor F proteins are cleaved intracellularly by furin-like proteases present in cells lining mucous membranes. The relative ease of intracellular cleavage allows virulent viruses to replicate in more cell types, with attendant widespread tissue injury, viremia and systemic disease.

Avian paramyxovirus serotype 1 virus initially replicates in the mucosal epithelium of the upper respiratory and intestinal tracts, which for lentogenic and enteric strains means that disease is limited to these two systems, with airsacculitis being most prominent. For virulent Newcastle disease viruses the virus quickly spreads after infection via the blood to the spleen and bone marrow, producing a secondary viremia that leads to infection of other target organs: lung, intestine, and central nervous system. Respiratory distress and dyspnea result from congestion of the lungs and damage to the respiratory center in the brain. Gross lesions include ecchymotic hemorrhages in the larynx, trachea, esophagus, and throughout the intestine. The most prominent histologic lesions are foci of necrosis in the intestinal mucosa, especially associated with Peyer's patches and cecal tonsil, submucosal lymphoid tissues, and the primary and secondary lymphoid tissues, and generalized vascular congestion in most organs, including the brain.

Virulent velogenic strains cause marked hemorrhage, in particular at the junctions of the esophagus and proventriculus, and proventriculus and gizzard, and in the posterior half of the small intestine. In severe cases, hemorrhages are also present in subcutaneous tissues, muscles, larynx, trachea, esophagus, lungs, airsacs, pericardium, and myocardium. In adult hens, hemorrhages are present in ovarian follicles. In the central nervous system, lesions are those of encephalomyelitis with neuronal necrosis.

Diagnosis

Because clinical signs are relatively non-specific, and because the disease is such a threat, the diagnosis of

Newcastle disease must be confirmed by virus isolation, RT-PCR, and serology. The virus may be isolated from spleen, brain, or lungs from dead birds, or tracheal and cloacal swabs from either dead or live birds, by allantoic sac inoculation of 9–10-day-old embryonating eggs. Any hemagglutinating agents detected can be identified by avian paramyxovirus serotype 1 virus-specific hemagglutination-inhibition tests or RT-PCR tests and subsequent sequence analysis. Determination of the virulence of virus isolates is essential. Immunofluorescence staining of tracheal sections or smears is rapid, although somewhat less sensitive. Demonstration of antibody is diagnostic only in unvaccinated flocks; hemagglutination-inhibition is the test of choice because of the rapidity of the test results. Commercial ELISA kits provide a convenient alternative, but most ELISA tests are only applicable for chickens and turkeys. These serological tests can also be used for surveillance of avian paramyxovirus serotype 1 viral infections in countries where the virus is enzootic, or to monitor vaccinal immunity. Knowing the flock vaccination history is critical in interpreting virological and serological results, because live-attenuated vaccines complicate the interpretation of positive test results for RT-PCR and serological assays in vaccinated flocks.

Immunity, Prevention, and Control

Antibody production is rapid after infection, and hemagglutination-inhibiting and virus-neutralizing antibody can be detected within 6–10 days of infection, peaks at 3–4 weeks, and persists for over a year. The level of hemagglutination-inhibiting antibody is an indirect measure of immunity. Neutralizing antibodies are directed against both the HN and F proteins. Maternal antibodies transferred via the egg yolk protect chicks for 3–4 weeks after hatching as they have a half-life of approximately 4.5 days. ImmunoglobulinG (IgG) is confined to the circulation and does not prevent respiratory infection, but it does block viremia; locally produced IgA antibodies play an important role in protection in both the respiratory tract and the intestine, although some IgG is secreted in the respiratory tract and provides some protection.

Because Newcastle disease is a notifiable disease in most developed countries, legislative measures constitute the basis for control. Where the disease is enzootic, control can be achieved by good hygiene combined with immunization, both live-virus vaccines containing naturally occurring lentogenic virus strains and inactivated virus (injectable oil emulsions) being commonly used. These vaccines are effective and safe, even in chicks. Live virus vaccines may be administered via drinking water or by aerosol, eye or nostril droplets, or beak dipping. The inactivated vaccines must be injected. Broiler chickens are vaccinated a minimum of twice, whereas long-lived chickens, such as laying hens, are revaccinated several times throughout their lives, with inactivated vaccines. Protection against disease can be expected approximately a week after vaccination. Birds vaccinated with live virus will excrete the vaccine virus for up to 15 days after vaccination, hence in some countries birds cannot be moved from vaccinated flocks until 21 days after vaccination. Inactivated vaccine, administered subcutaneously, is usually used for pigeons. New-generation vectored vaccines have been developed, and these would preclude the possibility of reversion of apathogenic vaccine strains and would not complicate the interpretation of diagnostic RT-PCR results in vaccinated birds.

HUMAN DISEASE

Newcastle disease virus can produce a transitory conjunctivitis in humans; the condition occurs primarily in laboratory workers and in members of vaccination teams exposed to large quantities of virus. Before vaccination was widely practiced, infections were reported in workers eviscerating poultry infected with virulent Newcastle disease virus. In developed countries, birds infected with Newcastle disease virus are not processed, but in village poultry and live markets of developing countries, Newcastle disease is common and may not preclude slaughter of infected birds. The disease has not been reported in individuals who raise poultry or consume poultry products.

OTHER AVIAN AVULAVIRUSES (AVIAN PARAMYXOVIRUSES 2–9)

Serologically distinct avulaviruses (avian paramyxoviruses 2–9) have been isolated from numerous species of birds, mostly turkeys with respiratory disease or asymptomatic wild waterfowl. However, the pathogenic significance of many of these viruses is uncertain. They commonly have been isolated from passerine and psittacine birds in import quarantine facilities, or from asymptomatic wild waterfowl during surveillance for avian influenza viruses. There are also additional, unclassified viruses that are not included in the avian paramyxoviruses 1–9 groupings.

MEMBERS OF THE SUBFAMILY *PARAMYXOVIRINAE*, GENUS *MORBILLIVIRUS*

Members of the genus *Morbillivirus* all utilize the same replication strategy and all lack neuraminidase activity. They cause severe but very different disease syndromes in their respective hosts.

RINDERPEST VIRUS

Rinderpest is one of the oldest recorded plagues of livestock. It most probably arose in Asia, and was described in the 4th century. Devastating epizootics of rinderpest occurred across Europe in the 18th and 19th centuries, and a massive epizootic spread throughout sub-Saharan Africa in the late 19th century (1887–1897), decimating populations of cattle and certain wildlife. The 1920 outbreak in Europe led to the founding of the Office International des Epizooties (OIE)—the World Organization for Animal Health—that today coordinates animal infectious disease authorities globally to regulate animal diseases and to facilitate science-based international trade. The historical impact of rinderpest was most eloquently summarized in 1992 by Drs Gordon Scott and Alain Provost when they described the disease as "*the most dreaded bovine plague known, belongs to a select group of notorious infectious diseases that have changed the course of history. From its homeland around the Caspian Basin rinderpest, century after century, swept west over and around Europe and east over and around Asia with every marauding army causing the disaster, death and devastation that preceded the fall of the Roman Empire, the conquest of Christian Europe by Charlemagne, the French Revolution, the impoverishment of Russia and the colonization of Africa.*"

The causative agent, rinderpest virus, was first shown to be a filterable virus in 1902. On the basis of phylogenetic analysis, it has been suggested that rinderpest virus is the archetype morbillivirus, speculated to have given rise to canine distemper and human measles viruses some 5000 to 10,000 years ago. As of 2008, there has been considerable and increasing optimism that rinderpest has been eradicated from domestic livestock worldwide, as a result of an intensive and coordinated global effort that involved active surveillance, animal culling and movement restrictions, and an intense vaccination program. If true, rinderpest will join smallpox as the only viral diseases to have been successfully eradicated.

Clinical Features and Epidemiology

Rinderpest is a highly contagious disease of cattle and other artiodactyls. The host range includes domestic cattle, water buffalo, yak, sheep, and goats. Domestic pigs can develop clinical signs and were regarded as an important virus reservoir in Asia. Among wild animals, wildebeest, waterbuck, warthog, eland, kudu, giraffe, deer, various species of antelope, hippopotami, and African buffalo are all susceptible, although there is a wide spectrum of clinical disease that is most severe in African buffalo, wildebeest, and giraffe and invariably mild or subclinical in several species of antelope and hippopotamus. It may well be that all artiodactyls are susceptible to infection, but not all will exhibit obvious clinical signs. Other species, including rodents, rabbits, and ferrets, are susceptible to experimental infection, but are unlikely to play any significant role in the epidemiology of natural infections.

The clinical features of individual outbreaks of rinderpest reflect the virulence of the infecting strain of virus and the susceptibility of the individual animal host. In its typical manifestation in cattle and other susceptible wild or domestic ruminant species, rinderpest is an acute febrile disease with morbidity in susceptible populations approaching 100% and mortality of perhaps 50% (range 25–90%). Some of the indigenous cattle breeds in Africa are highly susceptible to rinderpest, whereas other breeds experience lower mortality (less than 30%). After an incubation period of 3–5 days, there is a prodromal phase with rapid increase in temperature, decrease in milk production, labored breathing, and cessation of eating. This is followed by congestion of the mucous membranes of the conjunctiva and oral and nasal cavities, and an abundant serous or mucoid oculonasal discharge. Severe cases are characterized by extensive, typically coalescing, erosion and ulceration of the epithelial lining of the entire oral cavity; plaques of caseous necrotic debris overlie foci of epithelial necrosis and inflammation, and affected animals typically drool saliva because of the discomfort associated with swallowing. This is followed by a phase of severe bloody diarrhea and prostration caused by involvement of the gastrointestinal tract. Finally there is a precipitous drop in temperature, at which time affected animals may die from dehydration and shock. Young animals are predisposed to severe disease. Less severe disease is characteristic of infection of susceptible animals with specific virus strains, and inapparent infection invariably occurs within certain host species such as impala and hippopotamus. Disease also is often less severe in sheep and goats. These mild infections are characterized by reduced clinical signs and mucosal injury, little or no diarrhea, and considerably lower mortality.

Once established in a population, rinderpest virus causes a considerably milder disease. The attenuation of rinderpest in enzootic areas probably reflects both selection of less virulent virus strains with the highest potential for transmission, and immunity within populations of susceptible animals. The infection is maintained in enzootic areas in younger animals that become infected as their maternal immunity wanes. Rinderpest virus also can be maintained for long periods through subclinical infections in wildlife, which then can serve as a reservoir for infection of cattle. The virus rapidly can regain its virulence when it spreads from enzootic foci to cause epizootics in susceptible animal populations.

Rinderpest virus is spread in all the secretions and excretions of affected animals, in greatest quantities during the acute febrile stages of the disease. The virus is relatively labile in the environment, thus transmission in enzootic areas predominantly is by direct contact between infected and susceptible animals. Aerosol transmission also can occur,

and the virus can be spread by fomites. The virus can persist for several days in infected carcasses. Because infected cattle excrete large amounts of virus during the incubation period before the appearance of clinical signs, acutely infected but asymptomatic animals often introduced rinderpest virus into disease-free areas. The disease was also introduced into new areas by importation of subclinically infected sheep, goats, and possibly other ruminants and wildlife. Subclinically infected swine of any species may act as a source of infection for cattle, but only Asian breeds of swine and warthogs show clinical signs of rinderpest virus infection.

Pathogenesis and Pathology

After nasal entry via infected aerosols, rinderpest virus first replicates within mononuclear leukocytes in the tonsils and mandibular and pharyngeal lymph nodes. Within 2–3 days, virus is transported during leukocyte-associated viremia to lymphoid tissues throughout the body, as well as the epithelium lining the gastrointestinal and respiratory tracts. The virus utilizes the equivalent of human CD150 (signaling lymphocyte activation molecule) as a receptor, which is consistent with the cellular and tissue tropism of rinderpest virus, as this molecule is present on immature thymocytes, activated lymphocytes, macrophages, and dendritic cells. The virus also infects and replicates in endothelial cells and some epithelial cells, presumably through a CD150-independent pathway, causing multifocal necrosis and inflammation in a variety of mucous membranes.

Rinderpest virus infection triggers a rapid innate and acquired immune response, including a vigorous interferon response. However, a viral protein or proteins, most likely the P protein, block the interferon response through inhibition of the phosphorylation and nuclear translocation of STAT proteins (Figure 17.5). Profound lymphopenia occurs in infected animals as a consequence of virus-mediated destruction of lymphocytes in all lymphoid tissues, including the gut-associated lymphoid tissue (Peyer's patches). The immune cells that support replication of rinderpest virus also produce numerous potent immunoregulatory cytokines after appropriate stimulation. The production and release of these cytokines, coupled with severe virus-induced lymphopenia, probably is responsible for the profound but transient immunosuppression that very characteristically occurs in animals infected with rinderpest virus.

The profuse diarrhea that occurs in severely affected animals rapidly leads to dehydration and fatal hypovolemic shock. The lesions present in infected animals reflect the virulence of the infecting virus strain, and in severe, acute cases include: marked dehydration (sunken eyes, for example); disseminated erosions and ulcers throughout the mucosal lining of the oral cavity, esophagus, and forestomachs; diffuse hemorrhage and necrosis of the mucosa of the abomasum; focal congestion and hemorrhage in the mucosa of the intestinal tract, with hemorrhagic necrosis of Peyer's patches. Segmental vascular congestion within the mucosa of the large intestine can produce characteristic "zebra stripes." Hemorrhage and congestion can also occur in the mucosal lining of the urinary bladder and upper respiratory tract and trachea. Secondary bacterial pneumonias are common because of the transient but severe immunosuppression in infected animals. Histologic lesions include widespread necrosis of lymphocytes and multifocal epithelial necrosis; epithelial syncytia and intracytoplasmic and, less often, intranuclear eosinophilic inclusion bodies are characteristically present in affected tissues.

Diagnosis

In countries where rinderpest was enzootic, clinical diagnosis was usually considered sufficient. Rinderpest historically could be confused with other diseases causing mucosal congestion, erosions or ulcers, such as bovine viral diarrhea, malignant catarrhal fever, and, in the early stages, infectious bovine rhinotracheitis and foot-and-mouth disease. These diagnostic problems have largely been resolved with the development of specific PCR tests for all of these "look-alike" diseases. Quantitative (real-time) RT-PCR assays are now available for rinderpest virus that rapidly can distinguish it from the related peste des petits ruminants virus. Historically, virus isolation was done in a variety of different cell lines, routinely in primary bovine kidney cell cultures. Virus neutralization and, more recently, ELISA have been used to assess the prevalence of rinderpest virus infection in a given region, which has required that only unvaccinated animals be evaluated to assess the success of eradication programs.

Immunity, Prevention, and Control

Cattle that survive rinderpest virus infection have life-long immunity. Neutralizing antibodies appear 6–7 days after the onset of clinical signs, and maximum titers are reached during the 3rd and 4th weeks postinfection. With the advent of molecular typing, three distinct genetic lineages of rinderpest virus were defined, two from Africa and one from Asia. All strains belong to the same serotype, which permitted use of a vaccine that contained a single strain of virus. In recent times, lineage 3 was restricted to Asia, lineage 2 to East and West Africa, and lineage 1 to Ethiopia and Sudan. As of April 2007, there were no reports of rinderpest virus infection in any countries reporting to OIE, which includes all of Asia and Africa. Kenya became the last African country to report a self-declared free status. The basis of this report is that there has been no clinical disease in the past 2 years and that active vaccination has ceased. Surveillance must be maintained in order to insure that any unidentified wildlife reservoir does not re-establish infection in domestic livestock.

In rinderpest-free countries, veterinary public health measures were designed to prevent introduction of the virus. Importation of uncooked meat and meat products from infected countries was forbidden, and zoo animals were quarantined before being transported to such countries. In countries with enzootic rinderpest and where the disease had a high probability of being introduced, attenuated virus vaccines were used. Early rinderpest vaccine strains were produced by virus passage in rabbits (lapinized vaccine), embryonated eggs (avianized vaccine), or goats (caprinized vaccine). In the 1960s an attenuated virus vaccine produced in cell culture (Plowright vaccine or TCRV) was developed and has since been used throughout Africa in the program that now appears to have succeeded in eliminating the disease from the continent. This vaccine is efficacious because it induces life-long immunity and it is inexpensive to produce. In fact, it remains one of the best vaccines available for any animal disease, but it is thermolabile and requires a well-maintained "cold chain"—a difficult practical problem in many areas where rinderpest previously occurred. As the number of infected animals decreased, the use of vaccine was suspended in order to facilitate serological surveillance. This was necessary because the immune response to the vaccine was indistinguishable from the wild-type virus infections. Marker vaccines have been developed, but they have not been used widely, as rinderpest apparently has been eradicated with existing reagents and technology.

PESTE DES PETITS RUMINANTS VIRUS

Peste des petits ruminants is a highly contagious, systemic disease of goats and sheep that is very similar to rinderpest and caused by a closely related morbillivirus, peste des petits ruminants virus. The infection was first described in West Africa, but now occurs in sub-Saharan Africa, the Middle East, and the Asian subcontinent, including Nepal, Bangladesh, and Tibet. There are suggestions that this virus has recently moved into areas from which rinderpest virus was previously eradicated. Peste des petits ruminants virus has been grouped into four distinct lineages based on the sequence of the F protein. Regardless of lineage, all strains belong to a single serogroup. Lineages 1 and 2 occur in West Africa; lineage 3 in East Africa, the Middle East, and southern India; lineage 4 extends from the Middle East to Tibet. There is some correlation between virulence and lineage; for example, lineage 1 strains in West Africa are more virulent than lineage 2 strains from the same area.

Transmission of the virus is similar to that of rinderpest, and generally requires close contact with infected animals. Virus is excreted for several days before the onset of significant clinical signs, such that spread of the virus is enhanced with the co-mingling of animals. Wild animals are not believed to play a major role in the spread of virus.

The natural infection occurs in sheep and goats, with goats being more severely affected. Different breeds of goat show different morbidity rates, and young animals are more severely affected. Case fatality rates can be as high as 85% in goats, but rarely above 10% in sheep. Peste des petits ruminants virus is very similar to rinderpest virus, and cattle can be experimentally infected with both viruses; some putative cases of rinderpest may in fact have been peste des petits ruminants virus instead. In goats, a febrile response occurs at 2–8 days after infection. Clinical signs include fever, anorexia, nasal and ocular discharges, necrotic stomatitis and gingivitis, and diarrhea. Bronchopneumonia is a frequent complication. The course of the disease may be peracute, acute, or chronic, depending on strain of virus, age of animals and breed of host. The pathogenesis of the infection is probably similar or identical to that of rinderpest virus, with infection of mononuclear cells with a resulting viremia, leukopenia, and systemic infection, principally involving lymphocytes, macrophages, and the epithelial cells lining the alimentary tract. At necropsy, there are extensive erosions and necrosis in the mucosal lining of the oral cavity, esophagus, abomasum, and small intestine. Regional lymph nodes are enlarged and there typically is an interstitial pneumonia.

Diagnosis of the disease, aside from clinical signs, has shifted from virus isolation to quantitative RT-PCR tests. These tests can distinguish between peste des petits ruminants and rinderpest viruses, which has been critical in the rinderpest eradication program. Virus isolation in primary lamb kidney cells is still used to obtain isolates for molecular characterization and comparison. Virus neutralization tests are used to distinguish between antibodies induced in animals by peste des petits ruminants and rinderpest virus infections. A live-attenuated vaccine based on a lineage 2 virus isolate (Nigeria 75/1) is now the vaccine of choice. Rinderpest vaccine is no longer recommended to prevent peste des petits ruminants, because of the rinderpest eradication program.

CANINE DISTEMPER VIRUS

Canine distemper is a highly contagious acute febrile disease of dogs that has been known since at least 1760. Edward Jenner first described the course and clinical features of the disease in 1809; its viral etiology was demonstrated in 1906 by Carré. It is now comparatively rare in domestic dogs in many developed countries, being well controlled by vaccination. The clinical cases that do occur in developed countries invariably are in non-vaccinated or incompletely vaccinated dogs, especially those entering rescue shelters or adoption centers. The continued presence of canine distemper virus in heavily vaccinated dog populations in many countries might suggest that the virus has an alternative reservoir, perhaps in wildlife. Canine distemper virus has recently emerged

as a significant pathogen of the large species in the family *Felidae*. Beginning in 1994, thousands of African lions died in a succession of epizootics, with free-roaming canids (hyenas, feral dogs) being the most likely source of the virus.

Clinical Features and Epidemiology

The host range of canine distemper virus encompasses all species of the families *Canidae* (dog, dingo, fox, coyote, jackal, wolf), *Procyonidae* (raccoon, coatimundi, panda), *Mustelidae* (weasel, ferret, fishers, mink, skunk, badger, marten, otter), the large members of the family *Felidae* (lions, leopards, cheetahs, tigers), and the collared peccary (*Tayassu tajacu*). The highly publicized outbreaks of distemper in lions (*Panthera leo*) in the Serengeti National Park in Tanzania and cases in the Chinese leopard (*Panthera pardus japonensis*) and other large cats in zoos, have graphically confirmed the capacity of the virus to invade new hosts. In addition to the large cats, canine distemper virus has also caused high mortality rates in black-footed ferrets (*Mustela nigripes*), the bat-eared fox (*Otocyon megalotis*), red pandas (*Ailurus fulgus*), hyenas (genus *Hyaena*), African wild dogs (genus *Lycaon*), raccoons (genus *Procyon*), palm civets (*Paradoxurus hermaphroditus*), and Caspian (*Pusa caspica*) and Baikal (*P. sibirica*) seals. The threat of this virus to wildlife species can only be expected to increase with relentless human encroachment into traditionally undeveloped areas of the world.

At least seven distinct lineages of canine distemper are recognized worldwide, based on sequence analysis of the H gene: Asia-1, Asia-2, American-1, America-2, Arctic-like, European wildlife, Europe. Additional lineages probably will be identified in the future. The traditional vaccine strains of canine distemper virus—Snyder Hill, Onderstepoort, Lederle—are all included in the America-1 lineage; however, field strains of this lineage are not currently circulating in the canine population in North America, although a lineage America-1 virus recently was identified among raccoons in the United States. The European wildlife-like virus has also been isolated in North America, perhaps as a result of unregulated movement of dogs from Eastern Europe. Despite genetic differences amongst field strains of canine distemper virus, cross-neutralization studies show only minor antigenic differences that are not considered significant enough to warrant changes in the existing vaccines.

Clinical signs of canine distemper virus infection depend upon the strain of the virus, the host age and immune status, and levels of environmental stress. A significant proportion (estimated to be 50%) of infections are subclinical or so mild as not to require veterinary care. Dogs with mild disease exhibit fever, signs of upper respiratory tract infection, and become listless and inappetant. Bilateral serous ocular discharges can become mucopurulent with coughing and labored breathing, signs that are often indistinguishable from those of "kennel cough" (acute respiratory disease of canines). In severe generalized distemper, infected dogs first develop a fever after an incubation period of 3–6 days, but a second febrile response ushers in the more serious phase of the infection that coincides with systemic spread of the virus and accompanying profound leukopenia. Signs occurring at this time include anorexia, inflammation of the upper respiratory tract with serous or mucopurulent nasal discharge, conjunctivitis, and depression. Some dogs show primarily respiratory signs, whereas others develop gastrointestinal signs; respiratory signs reflect inflammation and injury to the upper respiratory tract and large airways, causing a productive cough; bronchitis and interstitial pneumonia follow. Gastrointestinal involvement is manifest by vomiting and watery diarrhea. The duration of disease varies, often depending on complications caused by secondary bacterial infections (Figure 17.6).

Profound central nervous system signs develop in some infected animals. Neurologic manifestations of distemper occur at 1–3 weeks after the onset of acute signs, but may also appear after apparent subclinical infection. There is no way to predict which dogs will develop neurological complications. Seizures (so-called chewing gum fits and epileptic seizures), cerebellar and vestibular signs, paraparesis or tetraparesis with sensory ataxia and myoclonus are common. Neurologic signs, whether acute or chronic, are usually progressive, which leads to a poor prognosis and surviving dogs may have permanent central nervous system sequelae. So-called old dog encephalitis is a rather poorly characterized chronic and slowly progressive neurologic disease caused by canine distemper infection in adult dogs that are not necessarily "old." Hyperkeratosis of foot pads and the nose occurs in some dogs with neurological disease, as a result of epithelial damage caused by the virus.

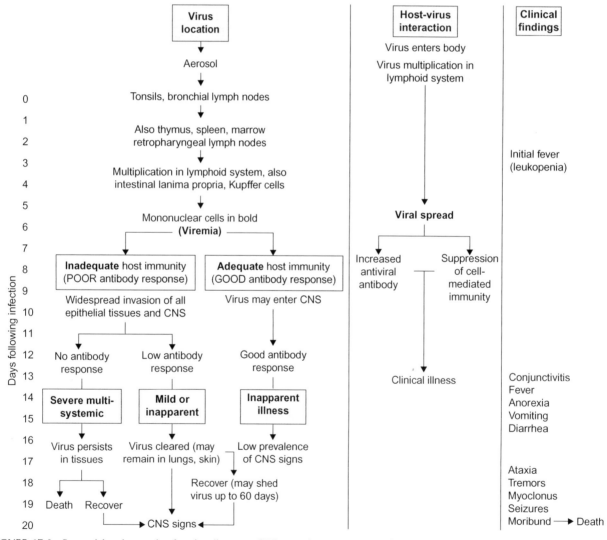

FIGURE 17.6 Sequential pathogenesis of canine distemper. CNS, central nervous system. [*From* Infectious Diseases of the Dog and Cat, *C. E. Greene, 3rd ed., p. 29. Copyright © Elsevier (2006), with permission.*]

Canine distemper virus is shed in all secretions and excretions from the 5th day after infection, which is before the onset of clinical signs, and continues, sometimes for weeks. Transmission is mainly via direct contact, droplet, and aerosol, as the virus is not stable in the environment. Young dogs are more susceptible to the disease than older dogs, with the greatest susceptibility being between 4 and 6 months of age, after puppies have lost their maternal antibody.

Pathogenesis and Pathology

Following aerosol respiratory infection, canine distemper virus first replicates within macrophages in the tissues of the upper respiratory tract, and it then quickly spreads to the tonsils and regional lymph nodes. Canine distemper, like other morbilliviruses, infects cells that express the equivalent of human CD150 (SLAM), which is present on thymocytes, activated lymphocytes, macrophages, and dendritic cells. The tropism of canine distemper virus for these cells explains the immunosuppressive effects of the virus, which probably reflect virus-mediated destruction of immune cells as well as induction of various immunomodulatory cytokines. After multiplication in regional lymph nodes, the virus enters the blood stream, where it circulates within infected B and T cells. Primary viremia is synchronous with the first bout of fever, and virus then is spread to lymphoid tissues throughout the body, including gut-associated lymphoid tissues, and fixed tissue macrophages such as Kupffer cells in the liver. Virions formed in these sites are carried by blood mononuclear cells during secondary viremia that coincides with the second peak of fever. Infection of epithelial cells in the lung, bladder, and skin occurs relatively late in the infection, through a CD150-independent mechanism of attachment that may follow direct interaction with infected lymphocytes. Epithelial cells do not possess CD150 (SLAM), and the receptor that facilitates virus entry into epithelial cells is yet to be defined. Infection of the central nervous system occurs relatively late in the course of infection, and only in dogs that do not develop protective immune responses sufficiently quickly to prevent this spread. Infection of neurons and glial cells also occurs through a CD150-independent mechanism.

Puppies with distemper develop pneumonia, enteritis, conjunctivitis, rhinitis, and tracheitis. The lungs are typically edematous; microscopically, there is bronchointerstitial pneumonia with necrosis of the epithelium lining small airways, and thickening of alveolar walls. Secondary bacterial bronchopneumonia is common as a consequence of both virus-mediated immunosuppression and inhibition of normal pulmonary clearance mechanisms. Lesions in the central nervous system of infected dogs with distemper are variable, depending on duration of infection and the properties of the infecting virus strain; these can include any combination of demyelination, neuronal necrosis, gliosis, and nonsuppurative meningoencephalomyelitis. Acidophilic inclusions may be present in the nuclei and cytoplasm of infected astrocytes, as well as in epithelial cells in the lung, stomach, renal pelvis, and urinary bladder (Figure 17.7). Canine distemper virus infection of neonates can result in failure of development of the enamel of adult teeth (odontodystrophy), and metaphyseal osteosclerosis in long bones.

Diagnosis

Clinical diagnosis of canine distemper can be complicated by the use of modified live vaccines. Cases of canine distemper can occur in recently vaccinated puppies, raising the obvious question of whether the signs are caused by the vaccine virus or a field strain. This question is not satisfactorily resolved

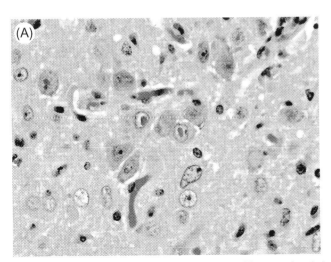 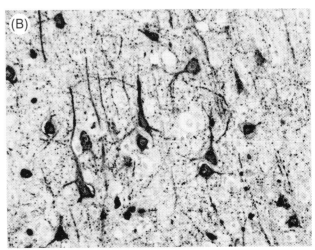

FIGURE 17.7 Canine distemper. (A) Intranuclear and intracytoplasmic inclusion bodies in the brain of an infected badger. (B) Immunohistochemical staining of canine distemper virus in the brain of a dog. *(Courtesy of R. J. Higgins, University of California, Davis.)*

with standard serological, virus isolation, or antigen detection tests. RT-PCR is now becoming a standard method of testing, but the distinction of field and vaccine viruses also requires very specialized RT-PCR assays that are not routinely available.

Laboratory diagnosis is necessary to exclude other diseases with similar clinical manifestations. Virus isolation can be achieved by co-cultivation of lymphocytes from suspect animals with cell lines expressing the CD150 (SLAM) molecule, which has eliminated the need to use activated mononuclear cells for isolation of field strains of canine distemper virus. After initial isolation, the virus can then be adapted to grow in primary dog lung cells or conventional cell lines, including Madin–Darby canine kidney or Vero. Immunohistochemical or fluorescent antibody staining methods are useful for demonstrating the presence of viral antigen in impression smears of the conjunctiva and skin biopsies (antemortem) or sections of lung, intestine, stomach, kidney, brain, and bladder tissue collected at necropsy (Figure 17.7). RT-PCR tests can be done on conjunctival swabs, blood mononuclear cells, any tissue sample that includes epithelium, and urine. The serological status of dogs can be assessed with virus neutralization assays, ELISA, or indirect fluorescent antibody tests.

Immunity, Prevention, and Control

Cell-mediated immunity is important in the protective immune response against morbillivirus infections in general. In human measles, persons with agammaglobulinemia can overcome the infection, but those with inherited or acquired deficiencies in their cell-mediated immune system are at extreme risk. However, those animals with any detectable neutralizing antibody are immune to reinfection, and immunity following morbillivirus infections is life-long.

Control of canine distemper virus infection is based on adequate diagnosis, quarantine, sanitation, and vaccination. The virus is very fragile, and susceptible to standard disinfectants. Thorough disinfection of premises, however, can be very challenging. Successful immunization of pups with attenuated canine distemper virus vaccines depends on the absence of interfering maternal antibody. The age at which pups can be immunized can be predicted from a nomograph if the serum antibody titer of the mother is known; this service is available in some diagnostic laboratories. Alternatively, pups can be vaccinated with modified live-virus vaccine at 6 weeks of age and then at 2- to 4-week intervals until 16 weeks of age, which is often now the standard practice. For treatment, hyperimmune serum or immune globulin can be used prophylactically immediately after exposure. Antibiotic therapy generally has a beneficial effect by lessening the effect of secondary opportunistic bacterial infections.

Standard modified live vaccines should not be used in species other than canids. Adverse reactions (disease) have occurred in other species, including red pandas and foxes. Inactivated (killed) vaccines previously were used to immunize zoo animals; however, these vaccines were often of marginal efficacy. The availability of a canarypox virus vectored vaccine containing only the H and F proteins of canine distemper virus has resolved this dilemma, as this product provides safe and effective immunization without ever exposing animals to live canine distemper virus. This product currently is used for immunization of endangered species such as giant pandas and black-footed ferrets in zoos in the United States, for instance.

MARINE (PHOCINE AND CETACEAN) MORBILLIVIRUSES

In 1988, a major die-off of harbor seals (*Phoca vitulina*) occurred in the North, Wadden, and Baltic Seas. Estimates of the number of dead animals ranged from 17,000 to 23,000. Animals initially showed a febrile response, with severe depression. The affected seals exhibited clinical signs similar to those of distemper in dogs, such as serous nasal discharge, conjunctivitis, gastroenteritis, cutaneous lesions, and neurologic signs. Lesions in affected seals included pneumonia, encephalitis, and ophthalmitis. The brains of affected seals had lesions consistent with viral encephalitis, with intracytoplasmic and intranuclear acidophilic inclusions. Pulmonary lesions were consistent with interstitial pneumonia. Lymphocyte depletion and necrosis were prominent in the spleen, bronchial lymph nodes, and Peyer's patches. Recovered seals had neutralizing antibodies to canine distemper virus. A morbillivirus was isolated from the affected seals, and genetic typing places this virus (phocine morbillivirus) in a separate species from canine distemper virus in the morbillivirus genus. A second epizootic occurred in 2002 that resulted in an estimated 30,000 deaths. The exact source of the virus causing these epizootics has not been definitively determined, but evidence suggests that other seals in which the virus is enzootic carried the virus to the affected region during a period of migration. Phocine morbillivirus is present in seal populations throughout the North Atlantic, and perhaps among those in some areas of the Pacific Ocean also.

An epizootic that resulted in the deaths of thousands of striped dolphins in the Mediterranean Sea began in 1990. A morbillivirus was isolated and typing indicated that it was a new species (cetacean morbillivirus virus) in the morbillivirus family, distinct from the previous marine isolate. In 1990, a virus was isolated from a harbor porpoise (*Phocoena phocoena*) in the Irish Sea showing similar signs to that of the harbor seals infected with phocine morbillivirus. This virus is also considered a cetacean morbillivirus. Retrospective studies on Atlantic bottlenose dolphins (*Tursiops truncatus*) that died between 1987 and 1988 along the east coast of North America showed evidence of morbillivirus infections. Since their identification, epizootics of disease in marine mammals caused by these viruses have occurred sporadically, and another major die-off of striped dolphin (*Stenella coeruleoalba*) occurred in the Mediterranean Sea in 2007. Recent sero-surveys indicate that cetacean morbillivirus infections occur in a wide variety of marine mammals in all areas of the world. Factors involved in virus transmission are unknown, as are the animal species that are responsible for maintaining enzootic infections.

MEASLES VIRUS

Measles (rubeola) is a disease of humans caused by a morbillivirus that is closely related to the morbilliviruses of animals. Measles virus is naturally infectious for several species of non-human primates, including gorillas, macaques, baboons, African green monkeys, colobus monkeys, squirrel monkeys, and marmosets. Infection is rare in wild populations, but may be common in laboratory animal colonies in association with human exposure. Most laboratory animal facilities are careful to exclude exposure of non-human primates to measles virus by vaccination of personnel (or clinical history of recovered measles virus infection). Clinical disease is relatively mild in most monkeys, with the exception of marmosets (family *Callitrichidae*) and colobus monkeys (genus *Colobus*), which may develop high mortality. Lesions include exanthematous rash, conjunctivitis, giant-cell pneumonia, and encephalitis. As in humans infected with measles virus, macaques (genus *Macaca*) may develop subacute sclerosing panencephalitis months or years after recovery from the acute infection. Marmosets may also develop gastritis and enterocolitis, with disseminated foci of necrosis in several other organs. Diagnosis is facilitated by recognition of characteristic syncytia and both intranuclear and intracytoplasmic inclusion bodies.

MEMBERS OF THE SUBFAMILY *PARAMYXOVIRINAE*, GENUS *HENIPAVIRUS*

Zoonotic henipaviruses have caused human deaths in Australia, Malaysia, Singapore, India, and Bangladesh. *Pteropus* species of fruit bats that are distributed throughout the Indo-Pacific region from Madagascar to the South Pacific islands are the known reservoir host of henipaviruses (Figure 17.8).

HENDRA VIRUS

In 1994, an outbreak of severe respiratory disease with high mortality occurred in thoroughbred horses stabled in Brisbane, Queensland, Australia. Two persons at the stable developed a severe influenza-like disease and one died. A new virus (Hendra virus) was isolated from both affected

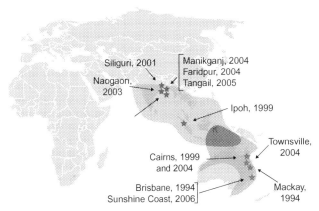

FIGURE 17.8 Locations of human deaths from zoonotic henipaviruses in the Indo-Pacific region.

horses and a human, and the syndrome was reproduced experimentally in horses. There have since been sporadic but continuing cases of this devastating disease in both horses and humans, including veterinarians who performed necropsies on affected horses. Serological surveillance confirmed that a similar or identical virus infected four species of fruit bats (flying foxes, suborder *Megachiroptera*) on the east coast of Australia, and Hendra virus ultimately was isolated from two species of fruit bat. Molecular analyses of the viruses isolated from horses, humans, and bats indicated a close relationship with viruses in the genus *Morbillivirus*, thus the initial designation of the virus as "equine morbillivirus." To avoid confusion with possible future isolates and not link the virus to a non-natural host, the virus designation was changed to Hendra virus to reflect the location of the first isolation, and Hendra virus has now been placed in a new genus, *Henipavirus*, of the subfamily *Paramyxovirinae*.

Clinical Features and Epidemiology

Hendra virus is maintained by enzootic, asymptomatic infection in certain species of fruit bat. The precise mechanism of virus transmission from bats to non-natural hosts such as horses and humans is uncertain, but probably is through environmental contamination by secretions or excretions from the bats (saliva, feces, urine, placental fluids). The sporadic nature of the outbreaks is probably the result of changes in the feeding behavior of the bats due to changes in food supplies or habitat incursions that facilitate close interaction of horses and bats.

Clinical signs exhibited by horses infected with Hendra virus include any combination of initial anorexia, depression, fever, and increased respiratory and heart rates, followed by respiratory or neurological signs. The clinical course is apparently short, with infected horses dying quickly after the onset of clinical signs. The incubation period in experimentally infected horses was from 6 to 10 days. Cats and guinea pigs, but not rabbits or mice, are susceptible to experimental infection, and cats develop a fatal pneumonia identical to that in horses.

Pathogenesis and Pathology

Affected horses often exhibit severe pulmonary edema, with copious thick, foamy, and hemorrhagic fluid in the airways. Pericardial effusion is also characteristic. Histologically, there is severe interstitial pneumonia, with protein-rich fluid and hemorrhage in the airspaces, dilated lymphatics, vascular thrombosis, and necrosis of the walls of small blood vessels. Vasculitis is limited to small arteries, arterioles, and capillaries, with viral antigen within endothelial cells and the tunica media of affected vessels. Syncytia are present in the endothelium of lung capillaries and arterioles. Cytoplasmic inclusion bodies within these syncytia were shown by electron microscopy to consist of massed viral nucleocapsids.

The finding that ephrin-B2, a transmembrane protein that is abundantly expressed on endothelial cells, is the functional receptor for the henipaviruses potentially explains the distribution of virus in the infected host. Like those of morbilliviruses, the Hendra virus *P* gene encodes proteins that interfere with interferon induction and signaling. This strategy of selective interference with host innate defenses very likely enhances the severity of the infection.

Diagnosis

The epidemiology, clinical signs and florid lesions of Hendra virus infection in horses are all distinctive, but the macroscopic lesions must be distinguished from those of African horse sickness in particular. Rapid diagnosis can be achieved using RT-PCR tests, and the virus also rapidly can be identified in tissues by immunofluorescence or immunohistochemical staining. Virus isolation can be accomplished in a variety of cell types, but Vero cells are generally preferred. Virus isolation should only be done in high-containment facilities, and any work involving live virus must be undertaken in a Bio Safety Level 4 (BSL-4) facility because of the devastating potential consequences of human exposure. Serological testing can be done by virus neutralization, but ELISA is much preferred because of safety issues pertaining to the requirement to use live virus in the neutralization assay.

Immunity, Prevention, and Control

Horses that survive Hendra virus infection develop very high titers of neutralizing antibodies to the virus, but although vaccines are in development they are not yet commercially available. Hendra virus very clearly is a most dangerous zoonotic pathogen that requires appropriate caution when its presence is suspected, and the availability of adequate biocontainment laboratory facilities for its diagnosis.

NIPAH VIRUS

In 1998–1999, there was an outbreak of acute encephalitis with high mortality in workers handling pigs in Malaysia. The morbidity and mortality in the pigs was not abnormally high, and there was some thought that this was an outbreak of Japanese encephalitis. The mortality rate in the first 265 identified human cases was 40%. A concurrent disease in the pigs was characterized as a febrile respiratory illness, with epistaxis, dyspnea, and coughing in young pigs; some older animals showed neurological signs such as ataxia, paresis, seizures, and muscle tremors. A morbillivirus was isolated from human cases and then from the affected pigs. The virus was antigenically related to Hendra virus, but subsequent sequence analysis identified a new species in the genus *Henipavirus*, now designated as Nipah virus.

Epidemiological investigations identified the source of the virus as fruit bats, as with Hendra virus. The virus occurs in several species of fruit bat in Southeast Asia, with infections being reported as far west as India. In experimentally infected fruit bats, virus can be detected by virus isolation or by RT-PCR in urine samples from the exposed bats. As with Hendra, the likely track of the infection is from the fruit bats to animals in agricultural facilities in close proximity to the feeding bats. The virus can easily be spread among the exposed pigs through the respiratory route. Workers handling the pigs or pig carcasses also became infected, and there is evidence of human-to-human spread. In Malaysia, the infection in pigs was known as "barking pig syndrome" because of characteristic coughing in the affected pigs. Virus can consistently be isolated from pharyngeal swabs from experimentally infected pigs by day 4 post infection, and the virus spread horizontally to control pigs. Cats can also be infected with Nipah virus and can transmit the virus to contacts.

The pathology of Nipah virus disease in pigs and humans is similar to that caused by Hendra virus. A prominent feature in the human cases was a vasculitis with endothelial cell damage, necrosis, and syncytial giant cells in the affected vessels; immunohistochemical staining confirmed that abundant viral antigen was present in endothelial and smooth muscle cells of the small blood vessels. Severe dysfunction of brain stem neurons occurs in humans with Nipah virus encephalitis, probably as a result of the strong tropism of the attachment G protein of Nipah virus for the ephrin-B3 receptor that is abundantly expressed on these cells. Naturally infected pigs developed tracheitis and bronchointerstitial pneumonia with hyperplasia of the airway epithelium. Sero-surveys indicate that many pigs have subclinical infections.

Nipah virus appears to be a more substantial threat to agriculture and humans than Hendra virus, in part because of the role of swine as amplifying hosts of Nipah virus.

Experimental vaccines have been developed that are efficacious, and rapid and sensitive diagnostic tests are available, including RT-PCR assays, and immunofluorescence and immunohistochemical staining assays to detect viral antigen. As with Hendra virus, immunoassays are routinely used for serological diagnosis because of the biosecurity issues with handling live Nipah virus.

OTHER HENIPAVIRUSES

Serological evidence exists of henipavirus infection of West African fruit bats (*Eidolon helvum*), suggesting that viruses that are identical or related to Nipah and Hendra viruses circulate in other regions of the world but in different bat reservoir hosts. Antibodies to henipaviruses also have been found in species of bats other than *Pteropus* in Madagascar.

MEMBERS OF THE SUBFAMILY *PNEUMOVIRINAE*, GENUS *PNEUMOVIRUS*

Viruses in the subfamily *Pneumovirinae* are genetically and antigenically distinct from those in the subfamily *Paramyxovirinae*, and they utilize somewhat different replication strategies. Most pneumoviruses lack both a hemagglutinin and a neuraminidase; rather, they utilize a G protein for cell binding. Viruses in the genus *Pneumovirus* are further distinguished from those in the genus *Metapneumovirus* on the basis of their sequence relatedness and differences in their genetic constitution.

BOVINE RESPIRATORY SYNCYTIAL VIRUS

Bovine respiratory syncytial virus was first detected in Japan, Belgium, and Switzerland in 1967, and was isolated soon thereafter in England and the United States. It is now known to occur worldwide in all bovine species as well as in sheep, goats, and other ungulates. The virus is related closely to human respiratory syncytial virus, and some monoclonal antibodies developed to detect the human virus also will detect the bovine equivalent. Caprine and ovine strains of respiratory syncytial virus are also recognized, and these perhaps represent, with bovine respiratory syncytial virus, a subgroup of ruminant syncytial viruses rather than different species.

In many settings the bovine virus causes inapparent infections, but in recently weaned calves and young cattle it can cause pneumonia, pulmonary edema, and emphysema. Infection also predisposes to other infections of the respiratory tract.

Clinical Features and Epidemiology

Bovine respiratory syncytial virus infection occurs most often during the winter months when cattle, goats, and sheep are housed in confined conditions. However, there have been substantial outbreaks in cow and calf herds in summer as well. The virus spreads rapidly, probably through aerosols or droplets of respiratory tract excretions. Reinfection of the respiratory tract is not uncommon in calves with antibody. Pre-existing antibody, whether derived passively from maternal transfer or actively by prior infection or vaccination, does not prevent virus replication and excretion, although clinical signs may be lessened. The virus persists in herds, most probably through continuous subclinical reinfections or in putatively inapparent virus carriers.

Inapparent infection of cattle is very common. Disease caused by respiratory syncytial virus infection is particularly important in recently weaned beef calves and young cattle, especially when they are maintained in closely confined conditions. Infection is characterized by a sudden onset of high fever, hyperpnea, abdominal breathing, lethargy, rhinitis, nasal discharge, and cough. Secondary bacterial pneumonia, especially that caused by *Mannheimia haemolytica*, is common. Outbreaks often occur after a sharp drop in temperature. In general, in outbreaks the morbidity is high but mortality is low, and animals that die are also often persistently infected with bovine viral diarrhea virus.

Pathogenesis and Pathology

In calves infected experimentally, the virus causes destruction of the ciliated epithelium of the airways in the lung, so that pulmonary clearance is compromised, which predisposes to secondary bacterial infections. At necropsy, there is interstitial pneumonia with emphysema that affects all lobes of the lungs. Secondary bacterial bronchopneumonia that affects the anteroventral aspects of the lung is common. Syncytia may be present in the airway epithelium lining the bronchi and bronchioles, as well as in alveolar macrophages and type II pneumocytes.

Protection against reinfection is short lived following natural infection, but the clinical signs in subsequent infections are less severe. Passive antibody is protective, in that the attack rate is less in 1-month-old calves than in older calves with no colostral antibodies. Calves immunized with formalin-inactivated vaccine preparations developed more severe lung injury following challenge infection with bovine respiratory syncytial virus than did control animals, and it has been proposed that the enhanced disease may be a consequence of a predominant T-helper 2 (Th2) cell response, with the preferential release of inflammatory cytokines in the absence of a CD8 T cell response. This abnormal Th2 cell response with eosinophilia can be reproduced by immunization with recombinant vaccines expressing only the G protein of the virus. This protein is one of the most unique among viral proteins as a result of its high degree of *O*-linked glycosylation, a property that may help evade immune surveillance and compromise efforts to develop an effective vaccine.

Diagnosis

Bovine respiratory syncytial virus infection is not reliably diagnosed by virus isolation, as virus frequently is complexed with antibody in cattle that already have developed an immune response. The virus can be isolated from appropriate samples using a number of bovine cell cultures. The presence of virus reliably can be detected in tracheal wash-derived cells by immunofluorescence staining with virus-specific monoclonal antibodies, and in tissue samples from necropsy cases. RT-PCR tests have also been developed for bovine respiratory syncytial virus, and these assays also have the inherent advantage of not being affected by the presence of neutralizing antibodies, although care must be exercised to consider the possible detection of virus from modified live vaccines. Virus neutralization assays can be used to detect neutralizing antibodies, and paired samples from the index case, in addition to age-matched herd mates, should be tested.

Immunity, Prevention, and Control

Although immunity is incomplete and transient following natural bovine respiratory syncytial virus infection of calves, vaccination remains the usual means of control. Several inactivated and attenuated virus vaccines are in current use. Efficacy data has been difficult to obtain because challenge models for cattle are not robust. There is anecdotal evidence in the United States suggesting that vaccination reduces the occurrence of severe outbreaks of disease associated with bovine respiratory syncytial virus infection; however, efforts are ongoing to develop more efficacious products, including vectored virus vaccines and the like.

PNEUMONIA VIRUS OF MICE

Pneumonia virus of mice was highly prevalent in mouse colonies before routine surveillance programs. This virus or related viruses also infect(s) rats, cotton rats (genus *Sigmondia*), hamsters (subfamily *Cricetinae*), gerbils, guinea pigs (*Cavia porcellus*), and dogs. It can be a clinically silent infection that is typically detected by sero-surveillance, generally by immunoassay (ELISA). It received its name when pneumonia developed in suckling mice following experimental serial passage, but natural disease occurs only in immunodeficient mice. Seropositive immunocompetent mice recover from infection without evidence of a carrier state. Pneumonia virus of mice is a clinically important infection in immunodeficient mice, such as nude and severe combined immunodeficient mice. Like Sendai virus, pneumonia virus of mice is non-cytolytic and infects respiratory epithelium and type II pneumocytes. However, pneumonia virus of mice virus tends to infect individual cells, rather than the entire respiratory epithelial population, so cellular immune responses do not result in recognizable necrotizing lesions that are typical of Sendai virus infection. T-cell-deficient mice develop progressive interstitial pneumonia that is difficult to differentiate from Sendai virus pneumonia in immunodeficient mice. Pneumonia virus of mice infection of marginally immune deficient mice (numerous types of genetic null mutant animals) may exacerbate pneumonias caused by either *Pneumocystis* spp. or bacterial infections.

MEMBERS OF THE SUBFAMILY *PNEUMOVIRINAE*, GENUS *METAPNEUMOVIRUS*

AVIAN RHINOTRACHEITIS VIRUS (METAPNEUMOVIRUS)

Avian metapneumovirus causes a variety of disease syndromes, depending on the bird species and virus type (types A, B, C, and D). The first infections were described in turkeys in South African in 1978. These infections were caused by type A viruses, and termed turkey rhinotracheitis. Later, infections caused by type B virus were described in turkeys in Europe. Infections by type A and B viruses causes upper respiratory disease in chickens, termed swollen head syndrome. Type C virus has been reported only in turkeys in the upper Midwest of the United States and in Muscovy ducks in France; and type D virus has been reported in turkeys in France. The currently preferred designation for avian metapneumovirus infections is "avian rhinotracheitis." Pheasants and guinea fowl with respiratory disease in the United Kingdom have also been infected with type A avian metapneumovirus.

In young turkeys the disease is characterized by inflammation of the respiratory tract, rales, sneezing, frothy nasal discharge, conjunctivitis, swelling of the infraorbital sinuses, and submandibular edema. Coughing and head shaking are frequently observed in older poults. These signs may be exacerbated by secondary infections. In turkey breeding operations, infections cause a decrease in egg production of up to 70%, and an increased incidence of prolapsed uterus from excessive coughing by affected birds. In hens, respiratory disease is milder than in young poults. Morbidity is often 100%; mortality ranges from 0.4 to 50% and is highest in young poults. Swollen head syndrome is a milder form of the disease that occurs in chickens, typically with co-infection by bacteria such as *Escherichia coli*. This disease is characterized by swelling of the infraorbital sinuses, torticollis, disorientation, and general depression, sometimes also with respiratory distress. In chickens, morbidity is usually less than 4% and mortality less than 2%.

In turkeys, the respiratory tract disease is characterized histologically by: increased glandular secretion, focal loss of cilia, hyperemia, and mild mononuclear mucosal inflammation within the turbinates during the first 2 days after infection epithelial destruction and intense mucosal inflammation on days 3–5; watery to mucoid exudate in turbinates from days 1–9. Tracheal lesions are generally milder, but in severe cases can include complete deciliation of the mucosal lining of the trachea within 4 days. Cytoplasmic eosinophilic inclusions occur in epithelial cells lining the airways and nasal cavities.

Diagnosis of both the turkey and the chicken disease is based most commonly on detection of specific antibodies on ELISA from non-vaccinated animals with recent history of respiratory disease, or detection of avian metapneumovirus genome by molecular tests such as RT-PCR in acute respiratory disease cases. Virus isolation is difficult, but can be achieved by serial passage in 6- to 7-day-old turkey or chicken embryos or in chicken embryo tracheal organ cultures. RT-PCR assays provide data on the subtypes of virus circulating in a given area. Attenuated virus vaccines and inactivated vaccines are available commercially for three of the four genetic subgroup types of avian metapneumovirus (A, B, and C), and appear to give cross-protection against the various strains.

As a curiosity, the only other species for which a metapneumovirus has been identified as a pathogen is humans.

UNCLASSIFIED MEMBERS OF FAMILY *PARAMYXOVIRIDAE*

BOTTLENOSE DOLPHIN (*TURSIOPS TRUNCATUS*) PARAINFLUENZA VIRUS

A paramyxovirus was isolated from a 19-year-old bottlenose dolphin with fatal bronchointerstitial pneumonia. Other significant findings were multifocal erosive and ulcerative tracheitis and laryngitis. Phylogenetic analyses indicated that the virus was most closely linked to bovine parainfluenza virus 3. A sero-survey confirmed that healthy dolphins from Florida and California had previously been exposed to this virus, suggesting that infections are common in bottlenose dolphins and that the virus may be involved in outbreaks of respiratory disease in marine mammals.

FER-DE-LANCE AND OTHER OPHIDIAN PARAMYXOVIRUSES

An apparently new epizootic disease of snakes was first reported in 1976 from a serpentarium in Switzerland. A paramyxovirus-like agent was isolated (Fer-de-Lance virus). Subsequently, similar viruses have been isolated from snakes, lizards, and turtles, thus Fer-de-Lance virus was the first isolate of what appears to be a whole new genus of reptile paramyxoviruses or ophidian paramyxoviruses. It has been proposed that viruses in this group be included in a new genus, *Ferlavirus*, with Fer-de-Lance virus being the type species.

Snakes infected with these viruses can develop abnormal posturing, regurgitation, anorexia, mucoid feces, head tremors, terminal convulsions, and high mortality. The lungs of affected snakes were congested, and histologic lesions included proliferative interstitial pneumonia with variable degrees of infiltration of mononuclear cells. Intracytoplasmic inclusions were present within epithelial cells of the airways. In the pancreas of several snakes, there were multifocal areas of necrosis. Immunohistochemical staining confirmed the presence of viral antigen at the luminal surfaces of pulmonary epithelium, and multinucleated cells within the pancreas.

Virus can be isolated using viper heart cells or Vero cells, but at reduced incubation temperatures (25–30°C). The ophidian paramyxoviruses hemagglutinate chicken red blood cells, which permitted the development of a serological test for screening of exposed animals. Virus can be detected by immunohistochemical staining of tissues from affected snakes, and by RT-PCR tests.

SALEM VIRUS

In 1992, an outbreak of febrile illness with limb edema occurred in horses at three race tracks in the Northeastern United States. A syncytium-forming virus was isolated from the blood mononuclear cells of one affected horse, and subsequent sequence analysis identified it as a member of the subfamily *Paramyxovirinae* that obeyed the "rule of six." This virus, however, did not segregate with viruses in the existing genera in the subfamily. The virus grows in a wide variety of cell cultures, but lacks either neuraminidase or hemagglutinating activity. Sero-surveys indicated that some 50% of horses in the region were seropositive, and sero-reactivity also was demonstrated with canine and porcine sera, but not that of ruminants. Dogs are susceptible to infection, and virus was isolated from them up to 1 month after infection. The pathogenic significance of Salem virus is uncertain, for both dogs and horses.

ATLANTIC SALMON PARAMYXOVIRUS

Atlantic salmon paramyxovirus has been associated with proliferative gill disease, which has a multifactorial etiology, in post-smolt farmed Atlantic salmon in Scandinavia. Sequence analysis of the entire genome indicates that the virus is most similar to viruses in the genus *Respirovirus*; however, the Atlantic salmon virus is not yet taxonomically classified, and it may represent a new genus within the subfamily *Paramyxovirinae*. Similar viruses frequently have been isolated from salmonids from the west coast of North America, but without any associated clinical disease.

Rhabdoviridae

Chapter Contents

The family *Rhabdoviridae* encompasses six genera of viruses that infect a broad range of hosts, including mammals, birds, fish, insects, and plants with some of the family members being transmitted by arthropod vectors. The family contains important animal and human pathogens, including rabies, vesicular stomatitis, and bovine ephemeral fever viruses, and several important rhabdoviruses of fish. There are also many largely unclassified rhabdoviruses that infect cattle, pigs, kangaroos, wallabies, birds, and reptiles; however, the pathogenic significance of most of these viruses remains uncertain.

Rabies is one of the oldest and most feared diseases of humans and animals—it was recognized in Egypt before 2300 B.C. and in ancient Greece, where it was well described by Aristotle. Perhaps the most lethal of all infectious diseases, rabies also has the distinction of having stimulated one of the great early discoveries in biomedical science. In 1885, before the nature of viruses was comprehended, Louis Pasteur developed, tested, and applied a rabies vaccine.

Vesicular stomatitis of horses, cattle, and swine was first distinguished from foot-and-mouth disease early in the 19th century—it was recognized as the cause of periodic epizootics of vesicular disease in livestock in the Western hemisphere. The disease was a significant problem in

artillery and cavalry horses during the American Civil War. The first large epizootic to be described in detail occurred in 1916 during the First World War; the disease spread rapidly from Colorado to the east coast of the United States, affecting large numbers of horses and mules and, to a lesser extent, cattle. Bovine ephemeral fever, another important rhabdovirus-induced disease was first recognized in Africa in 1867, and is now known to be widespread across Africa, most of southeast Asia, Japan, and Australia.

More recently, a number of rhabdoviruses in at least two different genera have been identified as the cause of serious losses in the aquaculture industries of North America, Europe, and Asia.

PROPERTIES OF RHABDOVIRUSES

Classification

The family *Rhabdoviridae* includes four genera that contain animal viruses: the genera *Lyssavirus*, *Vesiculovirus*, *Ephemerovirus*, and *Novirhabdovirus* (Table 18.1). Two additional genera include rhabdoviruses that exclusively infect plants: the genera *Cytorhabdovirus* and *Nucleorhabdovirus*.

Fenner's Veterinary Virology. DOI: 10.1016/B978-0-12-375158-4.00018-3

TABLE 18.1 Rhabdoviruses that Affect Animals

Genus/Virus	Geographic Distribution
Genus *Lyssavirus*	
Rabies virus	Worldwide except Australasia, Antarctica, and certain islands; recently eradicated from portions of Europe and Scandinavia
Mokola virus	Africa
Lagos bat virus	Africa
Duvenhage virus	Africa
European bat lyssaviruses 1 and 2	Europe
Australian bat lyssavirus	Australia
Genus *Vesiculovirus*	
Vesicular stomatitis Indiana virus	North, Central, and South America
Vesicular stomatitis New Jersey virus	North, Central, and South America
Vesicular stomatitis Alagoas virus	South America
Cocal virus	South America
Piry virus	South America
Chandipura virus	India, Africa
Isfahan virus	Iran
Pike fry rhabdovirus	Europe
Spring viremia of carp virus	Widespread
Genus *Ephemerovirus*	
Bovine ephemeral fever virus	Asia, Africa, Middle East, Australia
Genus *Novirhabdovirus*	
Infectious hematopoietic necrosis virus	North America, Europe, Asia
Viral hemorrhagic septicemia virus	Europe, North America, Asia
Snakehead virus	Southeast Asia
Hirame rhabdovirus	Japan, Korea

Individual species of rhabdovirus are distinguished genetically and serologically (Figure 18.1).

The genus *Lyssavirus* ('lyssa' meaning rage) includes rabies virus and closely related viruses, including Mokola, Lagos bat, Duvenhage, European bat lyssaviruses 1 and 2,

and Australian bat lyssavirus. Each of these viruses is capable of causing rabies-like disease in animals and humans. Certain terrestrial mammals are reservoir hosts of rabies virus, and bats are potential reservoirs of both rabies and the rabies-like viruses. The genus *Vesiculovirus* includes vesicular stomatitis Indiana and vesicular stomatitis New Jersey viruses, in addition to several similar viruses that also cause vesicular disease in horses, cattle, swine, and humans, and a number of rhabdoviruses isolated from eels, carp (spring viremia of carp virus), perch, pike, salmonids, and flounder that are also tentatively classified as members of this genus. The genus *Ephemerovirus* contains bovine ephemeral fever virus and other serologically distinct viruses that also infect cattle but are not pathogenic. The genus *Novirhabdovirus* contains the important fish pathogens, infectious hematopoietic necrosis virus and viral hemorrhagic septicemia virus.

Virion Properties

Rhabdovirus virions are approximately 45–100 nm in diameter and 100–430 nm long, and consist of a helically coiled cylindrical nucleocapsid surrounded by an envelope with large (5–10 nm in length) glycoprotein spikes. The precise cylindrical form of the nucleocapsid is what gives the viruses their distinctive bullet or conical shape (Figure 18.2). The genome is a single molecule of linear, negative-sense, single-stranded RNA, 11–15 kb in size. For example, the rabies virus (Pasteur strain) genome consists of 11,932 nucleotides that encode five genes in the order $3'$-N-P-M-G-L-$5'$: N is the nucleoprotein gene that encodes the major component of the viral nucleocapsid; P is a cofactor of the viral polymerase; M is an inner virion protein that facilitates virion budding by binding to the nucleocapsid and to the cytoplasmic domain of the glycoprotein; G is the glycoprotein that forms trimers that make up the virion surface spikes; L is the RNA-dependent RNA polymerase that functions in transcription and RNA replication. Some rhabdoviruses have additional genes or pseudogenes interposed. The glycoprotein (G) contains neutralizing epitopes, which are targets of vaccine-induced immunity; it and the nucleoprotein include epitopes involved in cell-mediated immunity. Virions also contain lipids, their composition reflecting the composition of host-cell membranes, and carbohydrates as side chains on the glycoprotein.

Rhabdoviruses are relatively stable in the environment, especially when the pH is alkaline—vesicular stomatitis viruses can contaminate water troughs for many days—but the viruses are thermolabile and sensitive to the ultraviolet irradiation of sunlight. Rabies and vesicular stomatitis viruses are inactivated readily by detergent-based disinfectants, and iodine-containing preparations are commonly applied as disinfectants for reducing or eliminating fish rhabdoviruses such as those that occur on the surface of living fish eggs.

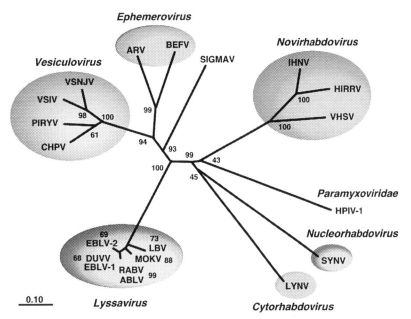

FIGURE 18.1 Family *Rhabdoviridae*: phylogenetic relationships based on a relatively conserved region of the N protein. Tree branch lengths are proportional to genetic distances. ABLV, Australian bat lyssavirus; ARV, Adelaide River virus; BEFV, bovine ephemeral fever virus; CHPV, Chandipura virus; DUVV, Duvenhage virus; EBLV, European bat lyssavirus; HIRRV, Hirame rhabdovirus; HPIV, human parainfluenza virus; IHNV, infectious hematopoietic necrosis virus; LBV, Lagos bat virus; LYNV, lettuce necrotic yellows virus; MOKV, Mokola virus; PIRYV, Piry virus; RABV, rabies vius; SIGMAV, Sigma virus; SYNV, Sonchus yellow net virus; VHSV, viral hemorrhagic septicemia virus; VSIV, vesicular stomatitis Indiana virus; VSNJV, vesicular stomatitis New Jersey virus. [*From* Virus Taxonomy: Eighth Report of the International Committee on Taxonomy of Viruses *(C. M. Fauquet, M. A. Mayo, J. Maniloff, U. Desselberger, L. A. Ball, eds.), p. 642. Copyright © Elsevier (2005), with permission.]*

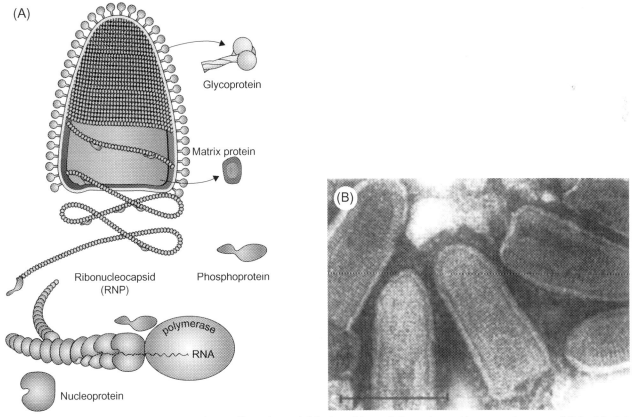

FIGURE 18.2 Family *Rhabdoviridae*. (A) Diagram illustrating a rhabdovirus virion and the nucleocapsid structure (courtesy of P. Le Merder). (B) Vesicular stomatitis Indiana virus showing characteristic bullet-shaped virions. [*A: From* Virus Taxonomy: Eighth Report of the International Committee on Taxonomy of Viruses *(C. M. Fauquet, M. A. Mayo, J. Maniloff, U. Desselberger, L. A. Ball, eds.), p. 623. Copyright © Elsevier (2005), with permission.]*

Virus Replication

Virus entry into host cells occurs by receptor-mediated endocytosis via coated pits, and subsequent pH-dependent fusion of the viral envelope with the endosomal membrane releases the viral nucleocapsid into the cytoplasm, where replication exclusively occurs (Figure 2.8). The viral glycoprotein G is solely responsible for receptor recognition and cell entry. Specific cell receptors have not clearly been identified for individual rhabdoviruses; several apparently non-essential (or redundant) receptors have been identified for rabies virus, including: neurotrophin receptor p75^{NTR}, a member of the tumor necrosis factor receptor family; the muscular form of the nicotinic acetylcholine receptor; neuronal cell adhesion molecule, a member of the immunoglobulin superfamily; and perhaps other components of the cell membrane such as gangliosides. Phosphatidyl choline is a proposed receptor for vesicular stomatitis virus, and fibronectin for viral hemorrhagic septicemia virus.

Replication first involves messenger RNA (mRNA) transcription from the genomic RNA via the virion polymerase (Figure 18.3). When sufficient quantities of the nucleocapsid (N) and phosphoprotein (P) have been expressed, there is a switch from transcription of mRNA to positive-sense antigenomes, which then serve as the template for synthesis of negative-stranded, genomic RNA. Using virion RNA as a template, the viral transcriptase transcribes five subgenomic mRNA species. There is only a single promoter site, located at the 3′ end of the viral genome; the polymerase attaches to the genomic RNA template at this site and, as it moves along the viral RNA, it encounters stop–start signals at the boundaries of each of the viral genes. Only a fraction of the polymerase molecules move past each junction and continue the transcription process. This mechanism, called attenuated transcription (or stop–start transcription, or stuttering transcription), results in more mRNA being made from genes that are located at the 3′ end of the genome and a gradient of progressively less mRNA from downstream genes $N>P>M>G>L$. This allows large amounts of the structural proteins such as the nucleocapsid protein to be produced relative to the amount of the L (RNA polymerase) protein.

Attachment of nucleocapsid protein to newly formed genomic RNA molecules leads to the self-assembly of helically wound nucleocapsids. Through the action of the matrix protein (M) protein, nucleocapsids are in turn bound to cell membranes at sites where the envelope spike glycoprotein is inserted. Virions are formed by the budding of nucleocapsids through cell membranes. Budding of rabies virus occurs principally from intracytoplasmic membranes of infected neurons, whereas the same process occurs almost exclusively on plasma membranes of salivary gland epithelial cells. Vesicular stomatitis viruses usually cause remarkably rapid cytopathology in cell culture, whereas the replication of rabies and bovine ephemeral fever viruses is slower and usually non-cytopathic, because these viruses do not shut down host-cell protein and nucleic acid synthesis. Rabies virus produces prominent cytoplasmic inclusion bodies (Negri bodies) in infected cells (Figure 18.4).

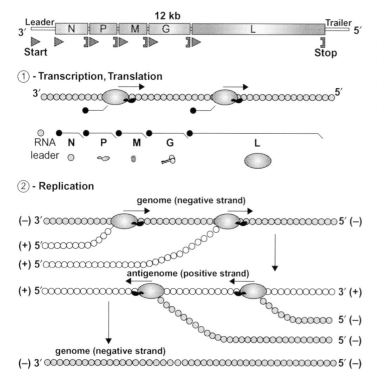

FIGURE 18.3 Genome structure of vesicular stomatitis virus and its mode of transcription (panel 1) and replication (panel 2). G, glycoprotein; N, nucleocapsid; P, phosphoprotein, M, matrix protein; L, RNA polymerase. [*From Virus Taxonomy: Eighth Report of the International Committee on Taxonomy of Viruses (C. M. Fauquet, M. A. Mayo, J. Maniloff, U. Desselberger, L. A. Ball, eds.), p. 627. Copyright © Elsevier (2005), with permission.*]

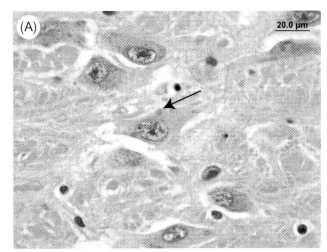

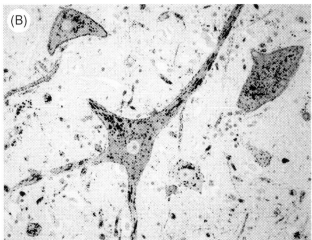

FIGURE 18.4 Rabies in a bobcat. (A) Cytoplasmic inclusions (Negri bodies) in neurons of an infected bobcat (arrow). (B) Immunohistochemical staining showing viral antigen. *(Courtesy of K. Keel, University of Georgia.)*

TABLE 18.2 Properties of Rhabdoviruses

Virions are enveloped, bullet shaped, 70 nm in diameter and 170 nm long (although some are longer, some shorter), and consist of an envelope with large spikes within which is a helically coiled cylindrical nucleocapsid

The genome is a single molecule of linear, negative-sense, single-stranded RNA, 11–15 kb in size

Cytoplasmic replication

Viral RNA-dependent RNA polymerase (transcriptase) transcribes five subgenomic mRNAs, which are translated into five proteins: (1) L, the RNA-dependent RNA polymerase (transcriptase); (2) G, the glycoprotein that forms the envelope spikes; (3) N, the nucleoprotein, the protein that associates with RNA to form the viral nucleocapsid; (4) P, a phosphoprotein that mediates binding of L protein to the nucleocapsid; (5) M, which associates with the viral nucleocapsid and lipid envelope

Maturation is by budding through the plasma membrane

Some viruses, such as vesicular stomatitis viruses, cause rapid cytopathology, whereas others, such as street rabies virus strains, are non-cytopathogenic

Defective interfering virus particles are commonly formed during rhabdovirus replication (see Chapter 2). These are complex deletion mutants with substantially truncated genomic RNA, which interfere with normal virus replication processes (Table 18.2). Defective interfering particles are proportionately shorter than infectious virions.

MEMBERS OF THE GENUS *LYSSAVIRUS*

RABIES VIRUS

Rabies virus can infect all mammals and infection virtually always results in death. The disease occurs or has occurred throughout extensive portions of the world (Figure 18.5), although certain regions have never reported domestic rabies (e.g., Japan, New Zealand) and others are now considered to be free of rabies after wildlife rabies eradication campaigns (e.g., Switzerland, France). Complicating the concept of countries having rabies-free status are situations in which rabies-related lyssaviruses that are transmitted by bats are apparently enzootic and human deaths from these agents occur (e.g., European bat lyssavirus 2 in Britain and Australian bat lyssavirus in Australia). Rabies is estimated to cause 35,000–60,000 human deaths worldwide annually, and an estimated 10 million people receive post-exposure treatments each year after being exposed to rabies-suspect animals. A large majority of human rabies cases still result from bites of rabid dogs, particularly in Africa and Asia. In contrast, wildlife rabies is now the major threat in North America, where skunks, raccoons, and foxes are all reservoirs, and in the portions of Europe where fox rabies is still important. The gray mongoose (*Herpestes auropunctatus*) is a significant reservoir of rabies in the Caribbean islands.

In many parts of the world, bat rabies represents a unique problem, as it occurs in areas where there is no other transmission of the virus. In the United States, bats have been the source of most human rabies cases. Further, an inordinate number of the most recent cases have been attributed to a genotype carried by the silver-haired bat (*Lasionycteris noctivagans*), a species that is uncommon and submitted infrequently for rabies diagnosis. It has been suggested that this viral genotype might have enhanced invasiveness, causing infection even after the most trivial, unrecognized bite. Similarly, bat rabies occurs with

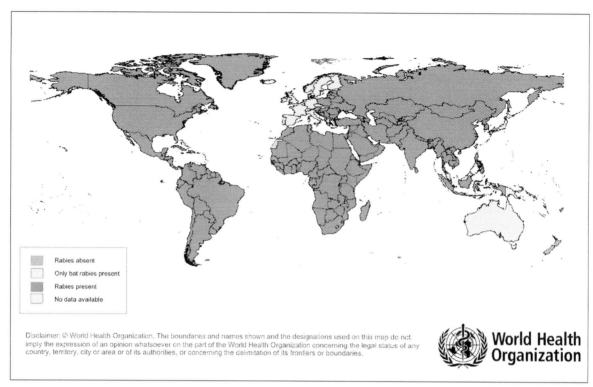

Rabies absent
Only bat rabies present
Rabies present
No data available

Disclaimer: © World Health Organization. The boundaries and names shown and the designations used on this map do not imply the expression of an opinion whatsoever on the part of the World Health Organization concerning the legal status of any country, territory, city or area or of its authorities, or concerning the delimitation of its frontiers or boundaries.

World Health Organization

FIGURE 18.5   Presence/absence of rabies worldwide in 2007. (*Courtesy of the World Health Organization.*)

some frequency in Europe. Bats also transmit a number of rabies-like viruses that cause sporadic cases of fatal human encephalitis. Rabies transmitted to cattle by vampire bats is important in Central and South America.

Clinical Features and Epidemiology

A variety of mammals, including dog, fox, wolf, jackal, raccoon, skunk, mongoose, and numerous species of bats, can serve as reservoir hosts of rabies virus that then transmit the virus to other mammals. Typically, the only risk of rabies virus transmission is by the bite of a rabid animal. In a substantial number of cases in North America, humans who have died of rabies did not recall any animal bite, and in most of these cases the rabies virus isolated was a bat variant virus. The likely explanation for most of these so-called cryptic cases of rabies is that transmission indeed resulted from the bite of a rabid bat, but the person did not recognize it because such bites can be rather nontraumatic and unnoticed, particularly by sleeping children or intoxicated individuals. In addition to transmission by bite, there have been several unfortunate incidents in which tissues from a person with undiagnosed, rabies virus infection were transplanted into other individuals, resulting in fatal infection in the transplant recipients. Transmission of rabies virus by aerosol has been reported in a few humans working in bat caves, but alternative

explanations (i.e., bat bites) cannot be excluded as the source of infection in these cases.

Different rabies viruses can be grouped into distinct genotypes, or variants, by either genome sequencing or reactivity against a panel of monoclonal antibodies. These genotypes reflect the evolutionary consequence of host preference: "raccoons-bite-raccoons-bite-raccoons," for example, and after an unknown number of passages the virus becomes a distinct genotype, still able to infect and kill other species, but transmitted most efficiently within its own reservoir host population. Thus, when spill-over does occur from a reservoir species, there rarely is sufficient fitness to sustain transmission in other species, although this unquestionably has occurred on occasion. In North America, several variants of terrestrial (i.e., not bat-associated) rabies virus are currently recognized from skunks, foxes, raccoons, and mongooses in Puerto Rico. In addition, there are numerous distinct genotypes carried by different species of bats. Phylogenetic analysis of rabies viruses has proven invaluable in epidemiologic investigations because it can identify spill-over events (cross-species transmission) and enable cases of human rabies to be attributed to bites from a particular animal.

The clinical features of rabies are similar in most species, but there is great variation between individuals. After the bite of a rabid animal, such as a bat or dog, the incubation period is usually between 14 and 90 days, but it may be considerably longer. Human cases have been described in which the last opportunity for exposure occurred some 2–7 years before the onset of clinical disease. In each of these distinctive human cases of long incubation, the infecting virus was identified as a dog variant (genotype). Similar data are not available for domestic animals, but an incubation period of 2 years has been reported in a cat.

There is typically a prodromal phase before overt clinical disease that often is overlooked in animals or is recalled only in retrospect as a change in temperament. Two clinical forms of the disease are recognized: *furious* rabies, and *dumb* (or paralytic) rabies. In the furious form, the animal becomes restless, nervous, aggressive, and often extremely dangerous as it loses fear of humans and bites at anything that gains its attention. The animal often cannot swallow water because of pharyngeal paralysis, giving rise to the old name for the disease, "hydrophobia." Other characteristic signs include excessive salivation, exaggerated responses to light and sound, and hyperesthesia (animals commonly bite and scratch themselves). As the encephalitis progresses, fury gives way to paralysis, and the animal presents the same clinical picture as seen in the dumb form of the disease. Terminally, there are often convulsive seizures, coma, and respiratory arrest, with death occurring 2–14 days after the onset of clinical signs. A higher proportion of dogs, cats, and horses exhibit fury than is the case for cattle or other ruminants or laboratory animal species.

Pathogenesis and Pathology

The proportion of animals that develop rabies after exposure depends on the dose and genotype of virus, the location and severity of the bite, and the species of animal involved (foxes, for example, reportedly have up to 10^6 infectious units of virus per ml of saliva). The bite of a rabid animal usually delivers virus deep into the musculature and connective tissue, but infection can also occur, albeit with less certainty, after superficial abrasion of the skin. From its entry site, virus must access peripheral nerves, which can occur directly, but in many instances virus is amplified by first replicating in muscle cells (myocytes). The virus invades the peripheral nervous system through sensory or motor nerve endings and virus binds specifically to the receptor for the neurotransmitter acetylcholine at neuromuscular junctions. Neuronal infection and centripetal passive movement of the virus within axons ultimately result in infection of the central nervous system. An ascending wave of neuronal infection and neuronal dysfunction then occurs. Virus reaches the limbic system of the brain, where it replicates extensively, leading to the fury seen clinically. Progressive spread within the central nervous system changes the clinical picture to the dumb or paralytic form of the disease. Depression, coma, and death from respiratory arrest follow.

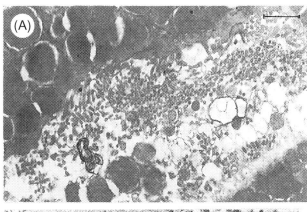

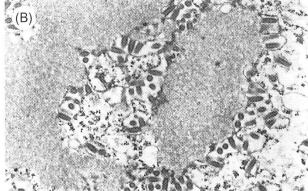

FIGURE 18.6 Rabies virus infection in the submandibular salivary gland and brain of a rabid fox. (A) Massive accumulation of virions "downstream" in the major salivary duct. (B) Infection in the brain. Bullet-shaped virions are budding on internal cellular membranes; the granular material is excess viral nucleocapsids forming an inclusion body, which by light microscopy is seen as a Negri body. In both the salivary glands and the brain the infection is noncytopathic, but in the brain nearly all virus is formed by budding on internal membranes of neurons and so is trapped, whereas in the salivary gland nearly all virus is formed by budding on the apical plasma membranes, where it is free to enter the saliva. Some reservoir host species can have 10^6 ID_{50} of rabies virus per ml of saliva at the time of peak transmissibility. Thin-section electron microscopy.

Late in the course of infection, rabies virus spreads centrifugally from the central nervous system through peripheral nerves to a variety of organs, including the adrenal cortex, pancreas, and, most importantly, the salivary glands. In the nervous system most virus is formed by budding on intracytoplasmic membranes; however, in the salivary glands, virions bud on plasma membranes at the apical (luminal) surface of mucous cells and are released in high concentrations into the saliva (Figure 18.6). Thus the saliva is often highly infectious at the time when virus replication within the central nervous system causes the infected animal to become furious and bite indiscriminately.

There are no characteristic macroscopic lesions in animals that die of rabies, although self-mutilation is common. The brains of animals with rabies exhibit variable inflammation and often only modest histological evidence of neuronal injury; the presence of eosinophilic intracytoplasmic inclusions (Negri bodies) in neurons is characteristic and diagnostic, these being especially common in neurons in the hippocampus and Purkinje cells in the cerebellum (Figure 18.4A). Ganglioneuritis occurs in some animals, and involves the Gasserian ganglion in particular. Widespread infection of neurons in the brains of affected animals can be confirmed by ultrastructural evaluation (electron microscopy) or immunohistochemical staining with rabies virus-specific antisera (Figure 18.4B). This remarkable paradox of lethal neurological dysfunction despite minimal target destruction in many rabid animals suggests that the primary neuronal lesion is functional rather than structural.

Diagnosis

The clinical manifestations of rabies are highly variable, and definitive diagnosis requires further laboratory testing. Negri bodies in the neurons of affected animals are characteristic of rabies, but not infrequently are difficult to identify. Laboratory diagnosis of rabies is done in most countries only in approved laboratories by qualified, experienced personnel. The most common request is to determine whether an animal known to have bitten a human is rabid. If rabies is suspected, the suspect animal must be killed and brain tissue collected for testing. Post-mortem diagnosis most commonly involves direct immunofluorescence (see Figure 5.4) or immunohistochemical staining to demonstrate rabies virus antigen in frozen sections of brain tissue (medulla, cerebellum, and hippocampus). Post-mortem diagnosis can in certain circumstances also be performed using RT-PCR assay to test for the presence of viral RNA in the brain of the suspect animal; this is done with primers that amplify both the genomic and mRNA sequences of the rabies virus. Antemortem diagnosis is only attempted in suspected human rabies cases, and is accomplished using either RT-PCR of saliva specimens or immunofluorescence staining of skin biopsy or corneal impression; in such cases, only positive results are of diagnostic value, as the choice of specimens for these procedures is never optimum and sites of infection may be missed.

Immunity, Prevention, and Control

Rabies virus proteins are highly immunogenic, and numerous different types of efficacious vaccines have been developed to protect humans and animals from rabies virus infection. In contrast, virus-specific responses are often not detected in infected animals during the stage of movement of virus from the site of the bite to the central nervous system, probably because very little antigen is delivered to the immune system as most is sequestered in muscle cells or within axons. However, infectious rabies virus is susceptible to antibody-mediated neutralization and clearance during this early stage of infection, hence the efficacy in exposed humans of the classical Pasteurian post-exposure vaccination, especially when combined with the administration of hyperimmune globulin. Immunologic intervention is effective for some time during the long incubation period because of the delay between the initial virus replication in muscle cells and the entry of virus into the nervous system.

Inactivated, live-attenuated and recombinant vaccines have been developed for the parenteral immunization of animals and humans against rabies. Original vaccines that incorporate nervous tissue containing inactivated virus cause immunologically mediated nervous disease in some individuals, and original live-attenuated vaccines that are propagated in embryonated duck eggs also induce allergic reactions in some immunized individuals. A considerable number of cell culture derived live-attenuated and inactivated vaccines are now available and, more recently, highly effective recombinant vaccines that express the rabies virus glycoprotein have been developed. Successful oral vaccination against rabies has been achieved using either live-attenuated or recombinant vaccines that are delivered in baits to target wildlife species. Recombinant vaccinia viruses that express the rabies virus glycoprotein have proven effective in immunizing foxes and raccoons, but a variety of other virus vectors now have been developed. The use of vaccine-containing baits has been used to control and even eliminate rabies from foxes in much of Europe, and regionally among coyotes, raccoons, and foxes in North America. The great merit of this approach over animal population reduction is that the eco niche remains occupied, in this case by an immune population.

The control of rabies in different regions of the world poses very different problems, depending on which reservoir hosts are present and the level of infection in such hosts.

Rabies-Free Countries

Rigidly enforced quarantine of dogs and cats before entry has been used effectively to exclude rabies from countries that were always free of the virus, or that recently eliminated the virus. The list of such countries is rapidly growing, with most being either islands or located on peninsulas. The presence of enzootic infection with rabies-like lyssaviruses clearly can complicate the designation of countries as rabies free. For example, rabies had never become enzootic in wildlife in the United Kingdom and was eradicated from dogs in that country in 1902 and again in 1922 after its re-establishment in the dog population in 1918. Since then, there have been no cases of classical rabies recognized in the United Kingdom, but the related European bat lyssavirus 2 has been isolated on several occasions from bats and was responsible for a fatal human infection in a bat biologist. Australia also is free of rabies, but Australian bat lyssavirus is enzootic in several areas and the cause of sporadic fatal human infections. Despite these sporadic cases of bat-associated lyssavirus infections, the maintenance of strict quarantine for imported dogs and cats is still key to preventing rabies virus from being introduced and becoming enzootic in terrestrial wild and domestic animals.

Rabies-Enzootic Countries

Enzootic dog rabies continues to be a serious problem in many countries of Asia, Africa, and Latin America, marked by significant domestic animal and human mortality. In these countries, very large numbers of doses of rabies vaccines are used and, although expensive to institute and maintain, there is a continuing need for comprehensive rabies control programs. For example, recent intensive dog vaccination programs in large cities have significantly decreased the number of rabies cases in Latin America, particularly Mexico. Control of rabies in enzootic regions is also complicated by the presence of wildlife reservoirs, such as the gray mongoose (*Herpestes auropunctatus*) in the Caribbean islands and numerous species of wild felids and canids in Africa. Similarly, vampire bat rabies is a problem for livestock industries and humans in parts of Latin America. There are three species of vampire bats, the most important being *Desmodus rotundus*. Control efforts have involved the use of vaccines in cattle, and the use of anticoagulants such as diphenadione and warfarin. These anticoagulants are either fed to cattle as slow-release boluses (cattle are very insensitive to their anticoagulant effect) or mixed with grease and spread on the backs of cattle. When vampire bats feed on the blood of treated cattle or preen themselves and each other to remove the grease, they ingest anticoagulant and later suffer fatal hemorrhage from vessels in their wings.

In Europe and North America, publicly supported rabies control agencies operate in the following areas: (1) stray dog and cat removal and control of the movement of pets (quarantine is used in epizootic circumstances, but rarely); (2) immunization of dogs and cats with appropriate vaccines so as to break the chain of virus transmission; (3) institution of programs to prevent and control rabies in wildlife, reflecting the important regional reservoir animal host(s); (4) laboratory diagnosis to confirm clinical observations and obtain accurate incidence data; (5) surveillance to measure the effectiveness of all control measures; (6) public education programs to assure cooperation.

European Countries

Dog rabies has been controlled or eliminated throughout Europe, and human cases have plummeted as a result. The control of rabies virus infection of wildlife species like the fox more recently has been achieved. Rabies was historically controlled in wildlife by animal population reduction by trapping and poisoning, a process that has been replaced by the immunization of wild animal reservoir host species, especially foxes, by the distribution of baits containing rabies virus vaccine. Fox rabies, the only enzootic rabies in much of Europe, recently has been eliminated or virtually eliminated in western Europe using this approach, and is increasingly being applied in eastern Europe.

North American Countries

The total number of cases of rabies in domestic animals in the United States has steadily declined since the introduction of rabies control programs in the 1940s and 1950s—programs that included widespread parenteral vaccination of domestic animals. These programs have eliminated the major canine variants of rabies virus from the United States and, very recently, a coyote-associated variant was eradicated by vaccination and regulations that prohibited the translocation of certain wildlife species. After peaking in the early 1990s, total number of animal rabies cases reported among wildlife in the United States has also shown an uneven but gradual decline. Reservoirs of rabies virus persist in the United States in fox, skunks, and raccoons, and in mongooses in Puerto Rico (Figure 18.7) Rabies also persists in red and arctic foxes (*Vulpes vulpes* and *Alopex lagopus*) in Alaska and Canada, although reports of rabid foxes have declined in Canada subsequent to the introduction of oral vaccination programs. Skunk rabies in central North America, from Texas to Saskatchewan, is the principal cause of rabies in cattle. Raccoons have been recognized as a major reservoir for rabies in the southeastern United States for more than 50 years, and raccoon-associated rabies has now spread over the entire eastern seaboard of North America, as well as across the Appalachian mountains into the Ohio Valley.

Human Disease

Public health veterinarians are called on regularly to provide advice on rabies post-exposure prophylaxis, pre-exposure vaccination, and other matters pertaining to the risk of rabies in humans. Furthermore, practicing veterinarians represent a major risk group for rabies virus infection in many areas of the world. Guidelines for post-exposure prophylaxis and human vaccination are available from local public health organizations, the World Health Organization (http://whqlibdoc.who.int/hq/1996/WHO_EMC_ZOO_96.6.pdf), or the United States Centers for Disease Control (www.CDC.gov). These guidelines are updated as new data and recommendations become available; those dealing with rabies issues should therefore consult these sources on a frequent basis.

The first step in dealing with a possible human rabies exposure is thorough cleansing of the wound; immediate

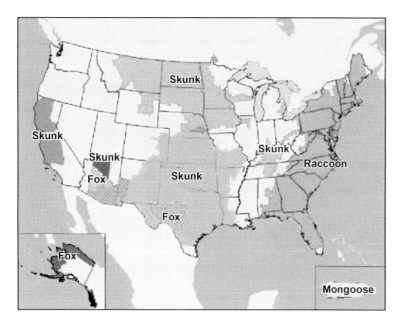

FIGURE 18.7 Distribution of major rabies virus variants among wild terrestrial animal reservoirs in the United States and Puerto Rico, 2008. *[From J. D. Blanton, K. Robertson, D. Palmer, C. E. Rupprecht. Rabies surveillance in the United States during 2008. J. Am. Vet. Med. Assoc. 235, 676–689 (2009), with permission.]*

vigorous washing and flushing with soap and water is crucial. The next step is an appraisal of the nature of the exposure. In a rabies enzootic area, if the individual has simply touched the suspect animal, treatment may not be recommended, whereas treatment should immediately be instigated if the individual has been scratched or bitten, or if skin abrasions are present. As this is a public health issue, local health officers should be contacted immediately when rabies exposure is suspected, so that proper treatment can be initiated and proper diagnostic testing be assessed for the suspect animal. Capture of the suspect animal for testing or quarantine is critical to the course of post-exposure treatment. If possible exposure involves a dog or cat, treatment may be stopped if the animal is determined to have been appropriately vaccinated, remains healthy throughout a 10-day observation period, or is euthanized and found to be negative by appropriate laboratory testing. When possible exposure involves any other domestic or wild animal, the animal is euthanized immediately and its brain examined using appropriate laboratory techniques. In the United States, because of recent experiences, more conservative recommendations have been made when exposure involves bats; in such situations the bat is treated as if rabid until proved negative by laboratory tests, and extra consideration is given to the possibility that exposure may have occurred even when a bite wound is not evident. In areas where there is little or no rabies, the decision to treat or not is adjusted accordingly, with extra consideration given to potential bat exposures, given the fact that bat rabies may occur in the absence of rabies in terrestrial species and the fact that rabies surveillance in bats is not commonly done. Exposure to rodents, rabbits, and hares seldom, if ever, requires specific antirabies treatment.

RABIES-LIKE VIRUSES AND BAT LYSSAVIRUSES

Bats are important reservoir hosts of rabies virus, but they also transmit a number of other zoonotic rhabdoviruses that cause sporadic cases of rabies-like disease. These viruses include several African viruses (Duvenhage, Lagos bat, and Mokola viruses) and European bat lyssaviruses (1 and 2). Australian bat lyssavirus was discovered in a black flying fox (fruit bat, *Pteropus alecto*) in 1996. This virus occurs along the entire east coast of Australia, and has been found in all four major species of flying fox and one species of insectivorous bat (*Saccolaimus flaviventrus*).

MEMBERS OF THE GENUS *VESICULOVIRUS*

VESICULAR STOMATITIS VIRUS

Vesicular stomatitis is a disease of cattle, pigs, and horses in the Americas that was historically important because of its significance in the differential diagnosis of foot-and-mouth disease, and the debilitating lameness it can cause in horses. More recently, however, the disease has been recognized as the cause of production losses in cattle, especially as more dairying is undertaken in warmer climates. The disease is caused by a group of antigenically related but distinct viruses, including vesicular stomatitis Indiana virus, vesicular stomatitis New Jersey virus, vesicular stomatitis Alagoas virus, and Cocal virus. Cocal virus was originally isolated in Trinidad and Brazil, and vesicular stomatitis Alagoas virus in Brazil; neither virus has been identified in North America.

Clinical Features and Epidemiology

The clinical features of vesicular stomatitis vary greatly among animals in a herd. Lesions develop quickly after an incubation period of 1–5 days. Excess salivation and fever often are the first signs of infection in cattle and horses, and lameness is often the first sign in swine. Vesicles that develop on the tongue, the oral mucosa, teats, and coronary bands of cattle rapidly rupture to leave extensive ulcers that quickly become secondarily infected. These lesions may cause profuse salivation and anorexia, lameness, and rejection of suckling calves. In horses, tongue lesions are most pronounced, sometimes progressing to ulceration of the entire tongue (Figure 18.8). In swine, vesicular lesions are most common on the snout and coronary bands. Lesions usually heal within 7–10 days without adverse sequelae.

Epizootics of vesicular stomatitis occur in North, Central, and South America, and portions of the Caribbean Basin. Epizootics typically occur annually or at intervals of 2 or 3 years in tropical and subtropical countries and at intervals of 5–10 years in temperate zones. Vesicular stomatitis New Jersey virus is the most common and has the widest distribution, with isolations as far north as Canada and as far south as Peru. Vesicular stomatitis Indiana virus has a similar wide geographical distribution but is encountered less frequently. Genomic analysis of large numbers of isolates of vesicular stomatitis New Jersey and vesicular stomatitis Indiana viruses indicates that each temperate zone epizootic is caused by a single viral genotype, suggesting spread from a common origin. For example, vesicular stomatitis Indiana isolates from the United States and Mexico always derive from a recent common ancestor. Epizootic isolates from different geographic areas, such as the temperate zones of North and South America, are distinct, indicating spatial genetic isolation. Isolates from different enzootic foci in the tropics are also distinct, but they reflect a more complex genetic diversity, including multiple phylogenetic lineages. For example, several genotypes of vesicular stomatitis Indiana virus co-exist in Costa Rica, Panama, and adjacent countries of South America. Within even small enzootic foci, these variants are maintained over extended periods of time. Enzootic foci of vesicular stomatitis Indiana and New Jersey viruses occur in southeastern Mexico, Venezuela, Colombia, Panama, and Costa Rica, mostly in wet lowland areas. In the United States, a band of enzootic vesicular stomatitis New Jersey virus infection formerly existed across the coastal plains of South Carolina, Georgia, and Florida; until very recently, only a single focus remained on Ossabaw Island, Georgia, but it now appears that the virus has also disappeared from this focus.

Several lines of evidence indicate that vesicular stomatitis viruses are naturally transmitted by biting insects, including the seasonal nature of epizootics and the seroconversion of caged animals during epizootics. Virus transmission by sandflies (*Lutzomyia* spp.) occurs in some tropical and subtropical areas, with transovarial transmission of the viruses in sandflies probably contributing to their perpetuation in enzootic foci—transovarial transmission is considered evidence of a long-standing evolutionary relationship between virus and vector. Sandflies have also been incriminated in maintaining the enzootic focus of vesicular stomatitis New Jersey that existed until recently on Ossabaw Island, Georgia. Virus isolations have also been made from *Simuliidae* (black flies), *Culicoides* (midges), *Culex nigripalpus* (mosquitoes), *Hippilates* spp. (eye gnats), *Musca domestica* (houseflies), and *Gigantolaelapsis* spp. (mites). In an extensive epizootic of vesicular stomatitis New Jersey that occurred in the western United States in 1982, many virus isolates were made from flies, mostly from the common housefly, *M. domestica*, but it remains uncertain what precise role these flies play in the epidemiology of the infection during epizootics. The manner by which vesicular stomatitis viruses are transmitted over long distances also remains controversial, despite years of study. In some instances, transport of infected animals has led to rapid spread of the disease. Vesicular stomatitis viruses can be stable in the environment for days—for example, on milking machine parts where transmission results in teat and udder lesions, in water troughs, in soil, and on vegetation where transmission results in mouth lesions.

Pathogenesis and Pathology

Vesicular stomatitis virus probably enters the body through breaks in the mucosa or skin, as a result of the minor abrasions caused, for example, by rough forage or by the bites of arthropods. There does not appear to be a substantial systemic, viremic phase of infection, except perhaps in swine and small laboratory animals. Localized viral infection of the epithelium of the mucous membranes of the oral cavity and the skin leads to intraepithelial edema and to the formation of fluid-filled vesicles that quickly ulcerate. Coalescence of these lesions often results in extensive ulceration, such that it is not uncommon for the entire epithelium of the tongue or teat to be sloughed (Figure 18.8). High titers of infectious virus are present, usually for a short time, in vesicular fluids and in tissues at the margins of lesions. From this source, virus may be transmitted by fomites, such as contaminated food, milking machines, and restraint devices. The virus may also be transmitted mechanically by arthropods. Despite the extent of epithelial damage, healing is usually rapid and complete.

Diagnosis

Vesicular stomatitis is clinically indistinguishable from other vesicular diseases of cattle and pigs, including foot-and-mouth disease. Vesicular lesions in horses are characteristic

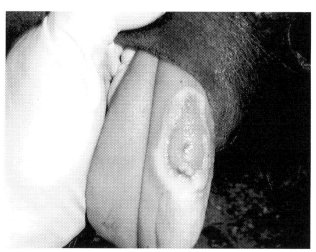

FIGURE 18.8 Extensive (craterous) ulcer in the tongue of a horse with vesicular stomatitis. *(Courtesy of R. Bowen, Colorado State University.)*

only of vesicular stomatitis. Virus can be recovered from vesicular fluids and tissue scrapings by standard virus isolation techniques in cell culture, or identified by RT-PCR assays. These procedures should be carried out in an authorized reference laboratory, because of the critical need to rapidly and accurately distinguish vesicular stomatitis from foot-and-mouth disease. Serologic testing, especially of cattle and horses, is often required for transport of animals or semen from enzootic areas or regions experiencing epizootics of vesicular stomatitis.

Immunity, Prevention, and Control

Infection with vesicular stomatitis virus induces a robust immune response. However, cattle with high levels of neutralizing antibodies are often susceptible to reinfection, suggesting that such antibodies have a limited protective effect. This may be explained by the restricted and localized replication of the virus within epithelium. There is little cross-protection between vesicular stomatitis New Jersey and vesicular stomatitis Indiana viruses.

Outbreaks of vesicular stomatitis can be explosive, but effective methods of control are poorly defined, as the epidemiology of the infection is uncertain and frequently there is little response even in the face of epizootics. Avoidance of pastures known to be sites of transmission may help avoid infection. Because of the potential for arthropod-borne transmission, fly control is often advocated, and animal quarantine and movement restrictions are frequently imposed. In temperate zones, epizootics occur at such infrequent intervals that concern wanes during inter-epizootic periods. Both inactivated and attenuated virus vaccines have been developed, but are not used widely.

Human Disease

Vesicular stomatitis is a zoonotic disease, and the causative viruses are transmissible to humans (typically, farmers and veterinarians) from vesicular fluids and tissues of infected animals. The disease in human resembles influenza, presenting with an acute onset of fever, chills, and muscle pain. It resolves without complications within 7–10 days. Human cases are not uncommon during epidemics in cattle and horses, but because of lack of awareness, few cases are reported. Human cases can be diagnosed retrospectively by serologic methods.

MEMBERS OF THE GENUS *EPHEMEROVIRUS*

BOVINE EPHEMERAL FEVER VIRUS

Bovine ephemeral fever, also called 3-day stiff-sickness, is an arthropod-transmitted disease of cattle and water buffalo that spans tropical and subtropical zones of Africa, Australia, the Middle East, and Asia. From these enzootic sites the disease extends intermittently into temperate zones, causing epizootics of variable severity. The disease has not been reported in North or South America or in Europe. Several closely related viruses can infect cattle, but do not cause disease.

Clinical Features and Epidemiology

Clinical signs of bovine ephemeral fever in cattle are characteristic, but all are not seen in an individual animal. Onset is sudden, and the disease is marked by a biphasic or polyphasic fever, with an immediate drop in milk production. Other clinical signs are associated with the second and later febrile phases; these include depression, stiffness, and lameness, and—less often—nasal and ocular discharges, cessation of rumination, constipation, and abortion. Infrequently, there is diarrhea and temporary or permanent paresis. Usually, recovery is dramatic and complete in 3 days (range 2–5 days). Morbidity rates often approach 100%, and the mortality rate in an outbreak is usually very low (less than 1%), but on occasion it can reach 10–20% in mature, well-conditioned beef cattle and high-producing dairy cattle. Subclinical cases occur, but their relative rate is unknown because antibody testing is confounded by intercurrent infections in the same areas by related but non-pathogenic rhabdoviruses.

Clinical disease is restricted to domestic cattle and buffalo, although a variety of other ruminants appear to be susceptible to subclinical infection. In enzootic areas, ephemeral fever is a seasonal disease that occurs in the summer and autumn, especially in the rainy season. Bovine ephemeral fever virus most probably is transmitted by arthropod vectors, although these are yet to be definitively characterized. Potential vectors include culicine and anopheline mosquitoes, and possibly *Culicoides* midges; both enzootic and epizootic spread is limited by the distribution of appropriate vectors.

Pathogenesis and Pathology

The pathogenesis of the disease is complex and probably reflects pathophysiologic and immunologic effects mediated by the release and activity of various inflammatory mediators. Injury to the endothelial lining of small blood vessels is central to the expression of bovine ephemeral fever, but there is no evidence that the virus causes widespread tissue destruction. In all cases, there is an early neutrophilia with an abnormal level of immature neutrophils in the circulation ("left shift"). There is an increase in plasma fibrinogen and a significant decrease in plasma calcium. Therapeutically, there is a dramatic response to anti-inflammatory drugs, and often to calcium infusion. Gross (macroscopic) lesions include serofibrinous polyserositis and synovitis, pulmonary and lymph node edema, and focal necrosis of selected muscles.

Diagnosis

Although the clinical and epidemiological presentations of bovine ephemeral fever are highly characteristic, laboratory diagnosis is difficult. The "gold standard" traditionally has been virus isolation by blind passage in mosquito (*Aedes albopictus*) cells or suckling mouse brain, but RT-PCR assays have been developed recently. A diagnostic increase in antibody titer can be detected by enzyme immunoassay, including blocking enzyme-linked immunosorbent assay (ELISA), by neutralization assays, which are virus specific, or by immunofluorescence or agar gel precipitin tests, which are cross-reactive with related rhabdoviruses.

Immunity, Prevention, and Control

Infection results in solid, long-lasting immunity. Because outbreaks tend to involve most animals in a herd, repeat clinical episodes usually involve young animals born since previous outbreaks. Prevention by vector control is impractical in the areas of the world where this disease is prevalent. In Japan, South Africa, and Australia, inactivated and attenuated virus vaccines are used. Problems with conventional vaccines stem from lack of potency—inactivated vaccines require more antigenic mass than it has been possible to achieve economically, and attenuated virus vaccines suffer from a loss in immunogenicity linked with the attenuation process. A recombinant baculovirus-expressed G protein vaccine has also been developed.

RHABDOVIRUSES OF FISH: GENERA *VESICULOVIRUS* AND *NOVIRHABDOVIRUS*

At least nine distinct rhabdoviruses in two different genera have been associated with economically important diseases in fish; specifically, viral hemorrhagic septicemia virus and infectious hematopoietic necrosis virus in the genus *Novirhabdovirus*, and spring viremia of carp virus, which is tentatively classified in the genus *Vesiculovirus*, are among the most significant pathogens of cultured and wild fish. These viruses, and additional fish rhabdoviruses, are distinguished by neutralization tests or sequence analysis. The viruses may be propagated in a variety of cell lines of fish origin and in some cases may also replicate in mammalian, avian, reptilian, and insect cells, although conditions for optimal growth vary substantially between individual viruses.

VIRAL HEMORRHAGIC SEPTICEMIA VIRUS

Viral hemorrhagic septicemia (*syn*. Egtved) is a systemic infection of several salmonid and a growing list of marine and freshwater fish that is caused by viral hemorrhagic septicemia virus. The infection may occur in fish of any age, resulting in significant mortality, and fish that survive may become carriers. There are acute, chronic, and subclinical forms of infection. Acute infections in rainbow trout (*Oncorhynchus mykiss*) occur within 30 days of first exposure and are characterized by lethargy, a spiral or flashing swimming pattern, darkened body color, pale gills, exophthalmia, and hemorrhages at the base of the fins. Mortality is generally greatest among young fish and can reach 100%. Subclinically and chronically infected fish may show no external signs, although virus tropism to the brain may result in a nervous form of the disease manifested by abnormal swimming behaviour.

Viral hemorrhagic septicemia virus can infect more than 60 species of freshwater and marine fish, and has been recognized in continental Europe, North America, Japan, and most recently in Iran. The virus is particularly troublesome in farmed salmonids in Europe, and at least 28 species of wild fish in the Great Lakes region of North America are susceptible to infection. There appears to be a single serotype with four subtypes (genotypes) that cluster into geographically specific topotypes. Three of the four genotypes occur in marine fish, which are the suspected source of the virus that adapted to infect rainbow trout in freshwater environments. The virus is readily transmissible to fish of all ages, and survivors of infection can become carriers that shed virus in urine and semen and on the surface of eggs. In aquaculture settings, virus transmission occurs by cohabitation or by fomites. The virus has been isolated from wild fish in waters receiving hatchery effluent, and in some cases hatchery outbreaks have been traced to infected wild salmonids in the water supply. Epizootic outbreaks and fish losses occur at water temperatures from 4 to 14°C. Both mortality and the proportion of fish that become virus carriers decreases as water temperatures approach or exceed 15°C.

Lesions of viral hemorrhagic septicemia in affected fish include hemorrhages in the eyes, skin, and gills, and at the bases of the fins. Internally, there may be ascites and hemorrhages in several organs. The liver is mottled and variably congested. Histopathologic lesions include multifocal necrosis and hemorrhage in several organs. Diagnosis is based on observation of typical signs of the disease and isolation of the virus with any of several regularly used cell lines of fish origin. Confirmation requires identification of the agent by antigen-based approaches, including fluorescent antibody, ELISA, or nucleic acid-based RT-PCR assays. Immunity develops among hatchery-reared rainbow trout that survive the infection. The virus induces interferon early in infection, before the appearance of anti-virus neutralizing antibodies in the serum. Attenuated and DNA vaccines have provided excellent protection in limited field trials, but none are commercially available, thus avoidance/exclusion is the principal method of control in enzootic regions. Among cultured populations of fish this includes use of certified virus-free stocks, surface disinfection of fertilized eggs, and the use of virus-free water supplies.

INFECTIOUS HEMATOPOIETIC NECROSIS VIRUS

Infectious hematopoietic necrosis is a disease of salmonid fish. Three principal genetic groups of infectious hematopoietic necrosis virus have been identified, which tend to segregate according to region of origin (topotype) and species of salmonid from which they are isolated. The individual diseases caused by specific virus strains such as the Oregon sockeye virus, Sacramento River Chinook virus, and a similar virus prevalent among cultured rainbow trout are associated with distinct genetic groups of infectious hematopoietic necrosis virus.

Infectious hematopoietic necrosis virus is enzootic in certain wild and hatchery fish populations of the west coast of North American from Northern California to Alaska. Sporadic outbreaks with significant losses occur in both salmon and trout hatcheries throughout the Pacific Northwest of North America, as well as continental Europe and the Far East (e.g., Japan, Korea, China, and Taiwan). Outbreaks usually involve juvenile fish at water temperatures from 8 to 15°C, with cumulative mortality reaching 50–90%. The virus may also cause significant losses among older salmonids in seawater (e.g., Atlantic salmon) or fresh water (e.g., rainbow trout). Survivors develop immunity to reinfection that is associated with the presence of virus-neutralizing antibodies in the serum. Anadromous salmonids

re-entering freshwater to spawn may shed large amounts of virus in urine and in ovarian and seminal fluids, in the absence of clinical signs of disease. In contrast, acute infections in juvenile fish are characterized by darkened body color, lethargy, pale gills indicating anemia, bilateral exophthalmia, distension of the abdomen as a result of the accumulation of ascites, and hemorrhages at the base of fins.

Diagnosis is based upon observance of typical clinical signs of the disease and isolation of the virus in cell lines of fish origin. Confirmation is obtained by virus identification with antigen-based approaches, including fluorescent antibody, enzyme immunoassays or nucleic acid-based approaches (RT-PCR or DNA probes). Control measures among cultured populations of fish are similar to those described for viral hemorrhagic septicemia. The disease has been successfully managed among Atlantic salmon populations reared in marine net pens along the west coast of North America by utilizing "all-in–all-out" stocking and harvesting strategies and by physical separations of the net pens. An efficacious DNA vaccine has been licensed for Atlantic salmon in Canada.

SPRING VIREMIA OF CARP VIRUS

Spring viremia of carp is a disease of cyprinid fishes (family *Cyprinidae*) that, as the name implies, occurs generally in the spring as water temperatures begin to increase into the range of 10–17°C. The disease is caused by a group of serologically and genetically distinct viruses that are further divided into four subgenogroups that display some, but not unique, geographic distribution. Once known as a disease principally among Eurasian populations of carp, more recent outbreaks among wild populations of carp and captive koi have occurred in China and North America. Although common carp are the principal species affected, the disease can also occur in other cyprinids, including crucian, silver, bighead, and grass carp, as well as goldfish, orfe, and tench. Outbreaks have also been reported in sheatfish (a silurid catfish). Losses are greatest, but not restricted to, fish less than a year of age. Lower water temperatures may protract the infection and mortality, whereas temperatures above 20°C (with some exceptions) may limit the disease and facilitate rapid clearing of the virus. Reservoirs for the virus are probably wild or cultured cyprinids that act as carriers that periodically shed the virus during periods of stress.

Fish with acute infections may show either no outward signs, or a range of non-specific clinical signs, including a distended abdomen with hemorrhagic ascites, petechial hemorrhages on the gills and skin, and an inflamed and protruding vent. During acute infection, the virus is shed from skin and gill lesions, as well as the urine and feces. Diagnosis is reliant upon isolation and identification of the virus. Confirmation is obtained by serum neutralization tests alone and, potentially, supplemental RT-PCR. Avoidance is the principal control measure, using methods analogous to those described for both viral hemorrhagic septicemia and infectious hematopoietic necrosis. These control measures can be supplemented with sound hygienic approaches, including regular disinfection of equipment used in ponds, pond disinfections, and prompt removal and appropriate disposal of dead fish. There are no approved vaccines for spring viremia of carp, although inactivated, live-attenuated, and DNA vaccines all have shown promise experimentally.

OTHER RHABDOVIRUSES OF FISH

Hirame rhabdovirus and snakehead virus are included in the genus *Novirhabdovirus*, along with infectious hematopoietic necrosis and viral hemorrhagic septicemia viruses, and are significant pathogens of fish in the Far East (Japan and Korea) and southeast Asia, respectively. Hirame rhabdovirus, the cause of a systemic hemorrhagic disease in hirame (a flounder-like flatfish) and ayu (a trout-like species), is a disease that resembles both viral hemorrhagic septicemia and infectious hematopoietic necrosis in salmonids. Snakehead virus has been isolated from both wild and cultured snakehead (*Channidae*) in southeast Asia, and is associated with an ulcerative disease; the virus probably has a role secondary to the oomycete *Aphanomyces invadans* in causing massive epizootics of ulcerative disease in snakehead. Both the hirame and snakehead viruses can be isolated in several cell lines of fish origin and identified by neutralization tests or nucleic acid-based methods (RT-PCR).

Pike fry rhabdovirus causes a disease similar to spring viremia of carp virus in hatchery-reared pike fry in Europe, where it is controlled primarily by isolation and by iodophor treatment of eggs to remove surface virus contamination. Rhabdoviruses with serologic properties similar to those of the pike fry rhabdovirus have been found in several species of cyprinids, including grass carp and tench. Serologic cross-reactions between spring viremia of carp and pike fry rhabdoviruses indicate that these agents are related.

Several rhabdoviruses, some apparently related to the novirhabdoviruses and others to the vesiculoviruses, have been isolated from eels. They are serologically distinct from other known fish rhabdoviruses and probably represent novel species. None of the eel viruses has been demonstrated to cause disease in the freshwater stages of eel, but certain isolates are pathogenic for rainbow trout fry. Other vesiculovirus-like agents have been isolated from perch, pike, grayling, European lake trout, and Swedish sea trout and starry flounder. Less characterized fish rhabdoviruses have been isolated from Rio Grande cichlids (*Cichlasoma cyanoguttatum*), Chinese perch (*Siniperca chuats*) and turbot (*Scophthalmus maximus*).

Filoviridae

Chapter Contents

In 1967, 31 cases of hemorrhagic fever, with seven deaths, occurred among laboratory workers in Germany and Yugoslavia who were processing kidneys from African green monkeys (*Cercopithecus aethiops*) that had been imported from Uganda. A new virus isolated from the tissues of these patients and monkeys was named marburgvirus, now the prototype member of the family *Filoviridae*. Nine years later, two epidemics of hemorrhagic fever with high mortality occurred, one in villages in the rain forest of Zaire (now the Democratic Republic of Congo) and the other in southern Sudan. A virus that was morphologically identical to, but antigenically distinct from, marburgvirus was isolated and named ebolavirus. Later, the viruses from Zaire and Sudan were found to be genetically distinct and are now designated ebolavirus, subtypes Zaire and Sudan. Since 1976, there have been regular epidemics of ebola hemorrhagic fever caused by three genetically distinct viruses [species Zaire, Sudan, and Côte d'Ivoire (Ivory Coast)]. In 1989 and 1990, monkeys imported from the Philippines into a quarantine facility in Reston, Virginia, were infected with another new filovirus species, now called Reston ebolavirus. Infected monkeys at the facility became ill, and many died. Four animal caretakers were infected, but there was no clinically apparent disease. This virus subsequently was identified in monkeys imported from the Philippines into Italy (1992) and Texas (1996). The infection of farmed pigs and their handlers with Reston ebolavirus was reported in the Philippines in 2008.

The member viruses of the family *Filoviridae* are intriguing for several reasons: (1) the viruses, although similar to other members of the order *Mononegavirales* (the viruses comprising the families *Paramyxoviridae*, *Rhabdoviridae*, *Filoviridae*, and *Bornaviridae*) in their genomic organization and mode of replication, are morphologically the most bizarre of all viruses; (2) the viruses have caused large outbreaks and therefore are recognized as having substantial epidemic potential; (3) the viruses cause a most devastating clinical disease in humans and non-human primates, including chimpanzees, gorillas, and macaques, with extremely rapid and florid tissue damage, and with a very high mortality rate; (4) although these infections are clearly zoonotic, much remains to be established regarding their epidemiology, but recent evidence indicates that species of fruit bats may be reservoir hosts of ebola- and marburgviruses. The viruses that cause these diseases are BioSafety Level 4 pathogens; they must be handled in the laboratory under maximum containment conditions to prevent human exposure.

PROPERTIES OF FILOVIRUSES

Classification

All non-segmented negative-sense RNA viruses share several characteristics: (1) a similar genome organization and roughly the same gene order; (2) a virion-associated RNA polymerase (transcriptase); (3) a helical nucleocapsid; (4) transcription of messenger RNAs (mRNAs) by sequential interrupted synthesis from a single promoter; (5) virion maturation via budding of preassembled nucleocapsids from the cellular plasma membrane at sites containing patches of viral glycoprotein spikes (peplomers). These characteristics and conserved ancient domains found in genomic nucleotide sequences support the notion of a common ancestry, as reflected in the establishment of the order *Mononegavirales*. Conserved domains in nucleoprotein and polymerase genes suggest that the family *Filoviridae* is related most closely to the genus *Pneumovirus* in the family *Paramyxoviridae*, rather than to the family *Rhabdoviridae* as might be expected from their similar, helically wound nucleocapsid structures.

Fenner's Veterinary Virology. DOI: 10.1016/B978-0-12-375158-4.00019-5

(A)

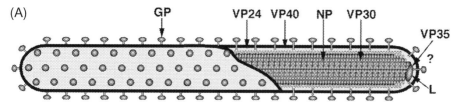

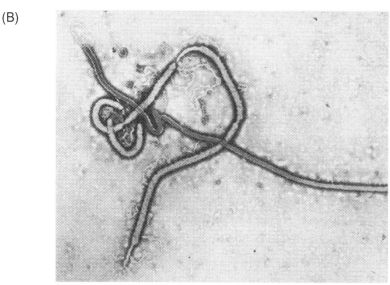

(B)

FIGURE 19.1 (A) Diagram of the cross section of a filovirus virion. GP, glycoprotein; VP40, matrix protein; VP30, polymerase co-factor; NP, nucleoprotein; VP35, phosphoprotein; VP24, membrane-associated protein; L, RNA polymerase. (B) Family *Filoviridae*, genus, *Ebolavirus*. Virions from diagnostic specimen cultured for 2 days in Vero cells. Negative-stain EM.

The family *Filoviridae* contains two genera, *Marburgvirus*, consisting of a single species, and *Ebolavirus*, with four recognized species (Sudan ebolavirus, Zaire ebolavirus, Reston ebolavirus and Côte d'Ivoire ebolavirus), with an additional recently characterized and tentatively named species, Bundibugyo.

Virion Properties

Filovirus virions are markedly pleomorphic, appearing as long, filamentous, sometimes branched forms, or as U-shaped, 6 shaped, or circular forms. Virions have a uniform diameter of 80 nm and vary greatly in length (particles may be up to 14,000 nm long, but have unit nucleocapsid lengths of about 800 nm in the case of marburgvirus and 1000 nm for ebolavirus). Virions are composed of a lipid envelope covered with trimeric glycoprotein spikes, surrounding a helically wound nucleocapsid (50 nm in diameter). They include at least seven proteins, including the RNA-dependent RNA transcriptase/polymerase (L), the surface glycoprotein (GP), the nucleoprotein (NP), the matrix protein (VP40), a phosphoprotein equivalent (VP35), a polymerase co-factor (VP30), and a membrane-associated protein (VP24) (Figure 19.1; Table 19.1). The genome is composed of a single molecule of negative-sense, single-stranded RNA, 19.1 kb in size, the largest of all negative-sense

TABLE 19.1 Properties of Filoviruses

Virions are pleomorphic, appearing as long filamentous forms and other shapes; they have a uniform diameter of 80 nm and vary greatly in length (unit nucleocapsid lengths of about 800 nm for Marburg and 1000 nm for Ebola virus)

Virions are composed of a lipid envelope covered with spikes surrounding a helically wound nucleocapsid

The genome is composed of a single molecule of negative-sense, single-stranded RNA, 19.1 kb in size

Infection is extremely cytopathic in cultured cells and in target organs of host

Cytoplasmic replication, large intracytoplasmic inclusion bodies, budding from the plasma membrane

RNA viruses. The gene order is: *3'-NP-VP35-VP40-GP-VP30-VP24-L-5'* (Figure 19.2). Genes are separated either by intergenic sequences or by overlaps—that is, short (17–20 bases) regions where the transcription start signal of the downstream gene overlaps the transcription stop signal of the upstream gene. Ebolavirus has three overlaps that alternate with intergenic sequences, whereas marburgvirus has a single overlap (Figure 19.2).

The glycoprotein forms homotrimeric surface spikes on virions and is important in binding host cells to initiate

Lake Victoria marburgvirus genome, 19.1 kb

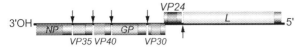

Zaire ebolavirus genome, 18.9 kb

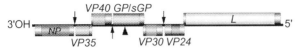

FIGURE 19.2 Genome organization of marburgvirus and ebolavirus. Adjoining genes are either separated from one another by an intergenic region (arrows) or overlap. The editing site of the GP gene of ebolaviruses is indicated by a black triangle. *GP*, glycoprotein; *L*, the RNA polymerase or transcriptase; *NP*, nucleoprotein; *sGP*, secreted glycoprotein; *VP35*, part of the polymerase complex; *VP40*, membrane-associated matrix protein; *VP30*, part of the virus transcription complex; *VP24*, a membrane-associated protein. *[From Virus Taxonomy: Eighth Report of the International Committee on Taxonomy of Viruses (C. M. Fauquet, M. A. Mayo, J. Maniloff, U. Desselberger, L. A. Ball, eds.), p. 647. Copyright © Elsevier (2005), with permission.]*

infection. Ebolaviruses also encode a second glycoprotein that is made in large amounts and is secreted extracellularly (sGP). The expression of secreted glycoprotein and glycoprotein (GP) involves transcriptional RNA editing of the glycoprotein mRNA by the viral polymerase. Expression of the full-length transmembrane-anchored glycoprotein requires the addition of a single non-templated adenosine residue via slippage of the polymerase along the viral genome template during RNA transcription. This additional adenosine residue alters the amino acid codon reading frame, and facilitates expression of the full length glycoprotein, including the hydrophobic transmembrane anchor domain. Without addition of this non-templated adenosine residue, the open reading frame is truncated to express the smaller secreted glycoprotein that is processed by the cell secretory pathway and excreted in high quantity. The role of this soluble glycoprotein in the pathogenesis of ebolavirus disease is unknown, but it may serve as some sort of immune decoy, minimizing the immune response to the virus. The secreted glycoprotein is also immunosuppressive, affecting the host response to infection. Other viral proteins, specifically VP24 and VP35, exert profound immunosuppressive effects through antagonism of the interferon type I response. Virions also contain lipids, their composition reflecting the composition of host-cell membranes, and large amounts of carbohydrates as side chains on the glycoproteins.

Viral infectivity is relatively stable at room temperature, but sensitive to ultraviolet and gamma irradiation, detergents, and common disinfectants.

Virus Replication

Filoviruses replicate well in cell cultures such as Vero (African green monkey kidney) cells. Infection is characterized by rapid cytopathology and large intracytoplasmic inclusion bodies (composed of masses of viral nucleocapsids). Virions enter cells by receptor-mediated endocytosis via clathrin-coated pits. The cell receptor for filoviruses has not definitively been identified, but virus molecules that promote attachment include dendritic cell adhesion molecule 3 and tyrosine kinase family receptors. Actin filaments and cellular microtubules are important in the entry process, as is proteolytic digestion of the viral glycoprotein by endosomal proteases. Virus replication occurs in the cytoplasm of infected cells.

Transcription is initiated at a single promoter site, located at the 3' end of the viral genome. Transcription yields monocistronic mRNAs—that is, separate mRNAs for each protein. This is accomplished by conserved transcriptional stop and start signals that are located at the boundaries of each viral gene. As the viral polymerase moves along the genomic RNA, these signals cause it to pause, and sometimes to fall off the template and terminate transcription (called stuttering or stop/start transcription). The result is that more mRNA is made from genes that are located close to the promoter, and less from downstream genes. This regulates the expression of genes, producing large amounts of structural proteins such as the nucleoprotein and smaller amounts of proteins such as the RNA polymerase. Replication of the genome is mediated by the synthesis of full-length complementary-sense RNA, which then serves as the template for the synthesis of virion-sense RNA. This requires that the stop/start signals needed for transcription be overridden by the viral polymerase—the immediate envelopment of newly formed viral-sense RNA by nucleoprotein seems to mediate this. Maturation of virions occurs via budding of preassembled nucleocapsids from the plasma membrane at sites already containing patches of viral glycoprotein (Table 19.1).

MARBURG AND EBOLA HEMORRHAGIC FEVER VIRUSES

Marburg and ebola viral hemorrhagic fevers are highly lethal and feared zoonotic diseases. The incidence of ebola hemorrhagic fever in West Africa has increased since the mid-1990s, although the basis of this apparent increase in not well understood and might reflect either increased reporting of outbreak events or a genuine increase related to increased exposure of humans and non-human primates to the virus reservoir.

Clinical Features and Epidemiology

Marburgvirus and ebolavirus subtypes Zaire and Sudan cause severe hemorrhagic fever in humans—it has been said that "the evolution of disease often seems inexorable and invariable." Following an incubation period of usually 4–10 days (extreme range 2–21 days for infection by Zaire ebolavirus),

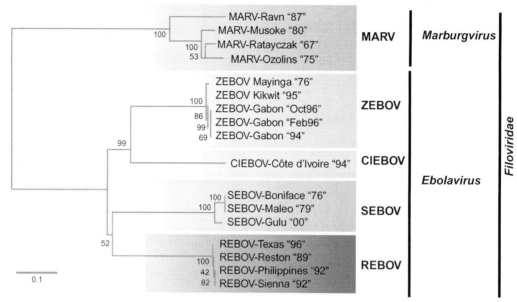

FIGURE 19.3 Phylogenetic tree showing the relationships among the glycoprotein genes of the filoviruses. CIEBOV, Côte d'Ivoire ebolavirus; MARV, Lake Victoria marburgvirus; REBOV, Reston ebolavirus; SEBOV, Sudan ebolavirus; ZEBOV, Zaire ebolavirus. *[From* Virus Taxonomy: Eighth Report of the International Committee on Taxonomy of Viruses *(C. M. Fauquet, M. A. Mayo, J. Maniloff, U. Desselberger, L. A. Ball, eds.), p. 652. Copyright © Elsevier (2005), with permission.]*

there is an abrupt onset of illness, with initial non-specific signs and symptoms including fever, severe frontal headache, malaise, and myalgia. There is a profound leukopenia, bradycardia, and conjunctivitis, and there may be a macropapular rash. Deterioration over the following 2–3 days is marked by pharyngitis, nausea and vomiting, prostration, and bleeding, which is manifested as petechiae, ecchymoses, uncontrolled bleeding from venipuncture sites, and melena. Abortion is a common consequence of infection, and infants born to mothers dying of infection invariably also die. Death usually occurs 6–9 days after the onset of clinical disease (range 1–21 days). The mortality rate has been very high: up to 80% with marburgvirus, 60% with Sudan ebolavirus, and 90% with Zaire ebolavirus. Convalescence is slow, and marked by prostration, weight loss, and often by amnesia for the period of acute illness. Death is usually attributed to hypovolemic shock, sometimes accompanied by disseminated hemorrhage. Human infections with Reston ebolavirus have so far been subclinical.

Non-human primates are, in general, highly susceptible to filovirus infections. Large outbreaks of lethal ebolavirus infection have been reported in wild populations of gorillas (*Gorilla gorilla*) and chimpanzees (genus *Pan*). In rhesus monkeys (*Macaca mulatta*), cynomolgus monkeys (*Macaca fascicularis*), African green monkeys (*Cercopithecus aethiops*), and baboons (*Papio* spp.) inoculated with marburgvirus or Zaire ebolavirus, the incubation period of 4–6 days is followed by an abrupt onset of clinical disease marked by petechiae, ecchymoses, hemorrhagic pharyngitis, hematemesis, melena, and prostration. Infection nearly always ends in death. The pathogenesis of filovirus infections is apparently similar in these non-human primates and humans.

Mice and guinea pigs are not highly susceptible to field isolates of filoviruses, but rodent-adapted strains of the viruses do induce uniformly lethal disease and have been utilized for testing vaccines and therapeutic agents.

The known geographic range of primary filovirus infections is tropical Africa, with the exception of Reston ebolavirus, which occurs in the Philippines. The fact that the ebolavirus subtypes that have caused human disease episodes have been different from each other makes it clear that a common source transmission chain extending across sub-Saharan Africa is not the case—rather, distinct virus subtypes from each site of human disease episodes have been responsible (Figure 19.3). However, genetic analyses of Zaire ebolavirus isolates obtained from human patients suggest that this virus has spread since 1976 from the northern Democratic Republic of Congo/southern Sudan to adjacent regions. Particular attention is now being focused on bats as reservoir hosts of these viruses, because several studies have found antibodies and viral nucleic acid in cave-dwelling fruit bats, suggesting that they may carry these agents.

The source of infection for index cases of ebolavirus and marburgvirus infections is rarely known, although there often has been an association with handling or butchering sick animals, including apes. Outbreaks among humans are propagated by direct contact with infected patients or their contaminated waste, and healthcare workers are at substantial risk of becoming infected. In some settings, particularly among infected monkeys, aerosol transmission of filoviruses appears to occur. Because of the high level of virus in blood, accidental needle sticks from

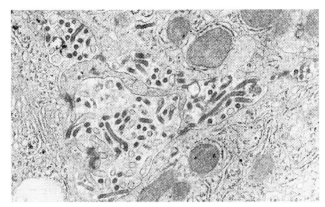

FIGURE 19.4 Liver from a *Cercopithecus aethiops* (African green) monkey inoculated with marburgvirus and killed at day 7 postinfection when clinically ill. This image depicts an area where hepatocytes are still intact; at this site, virions fill the intercellular space as a result of budding from plasma membranes. Thin-section electron microscopy. Magnification ×39,000.

infected patients or animals are very dangerous, and have been responsible for several laboratory-acquired infections.

Pathogenesis and Pathology

In experimentally infected rhesus, cynomolgus, and African green monkeys, filoviruses replicate to high titer in macrophages, dendritic cells, and endothelium. There is often extensive necrosis within target organs, especially the liver, and hemorrhage can be widespread and severe. Virus shedding from infected primates occurs from all body surfaces and orifices, including the skin and mucous membranes, and at sites of bleeding. Of all the hemorrhagic fever agents, filoviruses cause the most severe hemorrhagic manifestations and the most pronounced liver necrosis (the latter perhaps matched only by Rift Valley fever virus infection in target species). There is an early and profound leukopenia, followed by a dramatic neutrophilia with a left shift, and very little inflammatory infiltration in sites of parenchymal necrosis in the liver (Figure 19.4).

Lethal filovirus infections are associated with failures in both innate and adaptive immune responses. Macrophages are a principal site of virus replication and produce a host of pro-inflammatory cytokines that exacerbate systemic disease. Viral proteins VP35 and VP24 function as antagonists of the type I interferon response, an effect that abrogates the host response that would normally limit virus replication. Lymphocytes are not sites of virus replication, but infection is associated with extensive apoptosis of lymphocytes that is reflected in lymphoid depletion and profound peripheral lymphopenia. Additional deficits in mounting an adaptive immune response may result from failure in antigen presentation by infected dendritic cells.

Filovirus infection of macrophages, monocytes, and dendritic cells leads not only to dissemination of virus

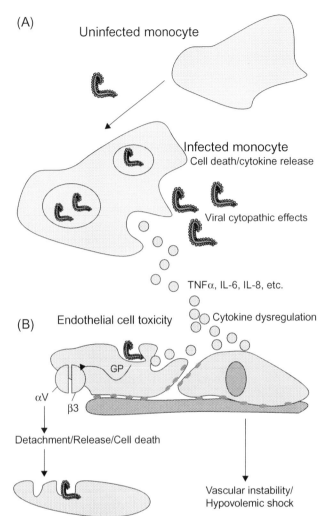

FIGURE 19.5 Host immune responses to ebolavirus and cell damage as a result of direct infection of monocytes and macrophages cause the release of cytokines [tumor necrosis factor α (TNFα), interleukins-6, 8 (IL-6, IL-8)] associated with inflammation and fever (A). Infection of endothelial cells also induces a cytopathic effect and damage to the endothelial barrier that, together with cytokine effects, leads to the loss of vascular integrity (B). Transient expression of ebolavirus glycoprotein (GP) in human umbilical vein endothelial cells or 293T cells causes a reduction of specific integrins (αV, β3; primary molecules responsible for cell adhesion to the extracellular matrix) and immune molecules on the cell surface. Cytokine dysregulation and viral infection may synergize at the endothelial surface, promoting hemorrhage and vasomotor collapse. *[From N. Sullivan, Z. Y. Yang, G. J. Nabel. Ebola virus pathogenesis: implications for vaccines and therapies. J. Virol. **77**, 9733–9737 (2003), with permission.]*

throughout the body, but also to secretion of a variety of inflammatory mediators such as tissue necrosis factor and interleukin-1 that have potentially profound effects on vascular permeability and coagulation. It is these vascular effects that contribute to hypovolemic shock and multi-organ failure in affected individuals (Figure 19.5). Disseminated intravascular coagulation is a common terminal event, which may in part be the result of hepatic necrosis and reduced synthesis of clotting factors.

Diagnosis

Diagnosis of filovirus infections has been based on virus isolation from blood or tissues in cell culture such as Vero (African green monkey kidney) cells, with detection of the presence of virus by immunofluorescence or electron microscopy. Diagnosis also can be based on the direct detection of viral antigen in tissues by immunofluorescence or antigen-capture enzyme-linked immunosorbent assay (ELISA), but reverse transcriptase-polymerase chain reaction (RT-PCR) assays are now routinely used for rapid diagnosis of filovirus infections. Serological diagnostics have been fraught with problems—indirect immunofluorescence suffers from many false positives, especially when used for sero-surveys of filovirus infection rates in captive monkeys. An immunoglobulin M capture ELISA has proven much more reliable than other serological methods, and has become the standard for human and primate serological diagnosis.

Immunity, Prevention, and Control

Considerable effort has been expended in development of filovirus vaccines. Early efforts showed inactivated virus vaccines to be largely ineffective. More recently, a variety of recombinant, vectored vaccines have been developed; for example, a single injection of a vesicular stomatitis virus vector that expresses the ebolavirus glycoprotein protected monkeys from a lethal challenge. Additional impediments to the development of efficacious vaccines include the lack of cross-protection between marburg- and ebolaviruses, and between different species of ebolavirus.

Filovirus disease prevention and control strategies have not been widely adopted in Africa. In contrast, the episodes in the United States and Italy involving Reston ebolavirus have refocused attention on the risk of importation of filoviruses into countries outside enzootic zones in West and Central Africa and the Philippines. Despite export prohibitions established by source countries for conservation purposes, large numbers of wild-caught monkeys are still imported into many countries, primarily for vaccine production and medical research. Today, most importing countries operate import quarantine facilities and adhere to international primate transport and import standards. These standards include testing for the presence of filoviruses, and protocols to prevent infection in primate facility workers. Similarly, guidelines are in place to minimize risk in caring for patients with filovirus hemorrhagic fever in hospitals in non-enzootic areas.

Bornaviridae

Chapter Contents

Borna disease is named for the town of Borna in Saxony, Germany, where, since around 1895 at least, devastating epizootics of a naturally occurring, infectious, usually fatal, neurological disease of horses and occasionally sheep have occurred. The viral etiology of the disease was established as early as 1925. Outbreaks of Borna disease sporadically have been described in horses in several European countries, notably Germany, Switzerland, and Austria. Cases of an apparently similar meningoencephalitis syndrome have been described amongst horses in North Africa and the Near East, but there is significant controversy as to whether or not Borna disease occurs outside Europe. Serological studies suggest that the causative virus, or its close relatives, has a very wide, perhaps worldwide, distribution. In addition to horses and sheep, cattle, goats, mules, donkeys, rabbits, cats, and South American camelids (llamas) have been described as having the infection, and there are unproven suggestions that infection of humans with Borna disease virus may be linked to specific neuropsychiatric illnesses. Genetically distinct strains of Borna disease virus have been incriminated recently as the cause of proventricular dilatation syndrome, a progressive and often fatal disorder of psittacine birds in particular.

PROPERTIES OF BORNA DISEASE VIRUS

Classification

Borna disease virus is the sole member of the genus *Bornavirus*, family *Bornaviridae*, order *Mononegavirales*. Strains of Borna disease virus segregate into at least two genetic types, based on sequence analysis, and related but genetically novel strains of the virus identified in birds with proventricular dilatation syndrome have been provisionally designated as avian bornaviruses.

Virion Properties

Borna disease virus virions are spherical, enveloped, about 90 nm in diameter and contain a core that is about 50–60 nm in diameter (Figure 20.1). The genome is a single molecule of negative-sense, single-stranded RNA, approximately 8.9 kb in size that encodes at least six different proteins (Figure 20.2). The major virion proteins include a matrix protein (M), glycoprotein (G), and nucleoprotein (N). The G protein expresses neutralization determinants of the virus. The remaining proteins are non-structural, and include the polymerase co-factor (P), the RNA-dependent RNA polymerase (L), and a small polypeptide (X) that is abundantly expressed in infected cells but absent in virus particles. The virus is sensitive to heat, acid, lipid solvents, and usual disinfectants (Table 20.1).

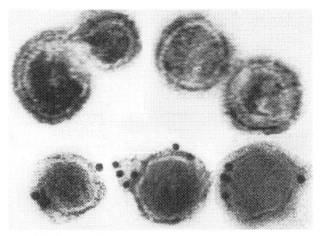

FIGURE 20.1 Family *Bornaviridae*, genus *Bornavirus*, Borna disease virus virions. Negative stain, immunogold label; because virions are so nondescript, specific antibody conjugated to gold microspheres was used to identify them. *(Courtesy of H. Ludwig.)*

Fenner's Veterinary Virology. DOI: 10.1016/B978-0-12-375158-4.00020-1

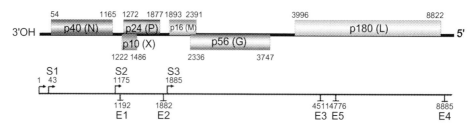

FIGURE 20.2   Genomic organization and transcriptional map of Borna disease virus. Open reading frames (ORFs) are represented by boxes in the top figure. The location of transcription initiation and transcription termination sites are indicated by S and E respectively. Numbers represent nucleotide positions on the genome. G(p56), glycoprotein; L, RNA polymerase; M(p16), matrix protein; N(p40), nucleoprotein; P(p24), phosphoprotein; X(p10), non-structural protein *[From* Virus Taxonomy: Eighth Report of the International Committee on Taxonomy of Viruses *(C. M. Fauquet, M. A. Mayo, J. Maniloff, U. Desselberger, L. A. Ball, eds.), p. 617. Copyright © Elsevier (2005), with permission.]*

TABLE 20.1   Properties of Borna Disease Virus

Virions are approximately 90 nm in diameter, enveloped with an inner core, 50–60 nm in diameter

The genome is a single molecule of negative-sense, single-stranded RNA, 8.9 kb in size

The genome has six main open reading frames encoding at least six proteins, including a glycoprotein and an RNA-dependent RNA polymerase

Virus transcription and replication take place in the nucleus

Infection in cell culture characteristically produces intranuclear inclusion bodies, and persistent infection of neurons is characteristic of infections of animals

Virus Replication

A broad range of cell types can be infected with Borna disease virus, including neurons and glial cells derived from several animal species. The viral G protein mediates attachment, and the virus enters susceptible cells via receptor-mediated endocytosis. The cellular receptor is uncharacterized. The virus uses a non-cytolytic replication strategy that results in virus persistence in cultured cells and infected animals. Borna disease virus differs from other members of the order *Mononegavirales* in that both transcription and replication occur in the host-cell nucleus.

Borna disease virus is also unusual in its transcriptional strategy (Figure 20.2). Three transcription initiation and four, possibly five, transcription termination signals have been identified in the viral genome and these differ from other negative-stranded viruses in the configuration of their initiation and termination signals, their intergenic regions, and overlaps at gene boundaries. The genome is transcribed into six primary transcripts, two of which are modified post-transcriptionally by cellular RNA splicing machinery to yield additional mRNA species. All mRNA species in cells infected with Borna disease virus are polycistronic, except that encoding the N protein. Several forms

of some Borna disease virus proteins are generated during replication, including two isoforms of the N protein and three of the G protein, including a full-length glycoprotein (GP-84/94) and two smaller glycoproteins that represent the N (GP-N) and C (GP-C) terminal subunits. Both GP-C and GP-N are present in infectious particles.

The N, P, and L proteins form the viral polymerase complex. They are all expressed in both the cytoplasm and the nucleus of infected cells. Only low numbers of infected cells express the G protein, in contrast to those expressing N and P, and expression of G protein is restricted to the endoplasmic reticulum and nuclear envelope. The M protein mediates particle assembly within the cytoplasm of infected cells.

BORNA DISEASE VIRUS

Clinical Features and Epidemiology

Natural infection with Borna virus has been described predominantly in horses and sheep in areas of central Europe, but cases have also been reported in other species. Experimentally, the host range is wide, from chickens to primates. For many years, Borna disease was considered sporadically enzootic only in certain areas of central Europe. However, seroepidemiologic investigations have shown that infection in horses is much more widespread. Antibodies have been found in approximately 12% of healthy horses in Germany, and a greater prevalence is found in enzootic areas and in stables with affected horses. Antibodies have also been found in horses in Asia, Australia, the Middle East, and the United States, although true Borna disease has not been unambiguously identified outside central Europe. The great majority of infections are clinically inapparent, and incidence of disease typically is low, even in enzootic areas.

The route of natural Borna disease virus infection of horses is uncertain, although oronasal transmission has been proposed on the basis of results from experimental infections of laboratory animals. The incubation period is highly variable, ranging from weeks to months, and the course of clinical Borna disease can be acute or protracted. Mortality is high in horses that develop neurological manifestations, whereas mildly affected animals may recover despite persistent infection within their nervous tissues. Affected horses may initially present with fever and behavioral changes that become increasingly worse, including depression, altered eating behavior, and head pressing. More advanced cases are characterized by profound neurological disturbances, including proprioceptive deficits and abnormal stance, and dysfunction of individual cranial nerves because of involvement of their respective nuclei. Early neurological signs are mainly attributable to dysfunctions in the limbic system, whereas, during later stages of the disease, dysfunctions of motor systems causing paralysis predominate. Ophthalmologic disorders including nystagmus, pupillary reflex dysfunction, and blindness may occur in advanced stages. The course of the disease is 3–20 days and usually ends in death; surviving horses usually have permanent sensory and/or motor deficits.

It remains uncertain whether or not Borna disease virus is a zoonotic pathogen. Serological and molecular virological investigations indicate that humans are infected with Borna disease virus, and—in several countries—specific antibodies or viral RNA have been identified in a substantial proportion of patients with behavioral or neuropsychiatric disorders. However, similar infections also have been identified in apparently normal human individuals.

There is compelling evidence that small mammals are the natural reservoir host of Borna virus, and the virus has been detected in the tissues of white-toothed shrews (*Crocidura leucodon*) in areas of Switzerland where Borna disease is enzootic.

Pathogenesis and Pathology

The most thoroughly investigated experimental model infection of Borna disease virus infection is in the rat. The intranasal route appears most likely to be responsible for natural infections, with virus passing intra-axonally to the olfactory bulbs of the brain from olfactory nerve endings. The virus then disseminates throughout the central nervous system. In rats, and perhaps other animals, there are substantial differences in pathogenesis, depending on when infection is initiated. Infection of newborn rats results in a persistent infection of the central nervous system as well as peripheral organs, but with minimal tissue injury or neurologic changes. In contrast, infection of adult rats of certain strains leads to severe lesions in the central nervous system, and marked behavioral changes. The virus replicates in both neurons and glial cells, and persistent infection of neurons is characteristic of Borna disease virus infection.

Infection does not elicit a protective immune response; rather, infection stimulates a cellular reaction that contributes to disease progression. Experimentally, whereas infection of adult immunocompetent animals regularly results

in disease, infection of neonatal or immunocompromised animals leads neither to encephalitis nor to disease, despite the persistence of the virus. Antibodies apparently do not contribute to disease pathogenesis; they lack neutralizing capacity, and adoptive transfer of immunoglobulins from infected animals to immunocompromised recipients does not induce pathological changes or disease.

Infection with Borna disease virus in horses and sheep induces a severe encephalomyelitis that principally affects the gray matter (polioencephalomyelitis); histologically, there typically is extensive perivascular cuffing with lymphocytes, macrophages, and plasma cells. Neuronal necrosis is not a feature, but distinctive eosinophilic intranuclear inclusions in neurons, called "Joest-Degen" bodies, are characteristic, even pathognomonic of Borna disease, although they cannot be demonstrated in all cases. Lesions are especially prominent in the gray matter of the olfactory bulb, basal cortex, caudate nucleus, and hippocampus. The retina typically also is involved in experimentally infected laboratory animals.

Diagnosis

Pre-mortem diagnosis of Borna disease is difficult, because several diseases can induce similar clinical signs in horses, including rabies, tetanus, equine herpesvirus 1 induced encephalomyelitis, protozoal encephalomyelitis, West Nile disease, and the equine alphavirus encephalitides. Diagnosis is usually confirmed by the demonstration of antibodies in the serum or, preferably, in the cerebrospinal fluid. This is performed routinely by indirect immunofluorescence, where persistently infected Madin–Darby canine kidney cells are used as substrate. Alternative serological tests include western immunoblotting and enzyme-linked immunosorbent assay.

Other methods are also used in reference laboratories. Virus isolation in sensitive cultured cells can be used to confirm infection. The presence of virus is usually detected by direct immunofluorescence. Enzyme immunoassay methods are sensitive and reliable if purified antigen is used and monoclonal antibodies are used for antigen capture. The reverse transcriptase-polymerase chain reaction (RT-PCR) has become a valuable tool for diagnosis—viral RNA may be detected in conjunctival or nasal secretions or saliva, and is more consistently detected in cerebrospinal fluid of affected horses than in their peripheral blood mononuclear cells. Post-mortem diagnosis relies on immunohistochemistry to demonstrate viral antigen in sections of brain with typical histologic lesions. The diagnosis then may be confirmed by virus isolation.

Immunity, Prevention, and Control

Although antiviral treatments have shown some promise in experimental studies, there currently is no specific treatment for animals with Borna disease. Similarly, although a number of inactivated, attenuated, and recombinant vaccines have been developed and tested to prevent Borna disease, none is commercially available.

Essential steps in the control of the disease are the identification and quarantine of carrier animals. The epidemiology of Borna disease virus infection also is poorly defined, including the mechanism of transmission of virus to horses and other animals from its reservoir in small mammals.

AVIAN BORNAVIRUS

Genetically distinct strains of Borna disease virus, provisionally designated as avian bornaviruses, recently have been implicated as the cause of proventricular dilatation disease, a devastating syndrome that affects many species of psittacine birds worldwide, including highly endangered species such as Spix's macaw (*Cyanopsitta spixii*). The virus has also been detected in canaries (*Serinus canaria*), a non-psittacine species. This disease was first recognized in the 1970s among macaws exported from Bolivia, and continues to cause incidents and outbreaks of disease in captive and free-living birds. The identification of bornavirus in these cases was achieved using microarray techniques that detected bornavirus RNA in infected tissue samples followed by full genomic sequence analyses of the virus that was detected. Proventricular dilatation disease recently was experimentally reproduced in cockatiels inoculated with avian bornavirus.

Affected birds present with signs of progressive neurological and/or gastrointestinal tract dysfunction, including weight loss, dysphagia, regurgitation, ataxia, and proprioceptive deficits. The disease is characterized by mononuclear (lymphocyte and plasma cell) inflammation within both the central and peripheral nervous systems. Involvement of the gastrointestinal autonomic nervous system is responsible for signs of gastrointestinal dysfunction, including paralytic dilatation of the esophagus and proventriculus. Bornavirus antigen can be detected within

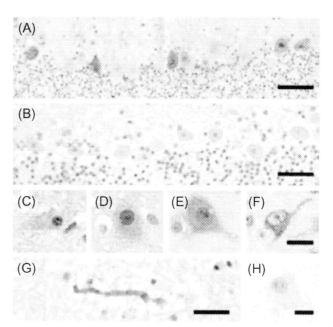

FIGURE 20.3 Avian bornavirus protein demonstrated by immunohistochemical testing in the central nervous system of birds with proventricular dilatation disease (PDD). (A) Within nuclei, cytoplasm, and dendrites of several Purkinje cells of the cerebellum; bar represents 50 μm. (B) Negative control: no immunoreactivity of Purkinje cells in a PDD-negative bird; bar represents 50 μm. (C–F) Different phenotypes of virus-positive neurons (bars represent 12.5 μm): (C) within neurons, viral protein expressed within intranuclear inclusion bodies; (D) diffusely within the nucleus, accompanied by faint cytoplasmic staining; (E) within both the nucleus and the cytoplasm, with more intense staining of intranuclear inclusion bodies; (F) exclusively within the cytoplasm, with the nucleus spared. (G) Within an axon in the white matter of the medulla oblongata; bar represents 25 μm. (H) Negative control: no immunoreactivity of a cerebral neuron in a PDD-negative bird; bar represents 12.5 μm. [*From H. Weissenböck, T. Bakonyi, K. Sekulin, F. Ehrensperger, R. J. T. Doneley, R. Dürrwald, R. Hoop, K. Erdélyi, J. Gál, J. Kolodziejek, N. Nowotny. Avian bornaviruses in psittacine birds from Europe and Australia with proventricular dilatation disease. Emerg. Infect. Dis. 15: 15. 1543–1549 (2009), with permission.*]

the nuclei of neurons of the central and peripheral nervous tissues of affected birds by immunohistochemical staining (Figure 20.3), and viral nucleic acid can be detected using virus-specific RT-PCR assay.

Orthomyxoviridae

Chapter Contents

The family *Orthomyxoviridae* includes viruses with genomes composed of several (six to eight) segments of single-stranded RNA. The most important members of the family are the influenza viruses, which are included in three genera (*Influenzavirus A, B,* and *C*). Influenza viruses that are pathogenic to domestic animals are included in the genus *Influenzavirus A*, whereas viruses in the two other genera (*B* and *C*) circulate continuously in humans. Influenza A viruses infrequently are transmitted from their animal hosts to humans, but human epidemics and pandemics caused by influenza A viruses typically have no animal involvement beyond the initial incursion. Continuing surveillance, therefore, is essential to identify and detect influenza A virus variants that are capable of infecting humans while they are still confined either to their animal host or to a limited number of human contacts.

Recent developments have advanced significantly the understanding of the biology of influenza viruses. First, the availability of rapid sequencing techniques has confirmed extensive genomic rearrangements between different influenza viruses. Secondly, the emergence of the highly pathogenic Eurasian–African H5N1 virus in southeast Asia in 1997 led to a worldwide surveillance program to track this virus because of its virulence to humans, but this surveillance activity also has identified other influenza viruses in many animal species. Lastly, the availability of a sensitive

and specific reverse-transcriptase-polymerase chain reaction (RT-PCR) assay that detects all influenza viruses has facilitated detailed surveillance without the need for virus isolation. Once a sample is identified as positive with this assay, the infecting virus rapidly can be further characterized by gene-specific RT-PCR assays to determine its hemagglutinin/neuraminidase subtype.

Although the original isolation of an influenza virus did not occur until 1930 (from swine), associated diseases previously had been recognized in both animals and humans. Indeed, human influenza was described by Hippocrates some 2400 years ago. Human pandemics have occurred throughout history, and the "Spanish flu" pandemic of 1918 was especially dramatic. The causative agent of fowl plague was recognized in the late 19th century as a filterable agent (i.e., virus), but was not determined to be caused by influenza virus until 1955. Fowl plague virus [i.e., high-pathogenicity avian influenza (HPAI) virus] was first isolated from wild birds in 1961—specifically, common terns (*Sterna hirundo*) in South Africa—but this highly lethal virus has since been rarely detected in wild birds. Low-pathogenicity avian influenza (LPAI) virus was first isolated from wild birds in 1972, and such low-virulence viruses are common in some species of wild birds. Aquatic birds (orders *Anseriformes* and *Charadriiformes*), especially ducks,

Fenner's Veterinary Virology. DOI: 10.1016/B978-0-12-375158-4.00021-3

TABLE 21.1 Distribution of Hemagglutinin (HA) Subtypes Between Different Birds (Class *Aves*) and Mammals (Class *Mammalia*)

HA Subtype	Host of Origin					
	Mammalia			Aves		
	Humans	Swine	Equines	Anserifonnes (e.g., Dabbling Ducks)	Charadriiformes and Procellariiformes (e.g., Shorebirds, Gulls, Seabirds)	Gallifonnes (Domestic Poultry)
H1	+	++		+	+	++[c]
H2	(++)[a]			+	+	+
H3	++	++	++	++	++	++[c]
H4		±		++	+	+
H5	±	±		+	+	++[b]
H6				++	+	+
H7	±	±	(++)[a]	+	+	++[b]
H8				±		±
H9	±	±		+	++	++
H10				+	+	+
H11				+	++	+
H12				+	+	±
H13				+	++	+
H14[c]				±		
H15[c]				±	±	
H16[c]					+	

±, sporadic; +, several reports; ++, most common.
[a]Previously common but now not reported.
[b]Both low-pathogenicity and high-pathogenicity viruses.
[c]Primarily swine influenza virus infections of domestic turkeys.
[From Avian Influenza (D. E. Swayne, ed.), p. 63. Copyright © John Wiley & Sons (2008), with permission.]

shorebirds, and gulls, are the essential reservoir hosts of low-pathogenicity influenza A viruses (Table 21.1). Influenza viruses replicate in the intestinal epithelium of these birds without producing overt disease, and are excreted in high concentrations in feces. The viruses efficiently are transmitted by the fecal–oral route, and migrating aquatic birds carry viruses between their summer and winter habitats, which may span continents. Feeding stops during the migrations provide further opportunity for spread of the viruses to contact populations, and facilitate the continuing process of evolution of these viruses.

Cross-species infections occur sporadically between birds and mammals, including swine, horses, mink, marine mammals, and humans (Figure 21.1). Incursions of influenza A virus from wild birds into domestic poultry occur much more frequently, but until recently most of these

events went undetected as the consequences were limited. There have been only a very limited number of outbreaks of influenza A virus infections in domestic poultry worldwide that resulted in high death losses or regulatory action to suppress the infection, such as the recent epizootic of Eurasian H5N1 virus infection. Domestic swine are considered an important intermediate ("bridge") host in those areas of the world where there is frequent contact between birds and swine, although the premise that swine are an essential intermediate host for the development of pandemic influenza virus strains has not been substantiated with the avian Eurasian–African H5N1 virus. Similarly, studies with the 1918 pandemic "Spanish flu" strain of influenza that was recovered by molecular means also do not show a linkage between this virus and swine influenza viruses.

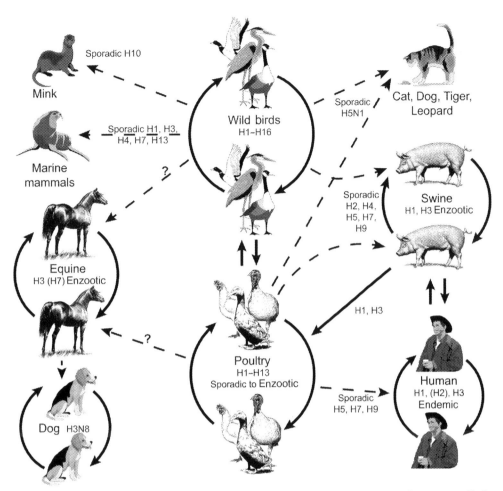

FIGURE 21.1 Interspecies transmission of influenza A viruses. Diagrammatic representation of the source and movement of influenza A viruses or their genes within avian and mammalian ecological and epidemiological situations. H, hemagglutinin subtype; those in ( ) were previously common but no longer are in circulation. *[From* Avian Influenza *(D. E. Swayne, ed.), p. 62. Copyright © John Wiley & Sons (2008), with permission.]*

Whole-genome sequencing of influenza viruses is now used for phylogenetic analyses, although the results vary, depending on which of the eight viral gene segments are compared. For instance, comparison of the hemagglutinin (*HA*) and neuraminidase (*NA*) genes shows no host-specific lineages because of gene reassortment. In contrast, analyses of the matrix protein gene (*M*) of field strains of influenza A virus show two major avian lineages (North American and Eurasian), two equine lineages, two gull lineages (North American and European), two swine lineages (North American and Eurasian) and a human lineage. Analysis of the *PB1* gene segregates human viruses between the North American swine and Eurasian avian groups. Predictably, there are exceptions such as an outbreak of equine influenza in China in 1989 that was caused by an H3N8 virus from a contemporary Eurasian avian source, whereas the classical H3N8 equine lineage has its origin from a North American avian lineage virus. Influenza A viruses from wild birds are very diverse, representing the entire breadth of the gene pool, and were believed at one time to be in evolutionary stasis. However, this dogma has been disputed as additional influenza viruses have been isolated from wild birds and sequenced, because there are continuing changes in all gene segments, with accumulation of amino acid changes, not only in mammalian (e.g., equine) and domestic poultry viruses, but also in viruses from wild birds. Similarly, changes also continue to accumulate in the Eurasian–African H5N1 viruses, perhaps as a result of circulation in a variety of wild and domestic birds, including species such as passerine birds that are not usually infected with influenza virus.

With renewed appreciation of the natural history of influenza viruses as "species jumpers," prevention efforts logically will continue to focus on those situations in which birds and mammals are maintained in close proximity and in which there are rapid changes in populations, such as live-animal markets that bring together a wide variety of birds such as chickens, ducks, turkeys, pheasants, guinea fowl, and chukars without proper movement controls, and with poor sanitation and housing. Surveillance also is required to enable rapid identification of the emergence of reassortant viruses. Although changes in agricultural practices that separate swine and domestic poultry production from aquatic birds can interrupt the evolutionary progression of some newly emergent influenza virus variants, such approaches are often difficult to enforce, and the potential threat of epidemics of human influenza that emerge from avian or mammalian reservoirs will persist.

The need for intensive surveillance for the emergence of novel influenza viruses was demonstrated dramatically in April 2009, with the appearance of a new pandemic strain of influenza A virus in Mexico. Instead of the widely anticipated emergence of a new pandemic virus based on the highly pathogenic Eurasian–African H5N1 influenza virus, this newly emergent virus had its origin in triple reassortant swine viruses (H1N1, H3N2, H1N2) that had been circulating in pigs in North America since the late 1990s. The novel feature of this new virus was an additional reassortment that replaced two gene segments (*NA* and *M*) of the North American swine virus with the respective segments of the Eurasian swine virus. The origin and the date of development of this novel H1N1 virus have not been definitively established, as the first indication of its existence was from human infections. Initial investigations were unable to detect the novel H1N1 infection in swine in the absence of contact with infected workers. This recent event further emphasizes the unpredictable evolution and emergence of influenza virus as a mammalian pathogen.

PROPERTIES OF ORTHOMYXOVIRUSES

Classification

The family *Orthomyxoviridae* comprises the genera *Influenzavirus A*, *Influenzavirus B*, *Influenzavirus C*, *Thogotovirus*, and *Isavirus*. The name of the family is derived from the Greek *myxa*, meaning mucus, and *orthos*, meaning correct or right. The name was intended to distinguish the orthomyxoviruses from the paramyxoviruses. *Influenza* is the Italian form of Latin, from *influentia*, "influence," so used because epidemics were believed to be caused by astrological or other occult influences. Influenza A viruses are common pathogens of horses, swine, humans, and domestic poultry throughout much of the world, but they also are the cause of sporadic or geographically limited infections and disease in mink, seals, whales, and dogs. Influenza B viruses are pathogens of humans, but there are two reports of influenza B virus infection in seals. Influenza C viruses infect humans and swine, and reassortants have been detected, but influenza C viruses rarely cause serious disease in either species. The thogotoviruses are tick-borne viruses that infect livestock and humans in Africa, Europe, and Asia, but their pathogenic significance remains conjectural. The sole member of the genus *Isavirus* is infectious salmon anemia virus, a highly fatal disease of marine-farmed Atlantic salmon.

A classification system was developed for influenza viruses because of the practical need to assess the risk represented by the emergence of new variant viruses, and

the need to determine herd or population immunity against previously circulating strains so that vaccine requirements can be assessed. The emergence of variant viruses depends not only on *genetic drift*—that is, point mutations (nucleotide substitutions, insertions, deletions), but also on *genetic shift*—that is, genomic segment reassortment. Previously, drift and shift in only the viral hemagglutinin and the neuraminidase were intensively monitored, but, with the advent of enhanced sequencing technology, other viral genes may assume more importance in assessing risk. In the current classification system, influenza A viruses are categorized into 16 hemagglutinin (H) and 9 neuraminidase (N) types. In naming virus strains, influenza virus species or type (A, B, or C), host (swine, horses, chicken, turkey, mallard, etc.), geographic origin, strain number, year of isolation and hemagglutinin and neuraminidase subtypes are included. The host of origin is not specified in viruses isolated from humans. Thus the full identification of an influenza virus looks like a secret code but is precise and informative. Examples of virus strain names include: A/equine/Miami/1/1963 (H3N8), the prototypic equine influenza virus 2; A/swine/Iowa/15/1930 (H1N1), the prototypic strain of swine influenza virus; A/Hong Kong/1/1968 (H3N2), the virus that caused the human pandemic of 1968; A/chicken/Scotland/1959 (H5N1), the first high-pathogenicity avian influenza virus of the H5 subtype.

Changes recently have been implemented in the nomenclature for Eurasian–African H5N1, and for other influenza A viruses as appropriate, because the linking of the isolates to a specific geographic location increasingly was confusing and uninformative. A numerical *clade* system has been adopted to better relate the evolutionary changes in these related H5N1 isolates over time; a *clade* is a taxonomic group comprising a single common ancestor and all descendants of that ancestor. For the Eurasian–African H5N1 virus, the reference isolate is A/Goose/Guangdong/1/1996 (H5N1). The initial outbreak viruses from Hong Kong from 1997 were included in a single clade with the prototype virus, based on the hemagglutinin sequence. However, since 2003 the viruses have spread to progressively more regions beyond China and have evolved into several independent but related clades. By 2008, 10 distinct genetic clades were recognized (0–9), and genetic diversity within individual clades that have several subclades have been recognized (2.1.3, 2.1.1, etc.) (Figure 21.2). This clade nomenclature system readily identifies the genetic linkage of the virus regardless of the geographic location, source of the isolate, or year of the isolate. The strain nomenclature system will continue to be maintained in repositories and be used to identify sequences deposited into databases such as GenBank.

Although any gene constellation and any combination of *HA* and *NA* genes can arise by genetic reassortment, only a limited range of combinations are recognized as important and naturally occurring subtypes responsible for animal infections: (1) enzootic H7N7 and H3N8 viruses (previously designated equine influenza viruses 1 and 2) that cause respiratory disease in horses; (2) enzootic H1N1, H1N2,

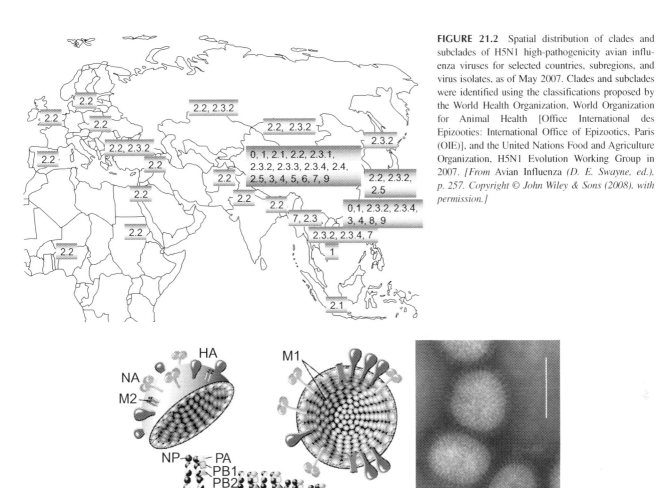

FIGURE 21.2 Spatial distribution of clades and subclades of H5N1 high-pathogenicity avian influenza viruses for selected countries, subregions, and virus isolates, as of May 2007. Clades and subclades were identified using the classifications proposed by the World Health Organization, World Organization for Animal Health [Office International des Epizooties: International Office of Epizootics, Paris (OIE)], and the United Nations Food and Agriculture Organization, H5N1 Evolution Working Group in 2007. [*From* Avian Influenza *(D. E. Swayne, ed.), p. 257. Copyright © John Wiley & Sons (2008), with permission.*]

FIGURE 21.3 (Left) Diagram of an influenza A virus virion in section. The indicated glycoproteins embedded in the lipid membrane are the trimeric hemagglutinin (HA), which predominates, and the tetrameric neuraminidase (NA). The enelope also contains a small number of M2 membrane ion channel proteins. The internal components are the M1 membrane (matrix) protein and the viral ribonucleoprotein (RNP) consisting of RNA segments, associated nucleocapsid protein (NP), and the PA, PB1, and PB2 polymerase proteins. (Right) negative contrast electron micrograph of particles of influenza A virus (*Courtesy of N. Takeshi*). The bar represents 100 nm. [*From* Virus Taxonomy: Eighth Report of the International Committee on Taxonomy of Viruses *(C. M. Fauquet, M. A. Mayo, J. Maniloff, U. Desselberger, L. A. Ball, eds.), p. 681. Copyright © Elsevier (2005), with permission.*]

and H3N2 viruses that cause influenza in swine; (3) sporadic H7N7 and H4N5 viruses that cause respiratory and systemic disease in seals; (4) sporadic H10N4 viruses that cause respiratory disease in mink; (5) historically endemic H1N1, H2N2, H3N2, and more recently sporadic or limited H5N1, H7N3, H7N7, and H9N2 viruses that cause respiratory disease in humans; (6) geographically restricted H3N8 and H3N2 viruses that cause respiratory disease in dogs; (7) nearly all genetic combinations occur in wild aquatic birds, but particular emphasis is placed on detection of H5 and H7 viruses in domestic poultry because they can be associated with the high-pathogenicity phenotype.

Virion Properties

Orthomyxovirus virions are pleomorphic, often spherical but sometimes filamentous, and 80–120 nm in their smallest dimension (Figure 21.3). They consist of a lipid envelope with large spikes surrounding eight (genera *Influenzavirus A*, *Influenzavirus B*, and *Isavirus*), seven (genus *Influenzavirus C*), or six (genus *Thogotovirus*) helically symmetrical nucleocapsid segments of different sizes (Table 21.2). For influenza A and B viruses, there are two kinds of glycoprotein spikes: homotrimers of the hemagglutinin protein and homotetramers of the neuraminidase protein. Influenza C viruses lack neuraminidase, and have only one type of glycoprotein spike that consists of multifunctional hemagglutinin-esterase molecules. Infectious salmon anemia virus (genus *Isavirus*) also has a hemagglutinin-esterase and an F protein. Regardless of the configurations, at least three functions are linked to the surface proteins: receptor binding, receptor cleavage, and membrane fusion. Virion envelopes are lined by the matrix protein, M1. on the inner surface of the lipid bilayer and are spanned by a small number of ion channels composed of tetramers of a second matrix protein, M2. Genomic segments consist of a molecule of viral RNA enclosed within a capsid composed of helically arranged nucleoprotein. Three proteins that make up the viral RNA polymerase complex (PB1, PB2, and PA) are associated with

---

TABLE 21.2　Properties of Influenza Virus

Five genera: *Influenzavirus A, Influenzavirus B, Influenzavirus C, Thogotovirus,* and *Isavirus*

Virions are pleomorphic, spherical, or filamentous, 80–120 nm in diameter, and consist of an envelope with large spikes surrounding six to eight helically symmetrical nucleocapsid segments of different sizes

The genome consists of linear negative-sense, single-stranded RNA, divided into six to eight segments, 10–14.6 kb in overall size

There are two kinds of spikes (influenza A & B virus); rod shaped, consisting of homotrimers of the hemagglutinin glycoprotein, and mushroom shaped, consisting of homotetramers of the neuraminidase protein

Transcription and RNA replication occur in the nucleus; capped 5′ termini of cellular RNAs are cannibalized as primers for mRNA transcription; budding takes place on the plasma membrane

Defective interfering particles and genetic reassortment occur frequently

---

the genomic RNA and nucleoprotein. The genome consists of six to eight segments of linear negative-sense, single-stranded RNA, and is 10–14.6 kb in overall size. The genome segments have non-translated regulatory sequences at both the 5′ and 3′ ends. The 13 nucleotides at the terminal 5′ end and 12 at the 3′ end are identical for each of the genomic segments and show partial inverted complementarity. This feature is essential for RNA synthesis.

Because of their lipid envelope, influenza viruses are sensitive to heat (56°C, 30 minutes), acid (pH 3), and lipid solvents, and are thus very labile under ordinary environmental conditions. However, infectious influenza A virus has been recovered after 30 days in cold lake water.

Virus Replication

Influenza virions attach to cells via the binding of their activated hemagglutinin to sialic-acid-containing receptors on the plasma membrane as depicted and described for influenza A virus (Figure 21.4). Different cells have different linkages of *N*-acetyl neuraminic acid (sialic acid) to a galactose residue, and the hemagglutinin recognizes these different linkages, which in turn determine the host range of the virus. The gut epithelium of ducks has a receptor with an α2,3 linkage (SAα2,3Gal), whereas the predominant influenza virus receptor in the upper respiratory tract of humans is an α2,6 linkage (SAα2,6Gal). There is also evidence that

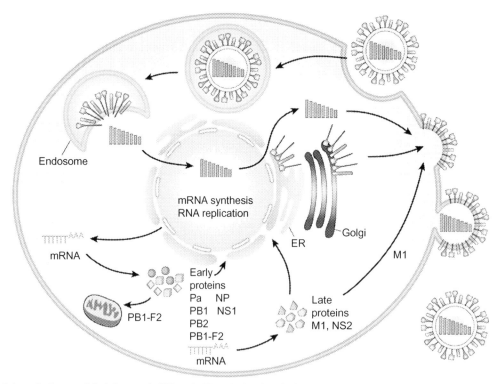

FIGURE 21.4　Schematic diagram of the influenza viral life cycle. ER, endoplasmic reticulum; M1, M2, matrix proteins; mRNA, messenger RNA; NP, nucleoprotein; NS1, NS2, non-structural proteins 1, 2; Pa, PB1, PB2, proteins of the viral RNA polymerase complex; PB1-F2, non-essential strain-dependent protein linked to virulence. *[From G. Neumann, T. Noda, Y. Kawaoka. Emergence and pandemic potential of swine-origin H1N1 influenza virus. Nature **459**, 931–939 (2009), with permission.]*

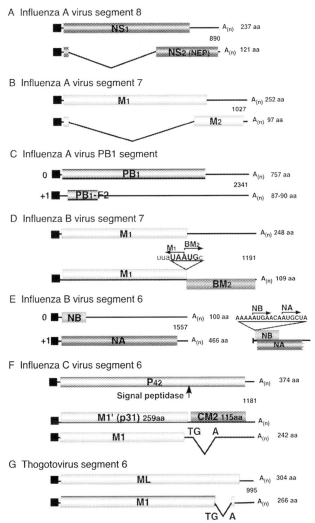

FIGURE 21.5 Orthomyxovirus genome organization. The genomic organization and open reading frames (ORFs) are shown for genes that encode multiple proteins. Segments encoding the polymerase, hemagglutinin, and nucleoprotein genes are not depicted as each encodes a single protein. (A) Inflenza A virus segment 8 showing NS1 and NS2 (NEP) mRNAs and their coding regions. NS1 and NS2 (NEP) share 10 amino-terminal residues, including the initiating methionine. The ORF of NS2 (NEP) mRNA (nt 529–861) differs from that of NS1. (B) Influenza A virus segment 7 showng M1 and M2 mRNAs and their coding regions. M1 and M2 share 9 amino-terminal residues, including the initiating methionine; however, the ORF of M2 mRNA (nt 740–1004) differs from that of M1. A Peptide that could be translated from mRNA3 has not been found *in vivo*. (C) Influenza A virus PB1 segment ORFs. Initiation of PB1 translation is thought to be relatively inefficient based on Kozak's rule, likely allowing initiation of PB1-F2 translation by ribosomal scanning. (D) Influenza B virus RNA segment 7 ORFs and the organization of the ORFs used to translate the M1 and BM2 proteins. A stop-start pentanucleotide, thought to couple translation between the two ORFs, is illustrated. (E) ORFs in Influenza B virus RNA segment 6, illustrating the overlapping reading frames of NB and NA. Nucleotide sequence surrounding the 2 AUG initiation codons, in the mRNA sense, is shown. Dark lines at the 5′- and 3′-termini of the mRNAs represent untranslated regions. (F) Influenza C virus mRNAs derived from RNA segment 6. The unspliced and spliced mRNAs encode P42 and M1, respectively. The cleavage of P42 by a signal peptidase produces M1′ (p31) and CM2. (G) Thogoto virus segment 6 showing M and ML. M is translated from a spliced mRNA with a stop codon that is generated by the splicing process itself, as in Influenza C virus M1 mRNA. ML is translated from the unspliced transcript and represents an elongated form of M with a C-terminal extension of 38 aa. The boxes represent different coding regions. Introns in the mRNAs are shown by the V-shaped lines; filled rectangles at the 5′-ends of mRNAs represent heterogeneous nucleotides derived from cellular RNAs that are covalently linked to viral sequences. (Modified from Cox and Kawaoka, 1998 and Lamb and Horvath, 1991). [*From* Virus Taxonomy: Eighth Report of the International Committee on Taxonomy of Viruses (*C. M. Fauquet, M. A. Mayo, J. Maniloff, U. Desselberger, L. A. Ball, eds.*), p. 683. Copyright © Elsevier (2005), with permission.]

binding affinity for the SAα2,6Gal glycan varies with the length of the oligosaccharide. Human-adapted H1 and H3 viruses show binding preference for long oligosaccharides present on epithelial cells in the upper respiratory tract, and mutations that affect this binding alter transmissibility. A single amino acid change in the hemagglutinin protein of the 1918 H1 Spanish flu virus at position 190 (E190D) changes binding preference from SAα2,3Gal to SAα2,6Gal.

Influenza viruses enter cells via receptor-mediated endocytosis. The low pH of the endosome triggers a conformational change in the hemagglutinin protein such that the hydrophobic domain of the HA2 trimer mediates fusion of the viral envelope with the endosomal membrane, releasing the RNA + nucleoprotein + polymerase proteins (RNP) into the cytoplasm. While in the endosome, the ion channel M2 tetramer transports protons into the virus particle to enable dissociation of the binding of M1 to the RNP complex, thus freeing it from the viral envelope (Figure 21.4). Amantadine and rimantadine inhibit virus replication by blocking the ion channel activity of M2. A unique feature of influenza virus is that all RNA synthesis takes places in the nucleus of the cell. This requires that the RNP, because of its size, be actively transported into the nucleus. Nuclear localization signals on the nucleoprotein interact with the nuclear transport machinery of the cells to transport the RNP into the nucleus.

As with all viruses with negative-sense RNA genomes, the genome of orthomyxoviruses serves two functions: as a template for the synthesis of messenger RNAs (mRNAs), and as a template for the synthesis of positive-sense replicative intermediate RNA, which is the template for progeny genomic RNA synthesis. Primary transcription involves an unusual phenomenon known as *cap snatching*: the viral endonuclease activity of PB2 cleaves the 5'-methylguanosine cap plus about 10–13 nucleotides from heterogeneous cellular mRNAs that are captured by PB2. These caps are then used by the virus as primers for transcription by the viral RNA polymerase (transcriptase; PB1). The viral mRNAs thus are capped and also become polyadenylated through transcription of five to seven "U" residues on the virion RNA. All orthomyxoviruses extend the coding capacity of their genomes by producing two proteins from one gene by using an alternative splicing mechanism. Influenza A virus uses splicing for gene segments 7 (M1 + M2) and 8 (NS1 + NEP/NS2) (Figure 21.5); influenza B virus uses gene segment 8 (NS1 + NEP/NS2); influenza C virus uses gene segments 6 (CM1 + CM2) and 7 (NS1 + NEP/NS2); thogotoviruses use gene segment 6 (M + ML); isavirus uses gene segments 7 and 8. (NS1 and NS2 [HEP] are defined as non-structural proteins while Ms, CMs and ML are membrane associated proteins.) Influenza B virus also uses a different strategy for gene segment 7, involving overlapping stop and start codons to generate two protein products. In certain influenza A virus strains, a PB1-F2 protein of 87–90 amino acids is generated by a +1 reading frameshift.

Viral protein synthesis occurs in the cytoplasm using cellular translation machinery. There is clear evidence for temporal regulation of gene expression, but the mechanism is unresolved. Early in infection, there is enhanced synthesis of nucleoprotein and NS1, whereas synthesis of hemagglutinin, neuraminidase, and matrix protein 1 is delayed. Nucleoprotein is required for replication of the virion RNA, and NS1 has been shown to inhibit the antiviral response triggered by the infection. Nucleoprotein must be transported to the nucleus to interact with the RNA to initiate replication.

Replication of genomic RNA segments requires the synthesis of full-length, positive-sense RNA intermediates, which, unlike the corresponding mRNA transcripts, must lack 5' caps and 3'-poly(A) tracts. Newly synthesized nucleoprotein binds to these RNAs, facilitating their use as templates for the synthesis of genomic RNAs. Late in infection, the matrix protein, M1, enters the nucleus and binds to nascent genomic RNA-nucleoprotein, thereby downregulating transcription and permitting export from the nucleus. NEP/NS2 bind the M1–RNP complexes, thus providing nuclear export signals and interaction with the nuclear export machinery that moves the RNP into the cytoplasm.

Virions are formed by budding, incorporating M1 protein and nucleocapsids that have aligned below patches on the plasma membrane in which hemagglutinin, neuraminidase, and matrix protein M2 have been inserted. In polarized cells, influenza virus buds from the apical surface of the cell. The hemagglutinin and neuraminidase proteins each contain transmembrane domains that associate with areas of the membrane enriched for sphingolipids and cholesterol that are designated *lipid rafts*. These lipid rafts have altered fluidity that appears to be critical for the budding process and infectivity of the mature virus particle. It was not known until recently by what mechanism one copy of each RNA segment was incorporated into each virion, but data now show that segment-specific packaging signals are contained in the initial protein coding region of each RNA segment. This mechanism provides specificity to the packaging process. As virions bud, the neuraminidase spikes (peplomers) facilitate the "pinching off" and release of virions by destroying receptors on the plasma membrane that would otherwise recapture virions and hold them at the cell surface.

For wild aquatic birds, the virus is shed in the feces and transmission is fecal–oral, but respiratory replication recently has been documented, indicating the potential for inhalational transmission. In poultry, replication is predominantly within the respiratory tract, but it also can occur in the intestinal tract, suggesting transmission may be by either ingestion or inhalation. In mammals, transmission is by aerosol, droplets, and fomites. The thogotoviruses are transmitted by ticks and replicate in both ticks and mammals. The isaviruses may be transmitted in water, with the gills of susceptible fish being the principal site of virus uptake and infection.

Molecular Determinants of Pathogenesis

The hemagglutinin protein of influenza A viruses is synthesized as a single polypeptide designated HA0. A key event in the history of influenza virus biology was the discovery that the hemagglutinin protein had to be cleaved post-translationally for the virus to be infectious, which established a clear link between cleavability of hemagglutinin and virulence. The avian viruses that were designated as highly pathogenic or high-pathogenicity avian influenza (HPAI) viruses had several basic amino acids at the hemagglutinin cleavage site or long insertions of amino acids, whereas those designated as low-pathogenicity avian influenza (LPAI) viruses contain a single arginine at a short cleavage site. The proteases that are capable of cleaving at the single arginine are tissue restricted, and access to the appropriate protease determines tissue tropism. In birds and mammals, epithelial cells within the respiratory and gastrointestinal tracts contain trypsin-like enzymes that can cleave the hemagglutinin of these LPAI viruses. Virus is produced in a non-infectious form and activation occurs extracellularly. In addition, certain respiratory bacteria, including normal flora, can secrete proteases that cleave the hemagglutinin of influenza A viruses. In contrast, in HPAI viruses, there are several basic amino acids at the cleavage site, which expands the range of cells capable of producing infectious virus, because cleavage can be mediated by the ubiquitous family of endopeptidase furins that are located in the *trans*-Golgi network. In this manner, the hemagglutinin is cleaved intracellularly and fully infectious virions are released from infected cells without any requirement for the extracellular activation that is necessary for LPAI virus strains. Thus continuous monitoring of the sequence at the cleavage site of circulating strains of LPAI viruses is used to identify hemagglutinin cleavage site mutations that might predict the emergence of highly virulent viruses. The HPAI viruses are not maintained in wild bird reservoirs, but arise following mutation in the hemagglutinin cleavage site of LPAI viruses.

As with most viruses, influenza viruses have developed mechanisms to counteract innate antiviral host defenses. NS1 is the key influenza virus protein responsible for blocking the response. Dimeric NS1 binds to double-stranded RNA, which is a potent interferon inducer. The exact mechanism by which NS1 blocks interferon responses is not known, but virus strains with mutations of NS1 are attenuated, and cells infected with these NS1 mutants contain increased levels of interferon response gene transcripts as compared with those infected with wild-type virus. The NS1 mutants are lethal to mice lacking interferon response genes, whereas infection is restricted in normal mice. Mutation of a single amino acid at position 42 (P42S) of NS1 greatly enhances virulence of influenza virus for attenuating the anti-interferon capability of NS1. In isaviruses it is the 7i protein that assumes the role of interferon antagonist, whereas in thogotoviruses it is the ML protein; the sites of action of these proteins in the antiviral pathway may be different.

The PB2 protein is a key component of the RNA transcription and replication process of influenza viruses, and may exert an important role in determining virulence and host range. The specific amino acid at residue 627 defines whether influenza A viruses grow well in mammalian cells, and whether or not the viruses are highly virulent to mice. In some human H3 and H5N1 viruses, a lysine at residue 627 enhances growth of the virus in mammalian cells, and this change from glutamic acid is selected when avian viruses successfully cross the species barrier.

In addition to changes in the glycoproteins in the viruses responsible for the human influenza pandemics of 1957 and 1968, there was also an exchange in the *PB1* gene. Furthermore, introduction of a *PB1* gene from a pathogenic virus into swine influenza virus increased the virulence of the reassortant. A novel protein that was generated by a +1 frameshift was mapped to the *PB1* gene. This protein, designated PB1-F2, localized to mitochondria in infected cells and induced apoptosis in monocyte/macrophages. Although PB1-F2 is dispensable for replication in cell culture and embryonated eggs, it can affect virulence of the virus in mice and, potentially, other mammals.

From the preceding, virulence of influenza viruses clearly can be multifactorial. Host range is determined by receptor specificity and cleavability of the hemagglutinin protein, as well as the activity of the PB2 protein. The PB1-F2 protein apparently contributes to the virulence phenotype of individual viruses, and NS1—and perhaps other proteins—interfere with innate host defenses. Studies in laboratory animals also show protracted alteration of innate immune responses mediated by pattern recognition receptors after influenza virus infection, and these alterations presumably can predispose affected animals to secondary respiratory infections.

MEMBERS OF THE GENUS *INFLUENZAVIRUS A*

EQUINE INFLUENZA VIRUSES

Although outbreaks of a respiratory disease in horses that probably was influenza have been described throughout history, including the so-called Great Epizootic of 1872 amongst horses in North America, the differentiation of equine influenza from other equine respiratory diseases was not definitively established until 1956, when influenza virus A/equine/Prague/1/56 (H7N7) (equine influenza virus 1) was isolated during an epizootic in central Europe. Subsequently in the United States, a second virus, A/equine/Miami/1/63 (H3N8) (equine influenza virus 2), was isolated in 1963. Since then, the disease has been reported in horses, and also in donkeys and mules, in virtually all parts of the world, although certain island countries, including Iceland and New Zealand, have maintained their freedom from infection.

Influenza is considered to be the most important cause of viral respiratory disease in horses. H3N8 virus has been identified in all recent outbreaks; the last outbreak caused by subtype H7N7 virus was in 1979 and it is now believed that the prototype H7N7 no longer circulates in equine populations. The H3N8 virus has undergone modest genetic drift since it was first isolated, and there are now discernible branches in the evolutionary tree: a Eurasian branch and an American branch. The American branch is further subdivided into Argentinean, Florida, and Kentucky sublineages. Both American sublineages also circulate in horses in Europe and Asia, but the Eurasian lineage has been detected in North America only once. Although only modest antigenic changes have occurred in the H3N8 virus over time, failure to upgrade vaccines to include currently circulating strains has resulted in significant outbreaks of respiratory disease. Continuing surveillance and isolation of new variants is necessary to optimize vaccine efficacy.

Clinical Features and Epidemiology

Influenza virus characteristically spreads very rapidly amongst susceptible horses, and causes disease of high morbidity 24–48 hours after infection. The clinical signs are the result of infection of the respiratory tract: there is reddening of the nasal mucosa, conjunctivitis, and serous; later, mucopurulent nasal discharge. The serous nasal discharge develops at the same time as a characteristic harsh, dry, paroxysmal cough that may persist for up to 3 weeks. Infected horses develop fever (39.5–41°C) lasting for 4–5 days and become inappetent and depressed. Mortality is rare, but prolonged fever in pregnant mares may result in abortion. Clinical diagnosis of acute cases is straightforward, but diagnosis in partially immune horses is more difficult, as the disease must be differentiated from other respiratory infections, including those caused by equine herpesviruses, equine adenoviruses, equine rhinitis viruses, and a variety of bacteria. Subclinical infections with virus shedding are frequently seen in vaccinated horses in which the immune response is weak or a poor match for the circulating virus. Secondary bacterial infections may occur, characterized by purulent nasal exudates and bronchopneumonia. In the absence of such complications, the disease is self-limiting, with complete recovery occurring within 2–3 weeks after infection.

Equine influenza viruses are highly contagious and are spread rapidly in stables or studs by infectious exudate that is aerosolized by frequent coughing. Virus is excreted during the incubation period and horses remain infectious for at least 5 days after clinical disease begins. Close contact between horses facilitates rapid transmission; however, contaminated clothing of stable personnel, equipment, and transport vehicles may also contribute to virus dissemination. Equine populations that are moved frequently, such as racehorses, breeding stock, show jumpers, and horses sent to sales, are at special risk. The rapid international spread of equine influenza is caused by the year-round transport of horses for racing and breeding purposes between Europe, North America, Japan, Hong Kong, South Africa, Australasia and elsewhere. Although clinical manifestations normally begin in the cold season, epizootics generally occur during the main racing season—that is, between April and October in the northern hemisphere.

The highly contagious nature of equine influenza virus was graphically illustrated in 2007, when an H3N8 virus (American lineage) spread amongst horses in Australia, a country that previously was free of the virus. From an initial incursion at a quarantine station in New South Wales, the virus spread within 3 months to some 10,000 premises in New South Wales and Queensland. The epizootic was controlled by movement restrictions and vaccination, but this extraordinary event emphatically confirmed the impact of equine influenza virus in an immunologically naïve population of horses.

Apart from one outbreak in China in 1989 that was derived from an avian source, equids are the only known source of equine influenza viruses. In 1989, a severe outbreak of H3N8 influenza A virus infection occurred in horses in northeastern China, with morbidity of 80% and mortality of 20%. In a second epizootic in the following year, morbidity was about 50%, but there was little or no mortality, probably because of the immune status of horses in the region. Of particular interest was the discovery that, although the causative virus had the same antigenic composition as viruses circulating among horses in other parts of the world, its genes were of recent avian origin. Serological studies indicated that the virus was not present in horses in China before 1989; thus it represents the transfer of an avian influenza virus to mammals without reassortment. This serves to emphasize that, however uncommon the emergence of new strains of influenza virus, ongoing surveillance is required to predict such events.

Pathogenesis and Pathology

Equine influenza viruses replicate in epithelial cells of the upper and lower respiratory tract. Infection causes destruction of the ciliated epithelial lining, which induces inflammation and subsequent formation of exudate and nasal discharge. The most important changes occur in the lower respiratory tract and include laryngitis, tracheitis, bronchitis, and bronchointerstitial pneumonia that are accompanied by pulmonary congestion and alveolar edema. Secondary infections may result in conjunctivitis, pharyngitis, bronchopneumonia and chronic respiratory disease. Fatal bronchointerstitial pneumonia was described amongst foals less than 2 weeks of age during the recent equine influenza epizootic in Australia; as this country previously was free of the virus, the epizootic occurred in an immunologically naïve population of horses. The severe disease encountered in these foals was attributed to lack of protection from colostral antibodies specific for equine influenza virus, rather than an infection with an unusually pathogenic virus.

Factors that contribute to innate resistance of horses include: (1) the mucus blanket that protects the respiratory epithelium, and the continuous beating of cilia that clears virus from the respiratory tract; (2) soluble lectins, lung surfactants, and sialoglycoproteins present in mucus and transudates that bind virions; (3) alveolar macrophages. If the horse has been infected previously, anti-hemagglutinin antibodies may intercept and neutralize the virus if the challenge virus is antigenically closely matched to the immunizing virus. Secretory immunoglobulin A is proposed to be the most relevant antibody in the upper respiratory tract, but serum-derived antibodies also provide protection. Levels of vaccine-induced serum antibodies as measured by single radial hemolysis correlate well with protection in challenged animals. In laboratory animal models, activated macrophages, natural killer cells, and virus-specific T cells are crucial to clearance of virus from the lower respiratory tract, as are interferon-γ and interleukin-2. Efforts to undertake similar studies in horses are complicated by the lack of necessary reagents.

Diagnosis

The clinical presentation of influenza in horses is very characteristic. In most laboratory settings, detection of equine influenza virus is achieved using RT-PCR assays. Nasal or oropharyngeal swabs taken early in the infection (within 3–5 days of onset of clinical signs) are the samples of choice, and virus need not be viable for detection by RT-PCR assay. Similar samples can be used for virus isolation, but the swabs should be placed in a virus transport medium to preserve infectivity. H3N8 viruses replicate in 10-day-old embryonated eggs, using either the amniotic or the allantoic route of inoculation and incubating at 35–37°C for 3–4 days, but a blind passage may be necessary to produce a detectable level of virus by standard hemagglutination tests. Isolation of the virus can be in cell culture systems. Madin–Darby canine kidney (MDCK) cells are preferred; trypsin must be included in the culture medium, because most cells lines cannot cleave the hemagglutinin protein, which is necessary for virus replication. Virus replication can be detected by the demonstration of hemagglutination activity in the harvested amniotic or allantoic fluid or cell-culture fluid by antigen-capture enzyme-linked immunosorbent assay (ELISA), or by RT-PCR assays. Isolates are now identified by hemagglutinin- and neuraminidase-specific RT-PCR assays or, less frequently, by hemagglutination-inhibition using a panel of subtype-specific reference antisera. Retrospective serologic diagnosis of equine influenza virus infection can be made using paired serum samples.

Outbreaks of respiratory disease in horses caused by influenza virus infection rapidly can be confirmed in the field (non-laboratory settings) using antigen-capture ELISA tests. Although these tests can be relatively insensitive in detecting infection of individual horses, they are very useful for rapid confirmation of epizootics.

Immunity, Prevention, and Control

Control of incursions of equine influenza virus into previously virus-free countries involves isolation and vaccination, as practiced during recent outbreaks in Australia and South Africa. Similarly, stables and racing facilities where equine influenza outbreaks occur should be quarantined. After all horses have recovered, cleaning and disinfection of boxes and stables, equipment, and transport vehicles is necessary.

Vaccination is extensively practiced in influenza virus enzootic countries. Vaccination was previously carried out exclusively with inactivated vaccines that now contain two different lineages of A/equine (H3N8) viruses, preferably including strains that match the prevalent field virus. Several vaccinations are necessary to achieve full protection of individual horses, although the optimal timing of booster immunizations is conjectural. The H7N7 equine influenza virus has been eliminated from most reformulated vaccines since 2000, when an OIE expert panel concluded that there was no epidemiological evidence to support inclusion of H7N7 in equine vaccines. A continuing concern with inactivated vaccines is their inability to induce a cellular immune response equivalent to that which occurs after natural infections. Various formulations have attempted to correct this problem, including the use of immunostimulatory adjuvants (oil- and polymer-adjuvanted preparations), Quil-A-based immune-stimulating complexes, DNA vaccines for use in prime-boost strategies, poxvirus-vectored vaccines, and a live-attenuated, cold-adapted virus vaccine. These approaches can induce a more durable immune response as compared with previous whole-virus and subunit vaccines. Commercially available canarypox virus vectored recombinant vaccines containing the hemagglutinin protein and an immune-stimulating complex have been demonstrated to produce a cellular immune response in horses. Recombinant canarypox virus vectored vaccines were used in the programs that successfully eradicated equine influenza from both South Africa and Australia.

A major potential problem with inactivated vaccines is their inability to provide a protective immune response for foals with maternally derived antibodies. Current recommendations are to withhold vaccination until at least 6 months of age. The canarypox virus vectored equine influenza vaccines can prime foals even in the presence of maternal antibody, which may afford enhanced protection of young animals.

Regardless of the vaccine type, regulatory agencies must develop flexible regulations that can allow rapid incorporation of new strains of virus into the vaccines in a manner similar to that adopted for human vaccines.

SWINE INFLUENZA VIRUSES

Swine influenza was first recognized and described in the north central United States at the time of the catastrophic

1918 pandemic of human influenza, and for a long time was reported only from this area, where annual outbreaks occurred each winter. The first isolation of swine influenza virus was by Richard Shope in 1930 (A/swine/Iowa/15/30 [H1N1]). Although the 1918 pandemic affected humans throughout Europe, swine influenza was not observed in Europe until the 1940s and 1950s in Czechoslovakia, the United Kingdom, and West Germany. The virus then apparently disappeared until 1976, when it reappeared in northern Italy and spread to Belgium and southern France in 1979; since then it has occurred in Europe rather regularly. However, the virus causing these more recent epizootics in swine was of avian origin, and closely related to a duck virus.

Two distinct variants of the H1N1 swine influenza virus now circulate in the world—specifically, the avian variant found in Europe since 1979, and the variant found in the United States that is similar to the original virus strain. Swine have also become infected with other types of influenza A virus, including human H3N2 strains in China, Europe, and North America, and reassortant H1N2 viruses have emerged that contain genes from both swine and human virus strains; there are even triple reassortants that contain genes from swine, human, and avian viruses. For example, a virus that caused a significant epizootic of respiratory disease in North American swine has: the *HA*, *NA*, and *PB1* genes from a human virus strain; *PB2* and *PA* from an avian strain; *NP*, *M*, *NS* from the classical swine virus (Figure 21.6). In China, H3N2 human-like virus, H3N2 double reassortants, and H3N2 triple reassortants have circulated in the pig population. Other combinations also exist, and novel reassortants may be develop frequently, as occurred with the emergence of the novel pandemic H1N1 virus in 2009. In addition, there is continuing accumulation of amino acid changes within the hemagglutinin proteins of circulating strains of swine influenza virus.

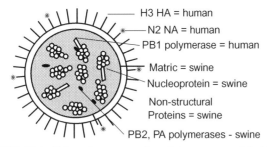

FIGURE 21.6 Schematic representation of the genotype of the H3N2 influenza A virus, Sw/NC/98, isolated from pigs in North America since 1997. This virus is a reassortant between human and classical swine influenza A viruses. HA, hemagglutinin; NA, neuraminidase. *[From C. W. Olsen. The emergence of novel swine influenza viruses in North America. Virus Res. 85, 199–210 (2002), with permission.]*

Pigs have been considered the "mixing vessel" for influenza virus because of their ability to become co-infected with both avian and human strains of influenza virus. Pigs possess both avian-type (SAα2,3Gal) and human-type (SAα2,6Gal) receptors. The reassortant influenza viruses that currently circulate in swine throughout the world support this intermediary role, although not all pandemic human influenza viruses are related to swine viruses. Curiously, although pigs can become infected with various avian viruses, enzootic swine viruses possess only the H1 or H3 hemagglutinins. The current Eurasian–African H5N1 avian virus can infect pigs, but replicates poorly.

Clinical Features and Epidemiology

After an incubation period of 24–72 hours, the onset of disease is abrupt, often appearing in many animals in a herd at the same time. There is fever (>42°C), with apathy, inappetence, huddling, and a reluctance to move, and signs of respiratory distress: paroxysmal coughing, sneezing, rhinitis with nasal discharge, labored breathing, and bronchial rales at auscultation. After 3–6 days, swine usually recover quickly, eating normally by 7 days after appearance of the first clinical signs. If sick swine are kept warm and free of stress, the course of disease is benign, with few complications and a case-fatality rate of less than 1%; however, some animals develop severe bronchopneumonia, which may result in death. Reproductive losses have occurred amongst pregnant sows infected with some H3 reassortant viruses. Although most pigs recover uneventfully, the economic consequences of swine influenza are considerable, in that sick swine either lose weight or their weight gains are reduced.

Outbreaks of swine influenza are observed mostly in late fall and winter, or after the introduction of new swine into susceptible herds. Infections can occur year-round in confinement swine facilities. Frequently, the disease appears simultaneously on several farms within an area; outbreaks are explosive, with all swine in a herd becoming sick at virtually the same time. The mechanism of the inter-epizootic survival of swine influenza virus has been a matter of intensive investigation for many years, but remains unsolved. Swine influenza virus clearly can become enzootic in large herds in which there is continuous infusion of newly susceptible animals, but there is no credible evidence of a true carrier state in any species infected with an influenza virus.

The novel 2009 pandemic strain of H1N1 influenza virus can infect pigs, but the associated clinical disease is mild. However, substantial economic losses have been incurred through the quarantine of infected herds because of public health concerns. As frequently occurs when zoonotic diseases appear, consumption of pork dropped substantially after the emergence of the "swine flu" virus in 2009, although there was no credible evidence of any risk to consumers.

Pathogenesis and Pathology

Swine influenza virus infection follows the typical pattern for respiratory viral infections: virus entry is via aerosol, and there is a rapid progression of the infection in the epithelium of the nasal cavity and large airways. Infection can progress to involve all airways in just a few hours. Animals develop bronchointerstitial pneumonia that is characterized by sharply demarcated lung lesions in the apical and cardiac lobes, with hyperemia, consolidation, and the presence of inflammatory exudates in airways. Histologically, epithelial surfaces are denuded, with accumulation of intraluminal debris within affected airways. There is collapse of adjacent airspaces, interstitial pneumonia, and emphysema.

Diagnosis

Swine influenza is characterized by sudden onset of highly contagious respiratory disease that may be confused with infectious diseases such as those caused by *Actinobacillus pleuropneumoniae* and *Mycoplasma hyopneumoniae*. Indeed, the gross lung lesions in swine with influenza can closely resemble those of swine with *M. hyopneumoniae* infection. For routine diagnosis, the RT-PCR test has replaced virus isolation, thanks to its speed and capability for automation. Isolation is still used to provide viruses for genetic analyses; isolations can be achieved using embryonated eggs or by cell culture using MDCK cells with a trypsin-containing overlay. Identification of the virus genotype is by hemagglutinin- and neuraminidase-specific RT-PCR tests with confirmation by sequence analysis of the amplified products, or with specific monoclonal antibodies. Virus can be detected in tissue samples by immunofluorescence or by immunohistochemistry. Serological tests (hemagglutination-inhibition and ELISA) can be used to detect infection of unvaccinated swine.

Immunity, Prevention, and Control

Swine influenza is controlled by vaccination and strict biosecurity measures that prevent introduction of the virus. Many commercial producers of swine now use an "all-in–all-out" system of production. In this type of facility, biosecurity may be sufficient to exclude influenza virus infection, provided there is reliable access to virus-free replacement stock. Vaccines can be used to control disease in facilities where exclusion is not practical. Because of the number of reassortant influenza viruses that currently circulate in the commercial swine population, vaccines are now being formulated with a minimum of two different viral antigens, and some with three. As with all influenza virus vaccines, the vaccines do not prevent infection, or even the shedding of virus following natural infection. For production facilities, the simple goal is to prevent significant clinical disease and the associated economic losses. Vaccination does confuse the interpretation of serological testing, either for diagnostic purposes or in seroprevalence studies.

Human Disease

Infection of humans with swine influenza virus can occur among abattoir workers exposed to virus-infected pigs, and may cause respiratory disease. Infection is otherwise rare, and person-to-person spread is limited. However, because of fears of another pandemic like that of 1918, swine influenza virus infections of humans are the subject of considerable public health concern. For example, the isolation of H1N1 swine influenza virus from military recruits at Fort Dix in the United States in 1976 led to a massive human immunization campaign in the United States. Many believe the response in 1976 was an over-reaction, but the emergence of the novel pandemic H1N1 in 2009 clearly validates concerns regarding zoonotic H1N1 influenza virus infections. Human infections have occurred with swine H3N2 reassortant viruses, but these infections have been restricted to the original source, and have not spread extensively between people.

AVIAN INFLUENZA VIRUSES

The devastating form of influenza in chickens known as "fowl plague" was recognized as a distinct disease entity as early as 1878, in Northern Italy. The disease spread rapidly in Europe and Asia, and was reported in both North and South America by the mid-1920s. The causative agent was isolated in 1901, but it was not identified as an influenza virus until 1955. In 1961, an outbreak of high mortality occurred in common terns (*Sterna hirundo*) in South Africa that provided the first evidence for direct involvement of wild birds in virus transmission. From the 1970s onward, avian influenza came into ecological focus when surveillance indicated the ubiquitous presence of asymptomatic viral infections in wild waterfowl and the risk that these birds pose to commercial chicken industries. A very large epizootic centered in the commercial industries of Pennsylvania in 1983–1984, which at the time cost approximately US $60 million to control (loss of an estimated 17 million chickens and turkeys), brought substance to this risk. Since 1955, there have been at least 27 outbreaks or epizootics of highly pathogenic avian influenza virus infection caused by distinct viruses (or virus lineages) in poultry and wild birds, with losses from disease or culling in excess of 500 million birds. All outbreaks were caused by mutants of low pathogenicity avian influenza viruses found in wild bird populations.

Avian influenza viruses are categorized, for international trade issues, as of either high or low pathogenicity.

The definitions (as found in the OIE *Terrestrial Animal Health Code* (2007), Chapter 2.7.12) are:

1. For the purposes of international trade, avian influenza (AI) in its notifiable form [notifiable avian influenza (NAI)] is defined as an infection of poultry caused by any influenza A virus of the H5 or H7 subtypes or by any AI virus with an intravenous pathogenicity index (IVPI) greater than 1.2 (or, as an alternative, at least 75% mortality) as described below. NAI viruses can be divided into highly pathogenic notifiable avian influenza (HPNAI) and low pathogenicity notifiable avian influenza (LPNAI):

   a. HPNAI viruses have an IVPI in 6-week-old chickens greater than 1.2 or, as an alternative, cause at least 75% mortality in 4- to 8-week-old chickens infected intravenously. H5 and H7 viruses which do not have an IVPI of greater than 1.2 or cause less than 75% mortality in an intravenous lethality test should be sequenced to determine whether multiple basic amino acids are present at the cleavage site of the hemagglutinin molecule (HA0); if the amino acid motif is similar to that observed for other HPNAI isolates, the isolate being tested should be considered as HPNAI;

   b. LPNAI are all influenza A viruses of H5 and H7 subtype that are not HPNAI viruses.

This standard was established because all outbreaks of HPAI have been caused by H5 or H7 viruses, and the presence of any H5 or H7 LPAI virus in a commercial rearing facility is cause for concern because of the inherent potential of these viruses to mutate to HPAI virus.

Clinical Features and Epidemiology

The disease caused in chickens and turkeys by HPAI viruses has historically been called "fowl plague." Today, the term should be avoided, except where it is part of the name of well-characterized strains [e.g., A/fowl plague virus/Dutch/27 (H7N7)]. Highly virulent strains of avian influenza A virus cause sudden death without prodromal symptoms. If birds survive for more than 48 hours (which is more likely in older birds), there is a cessation of egg laying, respiratory distress, lacrimation, sinusitis, diarrhea, edema of the head, face and neck, and cyanosis of unfeathered skin, particularly the comb and wattles. Birds may show nervous signs such as tremors of the head and neck, inability to stand, torticollis, and other unusual postures.

The LPAI viruses may also cause considerable losses, particularly in turkeys, because of anorexia, depression, decreased egg production, respiratory disease, and sinusitis. Clinical signs in chickens and turkeys may be exacerbated markedly by concurrent infections (e.g., various viral, bacterial, and mycoplasma infections), the use of live-attenuated virus vaccines, or environmental stress (e.g., poor ventilation and overcrowding).

Avian influenza virus is shed in high concentrations in the feces of wild birds, and can survive for long periods in cold water. The virus is introduced into susceptible flocks periodically by interspecies transmission—that is, between chickens and turkeys and from wild birds, especially wild ducks; thus facilities where wild birds have access facilitate this type of transmission. It is unclear how the many subtypes of avian influenza A viruses are maintained in wild birds from year to year; it is hypothesized that the viruses are maintained by circulation at low levels in large wild bird populations, even during migration and overwintering. Studies of wild ducks in Canada have shown that up to 20% of juvenile birds are already infected silently as they congregate before their southern migration. Avian influenza viruses have also frequently been isolated in many countries from imported caged birds, although such passerine and psittacine birds are not natural reservoirs of LPAI viruses and they probably only become infected after exposure to infected village poultry, especially domestic and captive ducks.

Live markets also may be critical to the epidemiology of influenza virus infections. The Eurasian–African H5N1 epizootic clearly confirms the risk associated with the mixing of domestic poultry with wild birds (particularly ducks), the potential for influenza viruses to be rapidly passaged through several species of birds, and unregulated movement of birds to and from markets. The first indication of a potentially new epizootic of avian influenza virus was the isolation of an HPAI virus from a goose in Guangdong, China, in 1996, with subsequent spread and outbreaks among poultry in Hong Kong in 1997, 2001, and 2002. In addition, this unique virus caused 18 human infections, with six deaths. Efforts to control the outbreak by depopulation and some vaccination with an H5N2 vaccine eliminated the disease and infection in Hong Kong, but by 2003 this H5N1 HPAI virus had spread to Korea, Japan, Indonesia, Thailand, and Vietnam. Wild water fowl infected with LPAI viruses normally show no clinical signs, and have been difficult to infect experimentally with HPAI viruses isolated before 1997. However, in 2002, waterfowl in two parks in Hong Kong developed neurological disease after infection with this Eurasian–African H5N1 virus. Furthermore, large cats in Thailand died after being fed infected poultry, which confirmed its unusual properties. The HPAI H5N1 virus that circulated in 2002 showed multiple gene reassortments and mutations as compared with the 1997 virus. In early 2005, HPAI H5N1 virus was isolated from dead wild birds in Qinghai Lake of central China and the virus then was detected in Mongolia, Siberia, Kazakhstan, and Eastern Europe later that year. This H5N1 HPAI virus was detected in most countries of Asia, Europe, and parts of Africa in 2006, although the "virus" has undergone many changes since the initial isolate from the goose in 1997 (Figure 21.7).

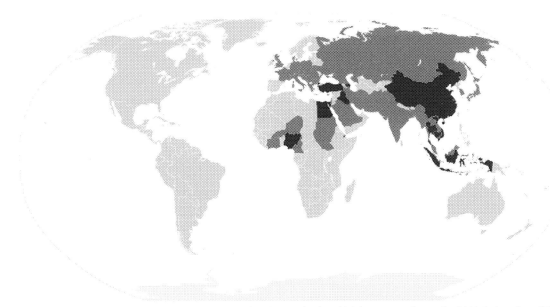

FIGURE 21.7 Global spread of H5N1 virus (May 2009). Dark red, countries in which humans, poultry and wild birds have been killed by H5N1. Light red, countries in which poultry or wild birds have been killed by H5N1.

Most strains of the virus are included in Clade 2.2, which includes viruses from Korea, Iran, Ghana, India, and Egypt.

The debate over the role of wild birds in the transmission of the Eurasian–African H5N1 virus continues, although it is abundantly clear that the virus is highly pathogenic for at least some species of wild birds. Legal and illegal trade in poultry and wild birds must also be carefully monitored, as a parrot imported into the United Kingdom died of an H5N1 infection in 2005. Intense surveillance for the Eurasian–African H5N1 virus has been initiated in Europe, North America, and elsewhere. In North America, initial emphasis has been on Alaska, western Canada, and the west coast of the United States, because of the overlapping migration routes of Asian and North American wild birds, but with expansion into the Mississippi and Atlantic flyways. Predictably, many LPAI H5 viruses have been identified in the course of these surveillance programs.

Pathogenesis and Pathology

The extraordinary virulence of some avian influenza virus strains reflects the properties of several viral gene products. A key pathogenic marker that is monitored with avian influenza viruses, particularly H5 and H7 viruses, is the amino acid sequence at the cleavage site of the hemagglutinin protein. Changes in the amino acid sequence can alter the rate of cleavage of the protein and drastically alter the virulence of these viruses. Most LPAI viruses have a single basic amino acid (arginine) at the cleavage site, with a glycosylation site that shields the cleavage site. Elimination of the glycosylation site, changes in the amino acids to basic

ones, insertions that open the cleavage site, and deletions that shift basic amino acids to the cleavage site all change cleavability and alter pathogenicity.

The phenomenon of hemagglutinin cleavage is a major determinant of the virulence of influenza viruses; however, other portions of the hemagglutinin protein, in addition to other gene products, also can contribute through their respective influences on virus binding and replication efficiency. There also is variation in the susceptibility or resistance of different bird species to individual HPAI virus strains. For example, A/chicken/Scotland/59 (H5N1) virus is more virulent for chickens, whereas A/turkey/Ontario/7732/66 (H5N9) virus is more virulent for turkeys. In nature, ducks historically have been refractory to infection with the most virulent HPAI viruses, but disease recently has been described following infection with Eurasian–African H5N1 virus that also causes disease in humans. However, despite millions of potential human exposures to infected birds carrying this virus, only some 400 hospital admissions and 254 deaths have been documented in 15 countries (as at January 2009). This suggests that, although highly fatal, human infections are rare with this H5N1 virus, and that the current Eurasian–African HPAI virus is principally a pathogen of birds and, to date, not a pandemic human virus.

The pathogenesis of avian influenza is quite different from that in mammals, in that virus replication occurs in the intestinal tract as well as the respiratory tract. In infections with the most virulent HPAI virus strains, there is viremia and multifocal lymphoid and visceral organ necrosis that result in pancreatitis, myocarditis, myositis, and encephalitis. Chickens and turkeys, which succumb after several days of illness, exhibit petechial hemorrhages and serous exudates in respiratory, digestive, and cardiac tissues. Turkeys may also have air sacculitis and pulmonary congestion. In all avian species, neutralizing antibodies are detectable within 3–7 days after the onset of disease, reaching a peak during the second week and persisting for up to 18 months.

Diagnosis

Clinical diagnosis is at best presumptive and only used during epizootics, because of the extreme variability in the clinical signs accompanying avian influenza virus infections in birds. Laboratory-based testing typically involves RT-PCR assay to detect the matrix protein (*M*) gene, as this is highly conserved in all strains of avian influenza viruses. Samples positive by this assay then are tested for specific *H5* and *H7* genes. If samples are *H5* or *H7* positive, sequence analysis is undertaken to determine the properties of the cleavage site. If several basic amino acids are detected at the cleavage site, then regulatory action is taken to eliminate the focus of infection. Virus isolation is used to obtain viruses for genetic analyses and for *in-vivo* pathogenicity tests; isolations are also performed for non-H5 or -H7 viruses, especially if there is any mortality associated with the sampled premise. Virus is best isolated from cloacal swabs (wild birds and poultry) and tracheal swabs (poultry). Specimens are inoculated into the allantoic cavity of 10–11-day-old embryonating eggs, or on to MDCK cells, and the presence of virus is indicated by hemagglutinating activity using chorioallantoic or cell culture fluids and chicken or turkey red blood cells. Isolates are routinely identified by gene-specific RT-PCR assays or with monospecific antisera using hemagglutination-inhibition (HI) tests. Infection of flocks can also be assessed using antibody tests such as agar gel immunodiffusion, ELISA tests, and hemagglutination-inhibition tests. The initial screening is with a broad serological test for influenza viruses (such as agar gel immunodiffusion or ELISA), followed by 16 different hemagglutination and nine neuraminidase inhibition tests for subtyping.

Immunity, Prevention, and Control

Control of avian influenza virus infections of domestic poultry is reliant on biosecurity, surveillance, and depopulation whenever HPAI viruses are detected. Biosecurity is critical to prevent potentially catastrophic economic loss as a result of epizootics of HPAI virus infections, and to prevent the evolution of H5 and H7 LPAI viruses to HPAI viruses by segregating domestic poultry from wild birds. Commercial facilities in southeast Asia that utilized appropriate biosecurity measures suffered no losses during the recent epizootic of H5N1 virus infection, whereas losses were substantial in those facilities that permitted the mixing of poultry with wild birds or those that had links to live poultry markets. Mixing of domestic and wild birds clearly also promotes evolution of the virus. Flocks that are found to be infected with HPAI viruses are depopulated, to prevent spread to other commercial facilities and to wild birds in the environment. Surveillance is used to monitor for the presence of H5 and H7 LPAI viruses in domestic poultry. These LPAI virus strains may cause some production losses, but the concern is that continued passage of the virus in domestic poultry can select for more virulent viruses. Depopulation of facilities infected with H5 and H7 LPAI virus is now routinely done to eliminate potential trade implications and concerns regarding the presence of avian influenza A virus.

Most countries with developed industries endeavor to prevent infection and limit outbreaks of avian influenza through a combination of biosecurity practices, including education of workers, quarantine, surveillance with appropriate diagnostic procedures, and rapid depopulation when indicated. Vaccination has not been used to control outbreaks of HPAI in most developed countries, because of the potentially negative impact on their ability to conduct international trade, which requires that expensive surveillance programs be instituted to identify any infected birds within the vaccinated population. In certain situations, principally those associated with H5 and H7 LPAI virus infections, vaccination in combination with strict quarantines can be used to prevent serious economic losses from depopulation without the opportunity to market meat or eggs. Uncontrolled vaccination will probably never be permitted in countries involved in international trade.

Human Disease

Avian influenza viruses are the original source of all human influenza A virus genes; however, direct infection of individual humans by avian influenza viruses is sporadic or rare. Among the avian influenza viruses, the Eurasian–African H5N1 HPAI viruses are unique in producing human infections and fatalities. The vast majority of these cases of H5N1 transmission to humans can be directly linked to contact with infected poultry, and a few instances are consistent with person-to-person spread, but only amongst individuals within very close proximity to one another. Although the highly pathogenic H5N1 virus has the requisite basic amino acids at the cleavage site, this property alone has not enhanced human-to-human transmission and the virus also does not replicate well in pigs. Thus additional changes clearly will have to occur if this virus is ever to cause the much anticipated next pandemic of human influenza.

CANINE INFLUENZA VIRUSES

In 2004, an outbreak of respiratory disease in a group of greyhounds in Florida resulted in the death of several dogs, some of which had remarkably severe hemorrhagic pneumonia. Comprehensive sequence analyses of an influenza virus, now known as canine influenza virus, which was isolated from one dog indicated the virus was from the H3N8 equine lineage. Serological surveys of greyhound populations throughout the United States showed very high seroprevalence rates for this H3N8 virus, consistent with a long history of respiratory disease outbreaks in racing greyhounds. The virus was isolated in dogs in New York State in 2005. Incursions into several other states subsequently were described, although the virus has spread very slowly and virtually all cases to date have involved dogs in kennels, animal shelters, or day-care centers. The virus is readily transmitted between intensively housed dogs.

The signs of influenza virus infection in dogs are similar to or indistinguishable from those of canine respiratory disease complex ("kennel cough"). The major difference is that up to 50–70% of dogs in a kennel may be affected with influenza, whereas kennel cough typically would affect fewer than 10% of the population. All ages and breeds of dog are susceptible. Recovery is usually uneventful, unless there is a secondary infection; the influenza virus infection destroys the ciliated epithelial cells of the respiratory tract, which greatly enhances the chances of a secondary bacterial infection. Greyhounds appear to be especially susceptible to influenza virus infection, but the pathogenesis of the severe hemorrhagic pneumonia that occurs in some infected individuals remains uncharacterized.

Canine influenza virus is continuing to evolve, as recent isolates exhibit an accumulation of amino acid changes in the hemagglutinin protein. Initial isolates had at least five amino acid changes in hemagglutinin, as compared with the current circulating equine influenza virus, H3N8.

Infection of hounds by equine influenza virus H3N8 has been detected in several instances in England and occurred during the recent equine influenza outbreak in Australia. However, the infections were limited, and there is no evidence that these were a result of canine influenza virus. These cases appear to be simply equine influenza virus infection in dogs. Canids have also shown a susceptibility to the Eurasian–African H5N1 virus. Dogs in the epizootic areas were seropositive for H5 antibodies, and dogs exposed to H5N1 virus experimentally became infected, shed virus, but showed no obvious clinical signs. An H3N2 virus of avian origin was isolated in Korea from dogs with significant clinical disease, and experimentally infected dogs shed high titers of virus and developed severe necrosis and inflammation of both the upper and lower respiratory tract. The latter study also confirmed the presence of receptors with an α2,3 linkage (SAα2,3Ga—avian) on cells lining the canine respiratory tract. All these instances highlight the fact that influenza virus infection in canines warrants continuing surveillance and virus characterization, to monitor the potential emergence of any highly pathogenic virus in canines.

HUMAN INFLUENZA VIRUSES

The relationship of animal influenza viruses to human infections has been described in the preceding sections, including the emergence of influenza A viruses from avian reservoirs. In general, epidemic human influenza is seldom maintained among animals, although there are exceptions. The pandemic H1N1 virus that emerged in 2009 can infect and be transmitted amongst pigs, but it is uncertain whether swine will become a natural reservoir for this virus. The 2009 H1N1 virus was also found to be transmitted from infected humans to domestic cats, dogs, and pet ferrets, with the occurrence of significant clinical disease in all species. Ferrets can be infected and transmit both human influenza A and B viruses; they are used as laboratory models for pathogenesis studies, because the associated disease closely mimics that in humans. Transmission of influenza virus from infected cats and ferrets to humans has yet to be described, but is likely, given the quantities of virus shed by infected ferrets. Non-human primates, including gibbons, baboons, and chimpanzees, can also be naturally infected with human influenza A virus, and many species of New World and Old World monkeys are susceptible to experimental infection.

MEMBERS OF THE GENUS *ISAVIRUS*

INFECTIOUS SALMON ANEMIA VIRUS

Infectious salmon anemia virus is the only member of the genus *Isavirus*. The virus has a segmented genome, with eight distinct segments that encode at least 10 proteins. One of the surface proteins (HE) is responsible for receptor binding and receptor destroying activity, whereas the other (F) is responsible for membrane fusion. The HE protein is not proteolytically processed, but the inactive F0 protein requires processing for the virus to be infectious (F0→F1 + F2). Because of the severity of the disease this virus causes in farmed salmon, the European Union includes it in its list of the most dangerous diseases of fish, and it is one of just 12 viral infections of fish that is reportable to the World Organization for Animal Health (OIE).

Since the recognition of infectious salmon anemia virus in 1984, outbreaks have been detected in coastal waters of many countries bordering the North Atlantic. The disease has its greatest impact on farmed salmon, but other fish may be susceptible to infection without showing signs. Wild Atlantic salmon (*Salmo salar*) appear to be resistant to clinical disease, whereas farmed Atlantic salmon can show 100% mortality rates. Initial reports from Chile described the presence of an atypical isavirus among farmed coho salmon (*Oncorhynchus kisutch*), but more typical outbreaks have since occurred among farmed Atlantic salmon in the region. Farmed rainbow trout and wild fish such as sea trout (sea-going brown trout) and Atlantic salmon that show no signs of disease are potential virus reservoirs.

The hallmark of the disease is a profound anemia, with hematocrit values less than 10% (normal value, approximately 40%). The severe form of the disease in infected fish is characterized by exophthalmia, pale gills, hemorrhagic ascites and hemorrhagic liver necrosis, and renal interstitial hemorrhage and tubular necrosis. Histological lesions include filamental arteriole congestion and lamellar telangiectasia (aneurisms) in the gills, diffuse sinusoidal congestion and erythrophagia in the spleen, and multifocal regions of congestion and hemorrhage in the pyloric ceca. In the highly sensitive farmed salmon, viremia develops, with the virus targeting blood cells, endothelial cells, and macrophage-like cells.

There is great variation in the mortality produced by infectious salmon anemia virus infections, which reflects host resistance and strain variation in the virus. Using the *HE* gene, isolates of infectious salmon anemia virus can be grouped into a North American lineage and a European lineage. The European lineage is further subdivided into genotypes based on viral virulence. In experimental infections of Atlantic salmon with the most virulent virus strains, death commences within 10–13 days after infection and continues for a further 9–15 days, ultimately yielding mortality rates greater than 90%. Moderately virulent viruses show mortality rates between 50 and 89% and protracted killing, whereas low virulent strains have mortality rates less than 50% in Atlantic salmon. However, experimentally infected coho salmon (a distantly related Pacific species) were resistant to the development of disease with all isolates of infectious salmon anemia virus. As with influenza A viruses, there does not appear to be a single viral protein that is always predictive of virulence. Interestingly, however, the esterase activity of the HE protein can dissolve the hemagglutination reaction with fish erythrocytes, with the exception of those from Atlantic salmon, the fish most severely affected by infectious salmon anemia virus infection. This enhanced binding is speculated to have a role in the severe anemia that develops in these fish. As with other orthomyxoviruses, infectious salmon anemia virus has at least one protein—7i—that is able to block the innate antiviral defense system. Infectious salmon anemia virus is a strong inducer of interferon response genes, but is insensitive to the actions of the interferon response.

The diagnosis of infectious salmon anemia virus infection is made on the basis of the characteristic gross and histopathologic lesions, immunofluorescence staining of tissue samples, isolation of virus using any of several cell lines, and RT-PCR assay. Because the presence of infectious salmon anemia virus has regulatory consequences, the tests and testing protocols that are acceptable for an official diagnosis may vary, but RT-PCR tests should become the standard because of their sensitivity and rapid turnaround time. Antibody tests to detect exposure to infectious salmon anemia virus have been developed, but have not been commonly applied. Control of infectious salmon anemia virus infections are complicated by the issue of dealing with fish in an uncontrolled environment in which the virus may be circulating in native wild fish without evidence of infection. Outbreaks have been managed through a combination of regulatory measures and husbandry practices, including restricted movements of fish between farms, enforced slaughtering, use of all-in–all-out programs at farms, and disinfection of slaughterhouses and processing plants. Inactivated whole-virus vaccine preparations provide partial protection, but their use is limited by difficulties associated with vaccine delivery to large numbers of fish and development of asymptomatic carrier infections of some vaccinated fish.

OTHER ORTHOMYXOVIRUSES

Thogotovirus and Dhori viruses respectively contain six or seven gene segments, but both viruses are included in the genus *Thogotovirus*. These viruses are transmitted between vertebrates by ticks. Thogotovirus infections of ticks, humans, and a variety of animals have been described in Africa and southern Europe. The range and species tropism of Dhori virus is apparently similar, but also includes India and eastern Europe. Dhori virus infection can cause a febrile illness and encephalitis in humans, but its significance as an animal pathogen is uncertain.

Bunyaviridae

Chapter Contents

The family *Bunyaviridae* is the largest virus family, with more than 350 member viruses included in five genera: *Orthobunyavirus*, *Hantavirus*, *Nairovirus*, *Phlebovirus*, and *Tospovirus*. The family name is derived from the place in Uganda where the prototype bunyavirus was isolated. The common features of the bunyaviruses pertain both to the nature of the virions and to their biological properties. Viruses in three genera (*Orthobunyavirus*, *Nairovirus, and Phlebovirus*) are maintained in arthropod–vertebrate–arthropod cycles (so-called arboviruses), which have specificity in regard to both arthropod vectors and vertebrate reservoir hosts. This specificity is the basis for the usually narrow geographic and ecologic niches occupied by each virus. Similarly, viruses in the genus *Tospovirus* can be transmitted between plants by thrips, and replicate in both thrips and plants. Viruses in the genus *Hantavirus* are an exception, in that they are maintained in vertebrate–vertebrate cycles without arthropod vectors; nevertheless, the hantaviruses also exhibit great specificity in vertebrate reservoir hosts, and therefore also have distinct geographic and ecologic niches (Table 22.1).

TABLE 22.1 Family *Bunyaviridae*: Major Pathogens of Animals and Humans

Genus	Virus	Geographic Distribution	Arthropod Vector	Target Host Species or Amplifier Host	Disease in Animals	Disease in Humans
Phlebovirus	Rift Valley fever virus	Africa	Mosquitoes	Sheep, cattle, buffalo, humans	Systemic disease, hepatitis, abortion	Flu-like illness, hepatitis, hemorrhagic fever, retinitis
Nairovirus	Nairobi sheep disease virus	Eastern Africa	Ticks	Sheep, goats	Hemorrhagic enteritis	Mild febrile illness
	Crimean-Congo hemorrhagic fever virus	Africa, Asia, Europe	Ticks	Sheep, cattle, goats, humans	Mild if any	Hemorrhagic fever, hepatitis

(Continued)

Fenner's Veterinary Virology. DOI: 10.1016/B978-0-12-375158-4.00022-5

TABLE 3.1 (Continued)

Genus	Virus	Geographic Distribution	Arthropod Vector	Target Host Species or Amplifier Host	Disease in Animals	Disease in Humans
Bunyavirus	Akabane virus	Australia, Japan, Israel, Africa	Mosquitoes, Culicoides	Cattle, sheep	Arthrogryposis, hydranencephaly	None
	Cache Valley virus	United States	Mosquitoes	Cattle, sheep	Arthrogryposis, hydranencephaly rarely	Very rarely congenital infection
	La Crosse and other California encephalitis group viruses	North America	Mosquitoes	Small mammals, humans	None	Encephalitis
Hantavirus	Hantaan virus	China, Russia, Korea	None	*Apodemus agrarius* (striped field mouse)	None documented	Hemorrhagic fever with renal syndrome
	Puumala virus	Scandinavia, Europe, Russia	None	*Clethrionomys glareolus* (bank vole)	None documented	Hemorrhagic fever with renal syndrome
	Seoul virus	Worldwide	None	*Rattus norvegicus* (Norway rat)	None documented	Hemorrhagic fever with renal syndrome
	Sin Nombre virus and other New World hantaviruses	The Americas	None	*Peromyscus maniculatus* (deer mouse) and other reservoir rodent species	None documented	Hantavirus pulmonary syndrome

Arthropod-borne bunyaviruses are transmitted by specific mosquitoes, ticks, midges, or biting flies, whereas the individual hantaviruses are disseminated by specific rodents. Bunyaviruses cause transient infection in their vertebrate hosts, whether mammal or bird, and life-long persistent infection in their arthropod vectors, whereas hantaviruses cause persistent infection in their rodent reservoir hosts. Most bunyaviruses never infect domestic animals or humans, but those that do can cause important diseases that vary from congenital fetal malformation to systemic "hemorrhagic fever" disease syndromes.

PROPERTIES OF BUNYAVIRUSES

Classification

The very large number and diversity of the bunyaviruses offer a considerable taxonomic challenge, and current nomenclature is confusing. Genomic features are used to define genera, particularly the organization of each RNA genome segment and the sequences of conserved nucleotides at the termini of each segment. Classical serological methods are used to classify these viruses further. In general, antigenic determinants on the nucleocapsid protein are relatively conserved, and so serve to

define broad groupings among the viruses, whereas shared epitopes on the envelope glycoproteins, which are the targets in neutralization and hemagglutination-inhibition assays, define narrow groupings (serogroups). Unique epitopes on envelope glycoproteins, also determined by neutralization assays, define individual virus species. With few exceptions, viruses within a given genus are related antigenically to each other, but not to viruses in other genera. The lack of adequate biochemical characterization of many named bunyaviruses confuses their precise classification.

Genetic reassortment occurs when cultured cells or mosquitoes are coinfected with closely related bunyaviruses, and this probably has been important in the natural evolution of these viruses. Within its particular ecologic niche, each bunyavirus evolves by genetic drift and selection; for example, isolates of La Crosse virus from different regions in the United States differ considerably, as a result of cumulative point mutations and nucleotide deletions and duplications. The evolution of La Crosse virus has also involved genome segment reassortment, and reassortant viruses have been isolated from mosquitoes in the field.

The bunyaviruses are assigned to five genera, four of which include viruses that infect animals and a fifth (the genus *Tospovirus*) that contains only plant viruses. A very substantial number of bunyaviruses have not yet been assigned to a genus or serogroup.

The genus *Orthobunyavirus* contains a large number of viruses that share common genetic features and are serologically unrelated to viruses in other genera of the *Bunyaviridae*. Most of these viruses are mosquito-borne, but some are transmitted by sandflies or *Culicoides* spp. The genus includes a number of pathogens of domestic animals and humans, including Akabane and La Crosse viruses and their relatives.

The genus *Phlebovirus* contains over 50 viruses, all of which are transmitted by sandflies or mosquitoes. The genus contains important pathogens, including Rift Valley fever virus and the sandfly fever viruses.

The genus *Nairovirus* contains a large number of viruses, most of which are tick-borne, including the pathogens Nairobi sheep disease and Crimean-Congo hemorrhagic fever viruses.

The genus *Hantavirus* also includes a substantial number of viruses, many of them relatively recently discovered. All are transmitted by persistently infected reservoir rodent hosts via urine, feces, and saliva; the same transmission pattern has occurred among rats in laboratory colonies. In humans, several of these viruses from Asia cause hemorrhagic fever with renal syndrome, whereas those from Europe are typically associated with a different and less severe disease syndrome designated "neuropathica epidemica." Some of the hantaviruses from the Americas cause a severe acute respiratory distress syndrome referred to as "hantavirus pulmonary syndrome."

Virion Properties

Morphological properties vary among viruses in the various genera, but bunyavirus virions are spherical, approximately 80–120 nm in diameter, and are composed of a lipid envelope with glycoprotein spikes, inside which are three circular ribonucleoprotein (RNP) complexes comprised of individual genome RNA segments associated with the viral nucleoprotein (Table 22.2; Figure 22.1). These RNP complexes are stabilized by a panhandle structure generated by non-covalent bonds between inverted palindromic sequences on the 3′ and 5′ ends of each RNA genome segment. The terminal sequences are identical for all three RNA segments within each virus species, and are critical for recognition by the viral polymerase for virus genome replication and initiation of virus mRNA transcription.

The genome of bunyaviruses is 11–19 kb and consists of three segments of negative-sense (or ambisense), single-stranded RNA, designated large (L), medium (M), and small (S). The RNA segments differ in size among the genera: the L RNA segment ranges in size from 6.3 to 12 kb, the M RNA segment from 3.5 to 6 kb, and the S RNA segment from 1 to 2.2 kb. The L RNA encodes a single large protein (L), the RNA-dependent RNA polymerase

TABLE 22.2 Properties of Bunyaviruses

Four genera infect vertebrates: *Bunyavirus*, *Phlebovirus*, and *Nairovirus*, all arthropod-borne; *Hantavirus*, non-arthropod-borne

Virions are spherical, enveloped, 80–100 nm in diameter

Virions have glycoprotein spikes but no matrix protein in their envelope

Three nucleocapsid segments with helical symmetry

Segmented negative-sense, single-stranded RNA genome; three segments—L (large), M (medium), and S (small)—that total 11–19 kb in size

The S segment of the genomic RNA of the member viruses of the genus *Phlebovirus* has an *ambisense* coding strategy

Capped 5′ termini of cellular RNAs cannibalized as primers for messenger RNA transcription

Cytoplasmic replication; budding into Golgi vesicles

Generally cytocidal for vertebrate cells, but non-cytocidal persistent infection in invertebrate cells

Genetic reassortment occurs between closely related viruses

(transcriptase). The M RNA encodes a polyprotein that is processed to form two glycoproteins (Gn and Gc) and, in some cases, a non-structural protein (NSm). The S RNA encodes the nucleocapsid (N) protein and, for members of the *Orthobunyavirus* and *Phlebovirus* genera, a non-structural (NSs) protein (Figure 22.2). The N and NSs proteins of viruses in the genus *Phlebovirus* are each translated from a separate subgenomic mRNA. The N protein is encoded in the 3′ half of the S RNA, and its messenger RNA (mRNA) is transcribed using genomic RNA as template. However, the NSs protein, occupying the 5′ half of the same S RNA molecule, is encoded in the reverse complementary sense, with the NSs mRNA being transcribed only after the synthesis of full-length viral genome RNA intermediates; thus the S segment RNA exhibits an ambisense coding strategy.

All bunyaviruses have at least four virion proteins (Figure 22.1), including two external glycoproteins (Gn, Gc), the L protein (transcriptase), and the N protein (nucleoprotein). Virions also contain lipids, with their composition reflecting the composition of host-cell membranes (principally derived from the Golgi membrane, but also cell-surface membrane) and carbohydrates as side chains on the glycoproteins. The Gn glycoprotein (formerly known as G2) is responsible for receptor binding of California serogroups bunyaviruses. The non-structural NSs protein of Rift Valley fever virus interferes with the innate host-cell antiviral response via inhibition of the cell signaling molecules (protein kinase and the transcription factor, TFIIH), leading to global suppression of the type I interferon response.

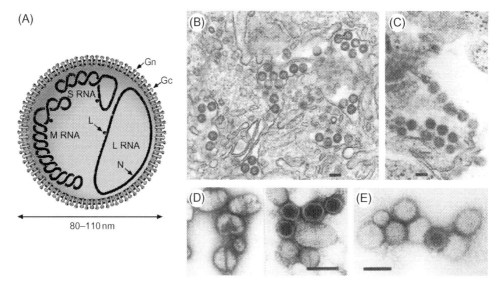

FIGURE 22.1 Diagrammatic representation of a bunyavirus virion in cross section. Family *Bunyaviridae*. (A) Gc, Gn, glycoproteins produced by processing of M RNA polyprotein; L, transcriptase encoded by L RNA; L, M, and S RNA, large, medium, and small RNA segments; N, nucleoprotein encoded by S RNA. (B) Hepatocyte of a rat infected with Rift Valley fever virus, showing virions budding in Golgi vesicles. (C) Thin section of mouse brain infected with California encephalitis virus, showing extracellular virions. (D) Negatively stained Hantaan virus virions, showing the pattern of spike placement in squares that is characteristic of all hantaviruses. (E) Negatively stained Rift Valley fever virus virions, showing the delicate spike fringe. Bars represent 100 nm. *[A: From* Virus Taxonomy: Eighth Report of the International Committee on Taxonomy of Viruses *(C. M. Fauquet, M. A. Mayo, J. Maniloff, U. Desselberger, L. A. Ball, eds.), p. 695. Copyright © Elsevier (2005), with permission. B–E all are reproduced from the 3rd edition of Veterinary Virology.]*

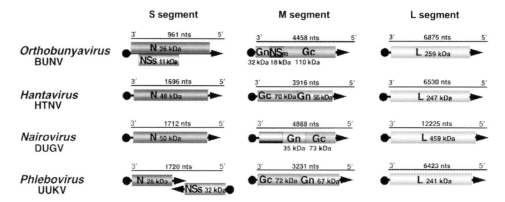

FIGURE 22.2 Coding strategies of genome segments of members of the family *Bunyaviridae*. Genomic RNAs are represented by thin lines (the number of nucleotides is given about the line) and mRNAs are shown as arrows (• indicates host derived primer sequence at 5′-end). Gene products, with their size (in kDa), are represented by solid rectangles. (Modified from Elliott, 1996). BUNV, Bunyamwera virus; DUGV, Dugbe virus; HTNV, Hantaan hantavirus; UUKV, Uukuniemi virus; Gc, Gn, glycoproteins produced by processing of M RNA polyprotein; L, transcriptase encoded by L RNA; L, M, and S RNA, large, medium, and small RNA segments; N, nucleoprotein encoded by S RNA; NSm, NSs, non-structural proteins encoded by M and S RNA, respectively. *[From* Virus Taxonomy: Eighth Report of the International Committee on Taxonomy of Viruses *(C. M. Fauquet, M. A. Mayo, J. Maniloff, U. Desselberger, L. A. Ball, eds.), p. 697. Copyright © Elsevier (2005), with permission.]*

The viruses are quite sensitive to heat and acid conditions, and are inactivated readily by detergents, lipid solvents, and common disinfectants.

Virus Replication

Most bunyaviruses replicate well in many kinds of cells, including Vero (African green monkey) cells, BHK-21 (baby hamster kidney) cells, and, except for hantaviruses, C6/36 mosquito (*Aedes albopictus*) cells. Except for hantaviruses

and some nairoviruses, these viruses are cytolytic for mammalian cells, but are non-cytolytic for invertebrate cells. Most of the viruses also replicate to high titer in suckling mouse brain.

Viral entry into its host cell is by receptor-mediated endocytosis; all subsequent steps take place in the cytoplasm. Cell receptors are not described for many bunyaviruses, but those that contribute to binding of the hantaviruses include $\alpha\beta$ integrins and other cell receptor proteins such as gC1qR/p32, which is expressed on endothelial cells, dendritic cells, lymphocytes, and platelets. Because the genome of the single-stranded, negative-sense RNA viruses cannot be translated directly, the first step after penetration of the host cell and uncoating is the activation of the virion RNA polymerase (transcriptase) and its transcription of viral mRNAs from each of the three virion RNAs. The exception, as noted earlier, is that in the genus *Phlebovirus* the 5′ half of the S RNA is not transcribed directly; instead, the mRNA for the NSs protein is transcribed after synthesis of full-length complementary RNA. The RNA polymerase also has endonuclease activity, cleaving 5′-methylated caps from host mRNAs and adding these to viral mRNAs to prime transcription (so-called cap snatching). After primary viral mRNA transcription and translation, replication of the virion RNA occurs and a second round of transcription begins, amplifying, in particular, the genes that encode structural proteins necessary for virion synthesis.

Virions mature by budding through intracytoplasmic vesicles associated with the Golgi complex and are released by the transport of vesicles through the cytoplasm and release by exocytosis from the apical and/or basolateral plasma membranes (Table 22.2).

MEMBERS OF THE GENUS *ORTHOBUNYAVIRUS*

AKABANE VIRUS

Akabane virus is best known for its teratogenic effects in ruminants, with seasonal epizootics of reproductive loss (embryonic/fetal mortality, abortion) and congenital arthrogryposis and hydranencephaly being well described in cattle in Australia, Japan, and Israel. The virus can cause similar reproductive losses and developmental defects in sheep and goats. Akabane virus and/or closely related viruses occur throughout much of Africa and Asia, in addition to Australia.

Clinical Features and Epidemiology

Akabane virus infection of non-pregnant ruminants typically is inapparent, but infection of pregnant cattle or sheep can lead to one of two outcomes: death of the fetus and abortion, or birth, sometimes premature, of progeny with congenital defects. Affected fetuses characteristically have extensive cavitary defects of the central nervous system (hydranencephaly) and severe musculoskeletal abnormalities (arthrogryposis), thus abortion or birth is often accompanied by dystocia. Fetuses born with hydranencephaly ("bubble brain") usually are unable to stand after birth; those less severely affected may manifest marked incoordination and a variety of other neurologic deficits.

Although the vectors of Akabane virus remain to be conclusively proven, it is believed that the virus is transmitted in Japan by *Aedes* spp. and *Culex* spp. mosquitoes, and in Australia by the midge, *Culicoides brevitarsis*. As Akabane virus is an arthropod-borne virus infection, its transmission is seasonal. The type and severity of clinical signs reflect the stage of gestation at which fetal infection took place, and in herds practicing year-round calving, the entire spectrum of lesions and outcomes can be observed.

Pathogenesis and Pathology

After the bite of an infected mosquito, the virus infects the pregnant ruminant (cow, goat, or sheep) without producing clinical signs, and reaches the fetus from the maternal circulation. The most severe fetal lesions in cattle result from infection at 3–4 months of gestation, and earlier in sheep and goats, when the central nervous system is developing. Fetal infection results in both encephalomyelitis and polymyositis, and virus replication within the developing central nervous system leads to destruction of the developing brain and subsequent hydranencephaly. In general, the earlier the virus reaches the developing cerebrum, the worse the teratogenic defect; in severe cases there is complete absence of the cerebral hemispheres, which are replaced by fluid-filled sacs. Arthrogryposis, the other highly characteristic manifestation of fetal infection with Akabane virus, is characterized by muscular atrophy and the abnormal fixation of several limbs, usually in flexion. Severely affected fetuses usually die and are aborted, whereas those alive at birth often must be euthanized.

Diagnosis

In enzootic areas, diagnosis of Akabane virus infection may be suggested by clinical, pathologic, and epidemiologic observations (seasonal occurrence), but most often by gross pathologic examination. Diagnosis is confirmed by the detection of a specific neutralizing antibody in serum collected from aborted fetuses or from newborn calves, kids, or lambs before ingestion of colostrum. Alternatively, diagnosis may be made by detecting an increase in antibody titer between paired maternal sera. Virus is difficult or impossible to isolate after calves, kids, or lambs are born, but can be recovered from the placenta, fetal brain, or muscle of animals taken before normal parturition by cesarean section or after slaughter of the dam. Virus isolation is carried out in cell cultures or by intracerebral inoculation of suckling mice.

Immunity, Prevention, and Control

Infection with Akabane virus induces lasting immunity, and outbreaks typically are seen outside the limits of recent past outbreaks. Imported naïve animals are also at risk. An inactivated virus vaccine produced in cell culture has proven safe and efficacious.

OTHER TERATOGENIC ORTHOBUNYAVIRUSES

A substantial number of viruses related to Akabane virus potentially can cause similar congenital abnormalities in ruminants, including Aino, Tinaroo, and Peaton viruses. Cache Valley virus, which is a member of another serogroup (Bunyamwera) within the genus *Orthobunyaviridae*, is the cause of sporadic outbreaks of arthrogryposis-hydranencephaly in sheep in the United States. Cache Valley virus is transmitted by mosquitoes.

LA CROSSE AND OTHER CALIFORNIA ENCEPHALITIS SEROGROUP VIRUSES

The California serogroup in the genus *Orthobunyavirus* includes at least 14 individual viruses, each of which is transmitted by mosquitoes and has a narrow range of vertebrate hosts and a limited geographic distribution. There is no evidence that there is any clinical disease associated with these viruses in animals other than humans. However, the infection in reservoir host animals and mosquitoes is the key to the understanding and prevention of the associated human diseases. The most important zoonotic pathogen in the California serogroup is La Crosse virus, which is maintained by transovarial transmission in *Aedes triseriatus*, a tree-hole-breeding woodland mosquito, and is amplified by a mosquito–vertebrate–mosquito cycle involving silent infection of woodland rodents, such as squirrels and chipmunks. The virus occurs throughout the eastern and midwestern United States; a closely related virus, snowshoe hare virus, occupies a similar niche in Canada. Most cases occur during the summer months in children and young adults who are exposed to vector mosquitoes in wooded areas. Humans are dead-end hosts, and there is no human-to-human transmission. The encephalitis caused by La Crosse virus is relatively benign compared with that caused by other encephalitis viruses, but it clearly can be devastating to individual patients: about 10% of children develop seizures during the acute disease and a few develop persistent paresis and learning disabilities. The mortality rate is less than 1%. It is now estimated that, annually, there are well over 100,000 human infections and at least 100 cases of encephalitis in the United States. This disease had been occurring regularly for many decades, long before the causative virus was identified.

OTHER ORTHOBUNYAVIRUSES

Infections of animals with other orthobunyaviruses clearly occur, although the pathogenic significance of many of these infections remains conjectural. Main Drain virus has been implicated as a sporadic and uncommon cause of encephalomyelitis in horses. Similarly, horses and other animals in enzootic regions are infected with California

serogroups viruses related to Jamestown Canyon virus, and Bunyamwera serogroups viruses related to Northway virus.

MEMBERS OF THE GENUS *PHLEBOVIRUS*

RIFT VALLEY FEVER VIRUS

Clinical Features and Epidemiology

Epizootics of Rift Valley fever in sheep, goats, and cattle have occurred at regular intervals in southern and eastern African countries from the time when intensive livestock husbandry was introduced at the beginning of the 20th century (Figure 22.3). An exceptionally devastating epizootic occurred in Egypt in 1977 and 1979, resembling the biblical description of one of the plagues of ancient Egypt. In addition to hundreds of thousands of cases in sheep and cattle, there were an estimated 200,000 human cases, with 600 reported deaths. In late 1997 and 1998, a major epizootic spread from Somalia through Kenya into Tanzania, causing the death of many thousands of sheep, goats, and camels, and more than 90,000 human cases, with some 500 deaths. This epizootic, considered the largest ever seen in eastern Africa, was blamed on exceptional rainfall as a result of an El Nino weather pattern. An extensive epizootic in Yemen and Saudi Arabia in 2000 was the first recognition of the disease outside Africa.

Rift Valley fever virus survives in enzootic regions of Africa in a silent infection cycle and emerges after periods of exceptionally heavy rainfall, to initiate disease epizootics (Figure 22.4). It was discovered in the late 1980s that the virus is transmitted transovarially among floodwater *Aedes* spp. mosquitoes; the virus survives for very long periods in mosquito eggs laid at the edges of usually dry depressions, called "dambos," which are common throughout grassy plateau regions. When the rains come and the dambos flood, the eggs hatch, and infected mosquitoes emerge and infect nearby wild and domestic animals.

In an epizootic, virus is amplified in wild and domestic animals by many species of *Culex* and other *Aedes* mosquitoes. These mosquitoes become very numerous after heavy rains or when improper irrigation techniques are used; they feed indiscriminately on viremic sheep and cattle (and humans). A very high level of viremia is maintained for 3–5 days in infected sheep and cattle, allowing many more mosquitoes to become infected. This amplification, together with mechanical transmission by biting flies, results in infection and disease in a very high proportion of animals and humans at risk. In its epizootic cycles, Rift Valley fever virus is also spread mechanically by fomites and by blood and tissues of infected animals. Infected sheep have a very high level of viremia, and transmission

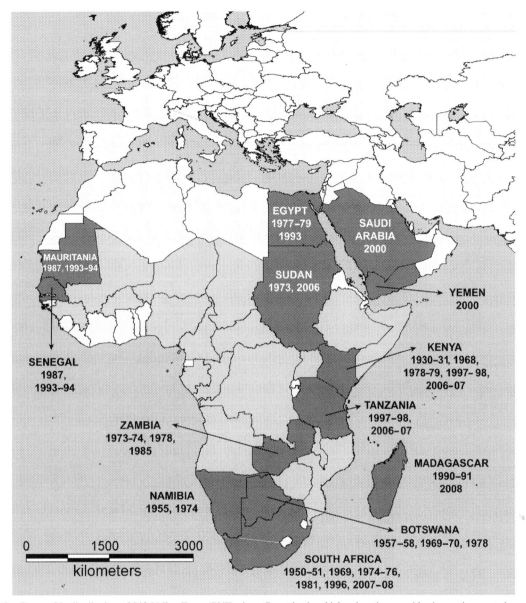

FIGURE 22.3 Geographic distribution of Rift Valley Fever (RVF) virus. Countries in which epizootics or epidemics are known to have occurred are indicated in red with the date of each outbreak. Countries with evidence of low-level enzootic activity (antibody prevalence or occasional RVF virus isolation) are indicated in pink. To convert kilometers to miles, multiply by 0.625. [*From B. H. Bird, T. G. Ksiazek, S. T. Nichol, N. J. MacLachlan. Rift Valley fever virus. J. Am. Vet. Med. Assoc. 234, 883–893 (2009), with permission.*]

at the time of abortion, via contaminated placentae and fetal and maternal blood, is a particular problem. Abattoir workers and veterinarians (especially those performing necropsies) are often infected directly.

The capacity of Rift Valley fever virus to be transmitted without the involvement of an arthropod vector raises concerns over the possibility for its importation into non-enzootic areas via contaminated materials, animal products, viremic humans, or non-livestock animal species. Once it is established in previously free regions, it would be difficult or impossible to eradicate the virus, because of the many mosquito species capable of efficient virus transmission and the phenomenon of transovarial transmission.

For example, experimental mosquito transmission studies have shown that more than 30 common mosquitoes in the United States could serve as efficient vectors.

The incubation period is short in animals infected with Rift Valley fever virus—typically less than 3 days. Infected sheep develop fever, inappetence, mucopurulent nasal discharge, and bloody diarrhea. Under field conditions, 90–100% of pregnant ewes abort ("abortion storm") and there is a mortality rate of 90% in lambs and 20–60% in adult sheep. The clinical disease and outcome are similar in goats. In cattle the disease is somewhat less severe, with mortality rates in calves and cows of 10–30%, but 90–100% of pregnant cows may abort. A variety of other animals can

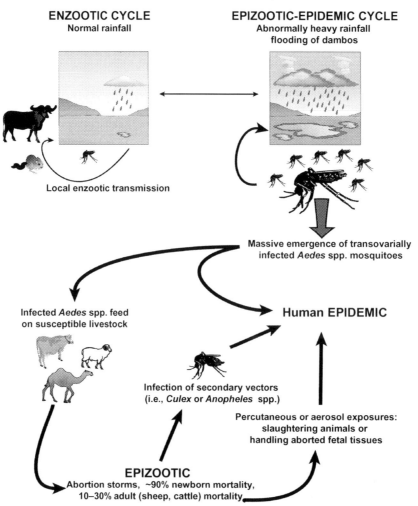

FIGURE 22.4 Enzootic and epidemic-epizootic transmission cycles of Rift Valley Fever (RVF) virus. In the enzootic transmission cycle (top left panel), wildlife (e.g., African buffalo species) are potential maintenance hosts. In the epidemic-epizootic transmission cycle (remainder of figure), live-stock amplification hosts and secondary bridge vectors are involved. *[From B. H. Bird, T. G. Ksiazek, S. T. Nichol, N. J. MacLachlan. Rift Valley fever virus. J. Am. Vet. Med. Assoc. 234 , 883 – 893 (2009), with permission.]*

be infected (camels, dogs, cats) but, unless they are very young, rarely develop serious clinical disease (Figure 22.5).

Rift Valley fever virus is zoonotic and causes an important human disease that occurs coincidentally with outbreaks in sheep, cattle, and camels. The human disease begins after a very short incubation period (2–6 days) with fever, severe headache, chills, "back-breaking" myalgia, diarrhea, vomiting, and hemorrhages. Usually the clinical disease lasts 4–6 days, followed by a prolonged convalescence and complete recovery. A small percentage of infected humans develop more severe disease, with liver necrosis, hemorrhagic pneumonia, renal failure, meningoencephalitis, and retinitis with vision loss. The case-fatality rate is about 1–2%, but in patients with hemorrhagic disease it may reach 10%. Vaccination can be used to prevent human disease, especially those most at risk, such as veterinarians, and livestock and abattoir workers.

All research and diagnostic procedures with Rift Valley fever virus are restricted to certain national laboratories. The virus is a BioSafety Level 3+ pathogen, and must be handled in the laboratory under strict biocontainment conditions, to prevent human exposure.

Pathogenesis and Pathology

Rift Valley fever virus replicates rapidly and to very high titer in target tissues. After entry by mosquito bite, percutaneous injury, or through the oropharynx via aerosols, there is an incubation period of 30–72 hours, during which virus invades the parenchyma of the liver and lymphoreticular organs. Extensive hepatocellular necrosis is common in terminally affected sheep. The spleen is enlarged and there are gastrointestinal and subserosal hemorrhages. Encephalitis, evidenced by neuronal necrosis and perivascular inflammatory infiltration,

(A) Infection and host response

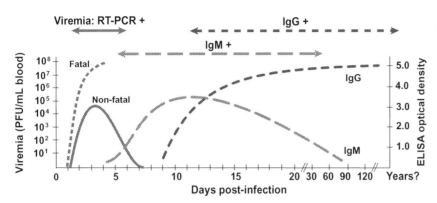

(B) Clinical signs—livestock

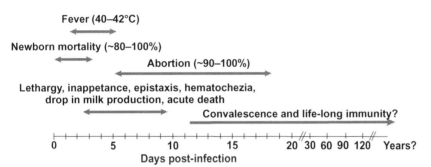

FIGURE 22.5   Generalized time course of viremia and antibody response against Rift Valley Fever (RVF) virus in livestock (A) and the development of RVF disease among livestock (B) and humans (C). In panel A, the intervals during which diagnostic testing involving nucleic acid-based (RT-PCR assays) and serologic (RVF virus-specific IgM or IgG) assays are appropriate are indicated in relation to the period of viremia. *[From B. H. Bird, T. G. Ksiazek, S. T. Nichol, N. J. MacLachlan. Rift Valley fever virus. J. Am. Vet. Med. Assoc. **234**, 883–893 (2009), with permission.]*

(C) Clinical signs—humans

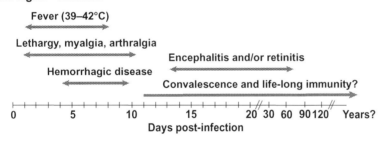

is a late event that occurs in a small proportion of animals surviving the hepatic infection. Hepatic necrosis, renal failure, and shock, sometimes with hemorrhagic complications, are the primary causes of death. In survivors, recovery is rapid and immunity is long lasting. Experimentally, the virus infects a wide variety of laboratory and domestic animals and is often lethal. In experimentally infected animals, the two most frequent syndromes are hepatitis and encephalitis.

Diagnosis

Because of its broad geographic distribution and its explosive potential for invading new areas where livestock husbandry is extensive, the laboratory confirmation of the presence of Rift Valley fever virus is treated as a diagnostic emergency. Rapid diagnosis is achieved using reverse-transcriptase-polymerase chain reaction (RT-PCR) assays, and can be confirmed by virus isolation by intracerebral inoculation of mice or in cell culture. The virus replicates in a variety of cell cultures such as Vero E6 and BHK-21 cells, and the virus is rapidly cytopathic and causes plaques. Nucleic acid sequencing and immunologic methods are used to prove the identity of isolates. Serologic diagnosis is by immunoglobulin (IgM) capture enzyme immunoassay on single acute sera, or by enzyme immunoassays, neutralization, or hemagglutination-inhibition assays on paired sera from surviving animals (Figure 22.5). Veterinarians and laboratory workers are at substantial risk during post-mortem examination of animals or processing diagnostic materials in the laboratory.

Immunity, Prevention, and Control

Control is based primarily on livestock vaccination, but vector control (via use of mosquito larvicides and insecticides) is also used during outbreaks. In addition, environmental management can be a useful control strategy, including assessment of the risk of creating new larval habitats (water impoundments, artificial dambos) in enzootic areas.

Attenuated-virus Rift Valley fever vaccines produced in mouse brain and in embryonated eggs are effective and inexpensive for use in sheep, but they cause abortions in pregnant ewes. Inactivated-virus vaccines produced in cell cultures avoid the problem of abortion, but are expensive. Both types of vaccines have been produced in Africa in large quantities, but to be fully effective vaccines must be delivered in a systematic way to entire animal populations, preferably on a regular schedule before the start of the mosquito season, or at least at the first indications of virus activity (as determined by sentinel surveillance). However, virus spread is so rapid in epizootics that it is difficult to administer enough vaccine rapidly enough. Even when vaccine is delivered quickly, there is often not enough time for protective immunity to develop. Thus disease control is expensive, rather ineffective, and very demanding in terms of fiscal and human resources—these realities have led to resistance to vaccination among farmers and ranchers in most areas of southern Africa. Several new vaccines are under development for use in both animals and humans, using recombinant DNA technology that allows for the differentiation of vaccinated from naturally infected animals (DIVA).

MEMBERS OF THE GENUS *NAIROVIRUS*

NAIROBI SHEEP DISEASE VIRUS

Nairobi sheep disease virus, a member of the genus *Nairovirus*, is highly pathogenic for sheep and goats. The virus is enzootic in eastern Africa, and closely related viruses occur in Nigeria (Dugbe virus in cattle), and in India and Sri Lanka (Ganjam virus in sheep and goats). The virus is not contagious among mammals; rather, it is transmitted by all stages of the brown ear tick, *Rhipicephalus appendiculatus*, in which there is transovarial and transstadial infection and very long-term carriage in adult ticks (up to 2 years). The vertebrate reservoir host of the virus remains unknown; the virus has not been found in wild ruminants or other animals in enzootic areas.

In Kenya, sheep and goats acquire the infection when they are transported from northern districts to the Nairobi area. After a short incubation period, there is high fever, hemorrhagic enteritis, and prostration. Affected animals may die within a few days, and pregnant ewes abort.

Mortality in sheep is 30–90%. Subclinical infections also occur, and recovered animals are immune. Diagnosis is made clinically and by gross pathologic examination; it may be confirmed by virus isolation and identification of isolates immunologically, or by simple immunodiffusion tests on tissue extracts utilizing hyperimmune virus-specific antisera. Control depends primarily on dipping to control the vector tick, which is also the vector of the economically important protozoan disease, East Coast fever. Both live-attenuated and inactivated vaccines are effective in preventing the disease in sheep.

The virus is not considered to be a significant human pathogen, although it was isolated from a person with a mild febrile disease. However, Nairobi sheep disease virus is a restricted animal pathogen; its importation or possession is prohibited by law or regulation by most national governments.

CRIMEAN-CONGO HEMORRHAGIC FEVER VIRUS

Crimean-Congo hemorrhagic fever virus, a member of the genus *Nairovirus*, is the cause of an important zoonotic disease (Crimean-Congo hemorrhagic fever) that had been recognized for many years in central Asia and Eastern Europe. There is no evidence of clinical disease in animals other than humans, but the infection in domestic animals is the basis for the overall importance of this disease. This virus is now known to be enzootic from western China, through Central Asia to India, Pakistan, Afghanistan, Iran, Iraq, Turkey, Greece, other countries of the Middle East, Eastern Europe, and most of Saharan and sub-Saharan Africa. In recent years, there have been repeated outbreaks of the disease in Turkey and the countries of the Persian Gulf, especially in connection with traditional sheep slaughtering and butchering practices. Crimean-Congo hemorrhagic fever is an emerging problem, with increasingly more cases being reported each year from many parts of the world, and increasing detection of antibody in animal populations. For example, in serosurveys, more than 8% of cattle in several regions of Africa have been shown to be seropositive.

The virus is maintained by a cycle involving transovarial and trans-stadial transmission in *Hyalomma* spp. and many related ticks. Larval and nymphal ticks become infected when feeding on small mammals and ground-dwelling birds, and adult ticks when feeding on wild and domestic ruminants (sheep, goats, and cattle). Infection in wild and domestic ruminants results in high-titer viremia that is sufficient to infect feeding ticks.

The disease in humans is a severe hemorrhagic fever. The incubation period is 3–7 days; onset is abrupt, with fever, severe headache, myalgia, back and abdominal pain, nausea and vomiting, and marked prostration. It is one of the most dramatic of all human hemorrhagic fevers, characterized by substantial hemorrhage within the subcutis and at mucosal surfaces lining the gastrointestinal and genitourinary tracts. There is also marked liver necrosis, and injury to both the myocardium and central nervous system; the case-fatality rate is commonly 15–40%. The disease affects primarily farmers, veterinarians, slaughter-house workers, butchers, and others coming in contact with livestock, forest-workers, and others coming in contact with infected ticks. The virus is also transmitted by direct contact with subclinically infected viremic animals—for example, during sheep docking, shearing, antihelminthic drenching, and veterinary procedures. The virus is also contagious, and can be transmitted from human to human, especially in hospitals.

Diagnosis is made by the detection of antigen in tissues (usually by immunofluorescence) or IgM antibody (by antigen-capture ELISA.) A recently developed RT-PCR assay is also valuable. Virus isolation has proven difficult: the virus is very labile, shipping of diagnostic specimens from usual sites of disease is often less than satisfactory, and all laboratory work must be performed under maximum containment conditions.

Inactivated vaccines have been developed and used in small-scale trials, but are generally not available. Prevention based on vector control is difficult because of the large areas of wooded and brushy tick habitat involved. One important prevention approach would be the enforcement, in endemic areas of Asia, the Middle East, and Africa, of occupational safety standards on farms and in livestock markets, abattoirs, and other workplaces where there is routine contact with sheep, goats, and cattle. Individual risk can be minimized in people living in endemic zones by avoiding tick bites through inspection of clothing and application of repellents.

MEMBERS OF THE GENUS *HANTAVIRUS*

The more than 20 member viruses of the genus *Hantavirus* comprise the only viruses in the family *Bunyaviridae* that are not arthropod borne. They are transmitted among rodents by long-term shedding in saliva, urine, and feces. Several of the viruses are zoonotic and the cause of severe human disease. Although there is overlap in the respective disease syndromes, four Old World (Asia and Europe) hantaviruses cause multisystem disease centered on the kidneys (*hemorrhagic fever with renal syndrome*), whereas several New World (the Americas) hantaviruses cause multisystem disease centered on the lungs (*hantavirus pulmonary syndrome*). The pathogenicity of some of the newly discovered viruses has not yet been determined. Some viruses also infect other mammalian species, such as horses, but this is uncommon and does not contribute to the life cycle of the viruses or to the risk of human disease.

One important aspect of the hantaviruses has been the level of difficulty surrounding their discovery. For example,

during the Korean war of 1950–1952, thousands of United Nations' troops developed a disease marked by fever, headache, hemorrhagic manifestations, and acute renal failure, with shock and substantial mortality of 5–10%. Despite intense research, the etiologic agent of this disease remained a mystery for 28 years until the prototype hantavirus, Hantaan virus (the name is derived from the Hantaan River in Korea), was isolated from the striped field mouse, *Apodemus agrarius*. Hantaviruses discovered since then have also been so difficult to isolate in cell culture or experimental animals that RT-PCR assays have become a key tool for obtaining diagnostic sequences from clinical specimens and rodent tissues. More than 200,000 cases of hemorrhagic fever with renal syndrome are reported each year throughout the world, with more than half in China. Russia and Korea report hundreds to thousands of cases; fewer are reported from Japan, Finland, Sweden, Bulgaria, Greece, Hungary, France, and the Balkan countries.

In 1993, a new zoonotic hantavirus disease was recognized in the southwestern region of the United States. The disease was manifest, not as hemorrhagic fever with renal syndrome, but rather as an acute respiratory distress syndrome. The virus responsible for the 1993 cases is now called Sin Nombre virus, and at least eight other hantaviruses have since been identified as causes of the pulmonary syndrome, including Bayou, Black Creek Canal, Andes, and Laguna Negra viruses. Cases of hantavirus pulmonary syndrome have been reported across the United States, and from Canada to Argentina. Other New World hantaviruses have been discovered recently, but their pathogenicity in humans has not yet been determined.

HEMORRHAGIC FEVER WITH RENAL SYNDROME (OLD WORLD) HANTAVIRUSES

The hallmark of hantavirus infection in rodent reservoir hosts is persistent, usually life-long, inapparent infection and shedding in saliva, urine, and feces. Human disease involves contact with contaminated rodent excreta, usually in winter when there is maximal human–rodent contact. In a landmark pathogenesis study, H. W. Lee inoculated the reservoir rodent, *Apodemus agrarius*, with Hantaan virus and followed the course of infection by virus titration of organs, serology, and immunofluorescence. Viremia was transient and disappeared as neutralizing antibodies appeared. However, virus persisted in several organs, including lungs and kidneys. Virus titers in urine and throat swabs were about 100 to 1000 times higher during the first weeks after inoculation than subsequently, and animals were much more infectious for cage mates or nearby mice during this period.

Four essential features define the global context of the disease hemorrhagic fever with renal syndrome (Table 22.1): (1) the viruses, *per se*; (2) their reservoir rodent hosts; (3) the locale of human cases; (4) the severity of human cases. At least four viruses are involved: Hantaan, Dobrava-Belgrade, Seoul, and Puumala viruses. Typically, the Hantaan and Dobrava-Belgrade viruses cause severe disease, with mortality rates of 5–15%. Seoul virus causes less severe disease, and Puumala virus causes the least severe form of the disease (mortality rate less than 1%), which is known in Scandinavia as "nephropathia epidemica." There are three disease locale patterns: rural, urban, and laboratory acquired. Rural disease is caused by Hantaan virus, which is widespread in China, Asian Russia, and Korea, and Dobrava-Belgrade virus in the Balkans and Greece. Rural disease is also caused by Puumala virus in northern Europe, especially in Scandinavia and Russia. Urban disease is caused by Seoul virus; it occurs in Japan, Korea, China, and South and North America. Each virus has a specific reservoir rodent host. For Hantaan virus this is the striped field mouse, *Apodemus agrarius*; for Dobrava-Belgrade virus it is the yellow-neck mouse, *Apodemus flavicollis*; for Seoul virus it is the Norway rat, *Rattus norvegicus*; and for Puumala virus it is the bank vole, *Clethrionomys glareolus*.

There is no evidence that there is any clinical disease in animals other than humans. The clinical course of severe hemorrhagic fever with renal syndrome in humans involves five overlapping stages—febrile, hypotensive, oliguric, diuretic, and convalescent—not all of which are seen in every case. The onset of the disease is sudden, with intense headache, backache, fever, and chills. Hemorrhage, if it occurs, is manifested during the febrile stage as a flushing of the face and injection of the conjunctiva and mucous membranes. A petechial rash may also appear. Sudden and extreme hypotension from vascular leakage can precipitate fatal hypovolemic shock, and patients who survive and progress to the diuretic stage show improved renal function but may still die of shock or pulmonary complications. The convalescent stage can last for weeks to months before recovery is complete. The disease in affected individuals is believed to have an immunopathologic basis, as virus-specific antibodies are present, usually from the first day that the patient presents for medical care.

Diagnosis is made by the detection of antigen in tissues (usually by immunofluorescence) or serologically by IgG and IgM capture ELISA. The IgM capture ELISA is the primary diagnostic tool in reference diagnostics centers, but RT-PCR assays are now available. Virus isolation is difficult: the viruses must be blind-passaged in cell culture (most commonly Vero E6 cells) and detected by immunologic or molecular means. Shipping of diagnostic specimens from sites of disease is often less than satisfactory, and all laboratory work on Hantaan and other highly pathogenic hantaviruses must be done under strict biocontainment conditions.

Several inactivated Hantaan virus vaccines have been developed and used in Asia. The key to preventing hantavirus infections is rodent control, including making homes and food stores rodent proof and removing dead rodents and rodent droppings from human habitations. However, control of the wide-ranging rodent reservoirs of Hantaan, Seoul, and Puumala viruses is not possible in most settings in which disease occurs; nevertheless, in some situations their entry into dwellings can be minimized.

There have been several instances in which wild rodents brought into laboratories, established colonies of laboratory rats, and even cell cultures derived from rats have carried or been contaminated with hantaviruses, and have led to virus transmission to animal caretakers and research personnel. Prevention of introduction of virus into laboratory rat colonies requires quarantined entry of new stock (or entry only of known virus-free stock), prevention of access by wild rodents, and regular serologic testing.

HANTAVIRUS PULMONARY SYNDROME (NEW WORLD) HANTAVIRUSES

Sin Nombre virus and other New World hantaviruses probably have been present for eons in extensive portions of the Americas inhabited by *Peromyscus maniculatus* and other reservoir rodent species; they were recognized in 1993 only because of the number and clustering of human cases of a very distinctive disease syndrome in the western United States. A great increase in rodent numbers after two especially wet winters and a consequent increase in pinyon seeds and other rodent food contributed to the number of human cases. The temporal distribution of human disease reflects a spring–summer seasonality (although cases have occurred throughout the year), again matching the behavior patterns of rodent reservoir hosts. Just as with Old World hantaviruses, each New World virus has a specific reservoir rodent host: Sin Nombre virus—the deer mouse, *P. maniculatus*; New York virus—the white-footed mouse, *P. leucopus*; Black Creek Canal virus—the cotton rat, *Sigmodon hispidus*; Bayou virus—the rice rat, *Oryzomys palustris*; and Andes virus—the long-tailed pygmy rice rat, *Oligoryzomys longicaudatus*.

Like the hantaviruses that cause hemorrhagic fever with renal syndrome, those that induce hantavirus pulmonary syndrome do not cause disease in their rodent reservoir hosts, but can induce severe disease in infected humans. The virus is shed in saliva, urine, and feces of rodents for at least many weeks, and probably the lifetime of the animal. Transmission from rodent to rodent occurs by close contact and from bite or scratch wounds. Transmission and human infection probably also occur by the inhalation of aerosols or dust containing infected dried rodent saliva or excreta.

Hantavirus pulmonary syndrome in humans typically starts with fever, myalgia, headache, nausea, vomiting, non-productive cough, and shortness of breath. As disease progresses, there is pulmonary edema, pleural effusions, and rapid disease progression, with death often following in hours to days. Recovery can be as rapid as the development of life-threatening clinical signs. Functional impairment of vascular endothelial integrity with subsequent hypovolemic shock is central to the pathogenesis of the disease. Lesions are those of the acute respiratory distress syndrome, with pulmonary congestion and edema and interstitial pneumonia. Person-to-person transmission appears to be rare, but has been confirmed in cases of Andes virus infection, and strict barrier nursing techniques are now recommended for management of suspected cases.

Increased capillary permeability, especially of the pulmonary vasculature, is central to the pathogenesis of hantavirus-induced pulmonary syndrome. However, although there is widespread hantavirus infection of endothelial cells in affected individuals, hantaviruses do not cause lytic infection. It is uncertain what causes this severe, often fatal increase in capillary permeability that results ultimately in hypovolemic shock, but virus-induced cytokine mediators probably contribute (so-called *cytokine storm*).

The clinical and hematologic findings of hantavirus pulmonary syndrome are characteristic, but the specific diagnosis is usually made by demonstrating antibodies to the infecting virus or one of its close relatives (typically using IgM capture ELISA). Isolation of the virus from patients is very difficult, but viral nucleic acid is readily detected by RT-PCR. Serological testing is usually performed to evaluate infection in reservoir rodent hosts, because of the biohazard associated with virus isolation.

Extensive public education programs have been developed to advise people about reducing the risk of infection, mostly by reducing rodent habitats and food supplies in and near homes, and by taking precautions when cleaning rodent-contaminated areas. The latter involves rodent-proofing food and pet food containers, trapping and poisoning rodents in and around dwellings, eliminating rodent habitats near dwellings, use of respirators, and wetting down surfaces with detergent, disinfectant, or hypochlorite solution before cleaning areas that may contain rodent excreta. Recommendations have also been developed for specific equipment and practices to reduce risks when working with wild-caught rodents, especially when this involves obtaining tissue or blood specimens: these include use of live-capture traps, protective clothing and gloves, suitable disinfectants, and safe transport packaging.

Arenaviridae

Chapter Contents

The fundamental determinant in the ecology of arenaviruses and their importance as zoonotic pathogens is their ancient co-evolutionary relationships with their reservoir rodent hosts. The risk of transmission of each virus to humans relates to the nature of the infection of its rodent host (usually persistent asymptomatic infection with life-long virus shedding), rodent population dynamics and behavior, in addition to human occupational and other risk factors that lead to exposure to virus-laden rodent excreta. The consequences of human exposure include some of the most lethal hemorrhagic fevers known: Lassa, Argentine (Junin virus), Bolivian (Machupo virus), Venezuelan (Guanarito virus), and Brazilian (Sabiá virus) hemorrhagic fevers. The viruses that cause these diseases are BioSafety Level 4 pathogens; they must be handled in the laboratory under maximum containment conditions to prevent human exposure.

The prototype arenavirus, lymphocytic choriomeningitis virus, has over many years played two disparate roles in comparative virology: wild-type strains of the virus are zoonotic pathogens and the subject of public health surveillance in some countries where they are enzootic, whereas laboratory strains have provided much of the conceptual basis for current understanding of viral immunology and pathogenesis.

PROPERTIES OF ARENAVIRUSES

Classification

The family *Arenaviridae* contains a single genus, *Arenavirus*, which is divided into two evolutionary subgroups based on genetic and serologic characteristics (Table 23.1). The first subgroup, the Old World arenaviruses, includes lymphocytic choriomeningitis virus, which is allied with the common house mouse, *Mus musculus*. This virus is now enzootic throughout the world because of global colonization by *Mus musculus*. Other Old World arenaviruses are associated with *Mastomys* spp. and *Praomys* spp. in Africa. The African viruses include Lassa virus, which produces severe disease in humans, and a few other viruses that infect humans but are not known to cause disease. The second subgroup includes the New World arenaviruses (also called the Tacaribe complex), which are associated with many different rodents in North, Central, and South America. This subgroup, which is further subdivided into three distinct clades, contains the important human pathogens Junin, Machupo, Guanarito, and Sabiá viruses, and several other viruses that are pathogenic for humans.

Virion Properties

Arenavirus virions are highly pleomorphic. Their size ranges from 50 to 300 nm, although most virions have a diameter of 110–130 nm (Figure 23.1). Virions are composed of an envelope covered with club-shaped spikes 8–10 nm in length composed of viral glycoproteins GP1 and GP2. Virions contain at least two circular helical nucleocapsid segments, each resembling a string of beads. The nucleocapsids are circular as a consequence of the genomic RNA forming "panhandles"—that is, non-covalent bonds

Fenner's Veterinary Virology. DOI: 10.1016/B978-0-12-375158-4.00023-7

TABLE 23.1 Natural History and Zoonotic Disease Potential of Arenaviruses

Virus	Natural Host	Geographic Distribution	Human Disease
Old World Arenaviruses			
Lymphocytic choriomeningitis virus	*Mus musculus*	Worldwide	"Grippe-like" disease, meningitis, meningoencephalitis
Lassa virus	*Mastomys natalensis*	West Africa	Hemorrhagic fever (Lassa fever)
Mopeia virus	*Mastomys natalensis*	Southern Africa	Infection, no disease
Mobala virus	*Praomys jacksoni*	Central African Republic	Infection, no disease
Ippy virus	*Arvicanthus* spp.	Central African Republic	Infection, no disease
New World Arenaviruses			
Junin virus	*Calomys musculinus, C. laucha, Akodon azarae*	Argentina	Hemorrhagic fever (Argentine hemorrhagic fever)
Machupo virus	*Calomys callosus*	Bolivia	Hemorrhagic fever (Bolivian hemorrhagic fever)
Guanarito virus	*Zygodontomys brevicauda, Oryzomys* spp.	Venezuela	Hemorrhagic fever (Venezuelan hemorrhagic fever)
Sabiá virus	Unknown	Brazil	Hemorrhagic fever (Brazilian hemorrhagic fever)
Tacaribe virus	Unknown, possibly *Artibeus* spp. bats	Trinidad	None, except for one laboratory-acquired case of systemic disease
Whitewater Arroyo virus	*Neotoma albigula*	United States	Hemorrhagic fever
Pirital virus	*Sigmodon alstoni*	Venezuela	Unknown
El-Arroyo virus	Unknown	United States	Unknown
Oliveros virus	*Bolomys obscurus*	Argentina	Unknown
Amapari virus	*Oryzomys goeldi, Neacomys guinae*	Brazil	None
Flexal virus	*Oryzomys* spp.	Brazil	None
Latino virus	*Calomys callosus*	Bolivia	None
Parana virus	*Oryzomys buccinatus*	Paraguay	None
Pichinde virus	*Oryzomys albigularis*	Colombia	None
Tamiami virus	*Sigmodon hispidus*	Florida, United States	None

between conserved complementary nucleotide sequences at the 3′ and 5′ ends of each RNA genome segment. The family derives its name from the presence within virions of cellular ribosomes, which, under thin-section electron microscopy, resemble grains of sand (*arena*, sand). The biological significance of this distinctive and unusual property remains uncertain. The genome of arenaviruses consists of two segments of single-stranded RNA, designated large (L) and small (S), approximately 7.5 and 3.5 kb in size, respectively. Virions may contain multiple copies of the two genome segments, often with more copies of the S RNA segment.

Most of the genome is of negative sense, but the 5′ half of the S segment and the 5′ end of the L segment are of positive sense; the term *ambisense* is used to describe this unusual genome arrangement, which is also

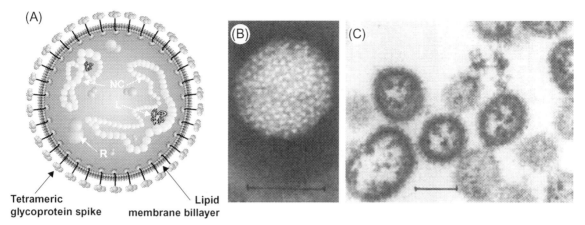

FIGURE 23.1 (A) Diagrammatic representation of virion structure, family *Arenaviridae*. L, L protein (RNA polymerase); NC, nucleocapsid; R, ribosome. *(Courtesy of A. Featherstone and C. Clegg.)* (B) Tacaribe virus, negative-stain electron microscopy. (C) Lassa virus—the presence of dense granules indicate the presence of non-functioning host-cell ribosomes within virions and is a characteristic of all arenaviruses; thin-section electron microscopy. Bars represent 100 nm. *[A: From* Virus Taxonomy: Eighth Report of the International Committee on Taxonomy of Viruses *(C. M. Fauquet, M. A. Mayo, J. Maniloff, U. Desselberger, L. A. Ball, eds.), p. 725. Copyright © Elsevier (2005), with permission.]*

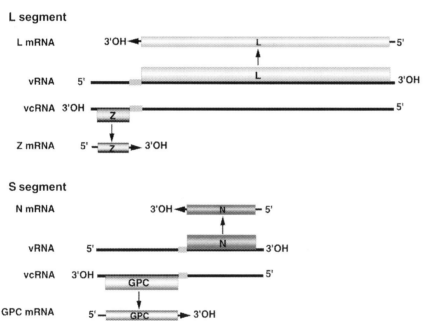

FIGURE 23.2 Organization, transcription and replication of the arenavirus L and S RNAs. Regions encoding the L, Z, GPC and N proteins are shown as boxes with arrow heads indicating the notional direction of translation. The intergenic regions separating the open reading frames (ORFs) are indicated by gray boxes. The sgRNAs which function as messengers are shaded grey. RNA transcription processes are indicated by solid arrows. (from V. Romanowski). GPC, glycoprotein precursor; L, RNA polymerase; N, nucleoprotein; vRNA, viral-sense RNA; vcRNA, viral complementary-sense RNA; Z, zinc-binding protein. *[From* Virus Taxonomy: Eighth Report of the International Committee on Taxonomy of Viruses *(C. M. Fauquet, M. A. Mayo, J. Maniloff, U. Desselberger, L. A. Ball, eds.), p. 727. Copyright © Elsevier (2005), with permission.]*

found in some members of the family *Bunyaviridae* (Figure 23.2). Specifically, the nucleoprotein (N) is encoded in the 3′ half of the complementary-sense S RNA, whereas the viral glycoprotein precursor (GPC) is encoded in the 5′ half of the viral-sense S RNA. The RNA polymerase (L) is encoded in the 3′ end of the complementary-sense L RNA and a zinc-binding protein (Z) is encoded in the 5′ end of the viral-sense L RNA. RNAs contain hairpin configurations between the genes (intergenic regions) that function to terminate transcription from viral and viral-complementary RNAs. The mRNAs are capped—5′-methylated caps are cleaved from host mRNAs by the viral RNA-dependent RNA polymerase (transcriptase), which also has endonuclease activity, and are added to viral mRNAs to prime transcription (so-called cap snatching).

The viruses are quite sensitive to heat and acid conditions, and are inactivated readily by detergents, lipid solvents, and common disinfectants.

Virus Replication

Arenaviruses replicate non-cytolytically to high titer in many kinds of cells, including Vero (African green monkey) and BHK-21 (baby hamster kidney) cells. Virus replication occurs in the cytoplasm. The viral spike glycoprotein attaches to a cell receptor, which can be transferrin receptor 1 for several New World arenaviruses and cell surface glycoproteins for lymphocytic choriomeningitis virus. Entry and endosomal uptake occur via either clathrin-dependent or clathrin-independent pathways,

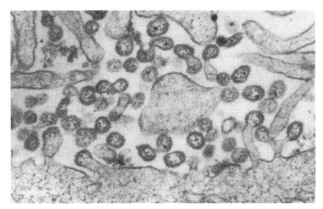

FIGURE 23.3 Prolific budding of Lassa virus from the plasma membrane of an infected Vero cell. Magnification: ×70,000.

perhaps depending on the individual species of arenavirus. Specifically, it is proposed that New World arenaviruses such as Junin virus utilize clathrin-mediated endocytosis, whereas Old World arenaviruses such as lymphocytic choriomeningitis and Lassa viruses utilize a clathrin-independent pathway. Because the genome of the single-stranded, negative-sense RNA viruses cannot be translated directly, the first step in replication is activation of the virion RNA polymerase (transcriptase). The ambisense coding strategy of the arenavirus genome means that only the nucleoprotein (N) and polymerase (L protein) mRNAs are transcribed directly from genomic RNA before translation (Figure 23.2). Newly synthesized polymerase and nucleocapsid proteins facilitate the synthesis of full-length, complementary-sense RNA, which then serves as template for the transcription of glycoprotein (GP) and zinc-binding protein (Z) mRNAs and the synthesis of more full-length, negative-sense RNA. Budding of virions occurs from the plasma membrane (Figure 23.3). Arenaviruses have limited lytic capacity, usually producing a carrier state in which defective-interfering particles are produced. After an initial period of active virus transcription, translation, genome replication, and production of progeny virions, viral gene expression is downregulated, and cells enter a state of persistent infection wherein virion production continues for an indefinite period but at a greatly reduced rate (Table 23.2).

OLD WORLD ARENAVIRUSES

LYMPHOCYTIC CHORIOMENINGITIS VIRUS

Lymphocytic choriomeningitis virus presents two major opportunities for zoonotic transmission. First, the virus causes human disease when, especially during winter months, infected wild mice invade dwellings and farm buildings, where the virus can be transmitted from dried, virus-laden excreta by aerosols or fomites. In this regard, lymphocytic choriomeningitis virus has been identified as a relatively common cause of aseptic meningitis in patients admitted to hospital, and significant numbers of inner-city residents may be seropositive to this virus. Secondly, the virus can become established in laboratory mouse or hamster colonies, where it then not only poses a zoonotic threat but also confounds research results dependent on virus-free animals or biological products derived from these animals. For example, infected mouse tumors have been implicated in infections of laboratory workers. More commonly, zoonotic transmission occurs from infected pet rodents, particularly hamsters. Mice and hamsters are the only species in which long-term, asymptomatic infection is known to exist, but guinea pigs, rabbits, rats, dogs, swine, and primates may also be infected.

Clinical Features and Epidemiology

The natural history of lymphocytic choriomeningitis virus involves an intimate co-evolutional relationship with its reservoir hosts, *Mus musculus* and related *Mus* species and subspecies throughout Europe and Asia. Wild mice, particularly *Mus musculus domesticus*, have colonized the entire world and, in so doing, have carried the virus to the New World, Africa, Australia, and other parts of the globe. Certain populations of New World and Old World species of wild rodents, including *Microtus*, *Apodemus*, and *Sciurus* spp., have been found to be seropositive, but it is unknown if they maintain an enzootic cycle similar to *Mus musculus*. Enzootic infections within wild *Mus musculus* populations depend upon vertical transmission from persistently infected female mice to their fetuses, with maintenance of this cycle from one generation to the next. The immunologically deficient and naïve fetus fosters entry and dissemination of the virus, which is non-cytopathic and exhibits pancytotropism for virtually all tissues. Infection of the developing thymus results in virus-specific immune tolerance. Mice that are infected in this way are otherwise fully immunocompetent, and harbor infection throughout their lives. Being selectively tolerant to the virus, mice persistently shed virus in their feces, urine, and saliva, and from other sites, thereby enhancing the opportunity for virus spread to unexposed mice, as well as zoonotic transmission. Mouse populations tend to be demographically distinct, and infection among disparate wild mouse populations is not uniform. Clinical signs of infection among enzootically infected wild mice are absent, and their reproductive fecundity is not altered.

When lymphocytic choriomeningitis virus was initially discovered in laboratory mice, it was enzootic within some colonies, but not widespread. Because of intensive surveillance for this virus, it is now rare in contemporary mouse populations. Laboratory mice are occasionally exposed to the virus through contact with wild and feral mice, and through iatrogenic contamination of mouse populations with experimental virus stocks and contaminated biological material, including transplantable tumors. Exposure of adult immunocompetent mice results in transient infection with seroconversion, but several incidents involving exposure of immunodeficient mice have resulted in zoonotic transmission. Enzootic infection of pet mouse populations and hamsters poses a much greater risk of human exposure. Unlike mice, hamsters are uniquely susceptible to persistent infection after natural exposure at all ages, with amplification of virus and very high zoonotic risk. Clinical disease is rare in hamsters, but infection of young hamsters may lead to growth retardation, failure to thrive, weakness, conjunctivitis, dehydration, occasional tremors, and prostration.

Clinical signs of lymphocytic choriomeningitis in mice depend on age, genetic background, route of infection, and immunological status at the time of infection. Most laboratory mouse strains infected *in utero* or during the first 48 hours after birth develop a persistent, apparently immunotolerant infection. This infection may be asymptomatic or, over the course of several weeks to a year, may become evident by weight loss, runting, blepharitis, and impaired reproductive performance. Terminal immune complex glomerulonephritis is a common result of the breakdown of tolerance. Animals infected peripherally after the first few days of life may overcome the infection or may show decreased growth, rough hair coat, hunched posture, blepharitis, weakness, photophobia, tremors, and convulsions over a period of weeks.

Lymphocytic choriomeningitis virus poses a particular threat to the golden lion tamarin (*Leontopithecus rosalia*), an endangered primate currently found only in a small area of Brazil. Lymphocytic choriomeningitis virus infection of tamarins or marmosets in zoological collections results in a disease called marmoset (callitrichid) hepatitis, which has threatened several captive breeding programs. The source of infection has usually been the practice of feeding the primates neonatal mice from enzootically-infected mouse populations. Amongst other species, guinea pigs are highly susceptible to interstitial pneumonia when naturally exposed to lymphocytic choriomeningitis virus.

Human infection may be asymptomatic or may present as one of three syndromes: (1) most commonly as an influenza-like illness with fever, headache, myalgia, and malaise; (2) less often as an aseptic meningitis; (3) very uncommonly as a severe encephalomyelitis. Rarely, intrauterine infection has resulted in fetal and neonatal death, as well as hydrocephalus and chorioretinitis in infants. Recently, a cluster of fatal human cases of lymphocytic choriomeningitis resulted from organ transplants into immunosuppressed recipients from an infected but undiagnosed donor. Because it is uncommon, nothing is done to prevent or control human exposure, except in laboratory animal facilities.

Pathogenesis and Pathology

Lymphocytic choriomeningitis virus is maintained in nature by persistent infection of mice, with life-long virus shedding in urine, saliva, and feces. Fetal infection occurs by transovarial and transuterine vertical transmission, resulting in non-cytolytic disseminated infection of the fetus, and immune tolerance. Tolerant infection may also arise when mice are infected postpartum as early neonates through milk, saliva, and urine. The mice effectively develop into reproductive adulthood, with subsequent transmission to the next generation within the population. However, as the mice age, their state of immune tolerance to the virus gradually deteriorates, resulting in development of a wasting syndrome known as "late disease," or "late-onset disease." Although the mice have selective depletion of virus-specific T cells, they progressively develop virus-specific antibody that is undetectable serologically because it is complexed with circulating antigen. This has been termed "split tolerance" and is probably attributable to natural and low-affinity antibodies that arise in the absence of T cell help. Mice with late disease develop glomerulonephritis, arteritis, and generalized lymphoid proliferation, with infiltration of several organs. These events are not likely to occur (or be observed) in wild mice, because their lifespan is short as a result of predation. Although lymphocytic choriomeningitis virus infects cells non-cytolytically, an additional pathogenetic characteristic of tolerant infection may be the loss of specialized cellular functions—for example, reduced neurotransmitter activity and reduced levels of growth and thyroid hormones. Reduced growth hormone synthesis may be associated with runting in young mice. These events have been the subject of experimental studies, but are not likely to be significant in natural infections.

Lymphocytic choriomeningitis virus earned its name by its ability to induce lymphocytic choriomeningitis (inflammation of the choroid and meninges) following intracerebral inoculation of non-human primates and other laboratory animals, including laboratory mice. This lesion has little practical significance in the natural infection, but has been extensively studied as an experimental model and therefore warrants discussion (Figure 3.14). The lesion that arises in the central nervous system occurs in immunologically competent hosts, and is the result of a CD8 T cell response to non-cytolytic infection of the meninges, ependyma, and choroid plexus. In the absence of a T cell response, lesions do not arise. When the virus is inoculated intraperitoneally, the host T cell response results in hepatitis, and T-cell-mediated lesions can arise in several other organs. Another feature of experimental inoculation of adult, immunocompetent mice may be the induction of persistent infection as a result of a state of immune exhaustion. Under these circumstances, usually arising from intraperitoneal inoculation, the virus initially targets dendritic cells of the spleen and lymphoid organs, with extension into the lymphoid tissues. As the mice mount a T cell response to infection, there is severe immune-mediated destruction and massive necrosis of lymphoid tissues. This results in a state of immune exhaustion (in contrast to immune tolerance), which favors persistent infection and wasting syndrome. These experimental scenarios are significantly influenced by virus strain, dose, route of inoculation, mouse age, and mouse genotype. Following natural routes of virus exposure, adult mice generally manifest an acute, transient infection, with seroconversion and recovery.

Diagnosis

Serosurveillance for lymphocytic choriomeningitis virus infection in laboratory rodents is most commonly performed using enzyme-linked immunosorbent assay (ELISA) or indirect immunofluorescence assays. This approach is useful when using sentinel mice or mice exposed to the virus as adults, but serology is not useful for detecting infection in enzootically infected, immune tolerant mice. Reverse-transcriptase-polymerase chain reaction (RT-PCR) is most useful for the screening of mice of unknown microbial status. Biological materials (tumors, cell lines, antibodies, serum) are a common source of introduction of virus into laboratory mouse populations, and should undergo RT-PCR or mouse antibody production testing before use in mice. This applies especially to hybridoma lines and embryonic stem cells. Virus is readily cultivated in a wide variety of mammalian cells, particularly Vero cells and BHK-21 cells. Virus typically produces minimal cytopathic effect, so cultures must be assayed for antigen by immunofluorescence, ELISA, or RT-PCR.

Immunity, Prevention, and Control

Exposure of adult, immunocompetent animals results in effective sterilizing immunity with seroconversion, but enzootically-infected mice are immunologically tolerant, and have no detectable circulating antibody. Surveillance and depopulation of infected colonies are the methods most commonly used for control of lymphocytic choriomeningitis in laboratory mice and hamsters. Valuable genetic stocks of research mice may be re-derived by cesarean section or embryo transfer, but with considerable difficulty because of the natural inclination of the virus toward vertical transmission. Alternate methods, including *in-vitro* fertilization or intracytoplasmic injection of sperm would be warranted if routine attempts at re-derivation fail. Well-established surveillance programs should be an institutional responsibility in order to protect, not only research, but also humans. Preventing infection of other susceptible animals, including humans, is based on eliminating or minimizing exposure to wild rodents and infected sources of pet rodents.

LASSA VIRUS

Lassa fever was first identified in 1969, amongst nurses at a missionary hospital in Lassa, Nigeria, and the causative virus, Lassa virus, was isolated from the blood of affected individuals. In succeeding years, Lassa fever was shown to be a prevalent zoonotic disease in West Africa, with an estimated 100,000–300,000 cases annually, and perhaps 5000 deaths. The reservoir of the virus is the mouse, *Mastomys natalensis*, one of the most commonly occurring rodents in Africa.

Clinical Features and Epidemiology

There is no evidence of clinical disease in animals other than humans; however, Lassa virus experimentally can induce fatal disease in several species of non-human primates and guinea pigs. Disease does not occur in the reservoir rodent host, *Mastomys natalensis*.

Lassa fever in humans is variable in its presentation, making it difficult to diagnose, whether in enzootic areas or in returning travelers. It usually starts with fever, headache, and malaise and progresses to sore throat, back, chest, and joint pain, vomiting, and diarrhea. In severe cases, there is conjunctivitis, pneumonia, myocarditis, hepatic necrosis and hepatitis, encephalitis, deafness, and hemorrhage; death occurs in about 20% of patients admitted to hospital, usually following cardiovascular collapse. Mortality is very high in pregnant women, and fetal loss is almost invariable.

Lassa fever has been imported to the United States and Europe on several occasions, by people returning from enzootic regions of Africa.

Pathogenesis and Pathology

Lassa virus infection in *Mastomys natalensis* is similar in character to lymphocytic choriomeningitis virus infection in mice, being persistent, with chronic shedding of virus in urine, saliva, and feces. Fatal cases of Lassa fever in humans are characterized by focal necrosis in the liver, spleen, and adrenal glands, but the mechanism of fatal disease is poorly characterized. The virus grows to high titer in dendritic cells and macrophages, and cytokines produced by these cells probably contribute to the vascular collapse and shock syndrome that characterizes fulminant Lassa fever ("cytokine storm"). The type I interferon response is critical to controlling the infection, and it is very likely that Lassa virus subverts this response in the dendritic cells and macrophages of infected humans, leading to unchecked virus production. Animal models of Lassa fever include infections of non-human primates, guinea pigs, hamsters, and marmosets. Experimentally infected rhesus monkeys develop anorexia, progressive wasting, vascular collapse, and shock, with death occurring at 10–15 days after infection. The pathophysiologic basis for the disease is not yet well characterized in either humans or relevant animal models.

Diagnosis

Diagnosis is now based on the demonstration of immunoglobulin M (IgM) antibodies using an IgM capture ELISA. Viral antigen may also be detected in liver tissue in fatal cases by immunofluorescence or ELISA, and viral nucleic acid readily is detected by RT-PCR assay. The virus also may be isolated from blood or lymphoid tissues using Vero cells.

Immunity, Prevention, and Control

Antibodies to Lassa virus are present in recovered humans and experimental animals, but they usually do not neutralize the virus in conventional neutralization assays and it is presumed that cell-mediated immunity is key to recovery and protection against reinfection. Nonetheless, passive immunotherapy may be beneficial for some infected patients. Several recombinant vaccines have shown promise in protecting non-human primates from Lassa fever, but these have not yet been developed to the point of use in the field.

Risk factors for human infection include contact with rodents (practices such as catching, cooking, and eating rodents), the presence of rodents in dwellings, direct contact with patients, and re-use of unsterilized needles and syringes. Political instability and ecologic changes account for much of the increasing occurrence of the disease in enzootic areas of West Africa, specifically the creation of temporary villages in which *Mastomys natalensis* populations can flourish. Demonstration projects have shown the value of rodent elimination in villages; however, these programs have been difficult to sustain.

NEW WORLD ARENAVIRUSES

Each of the four South American arenavirus hemorrhagic fevers occupies a separate geographic range, each is associated with a different reservoir host, and each represents an expanding zoonotic disease threat. The four viruses have similar natural histories: they cause persistent, lifelong infections in their reservoir rodent hosts, with long-term shedding of large amounts of virus in urine, saliva, and feces. The natural history of the respective human diseases is determined by the pathogenicity of the virus, its geographic distribution, the habitat and habits of the rodent reservoir host, and the nature of the human–rodent contact. Human disease is usually rural and often occupational, reflecting the relative risk of exposure to virus-contaminated dust and fomites. Several other rodent-borne arenaviruses have been identified in South America, including some that have been associated with human disease (Table 23.1). Changes in ecology and farming practices throughout the region have increased concerns over the potential public health threat posed by these viruses.

JUNIN (ARGENTINE HEMORRHAGIC FEVER) VIRUS

Argentine hemorrhagic fever, caused by Junin virus, was first recognized in the 1950s in a grain-farming region of Argentina. Farm workers most commonly are affected, which is explained by the behavior of the rodent hosts, *Calomys musculinus* and *Calomys laucha*. These rodents are not peridomestic, but rather occupy grain fields, exposing humans through contact with virus-infected dust and grain products. Virus is acquired through cuts and abrasions or through airborne dust generated primarily when rodents are caught up in harvesting machinery. Since the 1950s, the disease has spread to increasingly large areas, with associated potential exposure of increased numbers of people. There is a 3–5-year cyclic trend in the incidence of human cases, which exactly parallels cyclic changes in the density of *Calomys* spp.

MACHUPO (BOLIVIAN HEMORRHAGIC FEVER) VIRUS

Machupo virus emerged in Bolivia in 1952 among people attempting subsistence agriculture at the borders of tropical grassland and forest. By 1962, more than 1000 cases of Bolivian hemorrhagic fever had been identified, with a 22% case-fatality rate. *Calomys callosus*, a forest rodent and the reservoir host of Machupo virus, adapts well to human contact—invasion of villages resulted in clusters of cases in particular houses in which substantial numbers of infected rodents were subsequently trapped. Control of *Calomys callosus* in dwellings in the endemic area by trapping resulted in the disappearance of the disease for many years, but in the 1990s cases reappeared, again starting on farms and then moving into villages.

GUANARITO (VENEZUELAN HEMORRHAGIC FEVER) VIRUS

Venezuelan hemorrhagic fever was first recognized in rural areas of Venezuela in 1989, apparently as a consequence of clearing of forest and subsequent preparation of land for farming. Although there were some 100 cases in 1990–1991, fewer cases have been seen since then. An arenavirus, Guanarito virus, was isolated from cases and traced to a reservoir rodent host, the short-tailed cane mouse *Zygodontomys brevicauda*. In the same area another new arenavirus, Pirital virus, was isolated from the rodent *Sigmodon alstoni*; its association with human disease is uncertain.

SABIÁ (BRAZILIAN HEMORRHAGIC FEVER) VIRUS

Sabiá virus was isolated from a fatal case of hemorrhagic fever in São Paulo, Brazil, in 1990, but there have been very few cases documented since then. Rodents likely serve as the reservoir host, as with other New World arenaviruses.

Clinical Aspects of Junin, Machupo, Guanarito, and Sabiá Viruses

As with other pathogenic arenaviruses, the pattern of infection in reservoir hosts caused by the South American viruses differs with age, host genetic determinants, route of exposure, and virus entry, and the dose and genetic character of the virus. Transmission from rodent to rodent is horizontal, not vertical, and occurs through contaminated saliva, urine, and feces. Unlike lymphocytic choriomeningitis and Lassa viruses, Junin and Machupo viruses are pathogenic in their reservoir rodent hosts. Junin causes up to 50%

mortality among infected suckling *Calomys musculinus* and *Calomys laucha*, and stunted growth in others. Machupo virus induces hemolytic anemia and fetal death in its rodent host, *Calomys callosus*. Junin and Machupo viruses not only cause disease in their reservoir hosts, they also induce sterility in neonatally infected females, thereby minimizing their role in producing offspring that are chronic virus shedders. Complex cyclic fluctuations in infection rates and population densities are believed to be a consequence of this. Virtually nothing is known about the pathogenesis of Guanarito or Sabiá virus infections in their reservoir hosts.

The South American arenaviruses induce typical hemorrhagic fevers in humans. Prominent features are hemorrhage, thrombocytopenia, leukopenia, hemoconcentration, and proteinuria; some cases culminate in fatal pulmonary edema, hypotension, and hypovolemic shock. Human-to-human transmission can occur via virus-containing blood or excretions, and isolation and barrier nursing are required to prevent nosocomial spread of the viruses to other patients and nursing staff. The pathogenesis of human infection with South American arenaviruses is poorly defined, but is probably similar to that of Lassa virus, with widespread, productive infection of dendritic cells and macrophages. Lesions in infected humans reflect circulatory shock, probably as a consequence of virus-mediated tissue injury and the activity of cytokines released from virus-infected macrophages and dendritic cells

Diagnosis of South American arenavirus infections is based on the demonstration of IgM antibodies using an IgM capture ELISA, or by immunofluorescence. Viral antigen may also be detected in liver tissue in fatal human cases, and the virus can be detected by specific RT-PCR assays or by isolation from serum or tissues using Vero cells.

An attenuated vaccine for Junin virus has been evaluated in endemic areas and found to be quite effective in preventing Argentine hemorrhagic fever, but vaccines are not widely available for protection against the other South American arenaviruses. For all these viruses, rodent eradication is the simplest potential control strategy, but is often not practical in the field.

Coronaviridae

Chapter Contents

The family *Coronaviridae* is included with the families *Arteriviridae* and *Roniviridae* in the order *Nidovirales*; viruses in these three families share a distinctive replication strategy. The family *Coronaviridae* comprises at least two genera. One, the genus *Coronavirus*, contains a substantial number of pathogens of mammals and birds that individually cause a remarkable variety of diseases, including pneumonia, reproductive disease, enteritis, polyserositis, sialodacryoadenitis, hepatitis, encephalomyelitis, nephritis, and various other disorders. Coronavirus and coronavirus-like infections have been described in swine, cattle, horses, cats, dogs, rats, birds, bats, rabbits, ferrets, mink, and various wildlife species, although many coronavirus infections are subclinical or asymptomatic.

In humans, coronaviruses are included in the spectrum of viruses that cause the common cold and, recently, severe acute respiratory syndrome (SARS), which is a zoonosis. The second genus, *Torovirus*, contains at least two viruses of animals: Berne virus, which was first isolated from a horse with diarrhea, and Breda virus, which was first isolated from neonatal calves with diarrhea. Berne virus neutralizing antibodies have been detected in sera of sheep, goats, rabbits, and mice, and torovirus-like particles have also been observed by electron microscopy in feces of swine, cats, turkeys, and humans. A nidovirus from fish—white bream virus, which is most closely related to the toroviruses—recently was proposed as the prototype member of a new genus, *Bafinivirus*.

Fenner's Veterinary Virology. DOI: 10.1016/B978-0-12-375158-4.00024-9

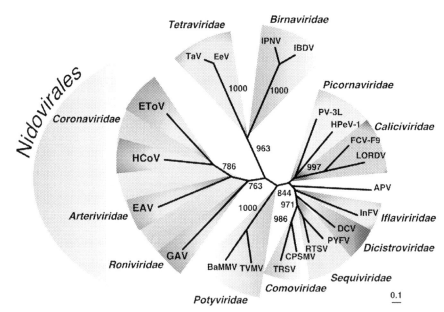

FIGURE 24.1   Phenogram showing the relationships of the RNA dependent RNA polymerases (RdRps) of the *Nidovirales* lineages with the virus families of the "Picornavirus-like" supergroup, *Tetraviridae* and *Birnaviridae*. APV, avian pneumovirus; BaMMV, barley mild mosaic virus; CPSMV, cowpea severe mosaic virus; DCV, Drosophila C virus; EAV, equine arteritis virus; EeV, *Euprosterna elaeasa* virus; EToV, equine torovirus; FCV-F9, feline calicivirus-F9; GAV, gill associated virus; HCoV, human coronavirus; HPeV-1, human parechovirus 1; IBDV, infectious bursal disease virus; InFV, infectious flacherie virus; IPNV, infectious pancreatic necrosis virus; LORDV, Lordsdale virus; PV-3L, poliovirus-3; PYFV, parsnip yellow fleck virus; RTSV, rice tungro spherical virus; TaV, *Thosea asigna* virus; TRSV, tobacco ringspot virus; TVMV, tobacco vein mottling virus. *[From Virus Taxonomy: Eighth Report of the International Committee on Taxonomy of Viruses (C. M. Fauquet, M. A. Mayo, J. Maniloff, U. Desselberger, L. A. Ball, eds.), p. 944. Copyright © Elsevier (2005), with permission.]*

PROPERTIES OF CORONAVIRUSES

Classification

Despite profound differences in virion structure and genome size, coronaviruses, toroviruses, arteriviruses, and roniviruses exhibit remarkable similarities in their genome organization and replication strategy. In infected cells, these viruses all utilize a distinctive "nested set" transcription strategy in which the expression of genes encoding structural viral proteins is mediated via a nested set of 3′ co-terminal subgenomic mRNAs. This unique strategy has been recognized by the establishment of the order *Nidovirales* (from the Latin *nidus*, nest), encompassing the family *Coronaviridae*, with two genera (*Coronavirus* and *Torovirus*), the family *Arteriviridae*, with one genus (*Arterivirus*), and the family *Roniviridae* containing invertebrate nidoviruses. Sequence analysis of the gene encoding portions of the viral RNA-dependent RNA polymerase (transcriptase) suggests that the member viruses of the order *Nidovirales* probably evolved from a common ancestor (Figure 24.1). Extensive genome rearrangements through heterologous RNA recombination have resulted in the variations seen—that is, viruses with similar replication and transcription strategies but disparate structural features.

The genus *Coronavirus* can be subdivided into at least three cluster groups on the basis of genetic and serologic properties, with subgroups in two of these (Table 24.1; Figure 24.2). Group 1a includes transmissible gastroenteritis virus of swine, porcine respiratory coronavirus, canine coronavirus, feline enteric coronavirus (feline infectious peritonitis virus), ferret and mink coronaviruses, and spotted hyena coronavirus. Group 1b includes certain human coronaviruses, porcine epidemic diarrhea virus, and bat coronavirus. Group 2a includes mouse hepatitis virus, bovine coronavirus, sialodacryoadenitis virus of rats, porcine hemagglutinating encephalomyelitis virus, canine respiratory coronavirus, and other human coronaviruses. Group 2b includes human SARS coronavirus and civet cat, raccoon dog, and horseshoe bat coronaviruses. Group 3 includes avian infectious bronchitis virus, turkey coronavirus, and several potential but still largely uncharacterized new species from ducks, geese, and pigeons. Further taxonomic subdivision of these viruses is likely in the future.

Viruses in the genus *Torovirus* are all apparently closely related and genetically distinct from coronaviruses; however, many toroviruses have yet to be fully characterized.

Virion Properties

Member viruses of the family *Coronaviridae* are enveloped, 80–220 nm in size, pleomorphic although often spherical (coronaviruses), or 120–140 nm in size and disc, kidney, or rod shaped (toroviruses). Coronaviruses have large (20 nm long) club-shaped spikes (peplomers) enclosing

TABLE 24.1 **Characteristics of Coronavirus and Torovirus Infections**

Coronavirus or Torovirus	Disease/Symptoms	Transmission/Diagnostic Specimen	Prevention/Control
Group 1a			
Feline enteric coronavirus (formerly feline infectious peritonitis virus)	Peritonitis, pneumonia, meningoencephalitis, panophthalmitis, wasting syndrome. Anorexia, chronic fever, malaise, weight loss, abdominal enlargement, CNS signs	Direct contact; fecal–oral route from maternal shedding. Feces, blood, body fluids	Attenuated (TS) vaccine. Interruption of transmission cycle, quarantine, high-level hygiene
Canine coronavirus	Mild gastroenteritis. Mild diarrhea	Ingestion by fecal–oral route. Acute feces; small intestinal sections or smears	Inactivated vaccine
Transmissible gastroenteritis virus of swine	Gastroenteritis. Watery diarrhea, vomiting, dehydration	Fecal–oral route. Acute feces; small intestinal sections or smears	Oral attenuated vaccine to pregnant sows. Good sanitation
Porcine respiratory coronavirus	Interstitial pneumonia. Mild respiratory disease or subclinical	Aerosols. Nasal swabs; trachea, lung sections	No vaccine available
Group 1b			
Porcine epidemic diarrhea virus	Gastroenteritis. Watery diarrhea, vomiting, dehydration	Fecal–oral route. Acute feces; small intestinal sections or smears	Oral attenuated virus vaccine (Asia) to pregnant sows
Group 2a			
Porcine hemagglutinating encephalomyelitis virus	Vomiting, wasting disease, encephalomyelitis. Anorexia, hyperesthesia, muscle tremors, emaciation	Aerosols, oronasal secretions. Nasal swabs, tonsil, lung, brain	Good husbandry, maintain immune sows. No vaccine available
Mouse hepatitis virus	Enteritis, hepatitis, nephritis, demyelinating encephalomyelitis. Various	Introduction of virus into a naïve colony: aerosols and direct contact. Target tissues, secretions	Depopulation. Preventive quarantine
Sialodacryoadenitis virus of rats	Inflammation and necrosis of salivary and nasolacrimal glands. Lacrimation, anorexia, weight loss, chromodacryorrhea	Direct contact, fomites, and aerosols. Nasopharyngeal aspirates, respiratory tissues	Depopulation and repopulation, preventive quarantine
Bovine coronavirus	Gastroenteritis, winter dysentery, shipping fever. Profuse or bloody diarrhea, dehydration, decreased milk, respiratory disease	Fecal–oral route, aerosols, respiratory droplets. Feces, large intestinal sections or smears, nasal swabs, lung sections	Maternal immunization: inactivated or attenuated vaccines; no vaccine for winter dysentery
Group 2b			
SARS coronavirus (humans)	Severe acute respiratory syndrome (10% patients). Fever, myalgia, diarrhea, dyspnea	Aerosol droplets, ?fecal–oral route. Nasopharyngeal aspirates, stools, serum	Quarantine, stringent isolation of patients
SARS coronavirus (civet cats, bats)	Subclinical?	Fecal–oral route. Feces	Testing and depopulation of animals in live markets

(Continued)

TABLE 24.1 (Continued)

Coronavirus or Torovirus	Disease / Symptoms	Transmission / Diagnostic Specimen	Prevention / Control
Group 3			
Avian infectious bronchitis virus	Tracheobronchitis, nephritis Rales, decreased egg production	Aerosols and ingestion of food contaminated with feces Tracheal swabs and tissue, cloacal swabs, cecal tonsils, kidney	Multivalent attenuated and inactivated vaccines available Good sanitation and testing
Turkey coronavirus, Bluecomb virus	Enteritis Diarrhea, depression, cyanotic skin	Fecal–oral route, aerosol Feces, intestinal sections or smears	Inactivated virus vaccine
Torovirus			
Breda virus (cattle)	Enteritis Diarrhea, dehydration	Fecal–oral route Feces, large intestinal sections or smears	No vaccine available

CNS, central nervous system; SARS, severe acute respiratory syndrome; TS, temperature-sensitive.

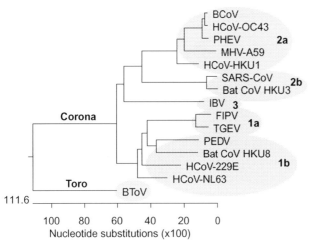

FIGURE 24.2 Phylogenetic analysis of relationship between different groups of coronaviruses (Corona) and toroviruses (Toro). The phylogenetic tree was constructed by the Clustal W method based on full-genome sequences. BCoV, bovine coronavirus; BToV, bovine torovirus; CoV, coronavirus; FIPV, feline enteric coronavirus (formerly feline infectious peritonitis virus); HCoV, human coronavirus; IBV, infectious bronchitis virus; MHV, murine hepatitis virus; PEDV, porcine epidemic diarrhea virus; PHEV, porcine hemagglutinating encephalomyelitis virus; SARS-CoV, severe acute respiratory syndrome coronavirus; TGEV, transmissible gastroenteritis virus. *(Courtesy of L. Saif and A. Vlasova, The Ohio State University.)*

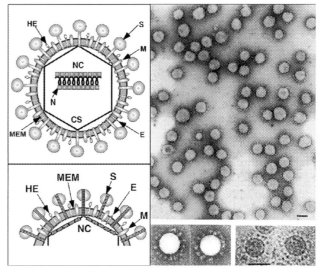

FIGURE 24.3 **Structure of coronavirus virions.** (Top left) Schematic diagram of virus structure; (Bottom left) Diagram of virion surface. (Top right) Electron micrograph of virus particles of transmissible gastroenteritis virus (TGEV) stained with uranyl acetate (top right) or sodium phosphotungstate (insert bottom left) showing the surfae of the virus particles. The spikes (peplomers) are better defined using sodium phosphotungstate. (insert bottom right) Cryo-electron microscopic visualization of unstained TGEV in vitreous ice. The particles contain an internal structure inside the viral envelope and well extended peplomers. MEM, lipid membrane; S, spike protein; M, large membrane protein, E, small envelope protein; HE, hemagglutinin-esterase; N, nucleocapsid protein; CS, core-shell; NC, nucleocapsid. The bars represents 100 nm. *[From Virus Taxonomy: Eighth Report of the International Committee on Taxonomy of Viruses (C. M. Fauquet, M. A. Mayo, J. Maniloff, U. Desselberger, L. A. Ball, eds.), p. 947. Copyright © Elsevier (2005), with permission.]*

what appears to be an icosahedral internal core structure within which is a helical nucleocapsid (Figure 24.3). Some coronaviruses also have a second fringe of shorter (5 nm long) spikes (hemagglutinin). Toroviruses also have large club-shaped spikes, but the particles are more pleomorphic and have a tightly coiled tubular nucleocapsid bent into a doughnut shape. By thin-section electron microscopy, torovirus nucleocapsids appear as kidney-, disc-, or rod-shaped forms.

The genome of the family *Coronaviridae* consists of a single molecule of linear positive-sense, single-stranded RNA, 27.6–31 kb in size for coronaviruses and 25–30 kb for toroviruses, the largest known non-segmented RNA viral

TABLE 24.2 Properties of Coronaviruses and Toroviruses

Virions are pleomorphic or spherical (genus *Coronavirus*) or disc-, kidney-, or rod-shaped (genus *Torovirus*); 80–220 nm (genus *Coronavirus*) or 120–140 nm (genus *Torovirus*) in diameter. Virions are enveloped, with large club-shaped spikes (peplomers)

Virions have an icosahedral internal core structure within which is a helical nucleocapsid (genus *Coronavirus*) or a tightly coiled tubular nucleocapsid bent into a doughnut shape (genus *Torovirus*)

The genome consists of a single molecule of linear positive-sense, single-stranded RNA, 25–31 kb in size; the genome is 5′ capped, 3′ polyadenylated, and infectious

Coronavirus virions contain three or four structural proteins: a major spike glycoprotein (S), transmembrane glycoproteins (M and E), a nucleoprotein (N), and, in some viruses, a hemagglutinin esterase (HE). Torovirus virions contain analogous proteins, but there is no E protein

Viruses replicate in the cytoplasm; the genome is transcribed, forming a full-length complementary RNA from which is transcribed a 3′ co-terminal nested set of mRNAs, only the unique sequences of which are translated

Virions are formed by budding into the endoplasmic reticulum and are released by exocytosis

genomes. The genomic RNA is 5′ capped and 3′ polyadenylated, and is infectious (Table 24.2).

The major virion proteins of the member viruses of the genus *Coronavirus* and *Torovirus* include a nucleocapsid protein (N, 50–60 kDa, 19 kDa for toroviruses) and several envelope/spike proteins: (1) the major spike glycoprotein (S, 180–220 kDa); (2) a triple-spanning transmembrane protein (M, 23–35 kDa); (3) a minor transmembrane protein (E, 9–12 kDa), which together with the M protein is essential for coronavirus virion assembly. Toroviruses lack a homolog of the coronavirus E protein, which may explain the structural differences between the coronaviruses and toroviruses. The secondary, smaller spikes, seen in some group 2 coronaviruses and in toroviruses, consist of a dimer of a class I membrane protein (65 kDa), a hemagglutinin esterase (HE) that shares 30% sequence identity with the N-terminal subunit of the HE fusion protein of influenza C virus. Sequence comparisons indicate that the *HE* genes of coronaviruses, toroviruses, and orthomyxoviruses were acquired by independent, non-homologous recombination events (probably from the host cell). Although there is no sequence similarity between the torovirus proteins and their counterparts in coronaviruses, they are similar in structure and function, and are related phylogenetically.

Virus neutralizing antibodies generated during natural infections are directed at the surface glycoproteins of coronaviruses and toroviruses, with the majority being conformational epitopes located at the N-terminal portion of the S protein. Cellular immune responses are principally directed toward the S and N proteins. Besides the canonical structural proteins, coronaviruses are unique among nidoviruses because their genomes encode (within differing regions) variable numbers of accessory proteins (four or five in most; eight in the SARS coronavirus) that are dispensable for *in-vitro* virus replication, but which increase virus fitness *in vivo*. The accessory proteins encoded by the SARS virus open reading frames 3b and 6, for example, are antagonists of innate immune responses, specifically interfering with the development of type I interferon responses; the specific roles of other accessory proteins are still largely unknown. The accessory proteins have homologous versions within coronavirus groups, but lack similarity with proteins in different groups. In group 2 coronaviruses, for example, the HE protein is considered an accessory protein, and mouse hepatitis virus HE-deletion mutants replicate like wild-type virus *in vitro*, but in mice they have an attenuated phenotype.

Virus Replication

The host spectrum of individual coronaviruses appears to be largely determined by the S protein, portions of which mediate receptor binding and virus cell fusion that occur at either the plasma membrane or within endosomes of susceptible cells. Individual coronaviruses utilize a variety of cellular proteins as receptors. Aminopeptidase N serves as a receptor for several group 1 coronaviruses, including feline enteric coronavirus (formerly feline infectious peritonitis virus), canine coronavirus, transmissible gastroenteritis virus and human coronavirus 229E. SARS and some other human coronaviruses utilize angiotensin converting enzyme 2. Mouse hepatitis virus utilizes carcinoembryonic antigen-related cell adhesion molecule 1 (CEACAM-1), and other group 2 coronaviruses utilize *N*-acetyl-9-*O*-acetyl neuraminic acid. The functional receptor for group 3 coronaviruses such as infectious bronchitis virus is undefined, although heparan sulfate and sialic acid residues may serve as non-specific attachment factors.

The strategy of expression of the coronavirus genome is complex (Figure 24.4). First, the viral RNA serves as messenger RNA (mRNA) for synthesis of the RNA-dependent RNA polymerase. The two large open reading frames (some 20 kb in total size) encoding the units of the polymerase are translated—the larger via ribosomal frameshifting—as a single polyprotein that is then cleaved. These proteins then assemble to form the active RNA polymerase. This enzyme is then used to transcribe full-length complementary (negative-sense) RNA, from which in turn are transcribed, not only full-length genomic RNA, but also a 3′ co-terminal nested set of subgenomic mRNAs. The nested set comprises up to 10 (differing in the various viruses) overlapping mRNAs that extend for different lengths from common 3′ ends and share a common 5′ leader sequence. They are

MHV

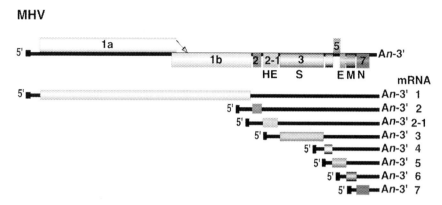

FIGURE 24.4 Structural relationship between mRNAs and the genomic RNA of coronaviruses. Thick lines represent the translated sequence. Thinner lines, untranslated sequences. The names below the boxes indicate the proteins encoded by the corresponding genes. An, poly A sequences; E, minor transmembrane envelope protein; HE, spike protein hemagglutinin esterase; M, transmembrane envelope protein; MHV, mouse hepatitis virus; N, nucleocapsid protein; S, spike glycoprotein. [*From* Virus Taxonomy: Eighth Report of the International Committee on Taxonomy of Viruses (*C. M. Fauquet, M. A. Mayo, J. Maniloff, U. Desselberger, L. A. Ball, eds.*), p. 952. Copyright © Elsevier (2005), with permission.]

generated by a leader-primed mechanism of discontinuous transcription: the polymerase first transcribes the noncoding leader sequence from the 3′ end of the complementary (negative-sense) RNA. The capped leader RNA then dissociates from the template and reassociates with a complementary sequence at the start of any one of the genes, to continue copying the template right through to its 5′ end. Only the unique sequence that is not shared with the next smallest mRNA in the nested set is translated; this strategy yields the various viral proteins in regulated amounts. Intergenic sequences serve as promoters and attenuators of transcription.

Torovirus transcription and replication apparently are similar to those of coronaviruses, except that there are no common 5′ leader sequences on the mRNAs. A puzzling finding is that subgenomic negative-sense RNAs complementary to the nested set of mRNAs are also present in torovirus-infected cells. The fact that these subgenomic RNAs contain 5′- and 3′-terminal sequences that are identical to those of genomic RNA implies that they may function as replicons.

The synthesis, processing, oligomerization, and transport of the several envelope glycoproteins of coronaviruses display some unusual features. For example, the envelope protein M, which in some coronaviruses contains *O*-linked rather than *N*-linked glycans, is directed exclusively to cisternae of the endoplasmic reticulum and other pre-Golgi membranes. As a result, virions bud only there and not from the plasma membrane. Virions are then transported in vesicles to the plasma membrane and are released by exocytosis (Figure 24.5). After their release, many of the mature enveloped virions remain adherent to the outside of the cell.

In addition to the accumulation of point mutations as a result of polymerase errors during transcription (genetic drift), genetic recombination occurs at high frequency between the

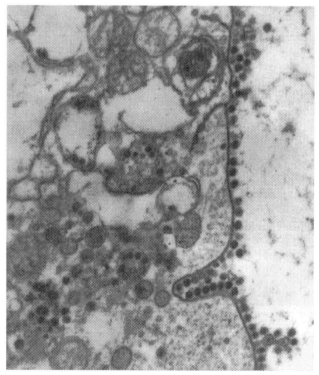

FIGURE 24.5 Mouse hepatitis virus infection in the duodenum of a 1-week-old mouse. Virions are transported to the plasma membrane from their site of formation in the endoplasmic reticulum in vesicles and are released by exocytosis. After their release, many virions remain adherent to the outside of the cell. Thin-section electron microscopy. Magnification: ×30,000.

genomes of different but related coronaviruses. This may be an important mechanism for the generation of the genetic diversity seen with these viruses in nature, and provides a constant potential source of new viruses with novel phenotypic properties, including host species tropism and virulence.

MEMBERS OF THE GENUS *CORONAVIRUS*

TRANSMISSIBLE GASTROENTERITIS VIRUS

Transmissible gastroenteritis is a highly contagious enteric disease of swine that occurs throughout much of the world. Porcine respiratory coronavirus arose from transmissible gastroenteritis virus through genetic deletions, and the respiratory virus now has superseded its enteric parent in many regions.

Clinical Features and Epidemiology

Clinical signs of transmissible gastroenteritis are most severe in very young piglets, and include vomiting, profuse watery yellow diarrhea, rapid weight loss, and dehydration. Most, often all, seronegative neonates succumb within a few days of infection with highly virulent strains of transmissible gastroenteritis virus, whereas death is uncommon in pigs infected after 2–3 weeks of age. Older growing and finishing swine often develop a transient, watery diarrhea, but vomiting is unusual. Infections of adult swine typically are asymptomatic, but in some outbreaks there is high mortality, and infected sows sometimes exhibit anorexia, fever, vomiting, diarrhea, and agalactia.

Transmissible gastroenteritis virus is highly contagious to swine of all ages. Dogs and cats have been experimentally infected with the virus, although their role in the epidemiology of infection is doubtful. Spread of transmissible gastroenteritis virus among farms occurs with the introduction of pigs excreting the virus or by mechanical vectors (fomites) such as contaminated vehicles, clothing, instruments, etc. Introduction of the virus into non-immune herds leads to explosive outbreaks, with epizootic spread among animals of all ages; mortality is very high in neonates. Disease is usually less severe in older animals. The epizootic terminates when no susceptible swine remain and no new animals are reintroduced, typically within a few weeks, although chronic or intermittent shedding has been described in some experimentally exposed sows. Another epidemiologic pattern occurs in intense production facilities where the farrowing system makes susceptible piglets available continuously. Enzootic infection and background immunity to transmissible gastroenteritis virus or related porcine respiratory coronavirus usually lead to low mortality and relatively mild disease that is most pronounced shortly after weaning, when maternally acquired immunoglobulin A (IgA)-based immunity has waned. Notably in Europe, virulent enteric transmissible gastroenteritis virus infections largely have been displaced by enzootic porcine respiratory coronavirus infections. Porcine respiratory coronavirus is a genetic variant of transmissible gastroenteritis virus with a deletion of variable size within the spike protein (see below), but which engenders strong immunity against transmissible gastroenteritis virus infection.

Pathogenesis and Pathology

Transmissible gastroenteritis virus enters the body by ingestion (fecal–oral transmission), and after an incubation period of 18–72 hours it causes clinical signs that vary according to the age of the animal infected. There are several reasons for the susceptibility of very young piglets: (1) their gastric secretions are less acidic than those of older animals and their milk diet buffers gastric acid, both of which are somewhat protective to the virus during its passage through the stomach; (2) renewal of enterocytes lining the intestinal villi from progenitor cells in the intestinal crypts is less rapid than in older pigs; (3) the neonatal immune system is naïve and not fully mature; (4) neonates are especially vulnerable to the electrolyte and fluid derangements that result from the maldigestion and severe malabsorption diarrhea that are characteristic of transmissible gastroenteritis in very young pigs. After virus passes through the stomach, the infection proceeds as a wave down the intestinal tract. The virus selectively infects and destroys the mature enterocytes lining the small intestinal villi, quickly resulting in profound shortening and blunting of villi, with consequent loss of the mucosal absorptive area (Figure 24.6). The destruction of enterocytes lining the villi leads to maldigestion because of the loss of critical digestive enzymes such as lactase and other disaccharidases, normally present in the microvillous brush border of villous enterocytes, that are responsible for digestion of milk. Thus destruction of villous enterocytes results in both malabsorption and maldigestion. The increased osmolarity of the intestinal contents from the presence of undigested milk results in further loss of water and electrolytes into the bowel lumen. The consequence is diarrhea, electrolyte imbalance leading to acidosis, and severe dehydration. Intestinal crypt epithelial cells remain uninfected, so recovery of the integrity and function of villi is rapid if the animal survives the infection; however, the proliferation of progenitor enterocytes in the crypts also increases intestinal secretion of fluid and electrolytes, which further exacerbates the diarrhea and metabolic pertubations that are characteristic of fulminant transmissible gastroenteritis.

Gross pathology (except for dehydration) is restricted to the gastrointestinal tract, and consists of a distended stomach that contains undigested milk, and flaccid, gas- and fluid-distended intestines. The destruction of villi, which can be seen when sections of intestine are submerged in isotonic buffer and viewed with a dissecting microscope, results in thinning of the intestinal wall (Figure 24.7).

Diagnosis

Mucosal impression smears or cryostat sections of intestine from neonatal piglets with acute disease can be stained for transmissible gastroenteritis virus by immunofluorescence or immunoperoxidase staining—these methods provide

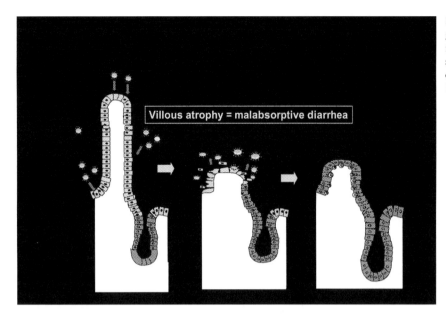

FIGURE 24.6 Pathogenesis of transmissible gastroenteritis. Schematic diagram showing viral infection and destruction of enterocytes lining small intestinal villi, leading to malabsorption diarrhea. *(Courtesy of L. Saif, The Ohio State University.)*

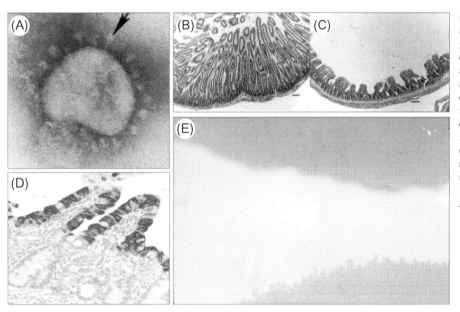

FIGURE 24.7 Pathogenesis of transmissible gastroenteritis. (A) Electron micrograph of causative virus, with prominent envelop spikes (arrow). Histologic appearance of small intestine of (B) normal piglet and (C) piglet with transmissible gastroenteritis. (D) Immunohistochemical staining showing selective viral infection of enterocytes lining the intestinal villi. (E) Mucosal surface of small intestine from (bottom) a normal suckling pig, and (top) a pig with transmissible gastroenteritis—note lack of villi. *(Courtesy of L. Saif, The Ohio State University, and N.J. Maclachlan, University of California.)*

rapid results. Antigen-capture enzyme-linked immunosorbent assay (ELISA) also can be used to detect transmissible gastroenteritis virus in the feces of infected pigs. Virus isolation can be done in porcine kidney, thyroid, or testicle cells; there is cytopathology, and isolates are identified with specific antisera, usually using an enzyme immunoassay. Serology using paired serum samples and either serum neutralization or enzyme immunoassay allows retrospective diagnosis and is also valuable in epidemiological investigations. However, none of these assays definitively differentiates transmissible gastroenteritis and porcine respiratory coronavirus infections; reverse-transcriptase-polymerase chain reaction (RT-PCR) assays using primers

targeting the deletion region of the porcine respiratory coronavirus *S* gene can be used to detect and differentiate the two viruses. Serological discrimination of prior infection with these two viruses can be accomplished using a blocking (competitive) ELISA incorporating monoclonal antibodies that recognize an antigenic site present in the S protein of transmissible gastroenteritis virus that is deleted in porcine respiratory coronavirus.

Immunity, Prevention, and Control

Oral vaccines have not proven highly effective, and better protection has been obtained when virulent virus has been orally administered to pregnant sows, thereby boosting lactogenic immunity in piglets. Maternal IgA antibodies, passed to piglets in colostrum and milk, provide protection against infection, whereas systemic IgG antibody does not. IgA antibodies are protected against proteolytic degradation in the intestine and provide immunity within the intestinal lumen. Lactogenic immunity is not stimulated by parenteral immunization, only by mucosal infection or immunization.

Control of transmissible gastroenteritis by exclusion of the virus from premises requires strict sanitation and management practices that eliminate all potential sources of the virus, including potentially infected or carrier animals, and which prevent reintroduction of the virus.

PORCINE RESPIRATORY CORONAVIRUS

The respiratory variant of transmissible gastroenteritis virus, porcine respiratory coronavirus, was discovered in 1986 when seroconversion was detected in swine herds in countries (e.g., Denmark) known to be free of transmissible gastroenteritis; the virus causing this disease pattern is a spike gene deletion mutant that has lost its enteric tropism. Instead, porcine respiratory coronavirus acquired a respiratory tropism and transmission pattern.

Clinical Features and Epidemiology

Porcine respiratory coronavirus infects piglets of all ages, causing subclinical or mild respiratory disease. Clinical signs may include mild fever with variable degrees of dyspnea, polypnea, and anorexia. Co-infection of pigs with other respiratory pathogens (bacteria, influenza virus, porcine reproductive and respiratory syndrome virus) or treatment with immunosuppressive agents accentuates porcine respiratory coronavirus infections and disease.

Porcine respiratory coronavirus now is enzootic in swine herds worldwide, spreading long distances by airborne respiratory transmission or directly by contact. Swine population density, distance between farms, and season all can influence the epidemiology of infection with this virus.

Pathogenesis and Pathology

The large 5' region deletion (621–681 nt in size) in the spike gene of porcine respiratory coronavirus probably accounts for the reduced virulence and altered tropism of this virus. Porcine respiratory coronavirus is spread by respiratory droplets and aerosols and, after infection, replicates in the tonsils, the mucosal epithelium of the nasal mucosa and airways of the lungs, and in both type I and II pneumocytes in alveoli. Virus-induced inflammation and necrosis in the terminal airways and airspaces manifest as bronchointerstitial pneumonia that can affect 5–60% of the lung, even in asymptomatic pigs. The severity of clinical signs and lesions vary, but infection is subclinical in many infected herds.

Diagnosis

Porcine respiratory coronavirus replicates to high titers in the lungs of infected swine, and the virus can be detected readily in nasal swabs. Laboratory diagnosis of porcine respiratory coronavirus infection utilizes the same assays as those described for transmissible gastroenteritis virus, and the two related viruses are only distinguished by virus-specific RT-PCR assays or highly specific competitive ELISA. The virus also can be isolated and grown in pig kidney or testicle cells.

Immunity, Prevention, and Control

There currently are no vaccines for prevention of porcine respiratory coronavirus infection, probably because most infections are so mild that there is little perceived need for a vaccine. Experimental and field studies suggest that repeated exposure of swine to porcine respiratory coronavirus results in high levels of both passive and active immunity to transmissible gastroenteritis, such that the latter disease has largely disappeared from porcine respiratory coronavirus enzootic herds in some countries.

PORCINE HEMAGGLUTINATING ENCEPHALOMYELITIS VIRUS

Porcine hemagglutinating encephalitis virus causes vomiting and wasting disease in susceptible piglets, and neurological disease in others. Vomiting and wasting disease was first reported in Canada in 1958, and serologic surveys indicate that the causative virus is common in many countries; however, disease is relatively infrequent, because neonatal pigs are often passively protected by colostral antibodies and subsequently develop age-related resistance to the disease.

Infection of adult swine usually is inapparent, and vomiting and wasting disease is a disease of piglets under 3 weeks of age suckling non-immune sows. The disease is characterized by repeated vomiting after feeding, depression, progressive emaciation, and death. In contrast to transmissible gastroenteritis, in vomiting and wasting disease diarrhea is not common. Infection also can lead to neurological signs similar to those of porcine polioencephalomyelitis, which is caused by a picornavirus; specifically, affected piglets may show a dog-sitting posture, paddling movements, opisthotonos, paralysis or convulsions, and death.

Porcine hemagglutinating encephalitis virus is spread by respiratory aerosols and multiplies first in the nasal mucosa, tonsils, lung, and small intestine; it then spreads to the central nervous system via peripheral nerves. Viremia is not important in the pathogenesis of this disease, neither is involvement of organs other than the nervous system. Infection of the vagal sensory ganglia is proposed to be responsible for the vomiting that characteristically occurs in affected animals, and the wasting component is attributed to viral infection of gastric myenteric plexuses leading to delayed emptying of the stomach.

A clinical diagnosis of porcine hemagglutinating virus encephalomyelitis may be confirmed by the isolation of virus in primary porcine kidney cell culture or in various pig cell lines; growth of the virus is detected by characteristic hemagglutination. Because no vaccines are available, good husbandry is essential for the prevention and control of the disease.

PORCINE EPIDEMIC DIARRHEA VIRUS

Porcine epidemic diarrhea is a diarrheal disease of piglets that has been described in Europe and Asia. The disease is clinically similar to transmissible gastroenteritis, but is caused by a different and less contagious coronavirus. Suckling piglets are unaffected in many outbreaks. The main clinical sign in young pigs is watery diarrhea, sometimes preceded by vomiting. Mortality can be very high (up to 80%). The virus also can cause diarrhea in growing and fattening pigs. Infection of adult swine is frequently asymptomatic, although diarrhea occurs sometimes. A diagnosis may be confirmed by the isolation of virus in primary porcine cell culture or Vero (African green monkey kidney) cells, by immunofluorescence or ELISA tests for porcine epidemic diarrhea virus antigens in intestine or feces, respectively, by RT-PCR assay to detect viral RNA, or by the demonstration of virus-specific antibodies in convalescent swine. Attenuated vaccines are available in some countries.

FELINE ENTERIC CORONAVIRUS AND FELINE INFECTIOUS PERITONITIS VIRUS

Feline infectious peritonitis was first described in the 1960s as a systemic and often fatal disease of cats. The pathogenesis of feline infectious peritonitis is complex and not fully characterized, despite intensive study. Feline enteric coronavirus infection is central to the pathogenesis of this disease, as the sporadic occurrence of feline infectious peritonitis is proposed to be the result of mutations of the enteric coronavirus during natural infection of cats, resulting in the emergence of a virus with an acquired tropism for macrophages. Although feline enteric coronavirus is classified in group 1a (Table 24.1), two serotypes of of the virus have been identified, both being able to cause

feline infectious peritonitis. The serotype 2 feline enteric coronavirus is a recombinant that includes portions of the genome of canine coronavirus. Both virus types can cause the two forms of feline infectious peritonitis, one that has a characteristic abdominal effusion (the "wet" form), and the other (the "dry" form) without abdominal effusion. Thus the pathologic manifestations are not solely a virus strain-specific property, as individual virus strains can cause either form of the disease in individual cats.

Clinical Features and Epidemiology

Feline infectious peritonitis is a common progressive, debilitating lethal disease of domestic and wild members of the family *Felidae*. Disease typically occurs in young or very old cats. The initial clinical signs are vague, and affected cats present with anorexia, chronic fever, malaise, and weight loss. Ocular and/or neurological manifestations occur in some individuals. In the classical wet or effusive form of feline infectious peritonitis, these signs are accompanied by progressive abdominal distention from the accumulation of a highly viscous fluid in the peritoneal cavity and rapid disease progression, with death typically within weeks to months. The dry or non-effusive form of the disease, with little or no peritoneal exudate, is more slowly progressive. The wet and dry forms of feline infectious peritonitis are different manifestations of the same infection, and both forms of the disease are characterized by foci of pyo-granulomatous inflammation in several organs.

The following is a proposed scenario of fatal feline infectious peritonitis. A kitten suckling a seropositive queen is protected by colostral antibody against enteric coronavirus infection during the first few weeks of life. As maternal antibody wanes, the kitten becomes infected during an episode of maternal feline enteric coronavirus shedding. The kitten now develops an active immune response, but in most cases not a sterilizing response, and a persistent viral infection of the gut with chronic fecal shedding is established. Virus and antibodies co-exist in the kitten, but the infection is modulated by an efficient cellular immune response that keeps infected macrophages and monocytes in check. The animal may remain healthy, but becomes susceptible to development of feline infectious peritonitis should it become stressed or immuno-suppressed. Viral mutants then emerge, with rapid selection and proliferation of macrophage-tropic mutants that cause the development of feline infectious peritonitis.

Pathogenesis and Pathology

The key initiating pathogenic event in feline infectious peritonitis is the productive infection of monocytes and macrophages by genetic variants (mutants) of the original enteric coronavirus. Experimentally, the virulence of strains of feline enteric coronavirus has been correlated with their capability of productive infection of cultured peritoneal macrophages, with avirulent isolates infecting fewer macrophages and producing lower virus titers than virulent isolates. Avirulent isolates are also less able to sustain virus replication and spread between macrophages. Mutations within the spike (S) and, potentially, other proteins alter the tropism of the ubiquitous avirulent feline enteric coronavirus to macrophages, which then allows the virus to spread and to cause feline infectious peritonitis. Affected cats typically produce a strong antibody response that is ineffective in eliminating the virus, and cellular immune responses are unable to prevent virus replication in macrophages.

The lesions in feline infectious peritonitis are characteristically centered on small blood vessels, and vascular injury and leakage are central to the pathogenesis of the wet form of the disease. However, there is uncertainty regarding the pathogenetic mechanisms involved, as there is increasing evidence that vascular injury is not simply the result of immune complex deposition in the walls of the affected vessels, as was once proposed. The central role of viral infection of macrophages, however, is clear, and perivascular clusters of virus-infected macrophages are characteristically present in the tissues of cats with both the wet and dry forms of feline infectious peritonitis. Despite the inability of macrophages to prevent virus from replicating in them, viral infection of macrophages probably leads to their activation, with production of inflammatory mediators including cytokines and arachidonic acid derivatives (leukotrienes and prostaglandins). These mediators probably contribute substantially to the disease process, as these host-response molecules induce changes in vascular permeability and provide chemotactic stimuli for neutrophils

and monocytes that further contribute to the inflammatory response. Both intravascular and recently emigrated monocytes and macrophages probably serve as new virus targets, thereby amplifying the infection further. The end result is enhanced local virus production, increased tissue damage, and a strong but ineffective host immune response.

Humoral immunity is not protective, but may actually enhance disease progression. Antibody-dependent enhancement of infection of macrophages is apparently mediated by neutralizing antibodies to the S protein, making vaccine development problematic. Cats that are seropositive to feline enteric coronavirus, either from natural infection or via purified IgG antibodies transfused into uninfected animals, develop an accelerated, fulminant disease when challenged experimentally with virulent feline enteric coronavirus (so-called feline infectious peritonitis virus). Clinical signs and lesions develop earlier, and the mean survival time is reduced as compared with seronegative cats.

The gross lesions of feline infectious peritonitis reflect one of the two forms of the disease. The wet form is characterized by the presence of variable quantities of thick, viscous, clear yellow peritoneal exudate, and the presence of extensive fibrinous plaque with numerous discrete gray-white nodules (from <1 to >10mm in diameter) in the omentum and on the serosal surface of the liver, spleen, intestines, and kidneys (Figure 24.8). Microscopically, these nodules are composed of aggregates of macrophages and other inflammatory cells (granulomas or pyogranulomas) that characteristically are centered on blood vessels, sometimes with necrosis of the wall of involved vessels. These lesions can occur in many tissues, but omentum and peritoneal serosa, liver, kidney, lung and pleura, pericardium, meninges, brain,

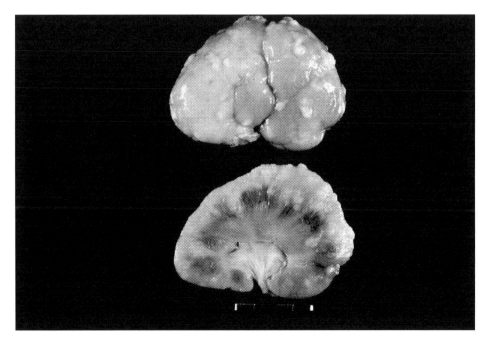

FIGURE 24.8 Feline infectious peritonitis. Granulomas disseminated throughout the kidney of an affected cat. (*Courtesy of N.J. Maclachlan, University of California.*)

and uvea are common sites. The lesions and pathogenesis of the dry form of feline infectious peritonitis are similar, but without the fibrinous polyserositis that characterizes the wet form, and discrete pyogranulomas form nodular masses within the parenchyma of affected organs. It is unknown what determines the form of feline infectious peritonitis that develops in an individual cat, neither is the relationship between the two forms well understood, as individual virus strains can cause either form in different animals.

Diagnosis

Serology utilizing indirect immunofluorescence or enzyme immunoassay generally shows cats with feline infectious peritonitis to have moderate to high antibody titers. Some cats with the disease remain seronegative or have only low antibody titers, however, whereas other cats with no clinical signs of disease may have high titers. Therefore, interpretation of serology data is frequently confusing, and surgical biopsy of affected organs not only confirms the diagnosis but also reveals the extent and stage of the disease. Immunohistochemistry can be used to obtain definitive confirmation of coronavirus infection of macrophages within the lesions in affected cats.

Immunity, Prevention, and Control

Feline infectious peritonitis is not controlled easily; control requires the elimination of the virus from the local environment, whether this is the household or the cattery. This requires a high level of hygiene, strict quarantine, and immunoprophylactic measures. Because kittens acquire the infection from their queens, early weaning programs have also been used in attempts to interrupt virus transmission.

The development of a safe and highly effective vaccine remains elusive, even with the availability of bioengineering approaches. The only commercially available feline infectious peritonitis vaccine contains a temperature-sensitive mutant virus. The vaccine is applied to the nasal mucosa to reduce virus replication and antibody formation. Under these conditions, a cellular immune response is favored, and some protection putatively is achieved. Vaccination of infected, seropositive adult cats is not effective.

CANINE CORONAVIRUS

A canine coronavirus that usually produces only a mild gastroenteritis in infected dogs was originally identified in 1971. More recently, strains of canine coronavirus have been identified with different properties; these include canine respiratory coronavirus and pantropic strains of the virus. Constant, continuing evolution of canine coronavirus, through accumulation of point mutations within the genome and genetic insertions or deletions, leads to the regular emergence of viruses with altered properties, including their tropism and virulence.

Enteric canine coronavirus infection is common in dogs worldwide, and epidemics of coronavirus enteritis have also been recorded in wild dogs. Similar or identical group 1 coronaviruses have been identified in foxes, raccoon dogs, and cats. The intestinal disease caused by canine coronavirus is similar to that caused by enteric coronaviruses in other species, with destruction of mature enterocytes lining the intestinal villi causing maldigestion, malabsorption, and subsequent diarrhea. Because there are many causes of diarrhea in dogs, clinical suspicion of canine coronavirus infection should be confirmed by laboratory-based procedures. The virus may be visualized by electron microscopy, and some but not all virus strains can be isolated in primary canine cell culture. Highly sensitive and specific RT-PCR assays have now been developed. Detection of antibody in the sera of pups is of limited value, because it may be of maternal origin and unrelated to the cause of the diarrhea. An inactivated vaccine is available for the control of canine coronavirus diarrhea, but its protective value is controversial.

Pantropic strains of canine coronavirus have been described as the putative cause of severe systemic disease in dogs that is characterized by pyrexia, anorexia, depression, vomiting, diarrhea, leukopenia, and neurological signs of ataxia and seizures. Coronaviruses that are genetically distinct from enteric canine coronaviruses, but that resemble bovine coronaviruses, have been detected with some frequency in the respiratory tract of dogs from Europe, North America, and Asia, sometimes in association with respiratory disease.

MOUSE HEPATITIS VIRUS

Mouse hepatitis virus includes a spectrum of mouse coronaviruses that may not necessarily cause hepatitis. These viruses vary widely in their tissue tropism. One end of the spectrum consists of enteric coronaviruses, which have selective tropism for enteric epithelium. Historically, enterotropic mouse hepatitis virus was given the name "lethal intestinal virus of infant mice" (LIVIM). The other end of the spectrum consists of polytropic coronaviruses, which have primary tropism for upper respiratory epithelium, and secondary tropism for a wide variety of cells or tissues, particularly vascular endothelium, lymphoid tissue, hemopoietic tissue, liver, and central nervous system. These viruses received the nickname of "hepatitis viruses" because of their common property of inducing hepatitis in experimentally inoculated mice. Thanks to their polytropism, these mouse hepatitis virus types replicate readily in a wide variety of cell types *in vitro*, whereas enterotropic strains of the virus do not, and also tend not to induce hepatitis. Thus, for many years, LIVIM was considered to be distinct from mouse hepatitis virus.

There are numerous laboratory strains of polytropic mouse hepatitis virus that grow readily *in vitro*, including MHV-JHM, MHV-S, MHV-A59, and MHV-3. These polytropic viruses have been extensively studied as models of neurologic disease and hepatitis, and form the basis of an expansive scientific literature. The enterotropic viruses are far more common in contemporary mouse colonies, but have received less experimental scrutiny. Common enteric strains of mouse hepatitis virus include MHV-S/CDC, MHV-Y, MHV-RI, and MHV-D. Despite the fact that mouse hepatitis virus strains are often named, the nomenclature is meaningless, because of the inherent property of these viruses constantly to mutate and recombine within mouse populations. Furthermore, although the distinction between enterotropic and polytropic is useful for understanding the biology of the virus, there is considerable overlap among isolates, and one group probably served as a progenitor for the other.

Clinical Features and Epidemiology

Enterotropic strains of mouse hepatitis virus tend to be highly contagious, and cause devastating epizootics in naïve mouse populations, with mortality approaching 100% among infant mice. Clinical disease is limited to infant mice, because susceptibility is determined by enteric mucosal proliferative kinetics. Thus enterotropic mouse hepatitis virus infection follows the features of neonatal enteric coronaviral enteritides in other species. Disease course is rapid, with pups dying from dehydration within 24–48 hours after introduction of the virus to a naïve breeding population. Older pups may be runted, and bloated with poorly formed feces, but often recover. Adults are susceptible to infection, but do not manifest clinical disease. Once the virus is enzootic within a population, clinical disease is no longer apparent, as pups are protected by maternal antibody during the period of age-related susceptibility. Polytropic strains of mouse hepatitis virus are generally less contagious, and tend to spread by direct contact among naïve mice. Outcome of infection with these viruses is highly variable, and dependent upon age, mouse strain, and virulence of the virus. Infant mice are susceptible to disease, because of an immature immune system. Clinical disease is often inapparent, but tends to be manifest as runting and neurologic signs, with reduced survival at weaning as a result of maternal cannibalism. When polytropic mouse hepatitis virus is enzootic within a population, clinical signs are absent among immunocompetent mice. In contrast, wasting disease, neurologic signs, and mortality may be observed in immunodeficient mice, particularly T cell deficient mice. A unique clinical presentation occurs in interferon-γ deficient mice, which develop abdominal distention as a result of polyserositis.

Host immunity to mouse hepatitis virus is virus-strain-specific, and directed toward the mutable S protein that constitutes the virion spikes. Immunocompetent mice mount an effective immune response to infection, with elimination of the virus and complete recovery. Duration of infection is therefore limited, except when mice with various types of immune perturbations are infected, in which case duration of infection varies. Mouse hepatitis virus has a reputation of being "latent" and "persistent," but neither is the case. Latency does not occur, but signs of infection are often subclinical. Persistence occurs within the context of the population, with constantly evolving mutants arising that are capable of reinfecting immune mice, thereby maintaining the virus in the population. In laboratory animal housing contexts, commercially obtained mice free of mouse hepatitis virus tend to be introduced to infected colonies on a weekly basis, which is the perfect interval for maintaining infection and observing disease. Vertical transmission is not a practical concern, but the virus can be introduced into a naïve mouse population through biological products (mouse serum, tissues, tumors, etc.). Polytropic mouse hepatitis virus can persistently infect cell lines, including ES cells, without cytopathic effect.

The significance of mouse hepatitis virus within laboratory mouse populations is not so much its overt pathogenicity; rather, it is its deleterious effects upon research. A wide variety of effects upon various physiologic parameters, particularly immune responses, have been documented. These research effects are often the only "clinical signs" of disease within an infected mouse population.

Pathogenesis and Pathology

Enterotropic strains of mouse hepatitis virus tend to selectively infect enterocytes, with minimal dissemination to other tissues, except mesenteric lymph nodes. The neonatal mouse bowel is poorly suited to deal with enterotropic mouse hepatitis virus infection, which induces rapid cytolysis of terminally differentiated enterocytes that line the intestinal villi. The intestinal mucosa of infant mice has shallow, slowly replicating crypt progenitors that are incapable of responding to the rapid cytolytic effects of the virus. Lesions consist of segmental epithelial necrosis, villus attenuation, and mucosal erosion. A diagnostic feature of enterotropic mouse hepatitis virus infection is prominent epithelial syncytia. Lesions are most likely to occur in the terminal small intestine, cecum, and proximal colon. As mice age, intestinal mucosal proliferative kinetics accelerate, allowing replacement of damaged mucosa. This is characterized by mucosal hyperplasia, which may contribute to clinical disease through malabsorption and increased mucosal secretion of fluid and electrolytes. Lesions are minimal in adult mice, which support ample virus replication, but the mucosa can compensate for the damage. Under those circumstances, lesions are limited to an occasional syncytium in the surface mucosa. Disease susceptibility among immunodeficient mice varies with the nature of the immune defect, but is also dependent on age and mucosal kinetics. Infection of adult immunodeficient nude mice, for example, may be clinically silent, with minimal enteric disease limited to a few epithelial syncytia.

Polytropic virus strains initially replicate in nasal respiratory epithelium. Dissemination depends upon the age of the mouse, the strain of the mouse, the immune status of the mouse, and the virus strain. Neurotropic strains may extend from the olfactory epithelium to the olfactory tracts of the brain without dissemination to other organs. More commonly, the virus will disseminate hematogenously to the pulmonary vasculature, with secondary viremia to other organs, particularly liver, hemopoietic tissues, and lymphoid tissues. Gut-associated lymphoid tissue may be infected, but enteric mucosa is often spared. Depending upon the genetic background of the mouse, susceptibility to polytropic mouse hepatitis virus can be illustrated at the cellular level *in vitro* (*intrinsic resistance*) or *in vivo*, in which several host factors may determine susceptibility (*extrinsic resistance*). Susceptibility to the MHV-A59 and MHV-JHM strains of mouse hepatitis virus, for example, has been linked to allelic variation of carcinoembryonic antigen-related cell adhesion molecule 1 (CEACAM1). SJL mice lack this susceptibility allele and are markedly resistant to infection with these virus strains. However, this explanation of susceptibility does not apply to all strains of mouse hepatitis virus or to all mouse genotypes.

Depending upon these various factors, lesions associated with polytropic mouse hepatitis virus are highly variable. Infection of adult immunocompetent mice with relatively avirulent strains of virus is often subclinical. When lesions are present, they consist of multiple foci of acute necrosis, and syncytia of parenchyma and vascular endothelium within lymphoid tissues, hemopoietic tissues (particularly spleen), liver, and brain. Lesions are particularly florid in immunodeficient mice, which develop progressively severe wasting disease with lesions that are strikingly apparent in liver, with foci of hemorrhage, necrosis, and nodular hyperplasia. Spleens are also enlarged as a result of extramedullary hemopoiesis. Central nervous system disease can arise directly through olfactory neural pathways (nasoencephalitis) or hematogenous infection, with necrotizing encephalitis. Infection involves neurons, glia, and endothelium, and surviving mice progress to demyelinating disease, which may be manifest as posterior paresis. This is most apt to be observed in chronically infected immunodeficient mice. As previously noted, mice deficient in interferon-γ may develop chronic polyserositis, which features prominent syncytia among infiltrating macrophages. Curiously, involvement of other organs or tissues (intestine, liver, etc.)

may be absent, suggesting that mice are able to clear infection partially from those tissues, but not macrophages.

Diagnosis

Mouse hepatitis virus infection of a mouse population can be detected retrospectively by serology. Strains of the virus are highly cross-reactive serologically, so antigen is typically prepared from polytropic strains of virus propagated from cell culture. Active infections can be diagnosed at necropsy, and virus can be detected by RT-PCR or cultured (especially polytropic strains). There is no practical point in defining virus strain for diagnostic purposes.

Immunity, Prevention, and Control

Mouse hepatitis virus is generally controlled by exclusion from pathogen-free mouse populations, or acquisition of mice free of the virus from commercial vendors. Control is approached by periodic serology of sentinel animals, re-derivation of incoming mice through cesarean section or embryo transfer, or quarantine and testing of mice. Infectious disease quality control and building-, room-, and cage-level containment are major areas of emphasis in maintaining research mice. Infected immunocompetent mice can be rid of infection by selective quarantine of adults without breeding for several weeks, commencing breeding of seropositive animals, and testing progeny (which will be transiently seropositive from maternal antibody). Because of the mutability of mouse hepatitis virus, this approach is not feasible on a room or population basis. Alternatively, mice can be "re-derived" by cesarean section and foster nursing on or embryo transfer into virus-free dams. This is the only option with immunodeficient mice, and special care is needed in testing the progeny to assure virus-free status. Once a mouse population is re-established as free of mouse hepatitis virus, stringent effort is needed to prevent reintroduction of virus. Conventionally housed mice cannot be maintained free of mouse hepatitis virus unless they are completely isolated from all other mice, including feral and wild mice (which are commonly infected).

SIALODACRYOADENITIS VIRUS

Like mouse hepatitis virus in mice, sialodacryoadenitis virus is represented by many strains of rat coronaviruses. So-called Parker's rat coronavirus is simply another isolate of sialodacryoadenitis virus. Although sialodacryoadenitis and mouse hepatitis viruses are closely related, they do not naturally cross the species barrier.

Sialodacryoadenitis virus is highly contagious within naïve rat populations. Primary tropism is to nasal respiratory epithelium, with secondary spread to lacrimal glands, salivary glands, and lung. The virus can induce disease in all ages of rat, but disease is most severe in young rats. Mortality may occur in suckling rats, complicated by failure to nurse as a result of the destruction of olfactory epithelium. Clinical features include nasal and ocular discharge, cervical swelling, photophobia, keratitis, and dyspnea. Lacrimal secretions surrounding the eyes are tinted with porphyrin pigment derived from affected retro-orbital Harderian glands. Lesions consist of necrotizing rhinitis, necrosis of salivary glands (excluding the sublingual glands, which are not affected) and lacrimal glands, periglandular edema, and interstitial pneumonia. Resolving lesions often feature marked squamous metaplasia, particularly in the Harderian glands. Infections are acute, with complete recovery, but permanent damage to the eye can arise indirectly from dysfunction of lacrimal glands (keratitis sicca) and inflammation in the filtration angle of the eye, resulting in hyphema, megaloglobus, and corneal ulcerations. Infection may contribute to anesthetic deaths, and predispose rats to secondary respiratory bacterial diseases. Immune-deficient rats are uncommon, but chronic wasting syndrome may occur in athymic nude rats, which succumb to progressive pneumonia.

Although rats are immune to reinfection with the homologous strain, they can be reinfected with novel strains of the virus. Sialodacryoadenitis virus infection is diagnosed by clinical signs and lesions, and retrospective diagnosis is accomplished by serology, usually utilizing cross-reacting mouse hepatitis virus antigen. Virus isolation, RT-PCR, and immunohistochemistry are available, but seldom used for diagnostic purposes. Although sialodacryoadenitis virus and mouse hepatitis virus are closely related, they do not naturally cross species barriers.

GUINEA PIG AND RABBIT CORONAVIRUSES

In juvenile European (*Orcytolagus*) rabbits, enteric coronaviruses induce disease that is characterized by intestinal villus attenuation, malabsorption, and diarrhea. Infection may predispose rabbits to, or be obscured by, the enteritis complex (dysbiosis). Rabbit coronavirus has been isolated, but not characterized. Another coronavirus infects rabbits asymptomatically, but experimental inoculation induces serosal effusion, right-sided heart enlargement, mesenteric lymphadenopathy, and multifocal necrosis of multiple organs. The "pleural effusion virus" was discovered as a contaminant of *Treponema pallidum*, which is maintained by intratesticular inoculation of laboratory rabbits. Little is known about the prevalence of either rabbit coronavirus, but enteric coronavirus is probably common.

Diarrhea and enteritis caused by a coronavirus has been reported in young guinea pigs, but its prevalence among guinea pig populations and its relationship to other coronaviruses are not known.

BOVINE CORONAVIRUS

Bovine coronavirus infections are associated with three distinct clinical syndromes in cattle: calf diarrhea, winter dysentery (hemorrhagic diarrhea) in adult cattle, and respiratory infections in cattle of various ages, including the bovine respiratory disease complex (shipping fever) in feedlot cattle. Coronaviruses were first reported as a cause of diarrhea in calves in the United States in 1973, and since then they have been recognized worldwide in association with the three clinical syndromes. The economic impact of respiratory disease and calf diarrhea is considerable.

Although many coronaviruses have restricted host ranges, group 2 coronaviruses such as bovine and SARS coronaviruses (Table 24.1) can infect other animal species, including wildlife. Bovine coronavirus is also closely related to the group 2 human coronavirus-OC43 that causes the common cold, and bovine coronavirus has been shown experimentally to infect dogs subclinically and to infect turkey poults, leading to fecal virus shedding, diarrhea, seroconversion, and transmission to contact controls. Genetically and/or antigenically related bovine coronavirus variants have been isolated from dogs with respiratory disease, humans with diarrhea, and captive or wild ruminants with intestinal disease similar to winter dysentery of cattle. The latter include Sambar deer (*Cerous unicolor*), waterbuck (*Kobus ellipsiprymnus*), giraffe (*Giraffa camelopardalis*), and white-tailed deer (*Odocoileus virgineanus*). Bovine coronavirus has also been linked to enteric disease in South American camelids. Interestingly, the human enteric coronavirus and wild ruminant coronaviruses both infected and caused diarrhea in experimentally exposed gnotobiotic calves, and the inoculated calves were subsequently immune to infection with bovine coronavirus.

Despite the different disease syndromes and apparent interspecies transmission of bovine coronavirus and its variants, only a single serotype of bovine coronavirus is recognized, and there is little sequence diversity between the wild ruminant coronaviruses and coronaviruses associated with the different disease syndromes in cattle. Furthermore, there are few common sequence differences to explain differences in host or tissue tropism.

Clinical Features and Epidemiology

Coronavirus-induced diarrhea commonly occurs in calves under 3 weeks of age after the decline of passively acquired antibodies, but disease can occur in calves up to 3 months of age. The severity of diarrhea and dehydration depends on the infecting dose as well as the age and immune status of the calf. Co-infections with other enteric pathogens such as rotavirus, torovirus, cryptosporidia, and enterotoxigenic *Escherichia coli* are common; their additive or synergistic effects increase the severity of diarrhea. Calf coronavirus diarrhea is often seasonal, being more common in winter in part because of the increased stability of the virus in the cold.

Bovine coronavirus has also been implicated as a cause of winter dysentery, a sporadic acute disease of adult cattle worldwide that is especially prevalent during winter months, as the name implies. Winter dysentery is characterized by explosive, often bloody diarrhea, accompanied by decreased milk production, depression, anorexia, and frequent respiratory signs. Morbidity rates range from 20 to 100% in affected herds, but mortality rates are usually low (1–2%). A similar winter dysentery syndrome associated with bovine coronaviruses variants occurs in captive and wild ruminants. This finding suggests that certain wild ruminants (deer, elk, caribou, etc.) that share common grazing areas with cattle could be a reservoir for coronavirus strains transmissible to cattle, or *vice versa*.

Bovine coronavirus causes mild respiratory disease (coughing, rhinitis) or pneumonia in 2–6-month-old calves. An epidemiologic study of calves from birth to 20 weeks of age confirmed both fecal and nasal shedding of coronavirus, with diarrhea prominent upon initial infection. The calves subsequently shed virus intermittently via the respiratory route, with or without signs of disease, suggesting that long-term mucosal immunity in the upper respiratory tract is ineffective in mediating virus clearance. As a consequence, coronavirus may recycle among cattle of all ages and regardless of their immune status, with sporadic nasal or fecal shedding from individual animals. Alternatively, new virus strains may be introduced when cattle from different sources are co-mingled, or from cohabiting wild ruminants.

Since 1993, bovine coronavirus has been incriminated as a precipitating cause of the bovine respiratory disease (shipping fever) complex. Both respiratory and enteric shedding of bovine coronavirus are common in affected feedlot cattle, peaking shortly after arrival at feedlots. Since its discovery, bovine coronavirus repeatedly has been identified in the lungs of feedlot cattle that died with bovine respiratory disease complex. Most feedlot cattle also seroconvert to bovine coronavirus within 3 weeks of arrival. Importantly, studies suggest that cattle arriving at feedlots with high serum titers of bovine coronavirus antibody were less likely to shed virus or to develop shipping fever. This observation suggests a role for serum antibodies in protection, or as an indicator of recent infection and active immunity.

Pathogenesis and Pathology

Concurrent fecal and nasal virus shedding persists for up to 10 days after coronavirus infection of calves. Coronavirus antigen is commonly detected in epithelial cells of both the upper respiratory and intestinal tracts, and occasionally in the lung. The pathogenesis of coronavirus enteritis in calves is similar to that caused by rotavirus, with the notable exception of extensive involvement of the large intestine by coronavirus. Disease occurs most commonly in calves at about 1–3 weeks of age, when virus exposure increases and antibody titers in the dam's milk begin to wane. The pathogenesis and consequences of enteric coronavirus infection of calves are similar to those previously described for transmissible gastroenteritis in piglets. The destruction of the mature absorptive cells lining the intestinal villi and mucosal surface in the large intestine leads to maldigestion and malabsorption, with rapid loss of water and electrolytes. The resultant hypoglycemia, acidosis, and hypovolemia can progress to circulatory failure and death, especially in very young animals.

The pathogenesis and lesions of winter dysentery of dairy and beef cattle resemble those of calf diarrhea, but often with marked intestinal hemorrhage and extensive necrosis of cells within the crypts of the large intestinal mucosa. Nasal and fecal shedding is more transient (up to 4–5 days). The anorexia and depression seen in dairy cattle with winter dysentery may explain the precipitous and sometimes prolonged decrease in milk production. The cause of the acute and often voluminous bloody diarrhea in some cattle is unexplained.

Both nasal and fecal shedding of bovine coronavirus can occur soon after cattle are transported to feedlots. Coronavirus infection is probably important in predisposing cattle entering feedlots to secondary bacterial infection that results in the characteristic shipping fever pneumonia—a severe, often fatal fibrinous bronchopneumonia caused by *Mannheimia haemolytica* biotype A, serotype 1 infection. Bovine coronavirus antigen also has been detected in epithelial cells of the upper (trachea, bronchi) and lower (terminal bronchioles and alveoli) respiratory tract of some affected cattle, but the precise role of coronavirus in precipitating the bovine respiratory disease complex awaits definitive characterization.

Diagnosis

Initially, the diagnosis of enteric bovine coronavirus infections was based on the detection of virus by electron microscopy, but cell culture isolation became a viable option when it was discovered that the virus could be grown when trypsin was added to the medium. For most bovine coronavirus strains, HRT-18 cells are optimal for primary isolation. Viral growth may be recognized by hemadsorption or cytopathogenic effects, and the presence of coronavirus confirmed by diagnostic tests. An array of assays is now available for detection of bovine (or variant) coronaviruses in cell culture or diagnostic specimens such as feces or nasal swabs, including ELISAs that incorporate monoclonal antibodies for antigen capture, immune electron microscopy using hyperimmune antiserum, and RT-PCR using bovine coronavirus or pan-coronavirus-specific primers to detect viral RNA. Post-mortem diagnosis is performed on acute fresh or fixed respiratory or intestinal tissues using hyperimmune antisera or monoclonal antibodies for immunofluorescence or immunohistochemical tissue staining.

Immunity, Prevention, and Control

Passive Immunity to Enteric Bovine Coronavirus Infections in Calves

Because coronavirus diarrhea occurs in young calves during the nursing period, maternal vaccination is required to provide immediate passive (lactogenic) immunity. Passive immunity to enteric viral infections in calves correlates with high levels of IgG$_1$ antibodies in colostrum and milk. In ruminants, IgG$_1$ antibodies are dominant in colostrum and milk and are selectively transported from serum. Most adult cattle are seropositive for antibodies to bovine coronavirus. Therefore, parenteral vaccination of mothers with adjuvanted inactivated bovine coronavirus vaccines effectively boosts IgG$_1$ antibody titers in serum and mammary secretions, to provide enhanced passive immunity to calves.

Immunity to Respiratory Bovine Coronavirus Infections

The correlates of immunity to respiratory coronavirus infections in cattle are not clearly defined. Data from epidemiological studies suggest that the serum titer of antibody to bovine coronavirus may be a marker for respiratory protection. In calves exposed in the field, and in feedlot cattle exposed upon entry, the serum magnitude of neutralizing or enzyme immunoassay antibody titer and the antibody isotype (IgG$_1$, IgG$_2$, IgA) were correlated with protection against respiratory disease, pneumonia, or coronavirus respiratory shedding. It is uncertain whether serum antibodies are correlates of protection, or whether they merely reflect prior enteric or respiratory coronavirus infection.

Available attenuated oral vaccines are not highly effective in preventing coronavirus-induced diarrhea in calves, because of interference by maternal antibodies and because vaccines typically do not have sufficient time to evoke protection of calves before the time of maximum risk. Attenuated or inactivated commercial vaccines are available to immunize the dam, thereby promoting increased antibody levels in colostrum and milk. Another alternative for dairy calves is to feed them colostrum and milk from hyperimmunized cows.

Currently, no vaccines are available to prevent winter dysentery or respiratory coronavirus infections. However, there are indications that the risk of shipping fever in cattle entering a feedlot is reduced if they receive intranasal vaccination with an attenuated enteric coronavirus vaccine.

SEVERE ACUTE RESPIRATORY SYNDROME CORONAVIRUS

In 2002, a new coronavirus emerged in China, associated with a severe acute respiratory syndrome (SARS) and substantial mortality in humans. The disease quickly spread globally before the epidemic was contained, in 2003, after more than 8000 cases and some 800 deaths in 29 countries. Patients infected with SARS virus initially presented with fever, general malaise, chills, and dry cough that progressed to diarrhea with fecal virus shedding, and about 30% of patients developed severe respiratory disease with interstitial pneumonia. Viral loads in nasopharynx, serum, and feces increased progressively to peak about day 10, and especially high viral loads in aerosols from some patients were correlated to superspreading events, an important but unexplained means of SARS virus transmission. Consistent with the clinical signs, SARS virus was detected mainly in intestine and lung, with infection of pulmonary type I pneumocytes and macrophages. The epidemic was contained by strict quarantine and sanitation methods, without the availability of vaccines or effective antiviral therapy.

A considerable and coordinated international effort led to the rapid cell culture isolation, genetic sequencing, and identification of an apparently new coronavirus as the causative agent of SARS. Both epidemiologic and genetic data suggest that SARS in humans is a zoonosis, and that SARS coronavirus evolved from a coronavirus that naturally infects a wildlife reservoir host. Individuals who were closely associated with live-animal markets in China were over-represented in initial cases of SARS, and SARS-like coronaviruses were isolated from clinically normal Himalayan palm civets (*Paguma larvata*) and a raccoon dog (*Nyctereutes procyonoides*) from live-animal markets. Although civets are susceptible to experimental infection with human SARS coronavirus, this virus was not detected in civets raised on farms, or in wild civets. Thus it was proposed that civets and raccoon dogs may amplify virus in wild-animal markets as intermediate hosts, but they probably are not the natural host reservoir for SARS coronavirus. Bats are now proposed to be the definitive reservoir hosts of SARS coronavirus, as enzootic infection of Chinese horseshoe bats with a remarkable genetic spectrum of SARS-like coronaviruses has now been established.

Changes in three genes were identified during the adaption of SARS coronavirus to humans, including the *S* gene, as related to adaptation to the human cell receptor (ACE 2) and in the accessory proteins encoded by open reading frames 3a and 8, which are of uncertain biologic significance. In 2004, SARS re-emerged in China and, judged by sequence data, the re-emerged SARS virus strains were more like civet viruses, suggesting that these cases represented new introductions from animals to humans.

The emergence of SARS was a sobering but timely reminder to the global biomedical community of the potential ramifications of "species jumping" of coronaviruses. It had been clearly shown previously that some animal coronaviruses were promiscuous in terms of their species specificity, but it was only when a zoonotic disease as devastating as SARS emerged that serious attention was given to the importance of this phenomenon. Importantly, SARS appears to have a relatively broad host range, in common with group 2a bovine coronaviruses, and experimental SARS coronavirus infection has now been described in rhesus macaques, ferrets, mice, cats, and hamsters. Despite their obvious importance, the determinants of host range specificity and interspecies transmission among coronaviruses remain largely undefined.

INFECTIOUS BRONCHITIS VIRUS

Infectious bronchitis was the term coined in 1931 to describe the principal clinical-pathological feature of a transmissible respiratory disease of poultry in the United States first reported in North Dakota. Infectious bronchitis virus was identified retrospectively as the cause of a disease that had been misidentified as high-pathogenicity avian influenza in New England and the upper Midwest during 1924–1925. The disease has now been identified worldwide and is one of the most important viral diseases of chickens. The virus is the prototype of the family *Coronaviridae*; there are many antigenic variants and serotypes as a consequence of mutations in its large genome.

Clinical Features and Epidemiology

The clinical presentation of infectious bronchitis depends on age, genetic background, and immune status of the bird at the time of infection, route of exposure, nutritional factors (especially levels of calcium in the diet), virulence of the virus strain, and the presence of stressors such as cold temperatures or secondary bacterial pathogens. Outbreaks may be explosive, with the virus spreading rapidly to involve the entire flock within a few days. The incubation period is typically brief: 18–48 hours. In chicks 1–4 weeks of age, virulent virus strains produce severe respiratory disease, with gasping, coughing, tracheal rales, sneezing, nasal exudate, wet eyes, respiratory distress, and, occasionally, swollen sinuses. Mortality in young chicks is usually 25–30%, but in some outbreaks can be as high as 75%. Less virulent strains cause fewer and milder respiratory signs, and lower morbidity and mortality rates. Infection of young female chicks may result in permanent hypoplasia of the oviduct that is evident later in life as reduced egg production and inferior quality eggs.

When the disease is uncomplicated by opportunistic bacterial superinfection, respiratory signs last for 5–7 days

and disappear from the flock in 10–14 days. High mortality can occur in broilers as a result of secondary infection with *Escherichia coli* or pathogenic mycoplasmas. Egg-laying chickens usually present with reproductive tract involvement that is manifest as a decline or cessation in egg production or, less consistently, respiratory disease. When laying resumes, many eggs are abnormal, including lack of calcified shell, thin shells, and shells with stipples, distortions, dimples, depressions, or ridging; eggs that should be colored are often pale or white, and egg albumen may be watery. In acutely infected birds, the kidneys can be pale and swollen, with urates distending the ureters, and in the chronic phase there can be atrophy of kidney lobules, with large calculi within the ureters (urolithiasis).

Infectious bronchitis virus spreads between birds by aerosol and by ingestion of food contaminated with feces. In the environment, the virus can survive on fomites for several days and possibly for weeks, especially at low environmental temperatures. Outbreaks of infectious bronchitis have declined in recent years as a result of the extensive use of vaccines; however, the disease may occur even in vaccinated flocks when immunity is waning, or upon exposure to variant viral serotypes. To minimize this risk, most poultry producers obtain 1-day-old chicks from maternal antibody-positive breeders and then spray-vaccinate them with live attenuated vaccine in the hatchery.

Pathogenesis and Pathology

The virus replicates to high titer first in the respiratory tract (ciliated epithelial cells); this is followed by viremia (within 1–2 days of infection), which distributes the virus to many organs. The virus can cause extensive damage to the ovaries, oviduct, and the kidneys. The intestinal tract is another site of primary infection, but damage usually is minimal.

Infectivity declines rapidly, and isolation of virus beyond 7 days after infection is uncommon (except from chicks). Rarely, virus has been reported to persist for up to 14 weeks in cecal tonsils, and has been recovered from the feces for up to 20 weeks after infection. Kidney and intestine are the likely sites of virus persistence.

The most frequent gross pathological finding is mucosal thickening, with serous or catarrhal exudate in the nasal passages, trachea, bronchi, and airsacs. In very young chicks, the main bronchi may be blocked with caseous yellow casts. Pneumonia and conjunctivitis are sometimes seen. In laying birds, ova can be congested and sometimes ruptured, with free yolk in the abdominal cavity. Desquamation of respiratory epithelium, edema, epithelial hyperplasia, mononuclear cell infiltration of the submucosa, and regeneration are seen in various combinations. Repair processes begin after 6–10 days, and are complete in 14–21 days. Some virus strains affect the kidney, causing interstitial nephritis, and some Asian strains of the virus cause enlargement of the glandular stomach (proventriculus), with ulceration and inflammation.

Diagnosis

Direct immunofluorescence staining of tracheal tissue smears is useful in the diagnosis of early cases before secondary bacterial infection has occurred. For virus isolation, embryonated eggs are inoculated via the allantoic sac route. Changes suggestive of the presence of a coronavirus include congestion of the main blood vessels in the chorioallantoic membrane and embryo stunting, curling, clubbing of down, or urate deposits in the mesonephros. Identification of virus in the chorioallantoic membrane is usually done by immunofluorescence or immunohistochemical staining, or in allantoic fluid by serological methods, nucleic acid analysis, or electron microscopy. Isolates are usually typed and subtyped by serological methods and nucleic acid analyses such as restriction length polymorphism, or genotype-specific RT-PCR assays.

Immunity, Prevention, and Control

Infection induces IgM, IgG, and IgA antibodies. In immune laying hens, the ovum begins to acquire IgG antibody (some of it virus specific) from the blood about 5 days before the egg is laid. As it becomes surrounded with albumen during passage down the oviduct, the ovum acquires both IgM and IgA antibodies, which are transferred into the amniotic fluid about halfway through development. During the last third of embryonation, IgG enters the circulation from the yolk; antibody can inhibit virus replication at this time. The chick hatches with a circulating IgG level similar to that of the hen. IgG antibody is metabolized with a half-life of approximately 3 days and may persist for 3–4 weeks. The virus may survive until passive immunity declines to a level at which it can replicate again, at which time the chicken mounts an active immune response. However, the correlates of active immunity to infectious bursal disease virus are less certain. Neutralizing antibodies can prevent virus dissemination from the respiratory tract and block secondary infection of the reproductive tract and kidneys. The adaptive transfer of CD8 T lymphocytes protects chicks against infectious bronchitis virus challenge, suggesting a role for cellular immunity as well in protection.

Attenuated virus vaccines are widely used to protect meat chickens. These vaccine viruses are derived by serial passage in embryonated eggs. They are administered in drinking water, by coarse spray, or by deposition on the conjunctiva (eye drops). The first vaccination is typically given in the hatchery when birds are 1 day old, and booster vaccination is given at 10–18 days. Passively acquired maternal immunity prevents respiratory infection and disease for the first 7 days. For layers or breeders, attenuated vaccines are used for priming, followed by killed oil-adjuvanted booster vaccines, often given repeatedly during the laying cycle. Vaccination breaks occur because of the variable presence of new antigenic variants and existence of several serotypes. Such variants will continue to emerge and spread, posing continuing problems for poultry producers.

Control of infectious bronchitis is difficult because of the presence of persistently infected chickens in some flocks and the continuing emergence of antigenically variant viruses. The domestic chicken is the primary and most important host, but infections and disease have been described in pheasants infected with a closely related coronavirus. Sporadic or individual cases of avian infectious bronchitis virus infection also have been described in peafowl, teal, partridge, and guinea fowl. Group 3 avian coronaviruses have been infrequently identified in graylag geese, mallards, pigeons, green-cheeked Amazon parrots, and Manx shearwater.

TURKEY CORONAVIRUS

Coronaviruses were first recognized in turkeys in the United States in 1951 and were associated with various enteric disease syndromes, variously termed "blue comb disease," "mud fever," "transmissible enteritis," and "coronaviral enteritis." The disease is present throughout the world, essentially wherever turkeys are raised. The virus can infect turkeys of all ages, but the most severe enteric disease is evident within the first few weeks of life. The onset is characterized by loss of appetite, watery diarrhea, dehydration, hypothermia, weight loss, and depression. Younger poults may die. The duodenum and jejunum are pale and flaccid, and the ceca filled with frothy, watery contents. The feces may be green to brown, watery, and may contain mucus and urates. The cloacal bursa is small (atrophic). Some turkeys may shed virus in their feces for up to 7 weeks, with virus transmission by the fecal–oral route. Turkey coronavirus infections also result in reduced egg production in breeder hens, and eggs may lack normal pigment and have a chalky shell surface. Interaction between turkey coronavirus and other agents (*E. coli*, astrovirus, etc.) accentuate the disease.

Only one serotype of turkey coronavirus is recognized. Turkey coronavirus is classified, along with other avian coronaviruses, in antigenic group 3. Although there is high sequence identity (85–90%) in the three major viral proteins (polymerase, M, and N) of turkey coronavirus and avian infectious bronchitis virus, their S proteins are quite different. Whether the latter divergence reflects altered enteric tropism, or adaptation to the turkey, is unclear. Recently, bovine coronavirus was shown experimentally to infect turkey poults, but natural cases have not been identified.

Turkey coronavirus can be isolated in embryonated eggs of turkeys and chickens using the amniotic route of inoculation. No licensed vaccines for turkey coronavirus are available. Treatment involves supportive care, and is not specific.

OTHER CORONAVIRUSES

Coronavirus infections have been described in a wide variety of other species, including humans, horses, bats, wild carnivores, rabbits, numerous species of birds, and wildlife, sometimes in association with enteric or respiratory diseases. An enteric coronavirus occurs in ferrets and mink, in association with outbreaks of enteritis. A related virus recently was incriminated as the cause of systemic pyogranulomatous inflammation resembling feline infectious peritonitis amongst ferrets in both Europe and North America.

MEMBERS OF THE GENUS *TOROVIRUS*

Toroviruses have been described in the horse (Berne virus), cattle (Breda virus), and turkeys. The equine and bovine toroviruses are serologically related. A torovirus of swine (porcine torovirus) that is genetically closely related to the equine and bovine viruses has been demonstrated only by molecular techniques, and has yet to be propagated in cell culture.

At least two serotypes of Breda virus are recognized (defined by hemagglutination-inhibition assays), with a third genotype suggested on the basis of sequence heterogeneity; there are two distinct genotypes of porcine toroviruses. A surprising feature of toroviruses is their sequence divergence and the presence of interspecies sequence homology, presumably acquired via homologous RNA recombination events. For instance, the M protein and S2 subunit (stalk) sequences are highly conserved (10–15% maximum divergence) among toroviruses, whereas the S1 subunit (globular top of the S protein involved in receptor binding) is more divergent (maximum 38% divergence), presumably as a consequence of selection pressure. The hemagglutinin esterase (HE) proteins that are also subject to immune pressure are the most highly divergent. The Berne virus lacks this protein, which is largely deleted. The N protein, which is usually highly conserved within coronavirus groups, shows less sequence divergence (20%) between Berne and Breda viruses and more divergence (35–37%) with porcine torovirus (genotype 2). Furthermore, the N protein genes of genotypes 2 and 3 Breda viruses appear to have been acquired from porcine torovirus genotype 1 strains, presumably through an RNA recombination event.

Clinical Features and Epidemiology

Little is known of the disease potential of Berne virus in horses, as only a single case has been described—this in a horse with diarrhea. Breda virus causes diarrhea in calves, and can be a serious problem in some herds. In swine, torovirus infection has been associated with post-weaning diarrhea. Torovirus infections of turkeys cause diarrhea, poor feed conversion, reduced weight gain (stunting), listlessness, and litter eating.

Torovirus infections are common. In cattle, 90–95% of randomly sampled cattle have antibodies. Antibody-positive cattle have been identified in every country in which tests have been done. Most adult horses in Switzerland possess neutralizing antibodies to Berne virus, which is also true for goats, sheep, pigs, rabbits, and some species of wild mice. Epidemiological surveys have indicated that torovirus infections are involved in two disease entities in cattle: diarrhea in calves up to 2 months of age, and winter dysentery of adult cattle in the Netherlands and Costa Rica. Nasal shedding of Breda virus in feedlot cattle has been reported, but without any clear association with respiratory disease in the infected animals.

Human toroviruses have been detected in stool samples, most commonly from diarrheic children, with prevalence rates of 22–35%. Their detection was based largely on the detection by electron microscopy of virus particles with characteristic torovirus morphology, but, more recently, viral antigen or RNA was detected by ELISA or RT-PCR, respectively, using Berne or Breda virus-specific reagents. Berne virus neutralizing antibodies are also detected in human sera. Sequence analysis of torovirus amplicons from human stool specimens revealed essentially identical sequences in the corresponding 3′-untranslated region with Berne virus and 9% divergence with Breda virus. However, the sequence of the torovirus *HE* gene from human stool samples was unique and divergent from that of other toroviruses. Additional studies of human toroviruses are needed to clarify their prevalence and relationships to animal toroviruses.

Pathogenesis and Pathology

Breda virus, the bovine torovirus, is pathogenic for newborn gnotobiotic and non-immune conventional calves; these animals develop watery diarrhea lasting for 4–5 days, with virus shedding occurring for another 3–4 days. Diarrhea is more severe in calves with a normal intestinal flora than in gnotobiotic calves. Histological lesions include necrosis of enterocytes with subsequent villous contraction (atrophy) from mid-jejunum to distal ileum, in addition to enterocyte necrosis in the large intestine. Epithelial cells lining both the intestinal crypts and villi are infected. Infection of the former may affect the severity and duration of diarrhea, as mucosal regeneration begins by division of crypt enterocytes. The germinal centers of the Peyer's patches become depleted of lymphocytes. There also is necrosis of dome epithelial cells, including M cells.

Diagnosis

Berne virus was originally isolated and then propagated *in vitro* using several types of equine cell, with subsequent manifestation of cytopathic effects. Recently, a bovine torovirus (Aichi/2004 strain) has been isolated in human rectal tumor (HRT-18) cells—the same cell line used for bovine coronavirus primary isolation.

Using immunofluorescence, Breda virus antigen can be detected in epithelial cells of the small intestine. Fluorescence is cytoplasmic, and is generally most intense in areas of the intestines with the least tissue damage. The mid-jejunum is the first site to be infected, with viral infection progressing down the small intestine and eventually reaching the large intestine. Given this course of the infection, tissue specimens must be obtained at several levels, and as early after the onset of diarrhea as possible. Torovirus particles also can be directly visualized in feces or intestinal contents, using electron microscopy. However, immune electron microscopy using hyperimmune antiserum is preferred for definitive identification of torovirus–antibody complexes, and to avoid potential confusion (misidentification) with coronaviruses or cellular debris. Serum neutralization, ELISA, and hemagglutination-inhibition assays (for bovine or porcine torovirus only) are available, using bovine torovirus or Berne virus from infected cell cultures as antigen, or Breda virus purified from the feces or intestinal contents of gnotobiotic calves. RT-PCR with primers targeting the S protein has been used to diagnose field infections in cattle, using nasal or rectal swab specimens or feces.

The turkey torovirus can be isolated in turkey embryos via the amniotic route of inoculation.

Immunity, Prevention, and Control

The seroprevalence of antibodies to Breda virus in adult cattle and colostrum-fed young calves (approximately 1 month old) is high (up to 90%). In the latter, this presumably reflects maternally acquired passive antibodies that have been shown to protect at least partially against Breda virus diarrhea, but not infection during the initial month of life. Maternal antibodies may delay active immune responses of calves to Breda virus, with late or low IgM and IgG serum antibody responses. Passive antibodies decline and calves become seronegative or exhibit low antibody titers by 4–7 months of age. At 6–8 months of age, all seronegative (100%) but fewer seropositive (57%) feedlot calves were susceptible to Breda virus infection, as demonstrated by fecal and nasal virus shedding and seroconversion. A surprising aspect of Breda virus infection in one study was a lack of IgA seroconversion. The authors attributed this to infection of M cells interfering with an active mucosal antibody response.

In view of the variable role of toroviruses as pathogens, vaccines have not been developed against them. For Breda virus, symptomatic treatment (electrolytes) may be needed to control dehydration in severely affected calves. Colostrum containing bovine torovirus antibodies may be used for prophylaxis. General hygiene, biosecurity, and good calf management practices (colostrum feeding immediately after birth) may reduce outbreaks or adverse effects of Breda virus infections in cattle.

Chapter 25

Arteriviridae and *Roniviridae*

Chapter Contents

Viruses within the families *Arteriviridae* and *Roniviridae* are included in the order *Nidovirales*, along with those in the family *Coronaviridae*. Viruses in these families have very different virion morphology, but the grouping reflects their common and distinctive replication strategy that utilizes a nested set of 3′ co-terminal subgenomic messenger RNAs (mRNAs). The family *Roniviridae* contains viruses that have been detected only in crustaceans, specifically, several genotypes of gill-associated and yellow head viruses. The name of the family *Arteriviridae* is derived from the disease caused by its type species, equine arteritis virus. Other arteriviruses include porcine reproductive and respiratory syndrome, lactate dehydrogenase-elevating, and simian hemorrhagic fever viruses (Table 25.1). The host range of arteriviruses is highly restricted, and all arteriviruses share the capacity to establish asymptomatic prolonged or persistent infections in their respective natural hosts; most can cause severe disease in certain circumstances.

PROPERTIES OF ARTERIVIRUSES AND RONIVIRUSES

Classification

Despite marked differences in their virion morphology, viruses in the families *Arteriviridae* and *Roniviridae*

TABLE 25.1 Arteriviruses of Animals

Virus	Host	Disease
Equine arteritis virus	Horse	Systemic influenza-like disease, arteritis, abortion, pneumonia in foals
Porcine reproductive and respiratory syndrome virus	Swine	Porcine reproductive and respiratory syndrome, systemic disease; abortion of sows or birth of stillborn or mummified fetuses; respiratory disease
Lactate dehydrogenase-elevating virus	Mice	Usually none, but the presence of the virus may confound research using infected mice
Simian hemorrhagic fever virus	Macaques	Systemic hemorrhagic disease, death

have a similar genome organization and replication strategy. The family *Arteriviridae* comprises a single genus, *Arterivirus*, which contains all member viruses, and the family *Roniviridae* contains a single genus, *Okavirus*.

Fenner's Veterinary Virology. DOI: 10.1016/B978-0-12-375158-4.00025-0

(A)

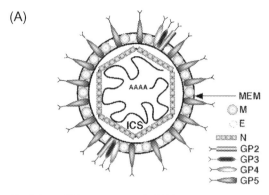

(B)

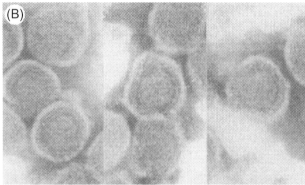

(C)

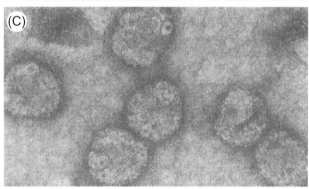

FIGURE 25.1 Family *Arteriviridae*, genus *Arterivirus*. (A) Schematic representation of an arterivirus particle. Seven virion-associated proteins have been identified in equine arteritis virus: N, nucleocapsid; M, membrane protein; GP5, major glycoprotein; GP2, GP3, GP4, minor glycoproteins; E, small integral envelope protein. MEM, lipid membrane; ICS, inner capsid space; AAAA, 3′ poly(A). *[A: From* Virus Taxonomy: Eighth Report of the International Committee on Taxonomy of Viruses *(C. M. Fauquet, M. A. Mayo, J. Maniloff, U. Desselberger, L. A. Ball, eds.), p. 965. Copyright © Elsevier (2005), with permission.]* (B) Lactate dehydrogenase-elevating virus and (C) equine arteritis virus virions; negative stain electron microscopy.

Virion Properties

Arterivirus virions are enveloped, spherical, and 45–60 nm in diameter, which is only about half the size of those of coronaviruses (Figure 25.1). In contrast to the nucleocapsids of coronaviruses and roniviruses, which are helical, arterivirus nucleocapsids are isometric, 25–35 nm in diameter. Whereas envelope glycoprotein spikes are prominent on coronaviruses and roniviruses, they are small and indistinct

on arterivirus virions. The genome of arteriviruses consists of a single molecule of linear positive-sense, single-stranded RNA, approximately 12.7–15.7 kb in size that includes 9–12 open reading frames (Figure 25.2). There are untranslated regions of 156–224 nt and 59–177 nt at the 5′ and 3′ ends of the genome respectively, and a 3′-poly(A) terminal sequence. Arterivirus virions include a single nucleocapsid protein, N, and six envelope proteins, designated E, GP2, GP3, GP4, GP5, and M. Of these, three minor envelope proteins (GP2, GP3, and GP4) form a heterotrimer, and the non-glycosylated triple-membrane spanning integral membrane protein, M, and the large envelope glycoprotein, GP5, form a heterodimer. The major neutralization determinants are expressed on GP5, although M protein exerts a conformational influence on GP5. Simian hemorrhagic fever virus is not as well characterized as the other arteriviruses, and its genome includes three additional open reading frames that may represent re-duplications of genes encoding structural viral proteins.

Ronivirus virions are approximately 150–200 nm × 40–60 nm, bacilliform, with rounded ends and prominent glycoprotein envelope spikes (Figure 25.3). Nucleocapsids have helical symmetry and a diameter of 20–30 nm. The genome consists of a single molecule of linear, positive-sense, single-stranded RNA approximately 26.2 kb in size that includes five long open reading frames, 5′- and 3′-untranslated regions, and a 3′-terminal poly(A) sequence. Virions consist of at least three structural proteins, and the envelope glycoproteins are cleavage products of a larger polyprotein precursor.

Virus Replication

Arteriviruses replicate in macrophages and a very limited number of other cell types within their respective hosts. The host range of arteriviruses is highly restricted, and the viruses typically grow *in vitro* only in cultured macrophages, macrophage cell lines, and a few other cell lines. Some arteriviruses effectively can subvert protective host innate immune responses, including apoptosis of infected macrophages and interferon signaling pathways.

The heterotrimer of envelope proteins GP2, GP3, and GP4 is responsible for cell tropism and receptor binding of equine arteritis virus, and arteriviruses appear to enter susceptible cells by a low-pH-dependent endocytic pathway. The receptors for most arteriviruses are uncharacterized; however, potential receptors involved in the attachment and internalization of porcine reproductive and respiratory syndrome virus include CD163 (a cellular protein in the scavenger receptor cysteine-rich superfamily), sialoadhesin (a macrophage-restricted surface molecule), and heparan sulfate glycosaminoglycans.

The two large open reading frames at the 5′ end of the arterivirus genome encode two replicase polyproteins that

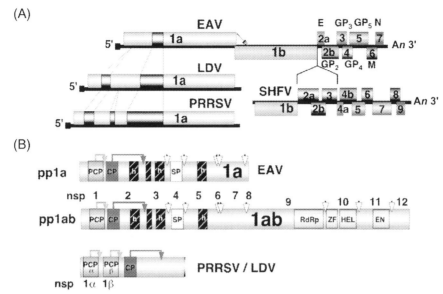

FIGURE 25.2 **Overview of arterivirus genome organization and replicase polyproteins.** (A) General genome organization. ORFs are represented by boxes. The proteins encoded by the equine arteritis virus (EAV) open reading frames (ORFs) are indicated. The 5′ leader sequence is depicted by a small black box; 3′ poly(A) tails are not shown. The arrow between ORF1a and ORF1b represents the ribosomal frameshift site. The grey boxes represent regions where porcine reproductive and respiratory syndrome virus (PRRSV), lactate dehydrogenase-elevating virus (LDV), and simian hemorrhagic fever (SHFV) contain major insertions compared to EAV. (B) Overview of proteolytic processing and domain organization of the EAV replicase polyproteins, pp1a and pp1ab, with differences in PRRSV and LDV indicated. Polyprotein cleavage sites are depicted with arrowheads matching the color of the proteinase involved. Abbreviations: PCP, papain-like cysteine proteinase; CP, nsp2 cysteine proteinase; SP, nsp4 chymotrypsin-like serine proteinase; h, hydrophobic domain; RdRp, RNA-dependent RNA polymerase; ZF, zinc finger; HEL, NTPase/helicase; EN, putative endoribonuclease. N, nucleocapsid; M, membrane protein; GP5 major glycoprotein; GP2, GP3, GP4, minor glycoproteins; E, small integral envelope protein. *[From* Virus Taxonomy: Eighth Report of the International Committee on Taxonomy of Viruses *(C. M. Fauquet, M. A. Mayo, J. Maniloff, U. Desselberger, L. A. Ball, eds.), p. 966. Copyright © Elsevier (2005), with permission.]*

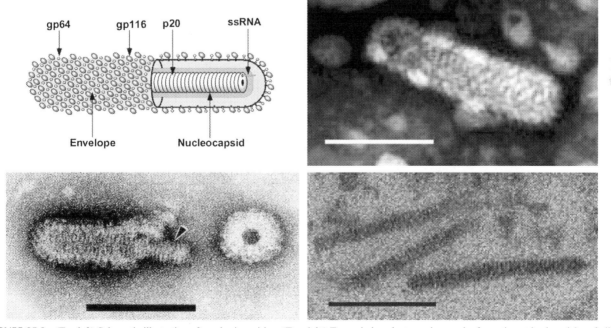

FIGURE 25.3 (Top left) Schematic illustration of an okavirus virion. (Top right) Transmission electron micrograph of negative-stained particles of gill-associated virus (GAV). (Bottom left). Transmission electron micrograph of partially disrupted yellow head virus (YHV) virion displaying the internal nucleocapsid and a ring-like structure which appears to be a disrupted virion in cross-section. (Bottom right) Transmission electron micrograph of cytoplasmic unenveloped nucleocapsids in a thin section of GAV-infected lymphoid organ cells. The bars represent 100 nm. (Courtesy of K. Spann, P. Loh, J. Cowley and R.J. McCulloch and reproduced with permission). p20, nucleocapsid; gp64, small spike glycoprotein; gp116, large spike glycoprotein; ssRNA, positive single-strand RNA *[From* Virus Taxonomy: Eighth Report of the International Committee on Taxonomy of Viruses *(C. M. Fauquet, M. A. Mayo, J. Maniloff, U. Desselberger, L. A. Ball, eds.), p. 975. Copyright © Elsevier (2005), with permission.]*

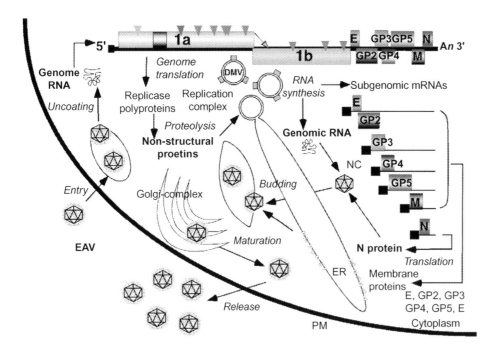

FIGURE 25.4 Overview of the life cycle of the arterivirus prototype equine arteritis virus (EAV). The genome organization, including replicase cleavage sites (arrowheads), is shown at the top of the figure. Abbreviations: ER, endoplasmic reticulum; PM, plasma membrane; DMV, double membrane vesicle; NC, nucleocapsid. N, nucleocapsid protein; M, membrane protein; GP5, major glycoprotein; GP2, GP3, GP4, minor glycoproteins; E, small integral envelope protein. *[From Virus Taxonomy: Eighth Report of the International Committee on Taxonomy of Viruses (C. M. Fauquet, M. A. Mayo, J. Maniloff, U. Desselberger, L. A. Ball, eds.), p. 969. Copyright © Elsevier (2005), with permission.]*

TABLE 25.2 Properties of Arteriviruses

Virions are spherical, 50–70 nm in diameter, with an isometric nucleocapsid and a closely adherent smooth-surfaced envelope with ring-like structures

The genome consists of a single molecule of linear, positive-sense, single-stranded RNA, 13–15 kb in size. Virion RNA has a 5′ cap and its 3′ end is polyadenylated; the genomic RNA is infectious

Replication takes place in the cytoplasm; the genome is transcribed to form full-length negative-sense RNA, from which is transcribed a 3′ co-terminal nested set of mRNAs; only the unique sequences at the 5′ end of each mRNA are translated

Virions are formed by budding into the endoplasmic reticulum, from where they are released by exocytosis

are expressed directly from viral genomic RNA through a ribosomal frameshifting mechanism. These replicase polyproteins are co- and post-translationally modified by viral proteinases into at least 12 non-structural proteins that mediate replication. The genes that encode the viral structural proteins are overlapping, and located in the 3′ end of the genome; they are expressed from a nested set of 3′ co-terminal subgenomic RNAs. These subgenomic RNAs all include a common 5′ leader sequence derived from the 5′-untranslated region of viral genomic RNA, at least one unique open reading frame encoding one or more structural virion proteins, and a common 3′-poly(A) tail. The individual open reading frames that are included in these subgenomic mRNAs reflect overlapping reading

frames contained in the 3′ end of the viral genome. It is believed that the subgenomic mRNAs are generated by discontinuous transcription that links non-contiguous portions of the viral genome, to produce negative-strand templates that are transcribed into positive-strand subgenomic mRNAs that are then translated into the individual virion proteins.

Arterivirus replication occurs in the cytoplasm of infected cells, although individual non-structural (nsp1) and structural (N) proteins selectively translocate to the nucleus. Viral RNA replication complexes localized in double membrane vesicles derived from the endoplasmic reticulum produce the genomic and subgenomic mRNAs (Figure 25.4). Viral nucleocapsids bud into the lumen of the endoplasmic reticulum and/or Golgi complex of infected cells, and from there move to the surface of the cell in vesicles and are released by exocytosis (Table 25.2).

The overall strategy for replication of roniviruses is similar to that of arteriviruses, but the structural proteins are expressed from a nested set of just two subgenomic mRNAs that each encode several proteins. The subgenomic RNAs also lack a common 5′ leader sequence derived from genomic viral RNA.

MEMBERS OF THE FAMILY *ARTERIVIRIDAE*, GENUS *ARTERIVIRUS*

EQUINE ARTERITIS VIRUS

Descriptions of a disease that very probably was equine viral arteritis were first published in the late 18th and

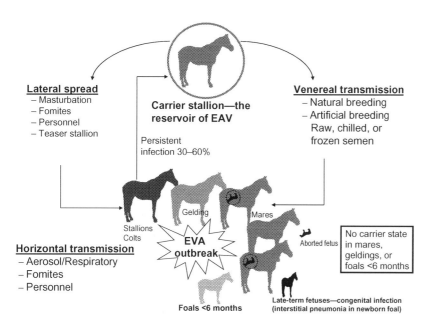

FIGURE 25.5 Natural transmission cycles of equine arteritis virus (EAV) in horses. *[From* Equine Infectious Diseases, *D. C. Sellon, M. Long, p. 156. Copyright © Saunders/Elsevier (2007), with permission.]*

early 19th centuries, with colloquial names such as "pink-eye," "infectious or epizootic cellulites," "influenza erysipelatosa," and "Pferdestaupe." Early investigators also recognized that apparently healthy stallions transmitted this disease to susceptible mares at breeding. The causative agent, equine arteritis virus, was first isolated in 1953 from lung tissue of aborted fetuses during an epizootic of abortion and respiratory disease on a breeding farm near Bucyrus, Ohio. Although serologic studies indicate that infection occurs worldwide, the incidence of both infection and overt disease varies markedly among countries and among horses of different breeds.

Clinical Features and Epidemiology

Most natural infections with equine arteritis virus are asymptomatic, and descriptions of fatal disease are based on experimental infections with highly horse-adapted laboratory strains of the virus. Nevertheless, relatively virulent field strains of equine arteritis virus periodically cause natural outbreaks of equine viral arteritis in horses. After an incubation period of 3–14 days, the onset of disease is marked by fever (greater than 41°C), leukopenia, depression, excessive lacrimation, anorexia, conjunctivitis, rhinitis and nasal discharge, urticaria of the head, neck, and trunk, and edema, which is most pronounced over the eyes (supraorbital), the abdomen, including the prepuce, scrotum, and mammary glands, and the hind limbs (often resulting in a stiff gait). Although naturally infected horses usually recover uneventfully, death as a result of rapidly progressive bronchointerstitial pneumonia occurs sporadically in young foals. Abortion is characteristic of infections of pregnant mares with particular strains of the virus, and infection of large numbers of susceptible

(unvaccinated) pregnant mares can lead to "abortion storms." Abortion generally occurs 10–30 days after infection and at any time between 3 and 10 months of gestation; it is linked closely with the late febrile or early convalescent phase of infection, but can occur even if no clinical signs are noticed.

Equine arteritis virus is spread by both the respiratory and venereal routes, respectively by aerosol from acutely infected horses or in the semen of persistently infected carriers stallions (Figure 25.5). The latter are the essential natural virus reservoir, and persistent infection occurs in some 30–70% of postpubertal colts and stallions. Carrier stallions are otherwise normal, and infection is confined to the reproductive tract during persistence. Virus is spread from carrier stallions exclusively via the venereal route; semen collected from persistently infected stallions and used in artificial insemination has been responsible for outbreaks of disease. Furthermore, genetic diversity is generated in equine arteritis virus during persistent infection of stallions. Persistent infection is maintained in the reproductive tract of individual stallions for variable intervals, from several weeks to life-long.

Pathogenesis and Pathology

Initial replication of equine arteritis virus takes place in alveolar macrophages and endothelial cells after aerosol respiratory infection of susceptible horses, and virus then rapidly spreads to the draining bronchial lymph nodes; subsequently it is disseminated via the blood stream. Although macrophages and endothelial cells are the principal sites of virus replication, the virus also productively infects selected epithelia, mesothelium, and smooth muscle of the media of arteries and the uterine wall. The clinical manifestations of equine viral arteritis reflect vascular injury. However, in the pathogenesis of vascular injury, the relative roles and importance of the direct involvement of viruses, as opposed to the involvement of virus-induced cytokines derived from macrophages and endothelial cells, are not clear. Strains of equine arteritis virus clearly differ in their virulence, including their potential to cause abortion, and in their ability to induce pro-inflammatory cytokine mediators.

The characteristic gross lesions of severe cases of equine viral arteritis in adult horses are edema, congestion, and hemorrhage. Pleural and pericardial effusion are characteristic of the fulminant disease caused by the highly pathogenic horse-adapted laboratory strain of equine arteritis virus, as is terminal disseminated intravascular coagulation, which leads to necrosis and hemorrhage in several organs. Foals with bronchointerstitial pneumonia develop marked pulmonary edema, with accumulation of protein-rich fluid in airspaces and lesions typical of acute respiratory distress syndrome. They also may develop pleural and pericardial effusion, and intestinal hemorrhage and necrosis. Aborted fetuses are usually expelled together with the placenta (fetal membranes) and without premonitory clinical signs. Aborted fetuses are typically autolyzed, and seldom exhibit characteristic gross or histologic lesions. Some may have excess fluid in the peritoneal and pleural cavities, and petechial hemorrhages in peritoneal and pleural mucosal surfaces.

The pathogenesis of the carrier state in stallions is poorly characterized. Virus concentrations are greatest in the accessory sex glands and in the vas deferens. The carrier state is testosterone dependent, as persistent virus shedding does not occur in either geldings or mares. Furthermore, persistently infected stallions that are castrated cease shedding virus in semen, whereas those supplemented with testosterone after castration continue to shed virus.

Diagnosis

Detection of equine arteritis virus in tissues samples and fluids can be achieved by either virus isolation or reverse-transcriptase-polymerase chain reaction (RT-PCR) assay. Virus isolation is routinely carried out in rabbit kidney cells. There can be marked variation in the amount of virus shed in the semen of individual stallions over time, and the highest quantities of virus are associated with the sperm-rich fraction of the ejaculate. Serum antibodies to equine arteritis virus are usually detected by virus neutralization assay, although several enzyme-linked immunosorbent assays (ELISAs) have been developed and partially characterized.

Immunity, Prevention, and Control

Despite its worldwide distribution, equine arteritis virus causes disease outbreaks only occasionally, with instances or outbreaks of abortion being especially devastating.

Epizootics occur where horses are congregated from several sources, such as at sales and shows, and on breeding farms. The virus readily is transmitted by horizontal aerosol spread during outbreaks, and likely sources of initial infection include susceptible mares that were recently bred to a carrier stallion. A high percentage of seronegative stallions and postpubertal colts infected during an outbreak will subsequently become persistently infected carriers of the virus. Identification of carrier stallions is central to control strategies, as only immune mares should be bred to these animals. Semen used for artificial insemination should be tested for the presence of virus, so that the use of contaminated semen can be restricted to immune mares. Furthermore, mares should be isolated after being bred to a carrier stallion, to prevent transmission to susceptible cohorts.

Virus neutralizing antibodies appear in serum within approximately 1 week after infection, coinciding with virus elimination from the circulation. There is only one known serotype of equine arteritis virus, and neutralizing antibodies prevent reinfection. Neutralizing antibodies persist for years after natural infection, and protection is long-lasting, if not life-long. Colostrum from immune mares moderates or prevents equine viral arteritis in young foals.

Immunization of horses with attenuated or inactivated virus vaccines can induce immunity, thus immunization of valuable breeding animals is justified. To prevent the establishment of persistent infections in stallions that will be used for breeding, vaccination of colts may be done at 6–8 months of age. This timing is important, because vaccination should be done after maternal antibody has waned but before puberty, to preclude any possibility of inducing persistent infection. The carrier state does not occur in colts exposed to equine arteritis virus before puberty. To prevent abortions, mares may be vaccinated before becoming pregnant.

During outbreaks, the spread of virus is best controlled by: (1) movement restrictions; (2) isolation of infected horses, followed by a quarantine period after recovery; (3) good hygiene, including assignment of separate personnel to work with infected and uninfected animals; (4) laboratory-supported surveillance.

PORCINE REPRODUCTIVE AND RESPIRATORY SYNDROME VIRUS

A previously unrecognized disease—initially designated as "mystery swine disease" in North America—appeared in pigs in North America in the 1980s, and subsequently in Europe. A virus identified as "Lelystad virus" was first isolated in the Netherlands and proven to reproduce the disease in 1991. Porcine reproductive and respiratory syndrome virus has since become a major pathogen in swine populations worldwide, and retrospective serological studies indicate the causative virus first appeared in the United States in 1979, Asia in 1985, and Europe in 1987. It has been speculated, but not proven, that this virus arose by the "species jumping," to swine, of the closely related lactate dehydrogenase-elevating virus from its natural host, the house mouse, *Mus musculus*. Field strains of porcine reproductive and respiratory syndrome virus are genetically heterogeneous, and there are distinct European and North American genotype lineages that share only some 60% sequence identity.

Clinical Features and Epidemiology

Porcine reproductive and respiratory syndrome virus infects only domestic and wild pigs. The disease is initially characterized by anorexia, fever, and lethargy. Clinically affected animals are hyperpneic or dyspneic, and exhibit transient hyperemia or cyanosis of the extremities. Nursery pigs have roughened hair coats and reduced growth rates. Infection of sows in early to mid gestation may have little adverse consequence, whereas infection of sows in late gestation frequently results in reproductive failure characterized by abortion, premature births, stillbirths, and mummified fetuses. Piglets that are born alive after *in-utero* infection are often weak and die quickly, typically with respiratory distress. Mortality in infected sows reflects the virulence of the infecting virus strain, but it can be high. Other types of infectious diseases are more common in herds with enzootic porcine reproductive and respiratory syndrome virus infection.

The virus is spread by direct contact, including pugilism, and the virus is shed from infected pigs in all secretions and excretions. Transplacental transmission also occurs commonly in fully susceptible sows.

Pathogenesis and Pathology

Porcine reproductive and respiratory syndrome virus replicates primarily in macrophages in the lungs and lymphoid tissues of infected pigs, although there also may be infection of endothelial cells, respiratory epithelium, and fibroblasts. Viremia begins within 24 hours of infection, and persists in some animals for several weeks in the presence of antibodies. The characteristic lesions of acute infection include lymph node enlargement and interstitial pneumonia, the severity of which reflects the virulence of the infecting virus strain.

Porcine reproductive and respiratory syndrome virus appears to utilize several novel mechanisms to subvert protective host immune responses to facilitate its replication, including: (1) inhibition of caspase-dependent apoptosis of infected macrophages; (2) suppression of the type I interferon response through blockade of the retinoic-acid-inducible

gene 1 (*RIG-1*) and interferon regulatory factor 3 (IRF3) signaling pathways; (3) use of decoy epitopes and extensive glycosylation of the N-terminal portion of the GP5 protein, both of which limit the impact of the neutralizing antibody response.

Diagnosis

Porcine reproductive and respiratory syndrome can be provisionally diagnosed on the basis of clinical signs and lesions in affected animals. The virus can be detected by RT-PCR assay, and, in the tissues of infected pigs, by immunohistochemical staining. The virus grows in swine lung macrophages and some, but certainly not all, virus strains grow well in an African green monkey kidney cell line (MA-104) and cotton rat lung cells. Serological diagnosis can be made using commercial ELISA.

Immunity, Prevention, and Control

Infected pigs develop a variable, but frequently weak, immune response to porcine reproductive and respiratory syndrome virus; however, recovered animals typically are immune to reinfection, indicating that immunity is effective and vaccination is feasible. Neutralizing antibodies are directed against epitopes on the N-terminal portion of GP5, and there is marked variation in the glycosylation of this region amongst field strains of the virus. The extent of glycosylation in this area probably affects the ability of antibodies to neutralize the virus, and the neutralizing antibody response of many infected pigs is both weak and slow to develop. Pigs also develop a cellular immune response to porcine reproductive and respiratory syndrome virus, but, despite these responses, virus clearance is delayed, leading to prolonged infection in some animals. It has been proposed that innate immune responses and the availability of susceptible populations of macrophages are major determinants of the outcome of primary infections of swine with the virus.

Control of porcine reproductive and respiratory syndrome virus in free herds is by exclusion, as the virus is spread between herds by the movement of infected swine or infective semen used in artificial insemination. It also is spread mechanically by fomites, and perhaps by long-distance aerosol. Once introduced, the virus spreads quickly in naïve swine populations; thus spread within herds is principally as a result of direct contact, and separation of pens markedly reduces the rate of transmission. Once established in a herd, enzootic infection is perpetuated by a cycle of transmission from sows to piglets *in utero* or through colostrum or milk, and by the regular introduction of new animals into the sow herd and the co-mingling of susceptible and infected pigs. Control in herds with enzootic infection is difficult, and usually achieved through a combination of vaccination and management strategies. Both live-attenuated and inactivated vaccines are commercially available, but vaccines are not infallible—perhaps because of the remarkable genetic variation amongst strains of the virus, and because of the uncertain nature of what constitutes a protective immune response. Furthermore, there is controversy regarding the potential transmission, circulation, and reversion to virulence of live-attenuated vaccine viruses.

LACTATE DEHYDROGENASE-ELEVATING VIRUS

Lactate dehydrogenase-elevating virus initially was identified in several laboratories in the early 1960s, during experiments using transplantable tumors in mice. The virus generally causes persistent infections that reveal themselves only by increased concentrations of numerous plasma enzymes, including lactate dehydrogenase. Presence of the virus in laboratory mice may confound experiments, as the infection can alter the immune response and thereby distort the results of immunological experiments.

Clinical Features and Epidemiology

Infected mice usually exhibit no clinical evidence of infection and live a normal lifespan, despite persistent life-long infection with the virus. The virus is spread between mice by direct contact, and especially by pugilism, through bite wounds. The virus also is contained in the secretions and excretions from infected mice, and may be disseminated by aerosol or ingestion to susceptible cohorts. The most likely source of infection in mouse colonies is by inoculation of mice with contaminated biological material such as transplantable tumors or cell lines.

Pathogenesis and Pathology

Lactate dehydrogenase-elevating virus replicates selectively in differentiated tissue macrophages in all strains of inbred laboratory mice. The virus rapidly achieves an extremely high-titered viremia by cytolytic infection of target macrophages in many tissues, including peritoneum, bone marrow, thymus, spleen, lymph nodes, liver, pancreas, kidneys, gonads, and so on, which quickly depletes this cell population. Persistent infection then follows in infected mice by selective infection of a renewable and continually generated subpopulation of macrophages. Virus-induced cytolysis of tissue macrophages delays the clearance of plasma enzymes such as lactate dehydrogenase, causing the characteristic increase in the concentrations of these enzymes in plasma.

Although infected mice develop antibodies to lactate dehydrogenase-elevating virus, they are ineffective in mediating virus clearance. Extensive glycosylation of the N-terminal portion of GP5, which expresses the neutralization determinants of lactate dehydrogenase-elevating virus, reduces the immunogenicity of this region, apparently by

blocking access of neutralizing antibodies to neutralization sites. Strains of the virus that lack some or all of these glycosylation sites are highly susceptible to antibody-mediated neutralization, and have altered tissue tropism; specifically, viruses lacking these glycosylation sites do not establish persistent infection, but are neurovirulent in immunosuppressed C58 and AKR mice. Interestingly, age-dependent poliomyelitis that occurs in these mice occurs because they express an endogenous retrovirus in several tissues, and co-infection of spinal cord ventral horn motor neuron cells with both lactate dehydrogenase-elevating virus and the endogenous retrovirus results in poliomyelitis and paralysis. These events do not occur under natural conditions, as they are unique to the nature of selected inbred strains of mice and their corresponding complement of endogenous retroviruses.

Diagnosis

Virus is most readily detected in tissues or biological products by RT-PCR, or by the mouse antibody production test. Plasma concentrations of lactate dehydrogenase are substantially increased in mice infected with this virus, with an 8–11-fold increase typically reached at 3–4 days after infection. Antibodies can be detected 1–3 weeks after infection, by either ELISA or immunofluorescence assays.

Immunity, Prevention, and Control

Mice infected with lactate dehydrogenase-elevating virus develop both cellular and humoral immune responses, neither of which are effective in mediating clearance of virus strains that have heterogenous glycosylation of the N-terminal portion of the GP5 ectodomain. Destruction and subsequent loss of the target macrophage population is the major factor in reducing viremia in early infection. Cytotoxic T lymphocyte responses disappear in the course of persistent infection, as a result of clonal exhaustion. Although antibodies are ineffective in preventing persistent infection, polyclonal B cell activation occurs during persistence, with formation of immune complexes. The combination of viral infection of macrophages, polyclonal B cell activation with immune complex formation, and clonal exhaustion of cytotoxic T cells modulates the immune capability of infected mice, which is the major concern regarding adventitious lactate dehydrogenase-elevating virus infection of laboratory mice.

Vaccines are not available, neither are they indicated, as control of lactate dehydrogenase-elevating virus infection in laboratory mice is by exclusion. Prevention of infection in mouse colonies can be accomplished by: (1) preventing entry of infected laboratory and wild mice or biological products; (2) use of barrier-specific, pathogen-free breeding and housing systems; (3) surveillance based on laboratory testing. The virus can be eliminated from contaminated cell lines or tumors by *in-vitro* culture or by passage through athymic nude rats, as either approach eliminates the source of susceptible mouse macrophages that the virus requires for its continued replication.

SIMIAN HEMORRHAGIC FEVER VIRUS

Simian hemorrhagic fever was first recognized in 1964, in both the United States and the former Soviet Union, in macaques imported from India. Nearly all infected animals died in these initial outbreaks. There have been remarkably few documented occurrences of this devastating disease since then, although, in the United States in 1989, there were epizootics at three primate colonies, resulting in the death of more than 600 cynomolgus macaques (*Macaca fascicularis*).

Serological studies indicate that subclinical simian hemorrhagic fever virus infection occurs in African cercopithecine monkeys, including Patas monkeys (*Erythrocebus patas*), African green monkeys (*Cercopithecus aethiops*) and baboons (*Papio anuibus* and *P. cyanocephalus*). Similarly, serological studies indicate subclinical or asymptomatic infection of Asian macaques in China, the Philippines, and Southeast Asia, probably with attenuated virus strains. In contrast, transmission of simian hemorrhagic fever virus from persistently infected African monkeys to Asian macaques (*Macaca mulatta, Macaca arctoides*, and *Macaca fasicularis*) results in acute, typically fatal hemorrhagic disease. Transmission occurs by direct contact, aerosol, and fomites, including contaminated needles. Epizootics in macaque colonies originate from accidental introduction of the virus from other primate species that are infected persistently without showing clinical signs.

The onset of disease in macaques is rapid, with early fever, facial edema, anorexia, dehydration, skin petechiae, diarrhea, and hemorrhages. Death occurs at between 5 and 25 days; mortality approaches 100%. Within a colony, infection spreads rapidly, probably via contact and aerosol. Lesions include hemorrhages in the dermis, nasal mucosa, lungs, intestines, and other visceral organs. Shock is suspected as the underlying cause of death. Like other arteriviruses, simian hemorrhagic fever virus replicates in macrophages, although there is much variation in the cellular tropism, immunogenicity, and virulence of individual virus strains in different species of monkey. Virus strains derived from African monkeys are highly infectious and fatal in macaques, whereas baboons and Patas and African green monkeys are persistently infected carriers of these viruses.

Vaccines are not available for simian hemorrhagic fever, and control is based on management practices, including species segregation to prevent transmission of the virus from persistently infected African monkeys, such as Patas monkeys, to macaques.

MEMBERS OF THE FAMILY *RONIVIRIDAE*, GENUS *OKAVIRUS*

The penaeid shrimp, *Penaeus monodon*, which occurs in Asia, Australia, and East Africa, is the principal aquatic invertebrate host for at least six genotypes of ronivirus. Two genotypes of the virus—designated yellow head virus (genotype 1) and gill-associated virus (genotype 2)—cause significant disease and mortality in cultured shrimp populations. The remaining genotypes have been identified in shrimp without specific disease signs.

YELLOW HEAD AND GILL-ASSOCIATED VIRUSES

Yellow head virus disease occurs in postlarval and subsequent stages of *P. monodon* as well as a wider range of juvenile penaeid and palemonid shrimp and krill. Infected shrimp cease feeding and congregate near the surface or corners of the pond. The disease is named because of the characteristic pale appearance of the cephalothorax as a result of yellowing of the underlying hepatopancreas, which is normally brown. Mortality up to 90% can occur after appearance of the disease. Shrimp with gill-associated virus infections also undergo an abrupt cessation of feeding and swimming near the surface, develop a reddened body, and may exhibit pink to yellow coloration of the gills. A wide range of tissues of both ectodermal and mesodermal origin are targets of yellow head virus, including the organ of Oka, which gives rise to the genus designation *Okavirus* used for the virus. Diagnosis of infections caused by roniviruses is best made from moribund shrimp from the pond borders. Stained preparations of gill filaments or hemolymph directly in the field may provide presumptive diagnoses, but standard fixation and processing for hematoxylin and eosin staining are used to identify characteristic 2-μm spherical basophilic inclusions in the cytoplasm of ectoderm- and mesoderm-derived tissues (e.g., lymphoid organ, stomach subcuticulum, and gills). RT-PCR, immunoblot, *in-situ* hybridization tests, and electron microscopy may be used to confirm presumptive diagnoses of these infections. The frequent presence of subclinical infections requires establishing that disseminated virus is associated with characteristic lesions in target tissues.

Vaccination or chemotherapeutic approaches to control are not available. Disinfection procedures, use of specific-pathogen-free seed stocks as demonstrated by RT-PCR screen, and use of water supplies confirmed to be free of virus are the major control methods that are used.

UNCLASSIFIED NIDOVIRUSES OF FISH

Additional unclassified nidoviruses have been identified among cyprinid fishes in Germany and the United States.

For example, an agent isolated from farmed juvenile fathead minnows (*Pimephales promelas)* in the United States was associated with disease. This virus induces up to 90% mortality among experimentally infected fathead minnows, but not in several other commercially important freshwater fish species, including channel catfish, goldfish, golden shiners, and rainbow trout. The agent is bacilliform (130–180 nm in length and 31–47 nm in diameter) as is characteristic of other nidoviruses, and the virus can be isolated using cell cultures of cyprinid fish origin. RT-PCR assays with generic and specific primer sets and sequencing of the amplified products confirms their relationship with other nidoviruses, and provides confirmation of the infection in fathead minnows.

Picornaviridae

Chapter Contents

Picornaviruses have played an important role in the respective histories of virology in both human and veterinary medicine. In 1897, Loeffler and Frosch showed that foot-and-mouth disease was caused by an agent that passed through filters that held back bacteria; this was the first demonstration that a disease of animals was caused by a filterable virus. Poliovirus, the cause of human poliomyelitis, was not identified until some 10 years later. Polioviruses, which are classified in the genus *Enterovirus*, and other picornaviruses were involved in key developments of virology, including the growth of viruses in cell culture, quantitative plaque assays, infectious clones of specific viruses, X-ray crystallographic analysis of virion structure at the atomic level, RNA replication, and viral protein synthesis. The development of poliovirus vaccines in the 20th century has greatly reduced the occurrence of human poliomyelitis,

a prevalent and often devastating disease that has been recognized since antiquity. Indeed, the advent of highly effective inactivated poliovirus vaccines has stimulated efforts to eradicate the disease from the human population, as was done for smallpox entirely from some countries.

In the second half of the 19th century and the first half of the 20th century, repeated rapidly spreading epizootics of foot-and-mouth disease resulted in great losses, as increasingly intensive systems of livestock production were developed in many countries. Producers demanded of their governments control programs to deal with these epizootics, as well as programs to prevent reintroductions. For example, in 1884, the United States Congress created the Bureau of Animal Industry within the Department of Agriculture. Its principal mission was to deal with foot-and-mouth disease and two other diseases, contagious bovine

Fenner's Veterinary Virology. DOI: 10.1016/B978-0-12-375158-4.00026-2

TABLE 26.1 Important Picornaviruses of Humans and Animals

Genus	Virus	Principal Species Affected	Disease
Aphthovirus	Foot-and-mouth disease viruses	Cattle, sheep, swine, goats, wildlife ruminant species	Foot-and-mouth disease
	Equine rhinitis A virus	Horses, camelids	Systemic infection with respiratory signs
	Bovine rhinitis B virus	Cattle	Mild respiratory
Cardiovirus	Encephalomyocarditis virus	Rodents, swine, elephants, primates, mammals in contact with rodents	Encephalomyelitis and myocarditis in swine and elephants; rarely in other species
	Theiler's mouse encephalomyelitis virus	Mice	Murine poliomyelitis
Enterovirus	Human enteroviruses A, B, C, and D	Humans	Aseptic meningitis, poliomyelitis, myocarditis
	Human rhinoviruses A, B, and C	Humans	Respiratory disease
	Swine vesicular disease virus	Swine	Vesicular disease
	Bovine enteroviruses (includes bovine rhinovirus 1, 3)	Cattle	Mild enteric and respiratory disease
	Simian enteroviruses	Primates	Usually asymptomatic infection
	Porcine enterovirus B (porcine enterovirus 9, 10)	Swine	Usually asymptomatic infection
Erbovirus	Equine rhinitis B virus	Horses	Mild rhinitis
Kobuvirus	Bovine kobuvirus	Cattle	Possible enteritis
Teschovirus	Porcine teschovirus 1 (porcine enterovirus 1)	Swine	Polioencephalomyelitis
	Porcine teschoviruses 2–11 (porcine enteroviruses 2–7, 11–13	Swine	Usually asymptomatic, mild diarrhea, pericarditis
Tremovirus (proposed new genus)	Avian encephalomyelitis virus	Chickens	Encephalomyelitis
Avihepatovirus (proposed new genus)	Duck hepatitis A virus (duck hepatitis virus 1)	Ducks	Hepatitis

pleuropneumonia and hog cholera (classical swine fever). From its beginning, this agency pioneered the development of veterinarians with special skills in disease control. An extensive epizootic of foot-and-mouth disease in 1914 accelerated the creation of disease control programs and the training of more specialized veterinarians. Eventually, this evolved into the complex field- and laboratory-based systems needed to assure the freedom of domestic livestock industries from foreign animal diseases. Similar developments occurred in other countries with increasingly intensive livestock industries, in each case advancing the scope of the veterinary medical profession from its roots

in equine medicine and surgery. Paradoxically, despite the increasing global intensification of livestock production, and rapidly escalating risks of infectious disease outbreaks, support for many of these same critical programs has decreased in recent years.

PROPERTIES OF PICORNAVIRUSES

Classification

The family *Picornaviridae* is divided currently into eight genera: *Aphthovirus, Enterovirus, Teschovirus, Cardiovirus,*

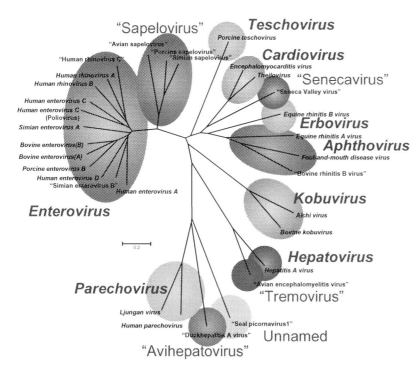

FIGURE 26.1 Unrooted neighbor-joining tree of the *Picornaviridae*, based on a comparison of the P1 capsid region. Proposed genera are not in bold. *[From N. J. Knowles, T. Hovi, T. Hyppia, A. M. Q. King, A. M. Lindberg, P. D. Minor, M. A. Pallansch, A. C. Palmenberg, T. Skern, G. Stanway, T. Yamashita, R. Zell. Taxonomy of Picornaviridae: Current Situation and Future Proposals. EUROPIC (2008)].*

Erbovirus, Kobuvirus, Hepatovirus, and *Parechovirus,* but it is likely that the number of genera will soon increase to 13. The former genus *Rhinovirus* was abolished in 2006, and the member rhinoviruses (99 serotypes of human rhinovirus, the major cause of common colds in people, and two of bovine rhinovirus) allocated to the genus *Enterovirus.* The process of re-classification reflects the development of rapid sequencing technology, along with the continuing identification of new picornaviruses, many from non-domestic species. Important member viruses of each genus are listed in Table 26.1; the phylogenetic relationships between representative members of each genus are shown in Figure 26.1. Updated information can be obtained from the International Committee on Taxonomy of Viruses (ICTV) website (http://www.ictv on line.org/).

An important difference between viruses in the various genera of picornaviruses is their stability at low pH; such differences were utilized in the classification of picornaviruses before molecular techniques were available. Specifically, the aphthoviruses are unstable below pH 7, whereas the enteroviruses, hepatoviruses, cardioviruses, and parechoviruses are stable at pH 3. However, other major differences were identified with the availability of complete genomic sequence data. All picornaviruses are single-stranded, positive-sense RNA viruses with a 5′-untranslated region (5′-UTR). The RNA is uncapped, but does have a viral protein (VPg) covalently linked to the 5′ end. There are major structural differences in the 5′-UTR among the genera of the picornavirus family: the length of the 5′-UTR in picornaviruses varies from approximately

500 to 1200 nt and contains one of four different internal ribosome entry sites (IRES). Cardioviruses, aphthoviruses, erboviruses, kobuviruses, teschoviruses, and the proposed sapeloviruses and senecavirus are also distinguished by the presence of a leader protein (L) encoded upstream of the capsid proteins (Figure 26.2). Foot-and-mouth disease virus is also unique in having three similar, but not identical, VPg proteins that are present in equimolar amounts among the virion RNAs. Equine rhinitis A virus, another member of the genus *Aphthovirus,* shares many genomic characteristics with foot-and-mouth disease virus, but its genome encodes only a single copy of the *VPg* gene.

Virion Properties

Picornavirus virions are non-enveloped, approximately 30 nm in diameter, and have icosahedral symmetry (Figure 26.3; Table 26.2). Virions appear smooth and round in outline in electron micrographs and in images reconstructed from X-ray crystallographic analyses. The genome consists of a single molecule of linear, positive-sense, single-stranded RNA, 7–8.8 kb in size. Both the 5′ and 3′ ends of the RNA contain untranslated regulatory sequences. The genomic RNA is polyadenylated at its 3′ end and has a protein, VPg, linked covalently to its 5′ end. Genomic RNA is infectious.

The atomic structure of representative viruses of most picornavirus genera has been solved. The virions are constructed from 60 copies each of four capsid proteins, VP1

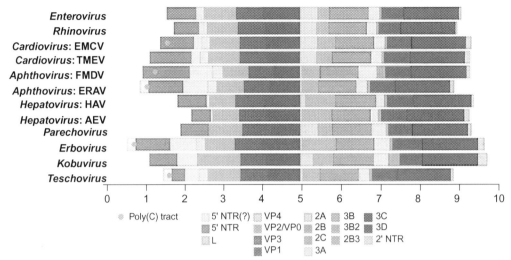

FIGURE 26.2 Genome structure and gene organization of selected members of the family *Picornaviridae*. Circles within the 5′-NTR indicate poly(C) tracts that are present in some members. The 1A gene products of many members are myristylated at the amino terminal glycine. The 5′-NTR is followed by a long ORF encoding the polyprotein, that is in turn followed by the 3′-NTR and a poly(A) tail. The eventual cleavage products of the polyprotein are indicated by vertical lines and different shading. The nomenclature of the polypeptides follows an L:4:3:4 schema corresponding to the genes (numbers) encoded by the L, P1, P2, P3 regions. The P1 region encodes the structural proteins 1A, 1B, 1C, and 1D, also referred to as VP4, VP2, VP3 and VP1, respectively. VP0 (1AB) is the intermediate precursor for VP4 and VP2 and in parechoviruses and kobuviruses it remains uncleaved. In all viruses 3C is a protease, in enteroviruses and rhinoviruses 2A is a protease, while in all viruses 3D is considered to be a component of the RNA replicase. Only foot-and-mouth disease virus encodes 3 VPg proteins that map in tandem. 2A, 2B, 2C, 2B3, 3A, 3B, 3B2, 3C, 3D, non-structural proteins; AEV, avian encephalomyelitis virus; EMCV, encephalomyocarditis virus; ERAV, equine rhinitis A virus; FMDV, foot-and-mouth disease virus; HAV, hepatitis A virus; L, leader protein; NTR, non-translated region; TMEV, Theiler's murine encephalomyelitis virus; VP0–4, viral structural proteins. *[From* Virus Taxonomy: Eighth Report of the International Committee on Taxonomy of Viruses *(C. M. Fauquet, M. A. Mayo, J. Maniloff, U. Desselberger, L. A. Ball, eds.), p. 759. Copyright © Elsevier (2005), with permission.]*

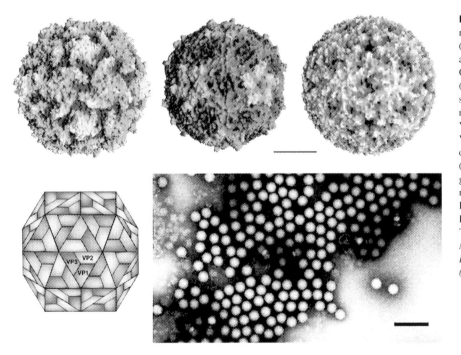

FIGURE 26.3 (Top) Pictures of picornavirus structures; poliovirus type 1 (PV-1) (Left), mengo virus (Center) and foot-and-mouth disease virus serotype O (FMDV-O) (Right). The bar represents 10 nm. (Images courtesy of J.Y. Sgro, with permission). (Bottom left) Diagram of a picornavirus particle. The surface shows proteins VP1, VP2 and VP3. The fourth capsid protein, VP4, is located about the internal surface of the pentameric apex of the icosahedron. (Right) Negative contrast electron micrograph of poliovirus (PV) particles. The bar represents 100 nm. (Courtesy of Ann C. Palmenberg). *[From* Virus Taxonomy: Eighth Report of the International Committee on Taxonomy of Viruses *(C. M. Fauquet, M. A. Mayo, J. Maniloff, U. Desselberger, L. A. Ball, eds.), p. 757. Copyright © Elsevier (2005), with permission.]*

(also designated 1D), VP2 (1B), VP3 (1C) (M_r approximately 30,000 for each), and VP4 (1A) (M_r 7000–8000), and a single copy of the genome linked protein, VPg (3B) (M_r variable). The exceptions to the four capsid protein rule are parechoviruses and kobuviruses, in which the VP0, a polyprotein that includes VPs 2–4, remains uncleaved. VP1, VP2, and VP3 are structurally similar to one another, each being composed of a wedge-shaped, eight-stranded β barrel and differing primarily in the size and conformation of the loops that occur between the strands and also in the

TABLE 26.2 Properties of Picornaviruses

Virions appear smooth and round in outline, are non-enveloped, ≈30 nm in diameter, and have icosahedral symmetry

The genome consists of a single molecule of linear, positive-sense, single-stranded RNA, 7–8.8 kb in size

Genomic RNA is polyadenylated at its 3′ end and has a protein, VPg, linked covalently to its 5′ end; genomic RNA is infectious

Virion RNA acts as mRNA and is translated into a polyprotein, which is then cleaved to yield some 11 or 12 individual proteins

Cytoplasmic replication

extensions of their amino and carboxyl termini. Amino acid substitutions correlating with antigenic variation occur in the surface-oriented loop regions. For foot-and-mouth disease virus, at least five antigenic sites have been identified. The VP1 proteins are located around the fivefold axes of icosahedral symmetry, and VP2 and VP3 alternate around the two- and threefold axes. The amino-terminal extensions of these three proteins form an intricate network on the inner surface of the protein shell. The small, myristylated protein, VP4, is located entirely at the inner surface of the capsid, probably in contact with the RNA.

In poliovirus and rhinovirus virions, the packing together of VP1, VP2, and VP3 results in the formation of a "canyon" around the fivefold axes of the virion. The amino acids within the canyon, particularly those on the canyon floor, are conserved, but the amino acids on the "rim" of the canyon are variable. For polio- and rhinoviruses, the conserved amino acids on the floor of the canyon form the points of attachment of the viruses to cell surface receptors. Changes on the rim of the canyon affect the binding affinity of the receptor. Beneath the floor of the canyon in picornaviruses is a hydrophobic pocket accessible from the surface via a small opening. This pocket is a target for chemotherapeutic drugs that may block capsid changes critical for effective receptor binding or RNA release. Foot-and-mouth disease viruses have a comparatively smooth surface, with no canyon structure. The attachment site for host-cell receptors is located on VP1, within the G–H loop. These sites have serotype and subtype antigenic specificities that differ among the various strains of foot-and-mouth disease virus. (See Chapter 1, Figure 1.5, for more information on capsid protein structure.)

The stability of picornaviruses to environmental conditions is important in the epidemiology of the diseases they cause, and in the selection of methods of disinfection. For example, if protected by mucus or feces and shielded from strong sunlight, most picornaviruses are relatively heat stable at usual ambient temperatures. Some enteroviruses,

for instance, may survive for several days, and often weeks, in feces. Aerosols of aphthoviruses are less stable, but under conditions of high humidity they may remain viable for several hours. Because of differences in their pH stability, only certain disinfectants are suitable for use against each virus; for example, sodium carbonate (washing soda) is effective against foot-and-mouth disease viruses, but is not effective against swine vesicular disease virus.

Virus Replication

Poliovirus, which in nature only infects humans and non-human primates, has been the principal model for studying the replication of RNA viruses. This model served as the basis for analyzing the replication pattern for all other picornaviruses, and deviations from this model have provided support for the continuing re-classification of the picornaviruses.

The cellular receptors for many picornaviruses are known, and are surprisingly diverse (Table 2.1). The receptors for polioviruses, coxsackie B viruses, and some human rhinoviruses are members of the immunoglobulin (Ig) superfamily. For other picornaviruses, many other cell surface molecules serve as receptors and co-receptors, including heparan sulfate, low-density lipoproteins, extracellular matrix-binding proteins, and integrins. Foot-and-mouth disease virus can use two different receptors, depending on the passage history of the individual virus strain; specifically, field strains of foot-and-mouth disease virus bind to integrins, whereas cell-culture-passaged virus can use heparan sulfate as a receptor, but this change in receptor specificity results in attenuation of the virus. Foot-and-mouth disease viruses can also enter cells via Fc receptors if virions are complexed with non-neutralizing IgG molecules. This pathway, termed the antibody-dependent enhancement of infection pathway, is of unknown significance, but may be important in the long-term carrier state that may occur in certain ruminants.

The pathway(s) following attachment of the virus to its receptor and the release of the virion RNA into the cytoplasm of the host cell varies among the picornaviruses. The specific pathways used may reflect the pH stability of the virions of picornaviruses in different genera. For poliovirus, its interaction with the cell receptor induces structural changes in the virion such that VP4 is released from the virion and the amino terminal of VP1 shifts from the interior of the virion to the surface. This amino terminal region is hydrophobic and participates in the generation of a "pore" in the cell membrane. It is proposed that the RNA from the virus particle gains access to the cytoplasm of the host cells through this membrane pore. The endosomal pathway of virus entry is not utilized by poliovirus, as indicated by the lack of inhibition of infectivity by drugs that block this pathway. For foot-and-mouth disease virus, the entry process is different, as the binding of this virus to its receptor does not induce changes in the virion structure, but simply functions as a docking mechanism; once bound to the receptor, the virus enters the cell through the endosomal pathway. Weak bases that increase the pH of the endosomes block replication of foot-and-mouth disease virus; low pH of the endosome induces the capsid to disassociate into pentamers, with release of the viral RNA. In contrast, poliovirus, which is stable at low pH, cannot utilize the low pH environment of the endosome for penetration and release of the virion RNA in the same manner as foot-and-mouth disease virus, which is sensitive to low pH.

After adsorption, penetration, and intracellular uncoating, VPg at the 5′ end of the RNA is removed from the virion RNA by cellular enzymes (see also Chapter 2, Figure 2.7). Picornaviruses have evolved a cap-independent mechanism of translation that permits normal cellular cap-dependent translation to be inhibited by viral gene products. Initiation of translation does not proceed by the well-established Kozak scanning model. Instead, ribosomal binding to viral RNA occurs in a region of the 5′-UTR of the genome known as the internal ribosome entry segment (IRES). This segment of the viral genomic RNA is folded into cloverleaf-like structures that bind specifically to host-cell proteins, which play key roles in initiating the synthesis of viral protein and RNA. The segment has been recognized as a determinant of the phenotype and neurovirulence of some viruses. At least four different IRES structures have been identified in the picornavirus family. All picornavirus genomes have a 3′-UTR and a 3′-poly(A) tail that is encoded by the virus rather than added by host-cell polyadenylation enzymes. The function of the poly(A) tails is not known, but removal of poly(A) tails from the virion RNA renders it non-infectious. It has been suggested that the 3′-UTR is involved in the regulation of RNA synthesis, but is not essential for infectivity.

The RNA genome of picornaviruses comprises a single open reading frame that is translated into a single polyprotein (Figure 26.2). The polyprotein is cleaved post-translationally by virus-encoded proteinases in a stepwise fashion to produce 11 or 12 proteins. Some of the intermediate cleavage products have functions vital to replication, in addition to the final products. The 5′-terminal region of the genome encodes the virion proteins VP4, VP2 (VP0), VP3, and VP1, in that order; the common designation of these proteins for foot-and-mouth disease virus is respectively 1A, 1B, 1C, and 1D. Seven of the genera or proposed genera of the family have a non-structural L protein at the 5′ end of the coding sequence. Foot-and-mouth disease virus has two initiation codons at the 5′ end of the genome, which results in two forms of the L protein. The function of the alternative forms of L is not known, but the two codons are strictly conserved in all isolates, and removal of the L coding region in foot-and-mouth disease virus produces an attenuated virus. The middle region of the genome of picornaviruses encodes non-structural viral proteins (designated 2A, 2B, and 2C) that exhibit protease activity in viruses

within some genera. The 3′ end of the genome encodes additional non-structural proteins 3A, 3B, 3C, and 3D. Protein 3C has invariably a protease activity, 3B is the virion protein VPg, and 3D is the core RNA polymerase.

Viral RNA synthesis takes place in a *replication complex*, which comprises RNA templates, the virus-coded RNA polymerase, and several other viral and cellular proteins, tightly associated with newly assembled smooth cytoplasmic membrane structures. Synthesis of the complementary strand is initiated at the 3′ terminus of the virion RNA and uses the uridylated protein, VPg, as a primer. The completed complementary strand in turn serves as a template for the synthesis of virion RNA. Most of the replicative intermediates found within the replication complex consist of a full-length complementary (negative-sense) RNA, from which several nascent plus-sense strands are transcribed simultaneously by viral RNA polymerase.

With the absence of a 5′ cap on picornavirus mRNAs, these viruses have evolved unique mechanisms for inhibiting the translation of cellular mRNAs. The 2A protease of poliovirus or the L protease of foot-and-mouth disease virus cleaves the eIF4G of the translation initiation complex in a manner that permits viral mRNA to be preferentially translated. Conversely, encephalomyocarditis virus blocks phosphorylation of a protein needed for translation of capped messages, and protein 3CD is transported to the nucleus, where it blocks cellular transcription. These types of disruption of cellular metabolism block antiviral responses by the cell and free the translation system to produce predominantly viral gene products. Thus picornavirus replication can be very efficient, producing new virions after an eclipse period of less than 3 hours at yields of up to 10^6 virions per cell. Picornaviruses do not have a defined mechanism of cellular exit, and large paracrystalline arrays accumulate in the infected cells (Figure 26.4).

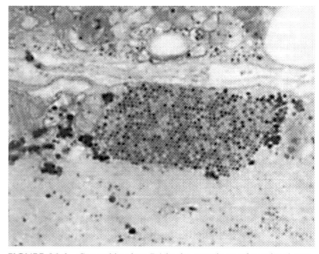

FIGURE 26.4 Coxsackie virus B4 in the cytoplasm of a striated muscle cell of a mouse, showing a typical large paracrystalline array of virions and associated destruction of contractile fibers. Thin-section electron microscopy. Magnification: ×67,000.

MEMBERS OF THE GENUS *APHTHOVIRUS*

The genus *Aphthovirus* now contains three species: foot-and-mouth disease virus, equine rhinitis A virus, and bovine rhinitis B virus (formerly bovine rhinovirus 2).

FOOT-AND-MOUTH DISEASE VIRUS

Clinical Features and Epidemiology

Foot-and-mouth disease is still a major global animal health problem, but its geographic distribution has diminished in recent years as control and elimination programs have been established in increasingly more countries (Table 26.3). Seven serotypes of foot-and-mouth disease virus have been identified by cross-protection and serologic tests; they are designated O, A, C, SAT 1, SAT 2, SAT 3, and Asia 1. At one time or another, these viruses occurred in most parts of the world, often causing extensive epizootics in domestic cattle and swine. Sheep and many species of wildlife are also susceptible. Mortality is typically low, but morbidity is high. Convalescence and virus shedding from affected animals may be protracted, and it is these features that make foot-and-mouth disease so important, especially when the

TABLE 26.3 Geographic Distribution of Foot-and-Mouth Disease[a]

Region	Virus Serotypes
South America	O, A, C
Africa	O, A, C, SAT 1, 2, 3
Asia, portions of the Middle East and Eastern Europe	O, A, C, Asia 1
Western Europe	Virus free (periodic epizootics)
North and Central America	Virus free
Caribbean	Virus free
Oceania	Virus free

[a]*Foot-and-mouth disease – free countries where vaccination is not practiced: Albania, Australia, Austria, Belarus, Belgium, Belize, Bosnia and Herzegovina, Brunei, Bulgaria, Canada, Chile, Costa Rica, Croatia, Cuba, Cyprus, Czech Republic, Denmark, Dominican Republic, El Salvador, Estonia, Finland, France, Germany, Greece, Guatemala, Guyana, Haiti, Honduras, Hungary, Iceland, Indonesia, Ireland, Italy, Japan, Korea (Rep. of), Latvia, Lithuania, Luxembourg, Macedonia, Madagascar, Malta, Mauritius, Mexico, Montenegro, Netherlands, New Caledonia, New Zealand, Nicaragua, Norway, Panama, Poland, Portugal, Romania, Serbia, Singapore, Slovakia, Slovenia, Spain, Sweden, Switzerland, Ukraine, United Kingdom, United States of America, Vanuatu.*
Countries having foot-and-mouth disease-free zones where vaccination is not practiced: Argentina, Botswana, Brazil, Colombia, Malaysia, Namibia, Peru, Philippines, South Africa.
Countries having foot-and-mouth disease free zones where vaccination is practiced: Argentina, Bolivia, Brazil, Colombia, Paraguay, Turkey.

virus is introduced into countries previously free of disease. Foot and mouth disease virus infection is still enzootic in much of Africa, Asia and the Middle East.

During the 19th century, foot-and-mouth disease was widely reported in Europe, Asia, Africa, and South and North America, and occurred on one occasion in Australia. From 1880 onward, the control of rinderpest and the improved husbandry in the livestock industries in Europe focused attention on foot-and-mouth disease. Its sequelae were found to be more important than the acute illness. In dairy herds, the febrile disease resulted in the loss of milk production for the duration of the lactation period, and mastitis often resulted in a permanent loss of more than 25% of milk production. For beef cattle, growth rates were reduced. Today, many countries have either eliminated foot-and-mouth disease through stringent eradication programs or have reduced its incidence greatly by extensive vaccination programs.

Historically, each virus type has been further subtyped on the basis of quantitative differences in cross-protection and serologic tests. Antigenic variation within a type occurs as a continuous process of antigenic drift, without clear-cut demarcations between subtypes. This antigenic heterogeneity has important economic implications for vaccine development and selection, as immunity acquired through infection or use of current vaccines is strictly type specific and, to a lesser degree, subtype specific. Difficulty in defining the threshold at which a new isolate should be given subtype status has always been problematic. For epidemiological purposes, isolates of foot-and-mouth disease virus within a given serotype are classified according to their *topotype* (topotype = geographic genotypes) (Figure 26.5). For serotype O, there are at least seven topotypes, reflecting the wide geographic distribution of this serotype from South America across Africa to Southeast Asia.

Foot-and-mouth disease virus infects a wide variety of cloven-hoofed domestic and wild animal species. Although the horse is refractory to infection, cattle, water buffalo, sheep, goats, llamas, camels, and swine are susceptible and develop clinical signs, and more than 70 species of wild mammals belonging to more than 20 families also are susceptible. In general, clinical signs are most severe in cattle and swine; however, outbreaks have been reported in swine while cattle in close contact with them did not develop clinical disease, such as occurred in Taiwan in 1997. Sheep and goats usually experience subclinical infections. Wild animals show a spectrum of responses, ranging from inapparent infection to severe disease and even death. However, with the notable exception of African buffalo, wildlife species are not linked to maintenance of foot-and-mouth disease virus in a given geographic region.

Cattle

After an incubation period of 2–8 days, there is fever, loss of appetite, depression, and a marked decrease in milk production. Within 24 hours, drooling of saliva commences,

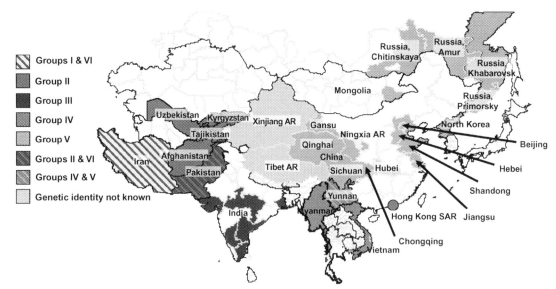

FIGURE 26.5 Origin (country and/or region) of isolates of foot-and-mouth disease virus serotype Asia 1 that were responsible for outbreaks in Asia during the period 2003–2007. The six different groups and their localities are indicated by different colors. AR, Autonomous Region; SAR, Special Administrative Region. *[From J. F. Valarcher, N. J. Knowles, V. Zakharov, A. Scherbakov, Z. Zhang, Y. J. Shang, Z. X. Liu, X. T. Liu, A. Sanyal, D. Hemadri, C. Tosh, T. J. Rasool, B. Pattnaik, K. R. Schumann, T. R. Beckham, W. Linchongsubongkoch, N. P. Ferris, P. L. Roeder, D. J. Paton. Multiple origins of foot-and-mouth disease virus serotype Asia 1 outbreaks, 2003–2007. Emerg. Infect. Dis. **15**, 1046–1051 (2009), with permission.]*

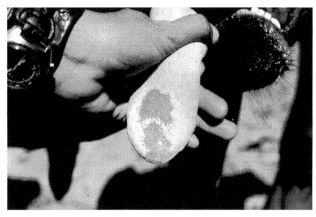

FIGURE 26.6 Ulcer from a ruptured vesicle in the tongue of a cow with foot-and-mouth disease. *(Courtesy of G. O'Sullivan, University of Minnesota.)*

and vesicles develop on the tongue and gums. The animal may open and close its mouth with a characteristic smacking sound. Vesicles may also be found in the interdigital skin and coronary band of the feet, and on the teats. The vesicles soon rupture, producing large, crater-like ulcers (Figure 26.6). Those on the tongue often heal within a few days, but those on the feet and within the nasal cavities often become infected secondarily with bacteria, resulting in prolonged lameness and a mucopurulent nasal discharge. In calves up to 6 months of age, foot-and-mouth disease virus can cause death through injury to the myocardium and myocarditis. The mortality in adult cattle is very low, but—even though the virus does not cross the placenta—cattle may abort, presumably as a consequence of fever in the affected cow, rather than infection of the fetus itself. Also, affected animals become non-productive or poorly productive for long periods. They may eat little for a week after the onset of clinical signs and are often very lame; mastitis and abortion further lower milk production. In enzootic areas, where cattle may have partial immunity, the disease may be mild or subclinical.

Swine

In swine, lameness is often the first sign of foot-and-mouth disease. Foot lesions can be severe, and may be sufficiently painful to prevent the pig from standing. Denuded areas between the claws usually become infected with bacteria; this causes suppuration and, in some cases, loss of the claw and prolonged lameness. Vesicles within the mouth are usually less prominent than in cattle, although large vesicles, which quickly rupture, often develop on the snout.

Other Animals

The clinical disease in sheep, goats, and wild ruminants is usually milder than in cattle and is characterized by foot lesions accompanied by lameness.

The recognition of foot-and-mouth disease as an important viral disease constraining efficient animal production in many parts of the world has resulted in intensive study of its epidemiology.

Countries Free of Enzootic Disease

In countries where foot-and-mouth disease either has not existed previously or has been eliminated, an epizootic can develop rapidly from introduction of virus on one farm. Within a short period, often measured in days rather than weeks, the outbreak can extend to so many farms that veterinary authorities have difficulty in controlling its spread, as occurred in the United Kingdom in 2001 with the introduction of the Pan Asia strain of the serotype O virus. Reasons for the rapidity of spread in such fully susceptible populations are the highly infectious nature of the virus, the production of high-titer virus in respiratory secretions, the large volumes of droplets and aerosols of virus shed by infected animals, the stability of virus in such droplets, the rapid replication cycle with very high virus yields, and the short incubation period.

Foot-and-mouth disease is spread rapidly within a locality by movement of infected animals and by mechanical transmission on items such as clothing, shoes, vehicles, and veterinary instruments. The excretion of virus for up to 24 hours before the onset of clinical signs means that virus dissemination may have occurred from a farm before any suspicion of disease is raised. The involvement of sheep or other animals that show minimal signs of infection may also contribute to rapid spread of the virus.

It was not until a dramatic epidemic of 1967–1968 in England, in which approximately 634,000 animals were slaughtered before the disease was successfully eradicated, that the possibility of long-distance airborne transmission was realized. Long-distance spread is dependent on wind direction and speed, and is favored by low temperature, high humidity, and overcast skies. Long-distance spread is therefore more likely to occur in temperate rather than tropical climates. With strict international movement controls of domestic food animals and their products, most introductions of foot-and-mouth disease virus to non-enzootic countries can be traced either to meat on the bone being fed to swine or, rarely, to long-distance spread of virus by aerosols. Molecular techniques are now available that enable rapid genotyping of viruses involved in new outbreaks, so that the source of the infection may be traced.

Countries with Enzootic Disease

The introduction of a virus type not present previously in a country may still cause an epizootic, because livestock will not have acquired immunity either through natural infection or through vaccination for the new serotype. For example, in 1961, the spread of SAT 1 from Africa through the countries of the Near East—where different serotypes of foot-and-mouth disease virus are enzootic—was more dramatic than any recorded spread of this type within Africa. In subtropical and tropical countries, with predominantly local breeds of cattle, the enzootic strains produce only mild disease in indigenous cattle, but cause severe disease in introduced European breeds. There is a greater variety of antigenic types in Africa and Asia than in Eastern Europe, the Middle East and South America and, in Africa

particularly, there is a large wildlife population that can become involved in the epizootiology. The African Cape buffalo (*Syncerus caffer*) is the natural host for serotypes SATs 1, 2, and 3 of foot-and-mouth disease virus. Transmission of virus occurs between African buffalo, but clinical disease has not been recorded; African buffalo do not appear to transmit the virus efficiently to domestic cattle.

Foot-and-mouth disease, more than any other disease, has influenced the development of international regulations designed to minimize the risk of introducing animal diseases into a country. Some countries have successfully avoided the introduction of foot-and-mouth disease by prohibiting the importation of all animals and animal products from countries where disease exists.

Pathogenesis and Pathology

The main route of infection in ruminants is through the inhalation of droplets, but ingestion of infected food, inoculation with contaminated vaccines, insemination with contaminated semen, and contact with contaminated clothing, veterinary instruments, and so on can all produce infection. In animals infected via the respiratory tract, initial virus replication occurs in the pharynx, followed by viremic spread to other tissues and organs before the onset of clinical disease. Virus excretion commences about 24 hours before the onset of clinical disease and continues for several days. Aerosols produced by infected animals can contain large amounts of virus, particularly those produced by swine, whereas sheep were relatively poor transmitters by aerosol of the O serotype of foot-and-mouth disease virus that caused the 2001 epizootic in the United Kingdom. Large amounts of virus are also excreted in the milk. The excretion of virus in high titer in droplets and in milk has significance for the control of disease.

Foot-and-mouth disease virus may persist in the pharynx of some animals for a prolonged period after recovery. Virus may be detectable for extended periods in cattle (perhaps up to 2 years) after initial exposure to infection; in sheep, for about 6 months. Virus persistence does not occur in swine. This carrier state has also been observed in wild animals, particularly the African Cape buffalo (*Syncerus caffer*), which is commonly infected with more than one of the SAT virus types, even in areas where foot-and-mouth disease does not occur in cattle.

The mechanisms by which the virus produces a persistent infection in ruminants are unknown. The virus is present in the pharynx in an infectious form: if pharyngeal fluids are inoculated into susceptible animals, the recipients develop foot-and-mouth disease. Attempts to demonstrate that carrier cattle can transmit disease, by placing them in contact with susceptible animals, have given equivocal results, but transmission of virus from persistently infected African Cape buffalo to cattle has been described.

TABLE 26.4 Differential Diagnosis of Vesicular Diseases Based on Naturally Occurring Disease in Different Domestic Animal Species[a]

Disease	Cattle	Sheep	Swine	Horse
Foot-and-mouth disease	S	S	S	R
Swine vesicular disease	R	R	S	R
Vesicular stomatitis	S	S	S	S
Vesicular exanthema of swine[b]	R	R	S	R

[a] R, resistant by natural exposure; S, susceptible by natural exposure.

[b] Now extinct in domestic swine, but virus occurs in marine mammals and possibly feral swine.

Diagnosis

Rapid diagnosis of foot-and-mouth disease is of paramount importance, especially in countries that are usually free of infection, so that control programs can be implemented as quickly as possible. Because three other viruses can produce clinically similar or indistinguishable vesicular lesions in domestic animals, confirmation by laboratory diagnosis is essential, although the history of the disease and the involvement of different species can be valuable pointers to the diagnosis (Table 26.4). Foot-and-mouth disease is a notifiable disease in most countries; thus, whenever a vesicular disease of domestic animals is seen, it must be reported immediately to the appropriate government authority.

Government officials collect specimens for diagnosis from animals with clinical signs; the exact procedure differs in different countries. Early in the infection, samples should include vesicular fluid, epithelial tissue from the edge of recently ruptured vesicles, blood (in anticoagulant), milk, and serum. In more advanced cases, esophageal/pharyngeal fluids collected with a probang (sputum) cup from ruminants should be submitted. Pharyngeal swabs from swine should also be collected. Typically, these samples are diluted immediately with an equal volume of virus transport medium containing a protein stabilizer such as 10% fetal bovine serum. A critical feature of the transport medium is a buffering system that can maintain the pH in the range 7.2–7.6. From dead animals, additional tissue samples may be collected from lymph nodes, thyroid, and heart. Samples should be chilled rapidly and moved to a diagnostic facility as quickly as possible. If a delay in transport is anticipated, samples should be frozen (preferably at $-70°C$).

A range of diagnostic tests is available for the differentiation of the vesicular diseases of livestock, including foot-and-mouth disease. Rapid differentiation of the agents causing vesicular disease is now available using multiplex reverse-transcriptase-polymerase chain reaction

(RT-PCR) assays, and PCR tests can also be used to identify specific serotypes of foot-and-mouth disease virus. The multiplex type of tests have the advantage of providing the identification of the "look-alike" disease agents when foot-and-mouth disease virus is not the etiological agent, which provides further confidence in the determination that the sample is truly negative for foot-and-mouth disease virus. An enzyme immunoassay (ELISA) is also available whereby a diagnosis can be made within a few hours, provided that vesicular fluid or tissues contain adequate amounts of antigen. This test can also be used to identify which of the seven types of foot-and-mouth disease virus is the cause of the disease.

Sensitive enzyme immunoassays are also available for specific antibody determinations. ELISA tests that detect antibodies to the non-structural proteins of foot-and-mouth disease virus have been developed in an attempt to distinguish animals vaccinated with killed vaccines from those naturally infected with the virus (DIVA). Virus neutralization assays have been a mainstay in the serological diagnosis of foot-and-mouth disease virus, but testing is complicated by the plurality of viral serotypes.

Cell cultures are used to isolate virus from clinical specimens in order to confirm the identity of the agent and to obtain virus isolates for genetic and antigenic analysis. Primary cultures of bovine, porcine, or ovine kidney are more sensitive than established cell lines such as BHK-21 or IB-RS-2 cells. Cell cultures are generally used to isolate the virus from tissues, blood, milk, and esophageal or pharyngeal fluids. The isolated virus is identified by ELISA, RT-PCR, or neutralization test.

Immunity, Prevention, and Control

Recovery from clinical foot-and-mouth disease is correlated with the development of a virus-specific antibody response. The early IgM antibodies neutralize the homologous type of virus and may also be effective against heterologous types. In contrast, the IgG produced during convalescence is type specific and, to varying degrees, subtype specific. Little information is available on the role of cell-mediated immunity in recovery from foot-and-mouth disease, but as in other picornavirus infections, it has been assumed to be of minor importance. Cattle that have recovered from foot-and-mouth disease are usually immune to infection with the same viral serotype for a year or more, but immunity is not considered life-long. Recovered animals, however, can be infected immediately with one of the other serotypes of foot-and-mouth disease virus and develop clinical disease.

The immunity following natural infection has stimulated attempts at developing an effective vaccine. As seen with natural infections, a vaccine strategy based on a single serotype will not work to control infections by the other serotypes. Even within a serotype, antigenic variation may make a vaccine less effective than is necessary to prevent infection. For cattle in which persistent or chronic infections occur, sterile immunity would be desirable, to be assured that vaccinated animals could not spread the infection, but sterile immunity is difficult to achieve with foot-and-mouth disease virus. Inactivated vaccines are used routinely in certain areas, to control the infection rather than to achieve eradication. Although current vaccines are not perfect, vaccination coupled with movement controls can be effective.

For countries such as Australia, Canada, the United Kingdom, and the United States that have a recent history of freedom from foot-and-mouth disease, cost–benefit analyses justified a "stamping out" policy whenever disease occurred. This was based on slaughter of affected and exposed animals, and rigid enforcement of quarantine procedures and restrictions on movement out of the quarantine area. This was the policy used in the 2001 outbreak in the United Kingdom. The destruction of millions of uninfected animals, partly as a result of the lack of food in the quarantine areas, made the cost in terms of public support too high to continue such a policy. Accordingly, new control procedures have been developed using emergency vaccination in the affected areas to stop the spread of the virus. Serological tests based on detection of antibodies to non-structural proteins will be used to discriminate between vaccinated and infected animals (DIVA) for movement control purposes. Vaccinations would cease with the end of the epizootic.

Human Infections

The rather rare human infections with foot-and-mouth disease virus are often subclinical, whereas others produce signs that resemble infections in animals. Clinical signs include fever, anorexia, and vesiculation on the skin and/or mucous membranes. There may be primary vesicular lesions at the site of virus exposure (e.g., skin abrasions) and secondary vesicular lesions in the mouth and on the hands and feet. Most cases reported over the years have been in persons in close contact with infected animals, and in laboratory workers. Laboratory diagnosis is required to confirm human cases. Prevention of human infection is based on control of the disease in animals and use of BioSafety Level 2 practices and equipment in laboratory facilities.

EQUINE RHINITIS A VIRUS

Equine rhinitis A virus (formerly equine rhinovirus 1) infection is prevalent in horses. The causative virus has physicochemical properties (e.g., acid lability) unlike those of human rhinoviruses, but similar to those of foot-and-mouth disease viruses. Infection of horses by equine rhinitis A virus can produce an acute upper respiratory infection 3–8 days after infection, with clinical signs including nasal discharge, pharyngitis, lymphadenitis, and cough. Virus can be detected in nasal secretions, blood, feces, and urine. Shedding of virus in urine can be prolonged. Seroprevalence studies indicate that, in older horses, some 50–100% have been infected with the virus previously, although many infected animals show no clinical signs.

Recently, it was found that equine rhinitis A virus can infect New and Old World camelids, and that this infection can result in abortion. In addition, infection of New World camelids can produce a wasting syndrome in which the animals become hyperglycemic, perhaps because of virus-induced destruction of islet cells of the pancreas. Similar infection of pancreatic islet cells has been described in goats infected with foot-and-mouth disease virus.

MEMBERS OF THE GENUS *ENTEROVIRUS*

In 2006, a new classification scheme was approved by the ICTV that significantly changed the member viruses in the genus *Enterovirus*. The genus *Rhinovirus* was dissolved, with member viruses becoming species within the genus *Enterovirus*. In addition, viruses previously designated as porcine enteroviruses (PEV) are now distributed among three genera: PEVs 1–7, and 11–13 are now in the genus *Teschovirus*; PEVs 9, and 10 remain in the genus *Enterovirus*; PEV 8 is proposed to be in a new genus, *Sapelovirus*, along with at least one avian picornavirus and three simian viruses. It is further proposed that other avian picornaviruses are classified within their own new genera.

Enteroviruses, like caliciviruses, are ubiquitous, and probably occur in all vertebrate species. However, only in swine and poultry do they cause diseases of economic significance. A number of enteroviruses have been recovered from swine, but only two cause diseases of importance: one causing swine vesicular disease, the major importance of which is its clinical resemblance to foot-and-mouth disease, and the other causing porcine polioencephalomyelitis (so-called Teschen/Talfan disease).

SWINE VESICULAR DISEASE VIRUS

Swine vesicular disease was first recognized in Italy in 1966, and since 1972 has been reported sporadically in other European and Asian countries. Italy remains the only country where the virus appears to be enzootic. Swine vesicular disease virus is genetically very similar to human coxsackievirus B5. It has been estimated that human coxsackievirus B5 first infected swine between 1945 and 1956, documenting an instance of a virus moving from humans to animals and establishing a new lineage.

Clinical Features and Epidemiology

There is no evidence that swine vesicular disease virus exists in any country without clinical disease being reported. Because of its resistance to low pH and ambient temperatures, the virus is transmitted easily between countries in infected meat. Various pork products that are prepared without heat treatment, such as salami, can harbor virus for several months. Fresh pork infected with swine vesicular disease virus can be an additional hazard within a country and delay eradication of disease, as infected carcasses may be placed unknowingly in cold storage for months or years; when released, such infected meat can give rise to new outbreaks.

At neutral pH and a temperature of 4°C, the virus has been reported to survive for more than 160 days without loss of titer. The conditions found on many swine farms are therefore conducive to gross and persistent contamination of the environment. Because the virus is so stable, it is extremely difficult to decontaminate infected premises, particularly where swine have been housed on soil. Disease is often detected by the sudden appearance of lameness in several swine in a herd. Affected swine have a transient fever, and vesicles appear at the junction between the heel and the coronary band then spread to encircle the digit. In severe cases, the swine are very lame and recovery is protracted. In about 10% of cases, lesions are found on the snout, lips, and tongue. Occasionally, some infected swine develop signs of encephalomyelitis, such as ataxia, circling, and convulsions. Subclinical infections also occur.

Pathogenesis and Pathology

Under natural conditions, swine can be infected by the fecal–oral route, with replication of the virus occurring predominantly in the gastrointestinal tract. Infection probably also occurs through damaged skin, particularly abrasions around the feet, and through the ingestion of infected garbage. Pigs placed into a virus-contaminated environment became viremic within 24 hours, and vesicle formation began by day 2 after exposure. Vesicles contain very high titers of virus and large quantities of virus are excreted in the feces, with virus being detected in feces up to 2 months after infection. Carrier animals have been detected rarely. Immunohistochemical staining of infected tissue sections showed strong staining of epithelial cells, with possible involvement of dendritic cells.

Diagnosis

Because swine vesicular disease cannot be differentiated clinically from the other vesicular diseases of swine, including foot-and-mouth disease, laboratory diagnosis is essential. A variety of rapid laboratory tests are available to distinguish the vesicular diseases. If sufficient vesicular fluid or epithelium is available, an ELISA can be used to detect antigen and establish a diagnosis within 4–24 hours. RT-PCR tests specific to swine vesicular disease virus can rapidly detect the virus in clinical material; however, multiplexed assays are gaining favor because this type of testing can identify specifically the agent causing the clinical event, rather than simply ruling out a single agent. Microarray assays are being developed for the same purpose, with the potential to screen for even more pathogens than can be detected by multiplex PCR assays.

Swine vesicular disease virus grows well in cultures of swine kidney cells, producing a cytopathic effect, sometimes as early as 6 hours after inoculation. The virus can also be isolated by the intracerebral inoculation of newborn mice, which develop paralysis and die.

Immunity, Prevention, and Control

Swine vesicular disease is not an economically important disease, and its significance historically was linked to its clinical presentation, which is similar to that of foot-and-mouth disease. With the advent of more rapid and reliable diagnostic testing, this cause of concern is lessening. Restriction of the movement of infected animals and meat products is the only available means to control swine vesicular disease, thus it is a notifiable disease and most affected countries have elected to eliminate the virus using slaughter programs.

Human Disease

Swine vesicular disease virus occasionally causes an "influenza-like" illness in humans. The fact that it is a zoonosis is consistent with its origin from human coxsackievirus B5.

BOVINE ENTEROVIRUS

Bovine enteroviruses and bovine rhinoviruses are ubiquitous in cattle populations, and both viruses were recently re-classified within the genus *Enterovirus*. There are two species and approximately 100 serotypes of human rhinovirus but, among domestic animals, rhinoviruses are recognized only in cattle. In cattle, three serotypes have been identified; these bovine rhinoviruses are unrelated antigenically to the human rhinoviruses. Bovine rhinovirus serotype 2 shares several distinctive features in common with foot-and-mouth disease virus, and has been moved to the genus *Aphthovirus*. The bovine rhinoviruses are highly host specific and have been isolated from cattle with mild respiratory disease similar to the common cold in humans.

Bovine enteroviruses have been grouped into two serotypes. The viruses are commonly found in healthy cattle, as well as in cattle with various clinical signs, thus their pathogenic significance remains conjectural.

SIMIAN ENTEROVIRUS

More than 20 picornaviruses have been identified from non-human primates. Many of the isolates have come from animals or tissues used for research purposes. As might be expected, some of the isolates show a high degree of sequence identity with viruses of human origin, and the zoonotic potential of these viruses has been noted. In one study from a primate center, 66% of fecal samples collected from animals with diarrheal disease were positive for a simian enterovirus. However, as with human enteroviruses, most simian isolates have come from healthy animals and the links to clinical disease are not strong.

MEMBERS OF THE GENUS *TESCHOVIRUS*

The porcine teschoviruses (also designated porcine enteroviruses 1–7, and 11–13) are a ubiquitous group of viruses found in most commercial swine herds. These viruses have been incriminated as potential causative agents of a wide variety of clinical diseases, including diarrhea, reproductive losses from stillbirths, fetal mummification, embryonic death, and infertility, and pneumonia, pericarditis, myocarditis, and polioencephalomyelitis. However, definitive proof of the causal role of porcine teschoviruses in most of these diseases is lacking, because of the frequent presence of several infectious agents, and the high rate of teschovirus infections in normal swine.

PORCINE TESCHOVIRUS 1

Porcine polioencephalomyelitis was first recognized in the town of Teschen—in what is now the Czech Republic—in 1930. The disease was described as a particularly virulent, highly fatal, non-suppurative encephalomyelitis in which lesions were present throughout the central nervous system. This severe form of the disease is still recognized, although less severe forms, referred to originally as Talfan disease in the United Kingdom and as endemic posterior paresis in Denmark, are more common and occur worldwide. Other porcine teschovirus serotypes (2, 3, 5) have also been detected in the outbreaks of the less severe disease.

Clinical Features and Epidemiology

Transmission of porcine teschovirus 1 is by the fecal–oral route. After an incubation period of 4–28 days, the initial signs include fever, anorexia, and depression, followed by tremors and incoordination, usually beginning with the hind limbs. Initially the limbs may be stiff, which is followed by paralysis and prostration, convulsions, coma, and death. There may be enhanced responses to touch and sound, paralysis of facial muscles, and loss of voice. In severe outbreaks the mortality may reach 75%. In milder forms of disease, the clinical signs are limited to ataxia associated with hind limb paresis, from which swine often recover completely in a few days.

Pathogenesis and Pathology

The pathogenicity of individual strains of porcine teschovirus 1 varies and the severity of the disease is also influenced by age, being most severe in young swine. The virus replicates initially in the alimentary tract and associated lymphoid tissues, followed by viremia and invasion of the central nervous system. Viremia apparently does not occur with viruses that do not produce central nervous system disease. Histologically, the lesions resemble those of other viral encephalomyelitides, with perivascular cuffing, neuronal degeneration, and gliosis. The extent of the lesions parallels the severity of clinical disease and, in extreme cases, involves the entire spinal cord, brain, and meninges.

Diagnosis

Polioencephalomyelitis caused by porcine teschovirus 1 must be differentiated from other viral encephalomyelitides, including pseudorabies, hemagglutinating encephalomyelitis, and rabies. Virus-specific RT-PCR assays are now used to detect the virus in clinical material, as well as to identify virus isolates. The porcine teschoviruses are isolated readily in porcine cell cultures, with neutralization assays being used for typing. Immunofluorescent or immunohistochemical staining of tissue specimens can also be used to diagnose porcine teschovirus infections.

Immunity, Prevention, and Control

Inactivated and attenuated virus vaccines, comparable to the Salk and Sabin vaccines for human poliomyelitis, are available commercially for prevention of porcine teschovirus 1 induced disease. Universal vaccination is not practiced, because control in intensive swine units is often achieved satisfactorily by quarantine and hygiene. In the event of an outbreak, ring vaccination with slaughter of the infected herd has been used to eliminate the infection. With the less severe forms of the disease, natural infection of the sows before breeding age has been used to control losses in the young swine.

MEMBERS OF THE GENUS *CARDIOVIRUS*

ENCEPHALOMYOCARDITIS VIRUS

Clinical Features and Epidemiology

The natural hosts of encephalomyocarditis virus are rodents. The virus is transmitted from rodents to many different animals, including humans, monkeys, horses, cattle, and swine. Severe epizootics of myocarditis, with fatalities, have occasionally been reported in swine and wildlife species, usually in association with severe mouse or, less commonly, rat infestations. There have been significant losses of elephants in the Kruger National Park in South Africa attributed to encephalomyocarditis virus infection. Animals in zoological parks appear to be more at risk, perhaps because of the opportunity for rodent contact, but perhaps also because of the enhanced surveillance of these animals. The virus frequently contaminates feed supplies as a result of rodent feces left by foraging rodents. In addition to myocarditis, swine herds often show reproductive losses due to encephalomyocarditis virus infections. The virus has been associated with non-suppurative meningoencephalitis in dogs and cats. Given the rather sporadic reports on encephalomyelitis virus infection in domestic and wild animals, it is likely that the associated disease is under-reported.

Pathogenesis and Pathology

Virus infection is by the oral route, with virus replicating in epithelial cells of the alimentary tract. Viremia has been detected within one day of an experimental infection of pregnant sows and lasted for 8 days. Virus has also been detected in feces for at least 7 days. In piglets infected with encephalomyocarditis virus, virus was isolated from all tissues by 2 days after infection. Histologically, infected animals showed a multifocal or diffuse interstitial myocarditis and necrosis of cardiac muscle cells and Purkinje fibers. Infected animals also had a necrotizing tonsillitis and an interstitial pancreatitis highlighted by mononuclear cell infiltrates. By immunohistochemical staining, viral antigen was localized to cardiac muscle cells in addition to the endothelial cells of cardiac vessels. In the tonsils and pancreas, antigen was localized to epithelial cells, macrophages, and fibroblasts.

Diagnosis

Laboratory testing is required to confirm encephalomyocarditis virus infections in animals. Viral antigen can be detected in tissue by immunofluorescence or by immunohistochemistry, and the virus itself can be isolated on numerous cell lines, including Vero cells and cells of mouse origin. RT-PCR testing is not commonly applied, but it can be used to identify an agent isolated from clinical cases. Infection does induce a strong serum neutralizing antibody response that can be used in contacts or herd mates to define exposure to encephalomyocarditis virus.

Immunity, Prevention, and Control

Transmission of encephalomyocarditis virus is by rodent feces contaminating food supplies, feces in herd outbreak situations, and perhaps by eating of infected rodents. Eliminating rodents from feed supplies is a critical control point, particularly in swine operations. Because of losses in zoological parks, experimental vaccines have been developed that showed protection in elephants.

THEILOVIRUS

The species *Theilovirus* includes Theiler's mouse encephalomyelitis virus (TMEV), which is a common enteric virus of mice that can spread to the central nervous system, where it causes several neurological syndromes. There are two major serogroups of the virus, including GDVII (GDVII and FA viruses) and TO (TO, DA, and BeAn8386 viruses). Rats may be naturally infected with related viruses, including MHG and rat cardiovirus. Hamsters and guinea pigs may also be infected with mouse encephalomyelitis virus or serologically related viruses. Clinical disease has been reported only in mice, in which most infections are subclinical, but infected mice may rarely develop poliomyelitis, with posterior paresis. Clinical disease is most often associated with GDVII serotypes of the virus. Neurologic disease occurs very rarely, and depends upon virus strain, age of the mouse, and mouse strain. Involvement of the nervous system is presumed to be the result of viremia, and may result in acute encephalomyelitis and demyelinating myelitis. Demyelination is due to direct lytic infection of neurons and oligodendroglia, and to secondary immune-mediated destruction of infected cells. Mouse encephalomyelitis virus infects intestinal enterocytes, and is shed in the feces intermittently. Infection is typically persistent, and seropositive animals must be considered to be actively infected.

This virus can be an important problem in mouse colonies, where its presence can interfere with research programs. It is diagnosed along with other mouse viruses in the usual viral diagnostic panel. Diagnosis involves serology (hemagglutination-inhibition, neutralization, enzyme immunoassay), which may be supported by confirmatory virus isolation in murine cell culture. Control involves a high level of sanitation, diagnostic surveillance, and preventing feral rodents entering the colonies. Theiloviruses spread slowly among rodents, usually resulting in a low rate of seroconversion within an infected population. Murine theiloviruses cross-react serologically with encephalomyelocarditis virus, but the latter virus is rare in laboratory rodent populations.

MEMBERS OF THE GENUS *ERBOVIRUS*

EQUINE RHINITIS B VIRUS

The equine picornaviruses that were previously classified as rhinoviruses because of their acid lability are now classified in two genera: equine rhinitis A virus (equine rhinovirus 1) is included as a member of the genus *Aphthovirus*, whereas equine rhinitis B virus (equine rhinovirus 2) is now classified in the new genus *Erbovirus*, with three recognized serotypes (designated as equine rhinitis B viruses 1, 2, and 3) that are distinguished on the basis of their acid lability/stability, genetic sequences, and neutralization by type-specific antisera. Equine rhinitis B viruses can cause mild upper respiratory disease in horses, but their importance as pathogens has not been firmly established. The viruses have a worldwide distribution and the seroprevalence rates in non-isolated populations are high.

MEMBERS OF THE GENUS *KOBUVIRUS*

The genus *Kobuvirus* includes two species of picornavirus, Aichi virus and bovine kobuvirus. Aichi viruses have been associated with diarrheal disease of humans, with a strong link to the eating of shellfish. Bovine kobuvirus was first identified as a cell culture contaminant. Subsequent testing demonstrated a high seroprevalence of neutralizing antibodies in cattle (60%) in Japan. RT-PCR testing of fecal samples from calves with diarrhea in Thailand showed an infection rate of 8%. Bovine kobuvirus may represent one of the "small round viruses" seen by electron microscopy in fecal sample from cattle, but a causative link to disease has not been definitively established.

UNCLASSIFIED PICORNAVIRUSES

AVIAN ENCEPHALOMYELITIS VIRUS

Avian encephalomyelitis virus was originally classified in the genus *Enterovirus*. However, the virus was later reclassified, on the basis of limited sequence data, to a new genus, *Hepatovirus*, which contains only human hepatitis A virus. More recent data on the 5′-UTR structure and function shows that avian encephalomyelitis virus contains a type IV IRES similar to that of the flaviviruses and distinct from hepatitis A. Thus a new genus, *Tremovirus*, has

been proposed, to contain avian encephalomyelitis-like viruses.

Clinical Features and Epidemiology

Avian encephalomyelitis was first described in the New England states of the United States in 1930 and is now recognized worldwide. Its natural history parallels closely that of poliomyelitis of humans and polioencephalomyelitis of swine. Avian encephalomyelitis occurs in chickens 1–21 days of age, but the virus is not pathogenic in older chickens. There is only a single antigenic type, but strains vary in virulence. With the advent of vaccination of breeding birds, clinical disease is now rare. Avian encephalomyelitis virus produces relatively mild encephalomyelitis in Japanese quail, turkeys, pigeons, and pheasants; other avian species are susceptible following experimental infection.

High morbidity and mortality occur in young birds when avian encephalomyelitis virus is first introduced into a flock. The major mode of transmission is by a fecal–oral route, although transmission via the egg may occur in association with the brief viremic phase of the disease in laying hens. Eggs from infected layers show a reduced hatchability and increased loss of hatched chicks. Once the virus has become established in a flock, losses continue at a greatly reduced incidence, because maternal antibody provides protection for chicks during their critical first 21 days after hatching.

After an incubation period of 1–7 days after vertical transmission of avian encephalomyelitis virus, and approximately 11 days after horizontal transmission, disease occurs that is characterized by dullness, progressive ataxia, tremors (particularly of the head and neck), weight loss, blindness, paralysis, and, in severe cases, prostration, coma, and death. Birds allowed to recover have deficits of the central nervous system and are usually destroyed. Susceptible (seronegative) layers that become infected with the virus may show depressed egg production of 5–10%, but no overt signs.

Pathogenesis and Pathology

At necropsy, there are no obvious macroscopic lesions of birds with avian encephalomyelitis. Histological lesions typical of viral encephalitis, but not diagnostic of avian encephalomyelitis, are present throughout the central nervous system, without peripheral nervous system involvement. Lesions include disseminated non-purulent (mononuclear cell inflammation) encephalomyelitis and ganglionitis of the dorsal root ganglia. Central chromatolysis of neurons in the medulla oblongata is strongly suggestive of avian encephalomyelitis.

Diagnosis

The clinical signs and histopathologic lesions are suggestive of avian encephalomyelitis, and immunofluorescence staining of tissues from affected chicks is widely used for definitive diagnosis. The virus may be isolated either in cell culture or by inoculating, by the yolk sac route, 5–7-day-old embryonated hen eggs obtained from antibody-free hens; chicks are allowed to hatch and are observed for 7 days for signs of encephalomyelitis. Increasingly, RT-PCR assays will replace virus isolation. Assessment of the flock status can be made by various serological tests, but ELISA tests using purified or recombinant antigens are becoming the standard. Avian encephalomyelitis must be differentiated from Newcastle disease, as well as from a range of non-viral causes of central nervous system disease in chickens.

Immunity, Prevention, and Control

Control of avian encephalomyelitis can be achieved by either depopulation or vaccination. Attenuated virus vaccines administered in the drinking water are available. The vaccines are administered after chickens reach 8 weeks of age, but at least 4 weeks before the onset of egg laying, and are designed to provide protection for chicks during the first 21 days after hatching by ensuring that adequate levels of specific antibody are transferred from hens to progeny chicks. These vaccines are not administered directly to chicks, because they may not be sufficiently attenuated; in addition, there is insufficient time to provide protection for chicks hatched into a heavily contaminated environment. Inactivated vaccines are also available and are preferred when immunized birds are housed in close proximity to non-immunized chickens. Vaccines are also used to control avian encephalomyelitis in quail and turkey.

DUCK HEPATITIS

The clinical entity "duck hepatitis" can be caused by at least three different viruses: duck hepatitis viruses 1, 2, or 3. Duck hepatitis viruses 2 and 3 are now classified as astroviruses (family *Astroviridae*), whereas duck hepatitis virus 1 (duck hepatitis A virus) is classified as a picornavirus in a new proposed genus, *Avihepatovirus*.

Clinical Features and Epidemiology

Duck hepatitis was first recognized in 1945 among ducks reared on Long Island, New York. The agent isolated from these initial outbreaks is designated duck hepatitis virus 1. There was initially only one serotype of duck hepatitis virus 1 known, and duck hepatitis viruses 2 and 3 were identified when ducks immune to duck hepatitis virus 1 showed signs of hepatitis. Three serotypes of duck hepatitis A virus are now recognized. Duck hepatitis virus 3 is

apparently less virulent than duck hepatitis virus 1. Disease occurs in ducks younger than 21 days, after an incubation period of 1–5 days. Adult ducks show no signs of infection, and egg production is unaffected. The course of the disease in a clutch of ducks is often dramatically swift, occurring over a 3–4-day period, with a mortality rate approaching 100%. Affected ducks tend to stand still with partially closed eyes, fall to one side, paddle spasmodically, and die. There may be some diarrhea. In addition to ducks, goslings, pheasants, Japanese quail, turkey poults, and chicks of guinea fowl and quail, but not chickens, are susceptible to experimental infection.

Pathogenesis and Pathology

At necropsy, the liver is enlarged, edematous, and mottled with punctuate or ecchymotic hemorrhages. The spleen and kidneys also may be enlarged. Histologically, there is extensive hepatic necrosis. Cholangitis and proliferation of the bile duct epithelium occur in birds that survive the infection.

Diagnosis

The history, clinical signs, and characteristic necropsy findings are suggestive of duck hepatitis virus infection; immunofluorescence provides a rapid, definitive diagnosis. The virus may be isolated in cell culture (duck hepatocyte cultures) or by allantoic sac inoculation of 10-day-old embryonated duck (preferred) or chicken eggs. When subsequently candled, infected eggs often show characteristic greenish discoloration of the embryonic fluids, and most are dead within 4 days after inoculation. Serological testing of affected flocks has been of limited value. Duck hepatitis has to be differentiated from other causes of high mortality in young ducklings, including aflatoxicosis and salmonellosis.

Immunity, Prevention, and Control

Recovered ducks are immune. Hyperimmune serum has been used successfully to reduce losses during outbreaks. Attenuated virus vaccines are available commercially and are used according to the same principles as already outlined for avian encephalomyelitis vaccines. Vaccine is now used almost exclusively in breeders, to insure transmission of passive antibody to the progeny.

OTHER UNCLASSIFIED PICORNAVIRUSES

As more studies are undertaken in wildlife species, it is certain that new picornaviruses will be discovered. If past experience is a useful guide, many of these isolates will be difficult to link to clinical disease. For example, two picornaviruses have recently been identified from marine mammals: the first was isolated from 20 of 22 lung samples from dead harbor seals from northern Europe, and the second was isolated from tissue samples from ringed seals hunted in northern Canada; there was no evidence of disease in these latter animals. Sequence analysis of these novel virus isolates indicates that they probably constitute members of a new genus in the picornavirus family.

Picornavirus-like agents have been observed by electron microscopy from fish and, in some cases, isolated in cell culture from fish (unassigned picornaviruses from grouper, smelt, sea bass, turbot). A picorna-like virus has been identified by electron microscopy in the livers of young turkey poults with fulminating hepatitis, termed turkey viral hepatitis. However, definitive classification of the etiological agent by molecular analysis is lacking.

Caliciviridae

Chapter Contents

The family *Caliciviridae* includes a rapidly growing list of viruses that infect an ever increasing variety of animal species, with pathogenic caliciviruses typically causing either gastroenteritis or systemic disease in their respective hosts. Members of the family *Caliciviridae* are frequently difficult to isolate in cell culture, thus recently described caliciviruses were only identified after the advent of modern molecular technologies. Calicivirus infections have been identified in many animal species, including swine, birds, marine mammals, lagomorphs, rodents, monkeys, cattle, sheep, mink, cats, dogs, skunks, reptiles, fish, amphibians, and even insects, although the pathogenic significance of many of these viruses is currently uncertain.

Vesicular exanthema of swine is a disease of largely historical significance that was first recognized in southern California in 1932 and eradicated from domestic swine in the United States by 1956. Closely related caliciviruses have since been isolated from numerous species of marine mammals that occur throughout the northern Pacific Ocean, and are likely to have been the sources of swine infections. The major importance of vesicular exanthema of swine is that it mimics foot-and-mouth disease in swine. Feline calicivirus is a common cause of respiratory tract infection and disease in cats, and highly virulent systemic forms of the infection recently have emerged. Rabbit hemorrhagic disease first emerged in China in 1984 as an apparently new,

often fatal disease in domestic rabbits; this virus has since spread extensively and now is enzootic in rabbit populations in much of the world. A related calicivirus causes European brown hare syndrome. Recently, murine caliciviruses (noroviruses) have been discovered among laboratory mouse colonies. Infections are clinically silent, except in specific types of genetically altered (engineered) mice.

PROPERTIES OF CALICIVIRUSES

Classification

The family *Caliciviridae* comprises four genera, with a fifth proposed (Figure 27.1). All the genera include viruses that infect animals. The genus *Vesivirus* contains feline calicivirus and vesicular exanthema of swine virus, and close relatives that include the numerous San Miguel sea lion viruses, cetacean calicivirus, primate calicivirus, skunk calicivirus, bovine calicivirus, reptile calicivirus, and, tentatively, mink calicivirus. The genus *Lagovirus* contains rabbit hemorrhagic disease and European brown hare syndrome viruses. The genus *Norovirus* contains the type species, Norwalk virus, that is a very prevalent and important cause of explosive outbreaks of acute gastroenteritis in humans, and noroviruses that infect cattle, sheep, pigs, dogs, and mice recently have been described. The genus

Fenner's Veterinary Virology. DOI: 10.1016/B978-0-12-375158-4.00027-4

Sapovirus also contains viruses that have been linked to outbreaks of human gastroenteritis and it tentatively now contains a number of strains of porcine enteric calicivirus, some of which are antigenically similar to human isolates, and a mink enteric sapovirus. A currently unassigned group includes canine calicivirus, fowl calicivirus, bovine calicivirus strain NB, and walrus calicivirus.

The caliciviruses are genetically heterogeneous (Figure 27.1). Sequence analysis of the capsid gene has identified at least five distinct genetic groups in both the genus *Sapovirus* and the genus *Norovirus*. Genetic recombination between viruses in the different genera complicates typing, and potentially might facilitate interspecies transmission of recombinant viruses, including from animals to humans. Additional viruses unquestionably will be added to this group as additional species, particularly wildlife species, are investigated.

Virion Properties

Calicivirus virions are non-enveloped, 27–40 nm in diameter, and have icosahedral symmetry. The calicivirus genome consists of a single molecule of linear, positive-sense, single-stranded RNA, 7.4–8.3 kb in size. The 5′ end of the genome is capped by a covalently bound protein (VPg) and the 3′ end is polyadenylated. Virions are composed of 180 identical protein molecules (58–60 kDa) arranged in dimers forming 90 arch-like structural units, which in turn form 32 cup-shaped surface depressions that give the viruses their unique appearance (Figure 27.2; Table 27.1). Some caliciviruses, especially enteric caliciviruses, lack this characteristic surface structure and have a fuzzy appearance.

Calicivirus virions are composed of a single major capsid protein (VP1; 55–70 kDa) that is functionally divided

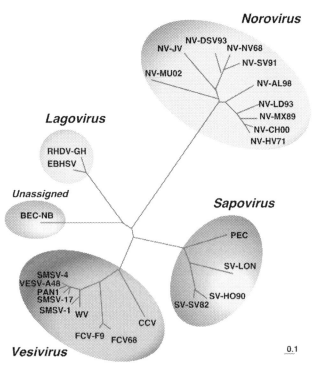

FIGURE 27.1 Phylogenetic relationships within the family *Caliciviridae*. Full length capsid amino acid sequences were used for the phylogenetic analysis and included representative strains from each genus in the family. NV, Norwalk virus; PEC, porcine enteric calicivirus; SV, Sapporo virus; CCV, cetacean calicivirus; FCV, feline calicivirus; SMSV, San Miguel sea lion virus; PAN, primate calicivirus; VESV, vesicular exanthema of swine virus; WV, walrus calicivirus; BEC, bovine enteric calicivirus; RHDV, rabbit hemorrhagic disease virus; EBHSV, European brown hare syndrome virus. [*From* Virus Taxonomy: Eighth Report of the International Committee on Taxonomy of Viruses (*C. M. Fauquet, M. A. Mayo, J. Maniloff, U. Desselberger, L. A. Ball, eds.*), p. 850. Copyright © Elsevier (2005), with permission.]

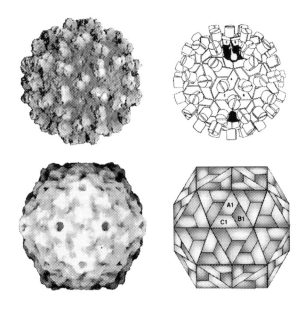

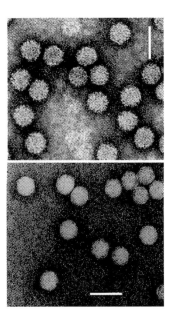

FIGURE 27.2 (Top left) Cyro-image reconstruction of recombinant Norwalk virus (NV)-like particles (rNV VLPs). (Top center) Cryo-image reconstruction of primate calicivirus. A set of icosahedral 5- and 3-fold axes is marked. (Courtesy of Prasad, B.V.V.). (Top right) Central cross-section of rNV VLPs. (Bottom left) Electronic rendering of Norwalk virus (Prasad et al., 1999). (Bottom center) Diagram representing a T = 3 icosahedral structure. (Bottom right) Negative stain electron micrographs of bovine calicivirus particles (Courtesy of S. McNulty). The bar represents 100 nm. [*From* Virus Taxonomy: Eighth Report of the International Committee on Taxonomy of Viruses (*C. M. Fauquet, M. A. Mayo, J. Maniloff, U. Desselberger, L. A. Ball, eds.*), p. 843. Copyright © Elsevier (2005), with permission.]

into S (shell) and P (protrusion) domains. As the name implies, the P domain is the most externally exposed; it is further subdivided into P1 and P2 subdomains. The P1 subdomain is formed by two non-contiguous regions with the P2 subdomain inserted in between. The P2 subdomain includes a 5′ hypervariable region, a conserved region, and a 3′ hypervariable region (Figure 27.3). Neutralization epitopes of feline calicivirus map to the hypervariable P2 subdomain, along with two linear B cell epitopes, suggesting that the P2 subdomain is the immunodominant region

of the calicivirus virion, and that changes in this region are responsible for antigenic variation. This same subdomain is implicated in receptor interactions that probably define host range and tissue specificity. Feline calicivirus also contains a minor virion protein (8.5–23 kDa) that is essential for the assembly of infectious virions. The lack of a lipid envelope makes this virus family resistant to inactivation by standard detergent-based disinfectants. They are relatively resistant to heat, but are inactivated at low pH.

Virus Replication

Since many of the members of the family *Caliciviridae* have not yet been propagated in cell culture, precise details of their replication cycles are uncertain. Caliciviruses infect cells via receptor-mediated attachment and clathrin-dependent endocytosis, and replication then occurs on the surface of membranous vesicles in the cytoplasm of infected cells. Feline junctional adhesion molecule (fJAM-A) is a functional receptor for the P2 domain of VP1 of feline calicivirus, whereas the cellular receptors for many other caliciviruses are yet to be defined.

Members of the genus *Vesivirus* readily replicate in a variety of cultured cells and cause overt cytopathology, probably from apoptosis of infected cells. Other factors may be required for virus replication in cell culture; for example, replication of porcine enteric calicivirus (genus *Sapovirus*) in porcine kidney cells requires the presence of bile acids that increase levels of cyclic AMP in the treated cells,

---

TABLE 27.1 Properties of Caliciviruses

Virions are non-enveloped, 27–40 nm in diameter, with icosahedral symmetry

Some virions have a characteristic appearance, with 32 cup-shaped depressions on their surface

Virions are assembled from one capsid protein (M_r 60,000)

Genome is composed of a single molecule of linear positive-sense, single-stranded RNA, 7.4–8.3 kb in size

Genomic RNA is polyadenylated at its 3′ end and has a protein linked covalently to its 5′ end; genomic RNA is infectious

Cytoplasmic replication. Genomic RNA and several subgenomic mRNAs are produced during replication; mature proteins are produced both by processing of a polyprotein and by translation of subgenomic mRNAs

---

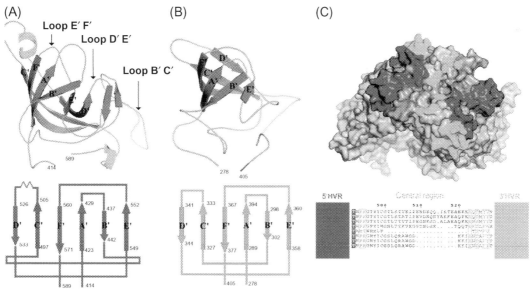

FIGURE 27.3 Structure of the P2 subdomain and mapping of the feline calicivirus (FCV) neutralizations sites. Ribbon representations (above) of the P2 subdomains in (A) San Miguel sea lion virus (SMSV) and (B) recombinant Norwalk virus (rNV), along with their respective topology diagrams (below). The β-strands are labeled from A′ to F′ in each case. The loops containing the FCV neutralization epitopes are indicated for SMSV. (C) Above: Surface representation of the A/B dimer as viewed from outside the capsid (approximately along the dimeric twofold axis), showing the N-terminal hypervariable region (HVR; red), central conserved region (blue), and C-terminal HVR (cyan). Below: Sequence comparison of the representative sequences from SMSV (top four sequences, corresponding to SMSV4, SMSV5, primate, and SMSV1), canine calicivirus, and FCV (bottom three sequences, corresponding to FCV6, FCV4, and FCV9) in the conserved region, flanked by the N-terminal and C-terminal HVRs showing host-dependent conservation. *[From R. Chen, J. D. Neill, M. K. Estes, B. V. V. Prasad. X-ray structure of a native calicivirus: structural insights into antigenic diversity and host specificity. Proc. Natl. Acad. Sci. U. S. A. **103**, 8048–8053 (2006), with permission.]*

Genomic RNA (7.4–8.3 kb)

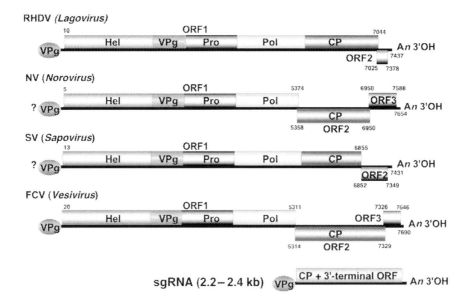

FIGURE 27.4 Genome organizations of viruses of the family *Caliciviridae*. The genomic organization and open reading frame (ORF) usage are shown for representative species (with strain indication shown in brackets) in the following genera: *Lagovirus*: rabbit hemorrhagic disease virus (RHDV); *Norovirus*: Norwalk virus (NV); *Sapovirus*: Sapporo virus (SV); and *Vesivirus*: feline calicivirus (FCV). Viruses in two genera (*Lagovirus* and *Sapovirus*) contain a large ORF1 in which the nonstructural polyprotein gene is continuous and in frame with the CP coding sequence. Some strains in the genus *Sapovirus* encode a third predicted ORF that overlaps ORF1 (not shown). Viruses in the other two genera (*Norovirus* and *Vesivirus*) encode the major structural CP in a separate reading frame (ORF2). The RNA helicase (HEL), protease (PRO), and polymerase (POL) regions of the genome are indicated. The linkage of VPg region of the genomes of representative viruses from the genera *Norovirus*, *Sapovirus*, and *Vesivirus* is shown by homology with the mapped VPg of RHDV. The shaded region of the ORF2 of the representative member of the genus *Vesivirus* illustrates the leader sequence (approximately 125 aa in length) of the precursor CP. Studies of FCV and RHDV have identified two major positive sense RNA molecules in infected cells. One RNA molecule corresponds in size to the full-length genome and the other, a subgenomic-sized RNA, is co-terminal with the 3′-end of the genome. The sgRNA is the template for translation of the major viral CP and the 3′-terminal ORF product that has been identified as a minor structural protein in FCV. CP, capsid protein; Hel, helicase; ORF, open reading frame; Pol, polymerase; Pro, protease; sgRNA, subgenomic RNA; VPg, genome-linked protein. *[From* Virus Taxonomy: Eighth Report of the International Committee on Taxonomy of Viruses *(C. M. Fauquet, M. A. Mayo, J. Maniloff, U. Desselberger, L. A. Ball, eds.), p. 845. Copyright © Elsevier (2005), with permission.]*

resulting in a downregulation of signal transducer and activator of transcription 1 (STAT1). This molecule (STAT1) is a key regulator of innate immunity and interferon response genes, and virus replication is enhanced in cells deficient in STAT1 and interferon receptor genes. Notably, clinical disease occurs in murine norovirus-infected, genetically engineered mice with STAT1 deficiency, but not in immunocompetent mice. The murine noroviruses are the first and only noroviruses to be successfully cultivated *in vitro*, and have therefore attracted much recent interest, because of the importance of human norovirus infections.

Individual caliciviruses utilize different strategies to generate the proteins essential for their replication (Figure 27.4). The genome of caliciviruses includes either two or three open reading frames, with the 5′ end of the genome encoding the non-structural proteins (helicase, VPg, protease, RNA polymerase) and the 3′ portion encoding the major and minor capsid proteins. The individual non-structural proteins are produced by post-translational proteolytic cleavage of the polyprotein encoded by open reading frame 1. In addition

to full-length genomic RNA, a subgenomic positive-sense RNA co-terminal with the 3′ end of the genome is present in infected cells, and VPg protein is covalently linked to the 5′ end of both the genomic and subgenomic RNA molecules. This protein binds initiation factors for the translation of the viral RNAs. The subgenomic RNA may function as a mechanism for the control of the level of translation of the structural proteins. Virions accumulate in the cytoplasm, either scattered as paracrystalline arrays or as characteristic linear arrays associated with the cytoskeleton. Caliciviruses have no defined method of egress and are released by cell lysis, probably after apoptosis of infected cells.

MEMBERS OF THE GENUS *VESIVIRUS*

VESICULAR EXANTHEMA OF SWINE VIRUS

Vesicular exanthema of swine is essentially an "extinct" disease that was eradicated from domestic swine in the United States by 1956; however, the viruses (San Miguel sea lion viruses) that caused the disease are still present in the marine environment. Furthermore, some feral swine along the Pacific Coast of North America are seropositive to the causative virus. The real importance of vesicular exanthema of swine is that its clinical signs and cutaneous lesions are indistinguishable from those of the three other vesicular diseases of swine, namely foot-and-mouth disease, swine vesicular disease, and vesicular stomatitis.

In addition to viruses isolated from swine, the taxonomic grouping of vesicular exanthema virus includes caliciviruses isolated from cattle, primates, reptiles, skunk, mink, and a variety of marine mammals (San Miguel sea lion viruses).

Clinical Features and Epidemiology

Vesicular exanthema of swine was transmitted by contact with infected pigs, and by contaminated feed that included virus-infected meat or offal. Vesicular exanthema is an acute, febrile disease of swine characterized by the formation of vesicles on the snout, tongue, and teats, within the oral cavity, and on the feet (between the claws and on the coronary band). Lameness typically is the first sign of the disease because of vesicle formation on the feet, with accompanying fever and, sometimes, diarrhea and failure to thrive. Pregnant sows often have aborted in outbreaks. Morbidity was often high in epizootics, but mortality low, and in uncomplicated cases recovery occurred after 1–2 weeks. However, high mortality was present in association with infection by some strains of the virus.

Pathogenesis and Pathology

The incubation period of vesicular exanthema is as short as 18–48 hours, followed by fever, lameness, rapid weight loss, and other signs of systemic infection; recovery is rapid and without sequelae. Following oronasal infection, the virus is disseminated and characteristically infects and replicates in squamous epithelium; lesions are limited to discrete regions of epithelia, with formation of vesicles and subsequent ulceration and epithelial sloughing, followed by rapid healing. Encephalitis and myocarditis also have been described in affected swine.

Diagnosis

In most countries, suspected cases of vesicular exanthema must be reported to regulatory authorities. Presumptive diagnosis is based on fever and the presence of typical vesicles, which rupture in 24–48 hours, forming erosions and ulcers. The diagnosis can be confirmed by virus isolation, various serologic tests, electron microscopy to demonstrate characteristic calicivirus particles, or by reverse-transcriptase-polymerase chain reaction (RT-PCR) assay. Vesicular exanthema of swine virus is antigenically heterogeneous, and nucleotide sequence comparisons among isolates of vesicular exanthema and San Miguel sea lion viruses confirm that the viruses clearly belong to the same genetic group within the genus *Vesivirus*, along with similar viruses from other species (Figure 27.1).

Immunity, Prevention, and Control

Convalescent swine are resistant to reinfection with homologous virus, but, because of the lack of cross-protection between the numerous antigenically distinct serotypes and strains of the causative virus, heterologous reinfection is possible. San Miguel sea lion viruses and vesicular exanthema of swine viruses are genetically similar, and inoculation of swine with San Miguel sea lion virus produces vesicular exanthema. There was a clear link between garbage feeding and natural outbreaks of the disease in swine, and inclusion of uncooked protein from marine mammal infected with San Miguel sea lion viruses apparently initiated outbreaks. The virus was readily transmitted horizontally between swine during outbreaks. Rigorous enforcement of infected herd quarantine, laws concerning the cooking of garbage, and a slaughter program all resulted in rapid eradication of the disease, although control was achieved without knowledge of the origin of the virus.

SAN MIGUEL SEA LION VIRUS

Marine caliciviruses were first isolated in 1972 from tissues of California sea lions inhabiting San Miguel Island. A considerable number of serologically distinct viruses are included in this group, including individual viruses capable of infecting virtually all species of marine mammal in the northern Pacific Ocean. Infection can lead to formation of oral vesicles in infected marine mammals, and vesicles on the flippers of pinnipeds (Figure 27.5), and virus has been isolated from aborted or premature sea lion pups. These viruses also can infect terrestrial mammals that eat the tissues of infected marine mammals. San Miguel sea lion viruses typically can be isolated in cell culture; RT-PCR assays are also useful, although the extensive genetic diversity of viruses within the group can potentially lead to false-negative results with this approach.

FELINE CALICIVIRUS

The feline caliciviruses are genetically heterogeneous, and the pathogenic significance of individual viruses is variable. These viruses are ubiquitous in cat populations worldwide.

Clinical Features and Epidemiology

Natural transmission of feline calicivirus occurs mainly by fomites, direct contact between cats, and occasionally over short distances by aerosol; the virus also can be passively carried to susceptible cats by human handlers. All felids are apparently susceptible to feline calicivirus infection. The virus has been isolated from a dog, and surveys suggest that feline calicivirus may also infect marine mammals.

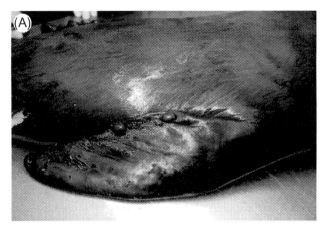
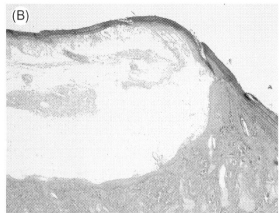

FIGURE 27.5 San Miguel sea lion virus infection. (A) Vesicles on the flipper of an affected animal. (B) Histological appearance of the vesicle, with fluid accumulation within the epidermis. *(Courtesy of K. Colegrove, University of California, Davis.)*

Feline calicivirus is initially shed in large amounts from infected cats, principally in oral secretions. Some cats continue to shed virus for extended periods, although most eventually eliminate the virus. In households or facilities containing large numbers of cats, strain variants may arise and reinfect cats that have cleared the original infecting virus. Genetic variants continually arise because of the error-prone replication process of RNA viruses, leading to the continuing emergence of viruses with different phenotypic properties such as virulence. The selective factors that lead to the periodic emergence of highly virulent systemic strains of feline calicivirus are undefined, although overcrowding as occurs in animal shelters may predispose to the emergence and spread of these viruses.

Feline calicivirus has long been recognized as a major cause of respiratory disease in domestic and wild felids that is characterized by acute conjunctivitis, rhinitis, tracheitis, pneumonia, and vesiculation and ulceration of the oral epithelium, including the tongue. Other common signs are fever, anorexia, lethargy, stiff gait, and sometimes nasal and ocular discharge. Morbidity is high in unvaccinated cats, but mortality is generally low, except in kittens infected with virulent strains that cause pneumonia.

Although there is just one serotype of feline calicivirus, there is considerable antigenic and genetic variation between strains. There is also marked variation in the virulence of individual strains of feline calicivirus. A highly virulent, systemic calicivirus disease with high mortality (30–60%) in adult cats emerged in 1998. Remarkably, adult cats that had been previously vaccinated suffered higher mortality rates after infection with these highly virulent systemic strains than did infected kittens. In addition to the characteristic oral ulcerations, rhinitis, and ocular discharge, cats infected with virulent systemic feline caliciviruses also exhibited subcutaneous facial and limb edema, icterus, alopecia, and striking ulceration of the nose, pinnae, and feet.

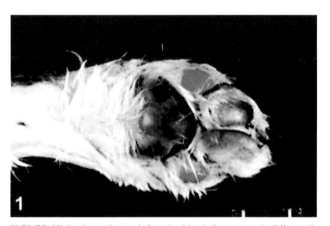

FIGURE 27.6 Paw of a cat infected with virulent systemic feline calicivirus. The epithelial lining of the footpads P2 and P5 have sloughed. There is peripheral ulceration at the pad–haired-skin junction of P4. *[From P. A. Pesavento, N. J. MacLachlan, L. Dillard-Telm, C. K. Grant, K. F. Hurley. Pathologic, immunohistochemical, and electron microscopic findings in naturally occurring virulent systemic feline calicivirus infection in cats. Vet. Pathol. 41, 257–263 (2004), with permission.]*

Pathogenesis and Pathology

The incubation period after infection is 2–6 days. Lesions in cats infected with less virulent virus strains are usually confined to the respiratory tract, oral cavity, and eyes. Interstitial pneumonia may occur in kittens infected with virulent strains of the virus. Oral ulceration is the most consistent sign of feline calicivirus infection. Ulcers begin as vesicles that quickly rupture; healing takes place over the subsequent 2–3 weeks. Oral ulcers also are characteristic of virulent systemic feline calicivirus infections, and typically involve the tongue, gingiva, and hard palate, but also may involve the nasal cavity, pinnae, and haired skin. Lesions in the footpads (Figure 27.6) range from mild hyperemia to sloughing of the entire pad. Pulmonary edema and parenchymal necrosis in the liver, spleen, and pancreas were additional features in experimentally infected cats, and the presence of feline calicivirus antigen within areas of epithelial necrosis in the skin, nasal, and oral mucosa and footpads, as well as lung and pancreas, has been confirmed by immunohistochemical staining. Infection of endothelial cells with subsequent vascular injury potentially explains the striking facial and limb edema.

Diagnosis

Presumptive diagnosis is based on clinical presentation; definitive diagnosis is based on isolation of the virus in feline cell culture; demonstration of viral antigens in the tissues of affected cats is by immunofluorescence, immunohistochemistry, or RT-PCR assay. The milder form of feline calicivirus infection may be difficult to differentiate clinically from feline rhinotracheitis caused by feline herpesvirus 1 (see Chapter 9), although these two viruses can readily be distinguished by available diagnostic assays.

Immunity, Prevention, and Control

Control of disease induced by feline calicivirus is reliant on vaccination and management procedures. Although there is only one serotype of feline calicivirus, current vaccines are an imperfect solution because of extensive viral antigenic heterogeneity. Cross-neutralization studies have clearly shown that there are substantial differences in the neutralization phenotypes of individual strains of feline calicivirus, whereas vaccines typically contain only a single virus strain. Multi-strain vaccines recently have been developed in an effort to prevent virulent systemic feline calicivirus disease. Modified live vaccines are proposed to be more effective than inactivated ones, but there are indications that live-attenuated vaccine viruses may circulate naturally in cats, with the potential for genetic variants to arise. Intranasal administration of live-attenuated vaccines is proposed to stimulate a more rapid immune response, which is especially critical in animal shelters.

The constant passage of virus between cats generates novel strains, as reinfection of previously exposed but uninfected cats can result in the selection and emergence of neutralization-resistant virus variants. Thus identification and isolation of shedding cats is important, as is decontamination of all potential sources of infection such as fomites. Caliciviruses are resistant to inactivation because of their lack of a lipid envelope; sodium hypochlorite solution is the most economical and effective means of inactivating the virus.

MEMBERS OF THE GENUS *LAGOVIRUS*

RABBIT HEMORRHAGIC DISEASE AND EUROPEAN BROWN HARE VIRUSES

In 1984 a new, highly infectious disease of the European rabbit, *Oryctolagus cuniculus*, was identified in China.

It was characterized by hemorrhagic lesions particularly affecting the lungs and liver, and was named "rabbit hemorrhagic disease." The disease killed nearly half a million rabbits in the first 6 months after its appearance, and by 1985 had spread throughout China. By 1988 the disease had spread throughout Europe and had reached North Africa, and it subsequently spread throughout much of the rest of the world, including the Americas. Spread sometimes was facilitated by intentional human intervention in an effort to reduce populations of feral rabbits, for example separately in Australia and New Zealand. Both feral and domestic (*O. cuniculus*) rabbits were affected, but all other species of mammals except the European hare appear to be resistant to infection. The disease was unknown in Europe before 1984; however, a very similar disease called "European brown hare syndrome" had been recognized in the early 1980s, affecting *Lupus europaeus* and subsequently some other *Lupus* spp. Rabbit hemorrhagic disease is caused by a calicivirus (genus *Lagovirus*) that is closely related to, but antigenically distinct from, the virus that causes European brown hare syndrome; however, the diseases caused by the two viruses are very similar in their respective hosts.

Clinical Features and Epidemiology

Rabbit hemorrhagic disease affects rabbits older than 2 months, typically causing explosive outbreaks of acute and severe disease, with mortality rates greater than 80% with certain virus strains. Notably, rabbits younger than 2 months do not develop clinical disease following infection. Infection principally is via the fecal–oral route between infected and susceptible rabbits. Onset of clinical disease can occur within 24–72 hours of infection, and the disease is often peracute, characterized by sudden death following a 6–24-hour period of depression and fever. Affected rabbits can have a serosanguineous or bloody nasal discharge and exhibit nervous signs, including incoordination, shaking, and terminal opisthotonos.

Pathogenesis and Pathology

At necropsy, lesions in affected rabbits include nasal hemorrhage, pulmonary congestion, edema, and hemorrhage, hemorrhages on the serosal surfaces of abdominal viscera, marked splenomegaly in some animals, and zonal (periportal to mid-zonal) necrosis of the liver that imparts an enhanced lobular pattern throughout the organ (Figure 27.7). Hepatocytes contain viral antigen as determined by immunohistochemistry, and virus particles readily are observed in infected cells by electron microscopy. Viral antigen also is present in macrophages in major organs, and in circulating mononuclear cells. The pathogenesis of the disease is linked to disseminated intravascular coagulation, presumably triggered by the extensive liver necrosis. Why young rabbits are resistant to expression of rabbit hemorrhagic disease is uncertain, because they are susceptible

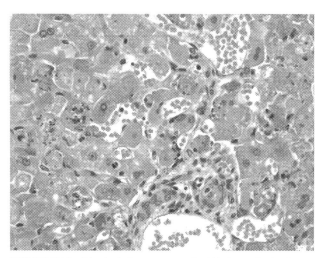

FIGURE 27.7　Histological appearance of rabbit hemorrhagic disease. Note extensive necrosis of hepatocytes. *(Courtesy of L. Woods, University of California, Davis.)*

to infection with the virus; it is possible that differences in the innate response of younger versus older rabbits might explain this profound difference in disease susceptibility.

Diagnosis

Rabbit hemorrhagic disease virus has yet to be grown in cell culture, but high concentrations of virus occur in tissues of infected rabbits and easily can be detected by immunofluorescence or immunohistochemical staining with specific antibodies. Antigens from infected tissue or from capsid protein expressed *in vitro* can be used to detect antibody from surviving animals, using enzyme-linked immunosorbent assay. Some strains of rabbit hemorrhagic disease virus hemagglutinate human erythrocytes, a property that can be used for a simple antibody detection test. RT-PCR assays for the detection of viral nucleic acid are routinely available.

Immunity, Prevention, and Control

Control of rabbit hemorrhagic disease in commercial husbandry units is based on the prevention of virus entry via fomites, infected wild rabbits, or insects. Vaccines to control the disease have been prepared as an inactivated homogenate of infected rabbit tissue mixed with adjuvant. Virus-like particles produced by recombinant DNA technology in baculovirus expression systems are effective as a vaccine after parenteral or oral administration, but are not yet available commercially because of economic limitations.

MEMBERS OF THE GENUS *NOROVIRUS*

MURINE NOROVIRUS

Clinical Features and Epidemiology

In 2003, a virus was isolated from immunocompromised mice that had the properties of viruses in the genus *Norovirus*. The virus initially was detected because of sporadic deaths in a colony of mice deficient in the *STAT1* and recombination-activating gene 2 (*RAG2*) genes. Both immune-deficient mice and wild-type mice are susceptible to oral infection, but virus replication is limited in immunocompetent mice as compared with *STAT1*-deficient mice. Phylogenetic analyses of isolates of murine norovirus confirm the presence of numerous virus strains within a single genetic group, and the duration of infection in immunocompetent mice varies depending on the infecting virus strain. Serological screening of mouse colonies has confirmed widespread infection, currently making murine norovirus the most prevalent known adventitious agent in research colonies.

Pathogenesis and Pathology

Disease in immunodeficient mice includes encephalitis, cerebral vasculitis, meningitis, hepatitis, and pneumonia, whereas infection of immunocompetent mice is clinically silent. The virus replicates in primary macrophage and dendritic cell cultures, as well as macrophage cell lines. Immunohistochemical staining of tissues from infected mice reveals antigen in Kupffer cells and marginal zones of the spleen. Virus can be readily isolated from mesenteric lymph nodes and feces, but intestinal tissue has not been examined for lesions or distribution of antigen.

Immunity, Prevention and Control

Virus-specific RT-PCR for analysis of feces, mesenteric lymph node, and small intestine, and enzyme immunoassays have been developed to screen research mouse colonies in an attempt to eradicate this emerging pathogen.

OTHER CALICIVIRUS INFECTIONS OF ANIMALS

Bovine and porcine viruses in the genera *Norovirus* and *Sapovirus* can produce diarrhea and anorexia in seronegative young animals. Noroviruses also recently have been described in sheep and dogs, and although these viruses probably have a global distribution, their importance as pathogens and their zoonotic relevance are uncharacterized currently. Calicivirus infections of wildlife have been described, including norovirus in a 4-week-old lion cub that died of severe hemorrhagic enteritis. Calicivirus was isolated from a lesion from the lip of a pigmy chimpanzee, and this same virus was re-isolated 6 months later from a throat swab from the animal, suggesting that this virus could persist, as does feline calicivirus. Putative calicivirus infections have been described in several other species, but their pathogenic significance, and in some instances their authenticity, is uncertain.

Astroviridae

Chapter Contents

Astroviruses were first described in 1975, when they were observed by electron microscopy in the feces of children with diarrhea. Astroviruses are currently second only to rotaviruses in importance as the cause of gastroenteritis in young children. Soon after the initial identification of astroviruses in children, similar viruses were demonstrated by electron microscopy in a variety of domestic animals, including cattle, sheep, deer, pigs, dogs, cats, mice, turkeys, chickens, and ducks; however, many of these still await detailed characterization. These viruses also have been identified in molluscan shellfish and insectivorous bats. Astroviruses appear to be ubiquitous in young animals, although they rarely, if ever, cause severe disease or death, except in birds.

PROPERTIES OF ASTROVIRUSES

Classification

The family *Astroviridae* comprises two genera, *Avastrovirus* and *Mamastrovirus*. The genus *Avastrovirus* includes three species of chicken astrovirus (avian nephritis viruses 1 and 2, and chicken astrovirus), duck astrovirus, and turkey astroviruses 1 and 2. The genus *Mamastrovirus* includes several human astroviruses (types 1–8), bovine astroviruses 1 and 2, feline astrovirus, mink astrovirus, ovine astrovirus, and porcine astrovirus (Table 28.1). Although there is extensive genetic heterogeneity among the members of the family, including strains of the same species, available sequence data confirm the host-specific segregation of these viruses. Astroviruses are so named because the surfaces of some particles have a distinctive five- or six-pointed star-like appearance (*astron*, star).

TABLE 28.1 Properties of Astroviruses

Virions are non-enveloped, with icosahedral symmetry, 28–33 nm in diameter

Some 10% of virions have characteristic five- or six-pointed stars on their surface

Genome is a single molecule of linear, positive-sense, single-stranded RNA, 6.4–7.4 kb in size. Genomic RNA is polyadenylated at the 3′ terminus and is infectious

A subgenomic mRNA is produced during replication; virion structural proteins are produced by translation of subgenomic mRNA, and processing and cleavage of precursor polyprotein(s)

Two genera: *Avastrovirus*, with three chicken (including avian nephritis viruses 1 and 2), one duck, and two turkey viruses; *Mamastrovirus*, with eight human, two bovine, one feline, one ovine, one porcine, and one mink viruses; viruses from different host species are unrelated antigenically

Virion Properties

Astrovirus virions are non-enveloped, 28–33 nm in diameter, and have icosahedral symmetry. As few as 10% of particles in negatively stained preparations have a five- or six-pointed star across their surface (Figure 28.1; Table 28.1); the remaining particles appear smooth. Size and shape can be affected by the strain of virus and the host cell in which it is propagated. The viral capsid proteins are all derived through cleavage of a single precursor, and the precursor capsid protein self-assembles into virus-like particles if expressed alone. It is proposed that the N-terminus region of the precursor capsid protein is responsible for packaging of viral RNA, and that the C terminus portion, which is highly variable, contains the neutralization determinants and is responsible for receptor binding. The genome consists of a single molecule of linear, positive-sense, single-stranded RNA, 6.4–7.4 kb in size, that includes three open reading frames (Figure 28.2). The 5′-RNA terminus has yet to be fully characterized as to whether it is covalently linked to a viral protein or has a 5′ cap. Both the 5′ and 3′ ends of the genome contain untranslated regions of variable length (strain dependent) and the 3′ end is polyadenylated. Viral infectivity is resistant to low pH, lipid solvents, and detergents, both ionic and non-ionic.

Virus Replication

Bovine, porcine, and human astroviruses can be grown in cell cultures, and avian astroviruses are propagated in either embryos or cell cultures. Most cell lines are not permissive for viral growth, but the human cell line, Caco-2, is permissive for the human astroviruses without host-cell

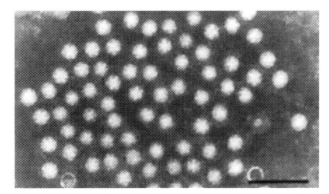

FIGURE 28.1 Family *Astroviridae*, genus *Astrovirus*. Typical virions with distinctive five- or six-pointed stars on their surfaces, as found in the feces of many different species of animals with diarrhea. Negative-stain electron microscopy. Bar represents 100 nm.

adaptation. Trypsin must be added to the growth medium in order to complete the virion maturation process during virus propagation in cell culture, except for the chicken astroviruses, which replicate efficiently in primary chicken kidney cells without trypsin. The C-terminal portion of the capsid protein is proposed to be responsible for cell binding, and thus determine cell tropism. The specific cell receptor(s) to which astroviruses bind has not been clearly identified, but preliminary studies have implicated the polio virus receptor (CD155) for one human astrovirus. Virus replication takes place in the cytoplasm, and mature virions can accumulate in the cytoplasm in crystalline arrays. Virions are released by cell lysis.

The astrovirus genomic RNA is infectious. It acts as a messenger RNA for the first two open reading frames (1a and 1b) that encode polyproteins that include the viral non-structural proteins. These first two open reading frames are transcribed through a frameshifting mechanism (Figure 28.2). The exact functions of all protein products of open reading frames 1a and 1b have not been defined, but a serine protease and an RNA-dependent RNA polymerase have been identified. Also encoded by this region are a nuclear localization signal and several (species dependent) transmembrane domains. The virion structural proteins are encoded by a second open reading frame at the 3′ end of the genome; during virus replication, a subgenomic 2.4 kb RNA that encodes the precursor capsid protein(s) is transcribed from this open reading frame. A VP90 protein is the precursor to the mature capsid proteins of human astrovirus and, through a series of caspase-like protease cleavages, VP90 is processed to a VP70 product that targets immature virions for release from infected cells. Once released into the intestinal tract, the capsid protein undergoes further processing by trypsin-like enzymes, to produce a fully infectious virus with three different capsid proteins, VP34, VP27, and VP25. This extracellular activation is critical to the creation of infectious virions.

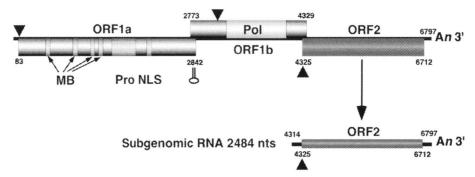

FIGURE 28.2 Genome organization and replication strategy of human astrovirus 1 (HAstV-1), A3′; poly(A) sequence at 3′ end of genome; MB, transmembrane helices; NLS, nuclear localization signal; nts, nucleotides; ORF, open reading frame; Pol, polymerase; Pro, protease; ▲, first methionine; ⬭, frameshift structure: numbers are nucleotide positions. [*From* Virus Taxonomy: Eighth Report of the International Committee on Taxonomy of Viruses (C. M. Fauquet, M. A. Mayo, J. Maniloff, U. Desselberger, L. A. Ball, eds.), p. 860. Copyright © Elsevier (2005), with permission.]

TURKEY ASTROVIRUS

Turkey astrovirus was first described in the United Kingdom in 1980 and in the United States in 1985. Once recognized, it was identified in some 80% of turkey flocks with enteric disease and was the most prevalent virus detected.

Clinical Features and Epidemiology

Astroviruses are associated with enteritis and stunting in turkey poults that typically are between 1 and 3 weeks of age. Clinical signs include diarrhea, listlessness, litter eating, nervousness, and stunting, but they are usually mild or moderate, with low mortality. However, a severe multifactorial variant disease entity termed "poult enteritis and mortality syndrome" also has been described that is characterized by additional features of dehydration, anorexia, immune dysfunction, and high death rates. Although astrovirus has been identified in turkeys with typical signs of this syndrome, all aspects of the syndrome have yet to be reproduced by experimental infection with any single agent.

Experimentally infected turkey poults may develop clinical signs within 2 days of inoculation, and shedding of virus may continue for several weeks. Clinical signs are variable, and depend somewhat on the infecting virus strain, but infected poults typically have reduced weight gain and exhibit watery to yellow-brown dropping without any evidence of blood. Shedding of virus can occur before the onset of clinical signs, which might explain the finding of virus in "clinically normal" birds.

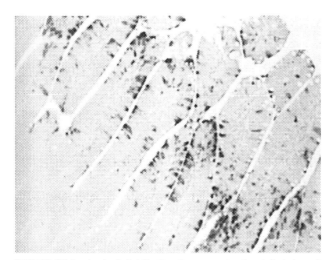

FIGURE 28.3 *In-situ* hybridization from an astrovirus-infected poult 24 hours after infection. Astrovirus primarily replicates in the enterocytes along the sides of the villi, and rarely in crypts. *[From* Diseases of Poultry *(Y. M. Saif, H. J. Barnes, J. R. Glisson, A. M. Fadly, L. R. McDougald, D. E. Swayne, eds.), 11th ed., p. 323. Copyright © 2003 Iowa State Press, Ames, IA, 2003, with permission.]*

Pathogenesis and Pathology

At necropsy, the intestines, especially the ceca, of infected birds are dilated and fluid filled. On histopathology, there is mild hyperplasia of crypt enterocytes but, unlike other enteric virus infections such as that caused by rotavirus, there is a lack of villous contraction (atrophy). Like rotavirus, however, replication of turkey astrovirus is restricted to the enterocytes lining the villi, with no significant involvement of crypt enterocytes (Figure 28.3). Inflammation is minimal or absent. Infected enterocytes may appear highly vacuolated and contain aggregates or crystalline arrays of virus particles. The mechanism(s) by which turkey astrovirus induces diarrhea remains uncertain, but the osmotic effect of undigested and unabsorbed disaccharides that accumulate because of virus-induced maldigestion probably contributes to retention of water within the lumen. In addition, the findings of recent studies suggest that the capsid viral proteins of astroviruses can themselves induce diarrhea and alter the integrity of the intestinal epithelial barrier.

Diagnosis

Astroviruses were originally detected by examination of feces or intestinal samples from affected birds using electron microscopy, but the small size and pH-dependent morphology of astroviruses often led to their mis-identification as only a "small round virus" or an "enterovirus-like virus." Visualization of virus aggregates using immunoelectron microscopy is necessary for accurate diagnosis, but astroviruses frequently are not detected in cases of mixed viral infections. The diagnostic sensitivity and specificity of testing for avian astroviruses increased substantially with the advent of reverse-transcriptase polymerase chain reaction (RT-PCR) assays; however, the genetic heterogeneity of turkey astroviruses requires that multiple primer pairs be utilized in these assays, to avoid false-negative results. There currently are two serotypes of turkey astrovirus, and the avian nephritis virus of chickens has also been detected in turkeys. An antigen-capture enzyme-linked immunosorbent assay was developed for turkey astrovirus and, although it is less sensitive than RT-PCR, its relative ease of use is ideal for assessing the infection status of flocks. Turkey astroviruses can be isolated in propagated in turkey embryos, but fail to grow in cell culture systems, even with the addition of exogenous trypsin.

Immunity, Prevention, and Control

There currently are two recognized serotypes of turkey astrovirus, but vaccines, chemotherapeutic agents, or other potential control measures have yet to be shown to be effective in eliminating infection. Astroviruses are resistant to inactivation by a variety of detergents, alcohol solutions, phenolics, and lipid solvents, and therefore environmental contamination is difficult to eliminate. Current control methods are based on thorough sanitation, followed by several weeks of "rest." Sourcing uninfected replacement birds is also critical.

AVIAN NEPHRITIS VIRUS

Avian nephritis virus was isolated in 1976 from the rectal contents of apparently normal 1-week-old chicks in Japan. The identity of the virus as an astrovirus was not confirmed until genomic sequence data became available. There currently are two serotypes of avian nephritis virus. Although chickens are the principal host of the virus, asymptomatic infection has been documented in turkeys. Chickens of all ages are susceptible to infection, but only young chicks manifest signs of disease, typically as runting syndrome or baby chick nephropathy. Virus is detected in feces within 2 days after infection, with peak virus shedding at 4–5 days. Infected birds die up to 3 weeks after infection.

Virus is widely disseminated in infected birds, with highest titers in kidney and jejunum, and lower titers in spleen, bursa, and liver. A transient diarrhea may occur, with a reduction in weight gain, the severity of which probably depends upon the infecting strain of virus, strain of chicken, and other factors. The kidneys of affected birds are swollen and discolored, and histological changes include necrosis of the epithelial cells lining the proximal convoluted tubules and lymphocytic interstitial nephritis. Crystalline arrays of virus particles in the cytoplasm of infected tubular epithelial cells appear as acidophilic granules on light microscopy. Viral antigens can be demonstrated by immunofluorescence staining in the jejunum, without obvious histological lesions.

Transmission of avian nephritis virus is by the oral route, but there is some evidence that the virus is passed vertically through the egg. The virus is resistant to most standard disinfectants. The distribution of avian nephritis viruses is poorly defined currently, due to the absence of obvious clinical signs in most infected birds and the lack of reliable diagnostic tests. The development and availability of RT-PCR tests will enhance diagnostic capability. There currently are no vaccines available to prevent avian nephritis virus infection of chickens.

OTHER ASTROVIRUSES

The typical outcome of astrovirus infection in young animals is a self-limiting gastroenteritis that usually goes undiagnosed. The majority of astrovirus infections are subclinical, especially in older animals. Mammalian astroviruses appear to be host restricted, so in settings where there is more than one animal species in close contact, infection is manifest as diarrhea in only one species. The incubation period is usually 1–4 days, followed by watery diarrhea lasting 1–4 days or more.

A rapidly fatal hepatitis in ducklings less than 6 weeks of age was reported in the United Kingdom in 1965, with mortality rates of up to 50%. Ducks from affected flocks were raised outdoors, which opens the possibility that the virus came from wildlife. The causative virus was originally designated as duck hepatitis virus 2 before its identity as an astrovirus was established, and the disease seems to have disappeared from commercial duck flocks, with last reports of the disease in the mid-1980s. A hepatitis syndrome in ducks with less than 30% mortality was originally described in Long Island, United States, and experimental infection studies have reproduced mild hepatic lesions that are more severe if the agent is given by the intravenous route. The etiology is an astrovirus distinct from duck hepatitis virus 2 and is named duck hepatitis virus 3. Originally, duck hepatitis virus 3 was misclassified as a picornavirus.

Nucleic-acid-based detection systems such as RT-PCR assays will greatly facilitate better characterization of the epidemiology of astrovirus infections and assist in more accurately defining their true pathogenic significance.

Togaviridae

Chapter Contents

Viruses included in the family *Togaviridae* possess a lipid envelope (or cloak: "toga") surrounding an icosahedral capsid. There are two genera within the family: specifically, the genera *Alphavirus* and *Rubivirus* (Table 29.1). The single member of the rubivirus genus is the exclusively human pathogen, rubella virus.

Alphaviruses are distributed worldwide, and several are important pathogens of humans and/or animals. With the notable exception of the salmonid alphaviruses, alphaviruses are maintained in an enzootic infection cycle that includes insect vectors and animal reservoir hosts.

Individual alphaviruses typically exist in geographically limited habitats defined by transmission cycles that involve specific mosquito and vertebrate hosts that contribute to virus persistence, geographic distribution, overwintering, and amplification. With the exception of chikungunya and perhaps Ross River viruses, domestic animals and humans are "dead-end" hosts that are not involved in primary enzootic transmission cycles in nature, although they can serve as critical amplifying hosts that contribute to geographic extension and disease outbreaks. For example, a mosquito–horse–mosquito transmission cycle is responsible

TABLE 29.1 Togaviruses that Cause Disease in Domestic Animals and Humans[a,b]

Virus	Arthropod Vector	Domestic Animal Host	Disease	Geographic Distribution
Eastern equine encephalitis virus	Mosquitoes	Horses (humans)	Encephalitis	Americas
Western equine encephalitis virus	Mosquitoes	Horses (humans)	Encephalitis	Americas
Highlands J virus	Mosquitoes	Horses	Encephalitis	Americas
Venezuelan equine encephalitis virus	Mosquitoes	Horses (humans)	Febrile disease, encephalitis	Americas
Getah virus	Mosquitoes	Horses	Febrile disease	Southeast Asia

[a] All viruses listed are members of the genus Alphavirus; the only member of the second genus, Rubivirus, is rubella virus, which infects only humans.

[b] The alphaviruses Sindbis virus, Semliki Forest virus, chikungunya virus, o'nyong-nyong virus, Igbo Ora virus, Ross River virus, Mayaro virus, and Barmah Forest virus also cause zoonotic human disease, rarely causing encephalitis, but often causing fever, malaise, and arthritis.

Fenner's Veterinary Virology. DOI: 10.1016/B978-0-12-375158-4.00029-8

for explosive spread during epizootics of Venezuelan equine encephalitis.

The host range for many alphaviruses is extensive, and may be restricted only by the feeding preferences of their insect hosts. Important alphavirus pathogens of vertebrate animals include eastern, western, and Venezuelan equine encephalitis and related viruses (the so-called equine alphavirus encephalitides), and Getah virus. Although the pathogenic significance to animals of other alphaviruses is largely undefined, particularly in wildlife species, several alphaviruses in addition to those just listed are important zoonotic pathogens: specifically, Sindbis virus and a group of viruses related to Semliki Forest virus, including chikungunya, o'nyong-nyong, Ross River, Barmah Forest, and Mayaro viruses. With regard to disease in mammals, alphaviruses can be classified into three groups: (1) those that cause neurologic disease (encephalitis); (2) those that cause a febrile illness with polyarthritis; (3) those that cause no apparent disease. In contrast to other alphaviruses, salmonid alphaviruses appear to infect only fish, without any requirement for an arthropod vector.

The first documented outbreak of apparent alphavirus-induced encephalitis occurred among horses in Massachusetts in 1831, although the likely causative agent, eastern equine encephalitis virus, was not isolated until 1933. Incidents and epizootics of encephalitis in horses caused by eastern equine encephalitis virus have since been described throughout much of the United States east of the Mississippi River, in addition to some mid-western states and the Canadian provinces of Quebec and Ontario. Eastern equine encephalitis still occurs commonly among horses in the eastern and, especially, the southeastern United States. Western equine encephalitis virus, the cause of a similar neurologic disease of horses, was first isolated from the brain of a horse in the San Joaquin Valley of California in 1931 by K. F. Meyer and colleagues, who quickly recognized the central role of mosquitoes in the virus transmission cycle, as well as the risk to humans. Extensive outbreaks of western equine encephalitis occurred throughout western North America until the middle of the 20th century, when the incidence of western equine encephalitis in horses declined precipitously after the advent of vaccination and has not occurred in recent years, despite limited virus circulation. In 1936, an epizootic of equine encephalitis occurred in Venezuela; the causative virus was not neutralized by antibodies to the two known viruses causing encephalitis in horses elsewhere in the Americas, and was named "Venezuelan equine encephalitis virus." These three equine encephalitis viruses initially were referred to as arboviruses because of their transmission by arthropods, and their further initial designation as "group A arboviruses" ultimately led to their current designation as alphaviruses.

PROPERTIES OF TOGAVIRUSES

All viruses in the family *Togaviridae* that are either animal pathogens or zoonoses are included in the genus *Alphavirus* (Table 29.1), thus only properties of alphaviruses will be described.

Virion Properties

Alphavirus virions are spherical, uniform in appearance, enveloped, and 70 nm in diameter. Virions consist of a lipid envelope with fine spikes surrounding an icosahedral nucleocapsid that is 40 nm in diameter (Figure 29.1). The spikes are composed of heterodimers of the E1 and E2 glycoproteins that are organized in a (T = 4) icosahedral lattice consisting of 80 trimers.

The genome is a single molecule of linear, positive-sense, single-stranded RNA, 11–12 kb in size (Figure 29.2). The RNA has a 5′-methylated nucleotide cap and its 3′ end is polyadenylated. The 5′ two-thirds of the genome encodes non-structural proteins; the 3′ one-third is not translated from genomic RNA, but is expressed from a subgenomic mRNA molecule that is transcribed from a full-length, negative-sense intermediate. The subgenomic mRNA encodes five proteins, including a nucleocapsid protein (C, M_r 30–33 kDa) and two envelope glycoproteins (E1 and E2, M_r 45–58 kDa). Some alphaviruses have a third envelope protein, E3 (M_r 10 kDa) which is a cleavage product of a precursor protein, PE2. Alphaviruses are relatively unstable in the environment, and are inactivated easily by common disinfectants and high temperature.

Virus Replication

Alphaviruses can replicate to very high titers and cause severe cytopathic changes in many kinds of vertebrate cells, including: Vero (African green monkey kidney), BHK-21 (baby hamster kidney), and primary chick and duck embryo cells. They also grow in, but do not cause cytopathic changes in, mosquito cells, such as C6/36, which are derived from *Aedes albopictus*. In mammalian and avian cells, infection causes a complete shutdown of host-cell protein and nucleic acid synthesis. In mosquito cells there is no shutdown, and cell division can continue, with the cells becoming persistently infected and continuously shedding virus.

Viral attachment to the host cell first involves interaction between the viral E2 glycoprotein and receptors on the cell surface. The broad host range of alphaviruses suggests that either E2 contains several receptor binding sites or the cell receptor is ubiquitous. Various lectins, integrins, and laminin have been identified as putative cellular receptors of individual alphaviruses. Once

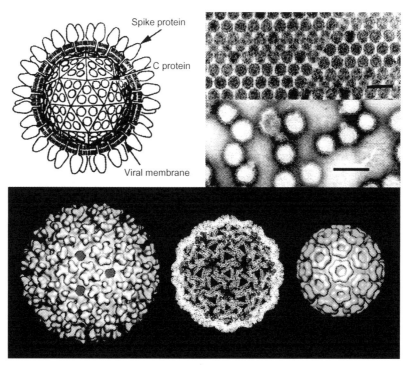

FIGURE 29.1 (Top panel–left). Diagrammatic representation of a Sindbis virus particle. The spike proteins on the surface represent the external portions of the E1+E2 heterodimers that associate to form trimers. C, capsid protein. (Upper right), Thin section of pelleted particles of Semliki Forest virus. (Lower right), Negative contrast electron micrograph of particles of Semliki Forest virus. (Bottom panel), Structure of Sindbis virus (SINV). (Left), Surface shaded view as determined by cryo-electronmicroscopy and image reconstruction. (Center), Surface view of SINV showing the organization of the E1 glycoprotein on the surface of the particle. (Right), Image represents the nucleocapsid core showing the pentameric and hexameric capsomeres (T = 4 icosahedron). *[From Virus Taxonomy: Eighth Report of the International Committee on Taxonomy of Viruses (C. M. Fauquet, M. A. Mayo, J. Maniloff, U. Desselberger, L. A. Ball, eds.), p. 999. Copyright © Elsevier (2005), with permission.]*

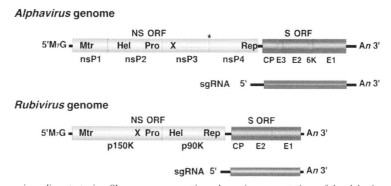

FIGURE 29.2 Togavirus genomic coding strategies. Shown are comparative schematic representations of the alphavirus and rubivirus genomic RNAs with untranslated regions represented as solid black lines and open reading frames (ORFs) as open boxes (NS-ORF = non-structural protein ORF; S-ORF = structural protein ORF). Within each ORF, the coding sequences for the proteins processed from the translation product of the ORF are delineated. The asterisk between nsP3 and nsP4 in the alphavirus NS-ORF indicates the stop codon present in some alphaviruses that must be translationally read through to produce a precursor containing nsP4. Additionally within the NS-ORFs, the locations of motifs associated with the following activities are indicated: (Mtr) methyl transferase, (Pro) protease, (Hel) helicase, (X) unknown function, and (Rep) replicase. The sequences encompassed by the subgenomic RNA (sgRNA) are also shown. CP, capsid protein; E1, 2, 3, envelope proteins; ns, non-structural proteins; An, poly(A) sequence; sgRNA, subgenomic RNA; M7G, 7-methylguanosine, p, precursor protein *[From Virus Taxonomy: Eighth Report of the International Committee on Taxonomy of Viruses (C. M. Fauquet, M. A. Mayo, J. Maniloff, U. Desselberger, L. A. Ball, eds.), p. 1001. Copyright © Elsevier (2005), with permission.]*

virions bind to the cell, the virus–receptor complex is endocytosed into coated vesicles using the clathrin-dependent pathway. The acidification of the vesicles causes a rearrangement of the E1–E2 dimer with the formation of an E1 trimer inducing fusion with the vesicle membrane with release of the nucleocapsid into the cytoplasm. Upon entry into the cytoplasm, the virion RNA has two main functions (Figure 29.3). The 5′ end of the genomic RNA serves as messenger RNA (mRNA) that, in some alphaviruses, is first translated to produce two polyproteins,

TABLE 29.2 Properties of Togaviruses

Two genera: *Alphavirus*, arthropod-borne viruses, and *Rubivirus*, rubella virus (an exclusively human pathogen)

Virions are spherical, uniform in appearance, enveloped, 70 nm in diameter, and consist of an envelope with fine glycoprotein spikes surrounding an icosahedral nucleocapsid, 40 nm in diameter

The genome is a single molecule of linear, positive-sense, single-stranded RNA, 9.7–11.8 kb in size; the 5′ end of the genomic RNA is capped, whereas the 3′ end is polyadenylated

Genomic RNA is infectious

The 5′ two-thirds of the genome encodes non-structural proteins; the 3′ one-third encodes the structural proteins, which are transcribed from a 26S subgenomic mRNA

Virions contain two (or three) envelope glycoproteins E1, E2, and E3, which form the spikes, and a nucleocapsid protein, C

Replication occurs in the cytoplasm, and maturation occurs via budding from the plasma membrane

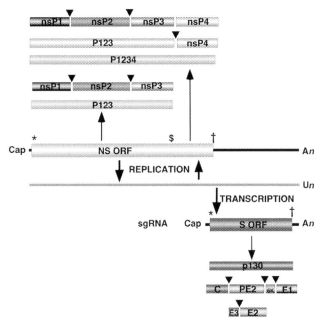

FIGURE 29.3 Genome organization, translation, transcription and replication strategies of Sindbis virus (SINV). The regions of the 11.7 kb genomic RNA and 26S subgenomic RNA (sgRNA) (dark lines) that code respectively for the non-structural (nsP) and structural proteins (colored boxes) are shown. Replication and transcription are indicated by thick arrows. The grey line is the replicative intermediate that is also the template for the sgRNA. E3 is a structural protein in some alphaviruses. Initiation codons are indicated by (*), termination codons by (†) and ($) (the latter is readthrough to produce P1234, hence nsP4 is cleaved off). Dark triangles represent nsP2 protease activity. (From Strauss and Strauss, 1994). C, nucleocapsid; ns, non-structural proteins; E, envelope proteins; NS ORF, non-structural protein open reading frame; p, precursor protein; PE2, precursor protein for E2; sgRNA, sub-genomic RNA; S ORG, structural proteins open reading frame. *[From Virus Taxonomy: Eighth Report of the International Committee on Taxonomy of Viruses (C. M. Fauquet, M. A. Mayo, J. Maniloff, U. Desselberger, L. A. Ball, eds.), p. 1002. Copyright © Elsevier (2005), with permission.]*

the larger of which is produced by a read-through of a weak stop codon. These non-structural proteins in their uncleaved and cleaved forms direct the synthesis of the template negative-sense RNA genome from the input virion RNA and then genomic-size plus-strand RNA, along with a subgenomic RNA (Table 29.2). The full-length plus-strand RNA is encapsidated into new virions, whereas the subgenomic RNA acts as message for the synthesis of the structural viral proteins. The structural proteins are expressed from the subgenomic RNA as a polyprotein that is then cleaved to form the individual proteins. In mammalian cells, nucleocapsids are assembled in the cytoplasm and move to the plasma membrane, where they align under patches containing viral glycoprotein spikes. Finally, virions are formed by budding of nucleocapsids through patches of plasma membrane that are studded with spike glycoprotein (Table 29.2). The budding process in insect cells may be localized to internal cellular membranes.

New World (eastern and Venezuelan equine encephalitis viruses) and Old World (Sindbis, Semliki Forest viruses) apparently utilize different mechanisms to interfere with the host interferon response, which is key to survival in infected animals. For Sindbis virus, the multifunctional non-structural protein, nsP2, inhibits host-cell transcription, whereas in Venezuelan and eastern equine encephalitis virus the nucleocapsid protein, C, inhibits RNA transcription. Host-cell macromolecular synthesis, including innate immune responses, is compromised by both mechanisms, thus enhancing the yield of infectious virus.

MEMBERS OF THE GENUS *ALPHAVIRUS* EQUINE ALPHAVIRUSES

EASTERN EQUINE ENCEPHALITIS VIRUS, WESTERN EQUINE ENCEPHALITIS VIRUS, HIGHLANDS J VIRUS, AND VENEZUELAN EQUINE ENCEPHALITIS VIRUS

Several closely related, mosquito-transmitted alphaviruses endemic in the Americas cause severe disease in horses and humans, and sometimes in other animal species. The most important of these are eastern, western, and Venezuelan equine encephalitis viruses. In addition to being closely related, these viruses share similar primary transmission cycles that involve mosquitoes and either birds or mammals as reservoir hosts.

Clinical Features and Epidemiology

Infection of horses with eastern, western, or Venezuelan equine encephalitis viruses produces a range of clinical manifestations that reflect the virulence of the infecting virus strain. Although the geographic range and epidemiological features of these three viruses are quite different, infections of horses can result in similar syndromes of neurological disease. These viruses are all zoonoses, and may infect other animal species, sometimes causing disease.

Equine encephalitic alphavirus infections of horses may be subclinical with only a transient fever, or may present with protracted fever, anorexia, tachycardia, and depression. Progressive systemic disease leading to death only occurs when the virus gains access to the central nervous system. After an incubation period of 4–6 days, affected horses develop high fever and signs of drowsiness and incoordination. The disease progresses rapidly to profound depression, typically with neurologic manifestations such an abnormally wide stance, hanging head, drooping ears, flaccid lips, irregular gait, wandering, and signs of encephalitis, including impaired vision, photophobia, inability to swallow, other reflex impairments, circling, yawning, and grinding of teeth. Constant head pressing against a corner of the stall or fence is a typical presentation. In terminal stages of disease, there is an inability to rise, paralysis, and, occasionally, convulsions. In horses, the case-fatality rate is high from North American (lineage I) eastern equine encephalitis virus infection (typically 50–90%), lower from western equine encephalitis virus infection (0–40%), and highly variable from Venezuelan equine encephalitis virus (epizootic types) infection (up to 80%). Mildly affected animals can recover slowly in a few weeks, but may have neurological sequelae (dullness, dementia); such horses have been referred to as "dummies."

Birds are critical to the enzootic transmission cycles of eastern and western encephalitis viruses. Alphavirus transmission to birds is primarily through mosquito bites, but, in pheasants, eastern equine encephalitis virus has been transmitted through feather picking and cannibalism.

Although the clinical signs of the equine alphavirus encephalitides are similar, the distribution and epidemiology of each is different.

Eastern Equine Encephalitis Virus

Eastern equine encephalitis virus is enzootic in eastern portions of North America, the Caribbean Basin, Central America, and along the northern and eastern coasts of South America. Eastern equine encephalitis virus is genetically heterogeneous, and there are at least four distinct lineages (I, IIA, IIB, and III) in the virus complex. The closely related group I viruses that occur in the United States, Canada, and the Caribbean are the most virulent to humans and horses. In contrast, infection of horses or humans with the more genetically diverse virus strains enzootic in Central and South America rarely results in significant clinical disease.

The virus is maintained in North America in resident birds in freshwater marshes by the ornithophilic mosquito, *Culiseta melanura*. This mosquito is responsible for amplification of the virus during the spring and summer by infecting and feeding on viremic wading birds, passerine songbirds, and starlings that are asymptomatically infected reservoir hosts of the virus (Figure 29.4). Outbreaks of encephalitis occur in humans and horses during the late summer and fall, when the virus is acquired by other species of mosquitoes, including those in the genera *Aedes* and *Coquillettidia* that serve as "bridge" vectors that transmit the virus from its enzootic infection cycle to humans and horses. Eastern equine encephalitis virus apparently overwinters within enzootic regions, including temperate regions such as the northeastern United States; however, the mechanism by which this is accomplished is uncertain. Conversely, there is evidence of repeated introductions of genetically distinct virus strains in other regions.

Virtually all bird species that have been tested are susceptible to eastern equine encephalitis virus infection, with variable pathogenic consequences. Passerine birds develop high-titer viremia, with minimal mortality. Clinical disease occurs primarily in pheasants, partridges, and turkeys, and small outbreaks have been reported in emus, whooping cranes, Pekin ducks, penguins, and egrets. Experimentally, young chickens have been infected, but only birds less than 14 days of age developed clinical signs. Pheasants typically develop encephalitis, with 50–70% mortality, whereas other birds (emus and turkeys) develop a viscerotropic disease, with necrosis of parenchymal organs, including heart, kidney, pancreas, liver, bursa, spleen, and thymus. Emus can develop remarkably high levels of viremia and mortality rates of 100%. Eastern equine encephalitis virus infection also has been reported in sheep, deer, goats, cattle, camelids, dogs, and pigs, sometimes with associated neurological signs and fatal meningoencephalitis.

Western Equine Encephalitis and Highlands J Viruses

Western equine encephalitis virus is distributed widely throughout the Americas, from Canada to Argentina. Infection was especially prevalent in the western regions of North America in the past, where there were substantial epizootics in horses and humans during the 1930s. However, the occurrence of western equine encephalitis has declined in both horses and humans in western North America in recent years. The vectors and reservoir hosts of western equine encephalitis virus probably are different in each of the ecological zones in which the virus is found; in western North America, the virus is maintained in an enzootic cycle involving passerine birds and *Culex tarsalis*,

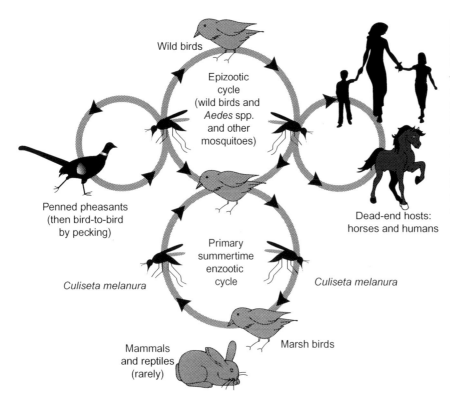

FIGURE 29.4 Transmission cycle of eastern equine encephalitis virus in North America. In wild birds, infection is asymptomatic, but in horses, pheasants, and humans, it is usually devastating, in many cases causing death, or neurological sequelae in survivors. The primary summertime enzootic cycle takes place mostly in freshwater marshes; the epizootic cycle is often centered in areas near such marshes. Although horses and humans are considered "dead-end" hosts from an epidemiological perspective, some horses produce viremia levels high enough to transmit virus to mosquitoes that feed on them. The mode of overwintering of this virus is unknown.

a mosquito particularly adapted to irrigated agricultural areas. The feeding pattern for *Culex tarsalis* changes from birds in spring and early summer to increasingly include mammals in late summer when mosquito populations peak, depending on climatic factors and irrigation practices. Other secondary mosquito vectors include *Aedes melanimon*, and *A. dorsalis*, which can facilitate a second cycle of infection and, along with *Culex tarsalis*, transmit virus to horses and humans. As with eastern equine encephalitis virus, the precise mechanism of overwintering of western equine encephalitis virus remains unknown. Chronic infections of birds have been demonstrated experimentally, but their role in natural overwintering of virus is uncertain.

Serosurveys have confirmed western equine encephalitis virus infection in various rodents, rabbits, bats, squirrels, ungulates, tortoises, and snakes, and non-avian species may be important reservoir hosts in parts of South America. Emus are susceptible to western equine encephalitis virus infection, but with considerably lower mortality rates than those associated with eastern equine encephalitis virus infection.

Genetic analysis suggests that western equine encephalitis virus arose through a recombination event between eastern equine encephalitis virus and a Sindbis-like alphavirus such as Aura virus, a non-pathogenic alphavirus found in Brazil and Argentina. Western equine encephalitis virus is genetically diverse, and epizootic strains of the virus generally exhibit enhanced virulence and neuroinvasiveness. North American strains are typically more virulent than the strains

that are enzootic in South America, with only sporadic reports of western equine encephalitis in horses and humans in South America. This suggests that there is minimal exchange of viruses between the continents.

Several closely related but distinct viruses have been isolated in North America, including Highlands J virus in the eastern United States. Highlands J virus is a very sporadic cause of encephalitis in horses, especially in Florida, and is also pathogenic to turkeys and partridges. Fort Morgan and related Buggy Creek viruses are western equine encephalitis-like viruses that are transmitted among swallows by their nest parasitic bugs, but are not considered pathogenic for either humans or horses.

Venezuelan Equine Encephalitis Virus

Viruses in the Venezuelan equine encephalitis antigenic complex (groups I–VI) occur in Central and South America; the exception is Everglades virus (group II), which is enzootic in Florida, infecting rodents and dogs. Enzootic virus strains occur in silent, stable transmission cycles primarily involving *Culex* (*Melanoconion*) spp. mosquitoes and a variety of small mammals (e.g., cotton rats, spiny rats, *Peromyscus* spp.) in tropical swamps in Central America and northern South America. Infections of domestic animals and humans with these virus strains rarely cause clinical disease, but subclinical infections are common, as demonstrated by serological surveys. Horses

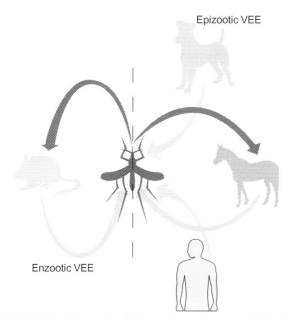

Epizootic VEE

Enzootic VEE

FIGURE 29.5 Life cycle of Venezuelan equine encephalitis virus (VEE). During the enzootic cycle, VEE is maintained in a sylvatic ecosystem with a rodent reservoir (spiny rat) and mosquito vector, generally *Culex* spp. (*Melanoconion*). On generation of an epizootic strain of VEE, multiple-vector species transmit the virus. The horse generates a sufficiently high-titer viremia to amplify the virus significantly. Several other terrestrial mammals also are susceptible to infection, and develop significant viremia (including human and dog). *[From* Equine Infectious Diseases, *D. C. Sellon, M. Long, p. 194. Copyright © Saunders/Elsevier (2007), with permission.]*

infected with these virus strains do not develop sufficient viremia to infect feeding mosquitoes.

Viruses within subtype I (IAB and IC) are virulent to horses and produce high-titered viremia in horses, donkeys, and mules. A common feature of all epizootics of Venezuelan equine encephalitis is that horses serve as efficient amplification hosts of the outbreak virus strain. Experimental infection of horses with the epizootic virus strains characteristically results in high-titered viremia that is sufficient to infect *Aedes* and *Psorophora* mosquitoes. Epizootic virus strains predominantly have been identified in Venezuela, Colombia, Peru, and Ecuador, where they cause major epizootics at approximately 10-year intervals. These viruses cause severe disease in all equid species, with survivors often having serious neurological sequelae.

Sequence analysis indicates that epizootic strains (IAB and IC) evolve from less virulent ID strains that are maintained in enzootic infection cycles between epizootics. Key substitutions that occur in the E2 glycoprotein during enzootic transmission lead to the periodic emergence of virulent epizootic strains (Figure 29.5). Two different changes may independently enhance transmission: one that increases the amount of virus produced by the mosquito vector, and another that produces high levels of viremia in the equine. It also has been suggested that use

of formalin-inactivated vaccines containing residual infectious virus may have been responsible for initiating some type IAB epidemics up until 1973.

Pathogenesis and Pathology

After virus entry via the bite of a mosquito vector, replication of the equine encephalitis alphaviruses occurs in cells near the entry site, including dendritic cells. Infected dendritic cells may then transport the virus to the regional lymph nodes. The resulting primary viremia allows virus to invade specific extraneural tissues, where further replication precedes high-titer secondary viremia. Virus replication occurs in immune cells, especially dendritic cells, and results in virus-mediated suppression of protective innate host responses. The magnitude and duration of the viremia are critical, because high-titer viremia facilitates infection of vector insects that feed on amplifying animal hosts, and also is necessary for the virus to gain access to the central nervous system. In the central nervous system, infection principally involves neurons, but other cells also are infected.

Most, if not all, alphaviruses are neurotropic, but neuroinvasiveness is a distinct property of certain strains; alphaviruses readily infect cultured neurons and cause neurological infection and damage if directly injected into the central nervous system. Encephalitis caused by naturally acquired alphavirus infections is the result of hematogenous spread of virus and subsequent entry to the central nervous system by one of several possible routes: (1) passive diffusion of virus through the endothelium of capillaries in the central nervous system; (2) virus replication in vascular endothelial cells and release of progeny into the parenchyma of the central nervous system; (3) virus invasion of the cerebrospinal fluid, with infection of the choroid plexus and ependyma; (4) carriage of virus in lymphocytes and monocytes, which may migrate into the parenchyma of the central nervous system. Characteristic histological features include widespread neuronal necrosis with neuronophagia, and intense perivascular infiltration of mononuclear inflammatory cells. The pathology of Venezuelan equine encephalitis in horses includes cellular depletion of bone marrow, spleen, and lymph nodes, pancreatic necrosis, and, in cases where the animal survives long enough, encephalitis.

In domestic birds, alphavirus infections produce similar signalment and lesions within susceptible hosts. In turkey hens, egg production will decrease precipitously and the few eggs produced will be small, devoid of shell pigment, and thin shelled. With eastern equine encephalitis virus and Highlands J virus, virus is isolated from oviducts, ovaries, and the eggs during the acute phase of infection. In addition, in young turkeys there is multifocal necrosis in heart, kidney, and pancreas, and lymphoid necrosis and depletion in thymus, spleen, and cloacal bursa. In partridges and pheasants, myocarditis and encephalitis are the most common lesions, whereas in whooping cranes (*Grus Americana*) and emus (*Dromaius novaehollandiae*), eastern equine encephalitis virus produces fulminating disease with necrosis of parenchyma in several visceral organs, but the central nervous system is spared or only mildly affected. In Pekin ducks, the lesions are limited to the spinal cord, resulting in posterior paresis and paralysis. Adult chickens are asymptomatically infected after natural or experimental exposure, and thus serve as public health sentinels for serological detection of alphavirus circulation in a geographic area. However, experimental infection in chicks younger than 2 weeks has produced myocarditis, and less frequently, encephalitis.

Diagnosis

The diagnosis of the equine encephalitides can be made by isolating the virus, or by detection of: (1) a virus-specific antibody response; (2) viral nucleic acid; (3) viral antigen in tissue samples. Immunoglobulin M (IgM) capture enzyme-linked immunosorbent assays are routinely used to detect alphavirus-specific IgM antibodies in individual serum and cerebrospinal fluid samples, because detection of IgG antibodies is not predictive of recent infection and may be confused with vaccine-induced antibodies in horses in enzootic areas. IgM antibodies are almost always detectable before the second week of infection. Where necessary, confirmation of positive IgM results can be achieved by evaluation of paired sera, using either virus neutralization or hemagglutination inhibition assays. The reverse transcriptase-polymerase chain reaction (RT-PCR) test has become a mainstay in diagnosing alphavirus infections, because it is rapid and detects viral RNA regardless of the presence of neutralizing antibodies. Viral RNA is detected for a longer period of time by RT-PCR than viremia is detected by virus isolation. Viral antigen can be detected either by fluorescent antibody staining or, more frequently, by immunohistochemical staining on formalin-preserved tissue samples, which has the advantage of achieving a diagnosis on samples that have an extended transit time to a diagnostic center.

The suckling mouse is a particularly sensitive host for virus isolation from clinical specimens (blood, brain), but this procedure has been largely replaced by cell culture procedures. Vero, BHK-21, and C6/36 (*Aedes albopictus* mosquito) cells all can be used for virus isolation. Isolation of viruses remains important in order to compare strains of viruses that might be circulating in any given area, which is especially important because enzootic and epizootic strains of Venezuelan equine encephalitis virus must be distinguished.

Immunity, Prevention, and Control

Immunity following alphavirus infection is probably lifelong. Immunization of horses with inactivated cell culture vaccines for eastern, western, and Venezuelan equine encephalitides is the basis of current immunization programs. These vaccines provide substantial, but not perfect, protection of immunized horses. Emus and other birds, including endangered whooping cranes, have also been successfully immunized with both western and eastern equine encephalitis vaccines. Horses typically are vaccinated annually each spring with either bi- or trivalent vaccine, after a primary immunization schedule of two doses 4–6 weeks apart. In areas where mosquitoes are active year round, foals are vaccinated at 3, 4, and 6 months of age, and at least annually thereafter. New-generation recombinant vectored vaccines, including replicon vaccines, also have been developed for potential use in humans and animals. In many areas, mosquito control programs are also in place to protect public health. Larval population management programs may be supplemented with aerial spraying of insecticides during emergency situations, such as during an epizootic or when an epizootic appears likely. Prohibition of the movement of horses is also used in the face of outbreaks, as equines are capable of transmitting the virus to new mosquito hosts.

Human Disease

Equine encephalitis alphaviruses are zoonotic and cause significant human disease. Eastern equine encephalitis virus infection in humans is characterized by fever, drowsiness, and neck rigidity. The disease may progress to confusion, paralysis, convulsions, and coma. The overall fatality rate among clinical cases is high (50–75%), and many survivors are left with permanent neurologic sequelae, such as mental retardation, epilepsy, paralysis, deafness, and blindness. Western equine encephalitis virus is usually less severe: a high proportion of infections are inapparent and the case-fatality rate is lower (3–10%) than with eastern equine encephalitis. Venezuelan equine encephalitis virus (epidemic types) causes a systemic febrile illness in humans, and about 1% of those affected develop clinical encephalitis. There is also abortion and fetal death when pregnant women are infected, and case-fatality rates as high as 20–30% have been reported in young children with encephalitis.

GETAH VIRUS

Getah virus (Sagiyama virus) is widely distributed in Asia, and the cause of abortions in pigs and systemic disease in horses. The virus appears to be transmitted by *Culex* mosquitoes, but both the maintenance cycle and the mechanism of transmission are poorly defined. The clinical signs in horses include depression, anorexia, fever, limb edema, urticarial rash, and swelling of submandibular lymph nodes. Some 40% of exposed horses developed clinical signs in the initial epizootic that was described in Japan in 1978, but seroprevalence rates of over 50% were found in horses not linked to the initial outbreak. Another outbreak occurred in India in 1990, and a serosurvey indicated that 17% of Indian horses had been infected with Getah virus. An inactivated vaccine was developed in Japan for use in equines.

OTHER ZOONOTIC ALPHAVIRUSES

In addition to the equine encephalitis alphaviruses, other alphaviruses cause zoonotic diseases that are important in various regions of the world, mostly in the tropics and subtropics. Semliki Forest virus is a mosquito-transmitted alphavirus that has been used extensively in biomedical research, although it rarely or never causes disease in naturally infected animals or humans. Fever, rash, and polyarthritis constitute a characteristic triad of clinical features in infections caused by Sindbis virus and other viruses related to Semliki Forest virus, specifically chikungunya, o'nyong-nyong, Ross River, Mayaro, Igbo Ora, and Barmah Forest viruses. The enzootic transmission cycles of several of these viruses remain poorly characterized.

CHIKUNGUNYA AND O'NYONG-NYONG VIRUSES

Chikungunya virus occurs throughout increasingly extensive portions of sub-Saharan Africa, the Indian subcontinent, and Southeast Asia. The virus recently caused a substantial epidemic throughout the Indian Ocean region, and has spread to southern Europe (Italy). The animal reservoirs of enzootic strains in Africa include species of non-human primates, whereas epidemic strains are transmitted among humans by *Aedes aegypti* and *Aedes albopictis*. O'nyong-nyong virus is a close relative of chikungunya virus that occurs in East Africa, where it is transmitted by *Anopheles* mosquitoes; however, the enzootic infection cycle remains uncharacterized. Both viruses cause severe and very painful polyarthritis, which lead to the African names of "chikungunya" and "o'nyong-nyong" that describe the agony of affected joints.

ROSS RIVER VIRUS

Ross River virus infection occurs in some coastal regions of Australia, New Guinea, and adjacent Pacific Islands. The virus is transmitted by species of both *Aedes* and *Culex* mosquitoes that breed in saltwater or freshwater marshes. The putative vertebrate reservoir hosts are large marsupials such as wallabies and kangaroos, but the reservoir hosts in large urban areas remain uncertain, as antibodies have been found in many animal species. The virus is an important cause of human disease in enzootic areas, and periodically is the cause of extensive human epidemics. A substantial proportion of infected individuals develop severe clinical signs, notably polyarthritis, but infection is rarely fatal. The

significance of Ross River virus as a veterinary pathogen remains a subject of conjecture, but there is speculation that it causes a disease in horses analogous to that in humans.

SINDBIS VIRUS

Sindbis virus originally was identified in Egypt, where it was first isolated in 1952. The virus occurs throughout much of the world, including Europe and Scandinavia, Africa, the Middle East, the Indian subcontinent, Southeast Asia, and Australia. A closely related variant, Aura virus, occurs in South America. The virus is transmitted by *Culex* mosquitoes among different species of birds, including migratory and game birds, which serve as amplifying hosts. Sindbis virus is typically transmitted to dead-end hosts such as humans by *Aedes* mosquitoes, and is a sporadic cause of polyarthritis, rash, and fever, although many infections are asymptomatic. There is considerable genetic diversity amongst the strains of Sindbis virus that occur worldwide, and some are apparently more virulent human pathogens than others.

SALMONID ALPHAVIRUSES

The first salmonid alphavirus was isolated in 1995, from farmed Atlantic salmon in Ireland and Scotland with pancreatic disease. The virus is now known as salmon pancreas disease virus or salmonid alphavirus 1. Several years later, another virus was identified as the cause of a "sleeping disease" in freshwater rainbow trout (*Oncorhynchus mykiss*) in France. This virus is known as sleeping disease virus or salmonid alphavirus 2. Another salmonid alphavirus (salmonid alphavirus 3) subsequently was identified in Norwegian farmed Atlantic salmon (*Salmo salar*).

Clinical Features and Epidemiology

The clinical signs associated with pancreatic disease in salmon may be a sudden onset of inappetence, lethargy, an increased number of fecal casts in the enclosures, increased mortality, and ill thrift. The affected fish may have difficulty maintaining position in the water, as a result of muscle damage. This inability to maintain posture can also result in erosions and ulcerations as the fish scrape against enclosure barriers. Fish affected by sleeping disease show a characteristic presentation of lying on their side at the bottom of the enclosure as if "sleeping." They also show swollen abdomens and bulging eyes (Figure 29.6).

Definitive detection of salmonid alphaviruses is currently restricted to Europe and Scandinavia; Ireland, England, France, Germany, Norway, Italy, and Spain in particular. Infection of salmon occurs in saltwater habitats, whereas rainbow trout are affected in freshwater. It is difficult to define the conditions that trigger a clinical event, other than stressors such as movement to new locations and high rates of growth. Pancreatic disease caused by salmonid alphavirus 1 is enzootic to virtually all rearing facilities in Ireland, and infections recur regardless of the time period between the introduction of a new generation of fish into vacant enclosures. This suggests either a significant reservoir of the virus in the sea water environment or the presence of the virus in the salmon in their freshwater rearing facilities. Vertical transmission of virus is unproven. Mortality rates for salmonid alphavirus infections are highly variable, and may depend upon the strain of fish, water temperature, and growth rate.

Pathogenesis and Pathology

Early studies confirmed that plasma, blood leucocytes, and kidney extracts could transmit salmonid alphavirus diseases, and that the time course of the disease was temperature dependent, with a faster progression at 14°C than at 9°C. Both salmonid alphaviruses 1 and 2 cause lesions in the pancreas, heart, and muscle in salmon or trout, although the severity of lesions in salmon is dependent on the strain of fish. The initial histological lesion noted for salmonid pancreatic disease, logically, was necrosis of the pancreas. However, subsequent studies also showed profound cardiomyopathy and skeletal myopathy (Figure 29.6). Time-course studies confirmed pancreatic necrosis during the very acute phase of the disease, with destruction of the acinar tissue with little or no inflammatory responses, whereas development of lesions in cardiac muscle was somewhat slower. The skeletal muscle lesions only appeared rather late in the course of infection, some 3–4 weeks after the pancreatic and heart lesions. Involvement of muscle accounts for the abnormal behavior of affected fish.

Diagnosis

The diagnosis of salmonid alphavirus infections is based on the clinical presentation and detection of characteristic lesions in affected fish. These viruses can be isolated *in vitro* using cell lines such as Chinook salmon embryo cells (CHSE-214) or rainbow trout gonad cells (RTG-2). However, virus isolation is complicated by the fact that the clinical course of infection is delayed, and the onset of clinical signs occurs only at 7–14 days after infection. By that time, virus titers are waning in the face of the host protective antiviral response, thus sampling of several fish is indicated. The presence of salmonid alphaviruses in a population can also be detected using serology based on virus neutralization assay, as there is sufficient cross-reactivity among the various salmonid alphaviruses identified to date. RT-PCR assay is now the test of choice for detection of salmonid alphaviruses. Sensitivity of this assay is not complicated by the presence of antibody, as is virus isolation, and viral RNA can be detected in tissue samples for at least 190 days

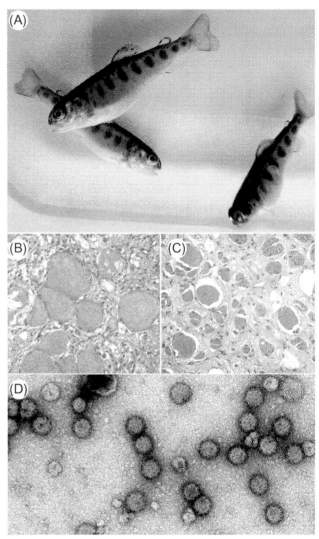

FIGURE 29.6 Infections with salmonid alphavirus 2 in rainbow trout. (A) Young rainbow trout with signs of sleeping disease, including failure to keep position in the water column, distended abdomens, and bilateral exophthalmos. (B) Skeletal muscle lesions during acute infection. (C) Skeletal muscle lesions during chronic stages of infection. (D) Partially purified and then negatively stained virions of salmonid alphavirus 2. *(A, B, C: Courtesy of J. Castric, Agence Française de Sécurité Sanitaire des Aliments. D; Courtesy of M. Bremont, Institut National de la Recherche Agronomique.)*

after infection, long after infectious virus can be cultured from the same tissues. This ability of RT-PCR to detect viral sequences months after the acute infection is useful in defining the exposure of populations to salmonid alphaviruses; however, caution should be exercised in ascribing disease causality merely on the basis of detection of viral RNA.

Immunity, Prevention and Control

Fish that recover from primary salmonid alphavirus infection are resistant to infection for at least 9 months, and the disease does not recur in naturally exposed fish that survive the infection. Neutralizing antibodies can be detected in the majority of infected fish by 14–16 days after infection, and in 100% of fish by 28 days. There is cross-protection between salmonid alphaviruses 1 and 2. Formalin-inactivated salmonid alphavirus vaccines can provide complete protection against challenge infection, but formulation of this type of vaccine in a combined product can be problematic. A genetically engineered modified-live vaccine also induced long-term protection in immunized fish; however a vaccine-mutant virus caused clinical disease.

Control programs are complicated by the lack of information regarding reservoirs of these viruses, and the epidemiology of their infections. Although direct transmission of the virus occurs between infected and uninfected fish, the potential role of vectors such as sea lice is currently unknown. Of potential relevance is the fact that an alphavirus distantly related to Semliki Forest virus was isolated from a louse collected from a southern elephant seal. Finally, although initial experimental trials with salmonid alphavirus suggest a potential role for vertical transmission of the virus, further studies to confirm this important pathway are required.

Flaviviridae

Chapter Contents

The family *Flaviviridae* comprises three genera (*Flavivirus*, *Pestivirus* and *Hepacivirus*), the members of which, although similar in genomic organization and physicochemical properties, are genetically distinct and biologically quite different (Table 30.1). The genus *Flavivirus* contains at least 70 viruses; several of which are of veterinary importance, including Japanese encephalitis, West Nile, louping ill, and Wesselsbron viruses. Some 30 members of this genus are arthropod-borne human pathogens, the causative agents of diseases varying from fevers with rash to life-threatening hemorrhagic fevers to encephalitis to hepatic necrosis. Members such as the four dengue viruses, West Nile virus, Japanese encephalitis virus, and several tick-borne encephalitis viruses rank among the most important human viral pathogens. The genus *Pestivirus* contains important veterinary pathogens, including bovine viral diarrhea virus, border disease virus of sheep, and classical swine fever virus. The genus *Hepacivirus* contains only the human pathogens, hepatitis C and the inappropriately named hepatitis G viruses.

Yellow fever virus, the prototype of the genus *Flavivirus*, was discovered in the course of investigating epidemic yellow fever. In Havana in 1900, Walter Reed, James Carroll,

and colleagues showed that the etiologic agent was a "filterable virus" and that it was transmitted by the mosquito, *Aedes aegypti*. Yellow fever was one of the great scourges of humankind during the 18th and 19th centuries, with epidemics repeatedly affecting coastal cities in the Americas, Europe, and West Africa. Following the discovery of the virus and its vector, mosquito eradication programs quickly eliminated the disease from cities in the western hemisphere. Hemispheric eradication was envisioned, but in 1932 the enzootic/zoonotic jungle cycle involving monkeys and jungle-canopy mosquitoes was discovered—a cycle that precludes eradication. The global significance and impact of other members of the genus are increasing, especially dengue, Japanese encephalitis and West Nile viruses.

Members of the genus *Pestivirus* occur worldwide as economically important veterinary pathogens. Classical swine fever (also known as hog cholera) was first recognized in Ohio in 1833; it has been conjectured that the virus might have emerged at that time by species jumping—that is, by a host-range mutation of another pestivirus. Early in the 20th century, as intensive swine production expanded, classical swine fever became a most important disease in developed countries—subsequent eradication programs

Fenner's Veterinary Virology. DOI: 10.1016/B978-0-12-375158-4.00030-4

TABLE 30.1 Flaviviruses that Cause Disease in Domestic Animals and Zoonotic Disease in Humans[a]

Virus	Host of Concern (Reservoir Host)	Arthropod Host (Mode of Transmission)	Disease in Domestic Animals (or Humans)	Geographic Distribution
Genus *Flavivirus*				
Japanese encephalitis virus	Swine, humans, horses (birds)	Mosquitoes: *Culex tritaeniorhynchus*	Abortion, neonatal disease (encephalitis)	Asia
Murray Valley encephalitis virus	Humans (birds)	Mosquitoes: *Culex annulirostris*	(Encephalitis)	Australia, New Guinea
St. Louis encephalitis virus	Humans (birds)	Mosquitoes: *Culex tarsalis*, *C. pipiens*	(Encephalitis)	United States, Canada, Central and South America
Wesselsbron virus	Sheep	Mosquitoes	Generalized infection, abortion	Africa
Dengue 1, 2, 3, 4 viruses	Humans (humans and monkeys)	Mosquitoes: *Aedes aegypti*, other *Aedes* spp.	(Fever and rash, arthralgia, myalgia, hemorrhagic fever)	Tropics worldwide
West Nile virus	Humans, horses, birds (birds)	Mosquitoes: *Culex* spp. (rarely ticks)	Fever, generalized disease, and encephalomyelitis	Africa, Middle East, North America, Central America, South America
Tick-borne encephalitis virus	Humans (rodents, birds, ruminants)	Ticks: *Ixodes* spp. and via ingestion of raw milk	(Encephalitis)	Europe, Russia, Asia
Omsk hemorrhagic fever virus	Humans (muskrats)	Ticks: *Dermacentor* spp.	(Hemorrhagic fever, gastrointestinal disease)	Central Siberia, Confederation of Independent States
Kyasanur Forest disease virus	Humans (monkeys, rodents)	Ticks: *Haemaphysalis* spp.	(Hemorrhagic fever, encephalitis)	India (Mysore)
Powassan virus	Small mammals	Ticks: *Ixodes* spp.	Encephalitis	Canada, United States, Russia
Louping ill virus	Sheep, horses, humans	Ticks: *Ixodes ricinus*	Encephalitis	Europe
Genus *Pestivirus*				
Bovine viral diarrhea virus	Cattle, calves	(Contact, congenital)	Mostly inapparent Congenital disease: generalized persistent infection, mucosal disease	Worldwide
Classical swine fever virus	Swine	(Contact)	Systemic disease Congenital disease	Worldwide, but eradicated in some countries
Border disease virus	Sheep		Congenital disease	Worldwide

[a]*The genus Hepacivirus contains hepatitis C virus, an important cause of human hepatitis.*

were so successful that today it is reintroductions of the virus, rather than enzootic infection, that attract attention. Bovine viral diarrhea was first described in New York in 1946 as an apparently new disease of cattle. Mucosal disease was described in 1953, and is another clinical entity caused by the same virus, but with markedly different severity and herd incidence pattern. Border disease originally was described in 1959 in sheep in the border region between Wales and England, and the infection still is common in intensive sheep production areas worldwide. Vertical transmission of border disease virus is characteristic of infection of pregnant ewes, and the resultant fetal abnormalities have given rise to colloquial names such as "hairy shaker disease" and "fuzzy lamb syndrome."

Hepatitis C virus was discovered in 1989 by a *tour de force* of modern molecular biology. Although the virus still

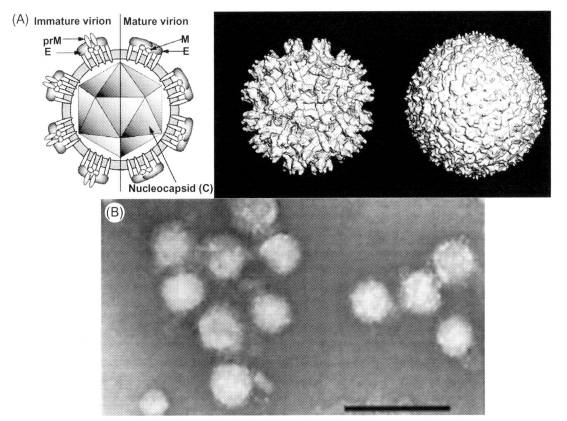

FIGURE 30.1 Family *Flaviviridae*, genus *Flavivirus*. (A) (Left), Schematic of immature and mature virion. (Center and right), Three-dimensional cryo-electron microscopic reconstructions of immature and mature particles of an isolate of Dengue virus. C, nucleocapsid protein; E, major spike protein; M, transmembrane protein; prM, precursor glycoprotein. (B) Central European tick-borne encephalitis virus. Negative-stain electron microscopy. Bar represents 100 nm. [*A: From* Virus Taxonomy: Eighth Report of the International Committee on Taxonomy of Viruses *(C. M. Fauquet, M. A. Mayo, J. Maniloff, U. Desselberger, L. A. Ball, eds.), p. 983. Copyright © Elsevier (2005), with permission.*]

has not been successfully grown in either cell culture or laboratory animals other than the chimpanzee, it has been completely sequenced and its diagnosis made routine using reagents produced with recombinant DNA technology. This success now serves as a model for the detection, characterization, and diagnosis of other uncultivable viruses.

PROPERTIES OF FLAVIVIRUSES

Classification

The genus *Flavivirus* includes the veterinary pathogens, Japanese encephalitis, West Nile, Wesselsbron, and louping ill viruses, in addition to many important human pathogens, including the dengue viruses (Table 30.1). Members of the genus are subdivided on the basis of their mode of transmission into four groups: (1) tick-borne viruses; (2) mosquito-borne viruses; (3) viruses with no known arthropod vector; (4) viruses with no known animal host. The mosquito- and tick-borne flaviviruses are maintained in nature in arthropod–vertebrate–arthropod cycles, whereas the non-arthropod-borne viruses are transmitted directly among bats or rodents.

The genus *Pestivirus* includes bovine viral diarrhea virus, border disease virus, and classical swine fever virus (hog

cholera virus). Genomic sequence analysis indicates that these three viruses are related very closely. Segregation of individual viruses can be difficult, and is based on sequence analysis, including that of the 5'-untranslated region of the genome, serological analysis with type-specific antisera, and host species of origin. Experimentally, the viruses have an overlapping host spectrum: swine fever virus can be transmitted to cattle; bovine viral diarrhea virus can infect swine, sheep, goats, New World camelids, and a variety of other wild and domestic ungulates, including deer, antelope, and buffalo; border disease virus infection rarely has been documented in cattle. A putative pestivirus of giraffe has been described, but is otherwise uncharacterized, and a highly pathogenic and genetically novel pestivirus in pigs (Bungowannah virus) recently was described in Australia.

Virion Properties

Virions are spherical, 50 nm (flaviviruses) or 40–60 nm (pestiviruses) in diameter, and consist of a tightly adherent lipid envelope that may display indistinct glycoprotein spikes, surrounding a spherical nucleocapsid with icosahedral symmetry (Figure 30.1; Table 30.2). The genome consists of a single molecule of linear, positive-sense, single-stranded RNA of approximately 11, 12.3, and 9.6 kb for flavi-, pesti-, and hepaciviruses, respectively. Flaviviruses contain a 5′-terminal cap structure, whereas pestiviruses and hepaciviruses do not.

The viral genome contains one long open reading frame encoding 10 or more proteins, which are created by co- and post-translational processing and cleavage of a single, large polyprotein (Figure 30.2). Virions contain three (genus

---

TABLE 30.2 Properties of Members of the Family *Flaviviridae*

Genera: *Flavivirus*, mostly arthropod-borne viruses; *Pestivirus*, non-arthropod-borne, includes several veterinary pathogens; *Hepacivirus*, human hepatitis C virus

Virions are spherical, 40–60 nm in diameter, and consist of a tightly adherent lipid envelope covered with indistinct spikes (peplomers) surrounding a spherical nucleocapsid

Genome is a single molecule of linear, positive-sense, single-stranded RNA, approximately 11 kb (flaviviruses), 12.3 kb (pestiviruses), or 9.6 kb (hepaciviruses) in size; 5′ end capped in flaviviruses, but not pestiviruses or hepaciviruses

Genomic RNA is infectious

Cytoplasmic replication; a single polyprotein is translated from genomic RNA; it is cleaved co- and post-translationally to yield eight or nine non-structural proteins and three or four structural proteins

Maturation occurs on intracytoplasmic membranes without evidence of budding

---

Flavivirus) or four (genus *Pestivirus*) structural proteins that are encoded in the 5′ end of the genome; the non-structural proteins are encoded in the 3′ end. Structural proteins of flaviviruses include: C, the nucleocapsid protein; prM, a precursor glycoprotein that is cleaved during virus maturation to yield M, the transmembrane protein; E, the major spike glycoprotein, which also is the major target for neutralizing antibodies. Pestiviruses have four structural proteins, including C, the nucleocapsid protein, and the E^{rns}, E1, and E2 envelope glycoproteins. There are seven or eight non-structural proteins, including NS5, the RNA-dependent RNA polymerase, and NS3, which has several functions, including helicase and protease activities, in addition to contributing to the RNA polymerase complex. NS2B and NS3 largely are responsible for cleavage of the polyprotein, and host-cell proteases are responsible for the remainder of this processing. Pestiviruses encode a unique non-structural protein, N^{pro}, that autocatalytically releases itself from the polyprotein; this protein is not essential for virus replication in cell culture, but modulates interferon responses in infected cells.

The viruses are inactivated easily by heat and by common disinfectants, and the lipid envelope is susceptible to organic solvents. However, the stability of swine fever virus in meat products and offal for weeks or even months has contributed importantly to its spread and reintroduction into previously virus-free areas.

Virus Replication

Members of the genus *Flavivirus* replicate well and cause cytopathic changes in many cell cultures: Vero (African

---

(A) ***Flavivirus* genome**

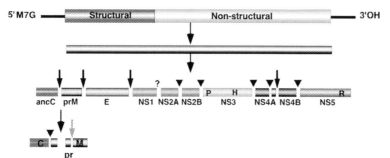

(B) ***Pestivirus* genome**

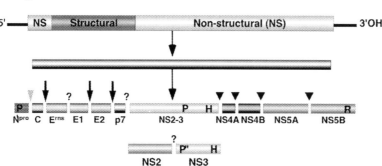

FIGURE 30.2 Genome organization and polyprotein processing of viruses in the genera *Flavivirus* and *Pestivirus*. At the top of (A) and (B) are the viral genomes with the structural and non-structural protein coding regions and the 5′- and 3′-non-coding regions (NCR). Boxes below the genomes indicate viral proteins generated by the proteolytic processing cascade. Arrows, arrowheads and "?" between the viral protein boxes represent protease cleavage sites. (A) *Flavivirus*. ancC, precursor capsid protein; C, capsid protein; prM, precursor membrane protein; M, membrane protein; E, envelope glycoprotein; NS, non-structural proteins; P, NS3 protease; H, NS3 helicase; R, RNA Polymerase. (B) *Pestivirus*. Npro, protease; C, capsid protein; Ernas, minor envelope protein with RNAse activity; E, envelope protein; p7, non-structural protein; NS, non-structural proteins; P, NS2-3(NS3) protease; H, helicase; R, RNA polymerase. *[From* Virus Taxonomy: Eighth Report of the International Committee on Taxonomy of Viruses *(C. M. Fauquet, M. A. Mayo, J. Maniloff, U. Desselberger, L. A. Ball, eds.), pp. 984, 990. Copyright © Elsevier (2005), with permission.]*

green monkey kidney), BHK-21 (baby hamster kidney), and mosquito (C6/36) and primary chick and duck embryo fibroblasts are commonly used for isolation and propagation of these viruses. Many flaviviruses infect and kill newborn and, in some cases, adult mice; indeed, most of the flaviviruses were first isolated in newborn mice.

Members of the genus *Pestivirus* generally replicate well in primary and continuous cell cultures derived from the principal host species—bovine viral diarrhea virus in bovine embryonic fibroblast or kidney cells. Border disease virus is best isolated in ovine cells, and classical swine fever virus in porcine lymphoid or kidney cells. Pestiviruses isolated from naturally infected animals are predominantly non-cytopathic in cell culture.

Cellular attachment of all members of the family *Flaviridae*, regardless of genus, appears to be mediated by ligands on the E glycoprotein(s), although cellular receptors have not been unambiguously identified. The viruses enter cells via receptor-mediated endocytosis and replication takes place in the cytoplasm. Flaviviruses only partially shut down protein and RNA synthesis of mammalian host cells. Infection commonly is accompanied by a characteristic proliferation of perinuclear membranes.

Replication involves the synthesis of complementary negative-sense RNA, which then serves as a template for positive-sense (genome-sense) RNA synthesis. The only viral mRNA is the genomic RNA—translation yields a single polyprotein that is cleaved and processed to form the various viral structural and non-structural proteins (Figure 30.2). For mosquito-transmitted flaviviruses, virion assembly occurs on membranes of the endoplasmic reticulum and plasma membrane in mosquito cells (Figure 30.3), but preformed capsids and budding are not seen. Instead, fully formed virions appear within the cisternae of the endoplasmic reticulum and are released via exocytosis or cell lysis.

MEMBERS OF THE GENUS *FLAVIVIRUS*: MOSQUITO-BORNE FLAVIVIRUSES

All members of the genus *Flavivirus* are serologically related. The mosquito-transmitted flaviviruses are subdivided, on the basis of neutralization assays, into at least seven serocomplexes that include approximately 40 individual flaviviruses, several of which are important pathogens of humans and animals. Dengue virus persists in a mosquito–human–mosquito transmission cycle, whereas the other mosquito-transmitted flaviviruses typically are amplified in a variety of animal species, with wild birds being important to the enzootic transmission cycle of many of these viruses.

JAPANESE ENCEPHALITIS VIRUS

Japanese encephalitis virus is the type virus of a distinct group (serocomplex) containing at least three other important pathogenic viruses: St. Louis encephalitis virus, Murray Valley encephalitis virus, and West Nile virus. Each is an important human pathogen, and both Japanese encephalitis and West Nile viruses also cause significant disease in domestic animals. A variety of animals, including swine, horses, dogs, bats, and reptiles, naturally are infected with Japanese encephalitis virus. Horses may develop fatal encephalitis similar to that caused by West Nile virus infection, whereas infection of swine is generally inapparent other than stillbirths and abortions after infection of pregnant sows.

Japanese encephalitis virus is an important mosquito-borne human pathogen in much of Asia and Southeast Asia, and the virus recently has extended its range to the Indian subcontinent, the Pacific islands, and northern Australia (Figure 30.4). Human disease is devastating.

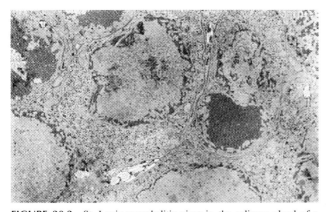

FIGURE 30.3 St. Louis encephalitis virus in the salivary gland of a *Culex pipiens* mosquito 26 days after infection. Massive amounts of virus, some in paracrystalline array, may be seen within the salivary space. Transmission to the next vertebrate host occurs when the mosquito injects its saliva (which contains anticoagulants) when taking a blood meal. Magnification: ×21,000.

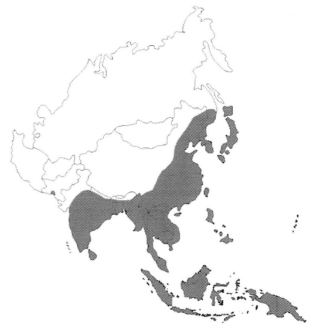

FIGURE 30.4 Distribution of Japanese encephalitis. *(Courtesy of Centers for Disease Control.)*

Although there are many inapparent infections, the case-fatality rate amongst symptomatic cases is 10–40%, and 40–70% of survivors have permanent neurologic deficits. The primary mosquito vector, *Culex tritaeniorhynchus*, develops in freshwater marshes and irrigated rice fields, and blood-feeds on birds, swine, and humans. Other species of *Culex* mosquito may be locally important vectors. Swine are abundant throughout much of Asia, and continuously provide new generations of susceptible hosts. The mosquito–swine and mosquito–bird transmission cycles both serve as efficient modes for virus amplification. In tropical areas, outbreaks occur at the end of the wet season, but sporadic cases occur throughout the year. In temperate zones, outbreaks tend to occur in late summer and early autumn, and subside with the onset of cold weather.

Control of Japanese encephalitis previously was achieved in Japan by intermittently draining rice fields to interfere with the development of *Culex tritaeniorhynchus*, removal of swine from areas of human habitation, and widespread vaccination of swine, horses, and children with an inactivated-virus vaccine produced in mouse brain. Inactivated virus and live-attenuated virus vaccines produced in cell culture have been used to reduce disease substantially in both humans and swine in enzootic areas of Asia, including China, Taiwan, and Korea. New-generation vaccines, including recombinant vaccines, are now being developed and evaluated because of the adverse side effects and increasingly limited use of existing vaccines.

WEST NILE VIRUS

West Nile virus historically was recognized as a cause of mild febrile disease in humans over large areas of Africa and the Middle East. There are two major genetic lineages (1 and 2) of West Nile virus; Kunjin virus is a variant of lineage 1 West Nile virus that is enzootic in Australia. During the 1990s, a virulent strain of lineage 1 West Nile virus emerged in the Middle East and invaded portions of Eastern Europe and subsequently the United States, causing extensive mortality in birds and fatal encephalitis in humans and horses. The virus has since spread throughout North America and into Central and South America, and is now a leading cause of human arbovirus encephalitis in the New World.

Clinical Features and Epidemiology

Throughout its range, West Nile virus is maintained in a mosquito–wild bird–mosquito cycle, with several species of *Culex* mosquitoes serving as vectors (Figure 30.5). Although more than 300 species of birds have been reported to be infected with West Nile virus, maintenance and amplification principally involve wild passerine birds and *Culex* mosquitoes. Some birds, especially corvids such as American crows (*Corvus brachyrhynchos*), jays, and yellow-billed magpies (*Pica hudsonia*), develop very high-titer viremia and suffer nearly uniform mortality after infection; monitoring of dead corvids can be a sensitive surveillance technique for monitoring arrival of the virus in new areas. In North America, species such as finches and sparrows, which exhibit variable mortality and comparatively low-titer viremia (as compared to corvids), may serve as primary maintenance and perhaps even amplification hosts of West Nile virus, whereas highly susceptible birds such as corvids and robins that invariably succumb to infection may be more important in explosive amplification of the virus during outbreaks. High mortality as a result of West Nile virus infection has also been observed on several occasions in a variety of raptors and in domestic geese, particular among young goslings. Other bird species, including many species of wild birds as well as chickens and pigeons, usually do not develop disease following infection, and develop a low-magnitude viremia that is insufficient to infect mosquitoes. Humans and other mammals, including horses, also

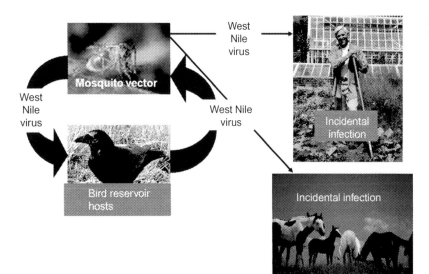

FIGURE 30.5 West Nile virus transmission cycle. *(Courtesy of Centers for Disease Control.)*

are "dead-end" hosts that are considered to be unimportant as virus reservoirs; however, serological surveillance of susceptible horses can be a highly sensitive method for detection of West Nile virus in a region.

Horses are the most important domestic animal affected by West Nile virus, but disease occurrence is dependent on the pathogenicity (neurovirulence) of the infecting virus strain. Infection of horses with lineage 2 strains of West Nile virus is common in much of sub-Saharan Africa, where these infections appear seldom to cause serious disease; however, neurovirulent strains exist of both lineages 1 and 2 of West Nile virus. The strain of lineage 1 West Nile virus that recently emerged in both Europe and the Americas is highly pathogenic in horses, and large numbers of horses were clinically affected during the North American epizootic. Affected horses show a variety of neurological signs, including depression, abnormalities in gait, head tremors, muscle fasciculations, weakness, ataxia, and recumbency. Somewhat fewer than 10% of infected horses develop neurological manifestations after infection with virulent lineage 1 West Nile virus, but mortality is high in those that do (up to 40%). As is the case with humans, the magnitude of viremia in infected horses is low, and unlikely to be sufficient to transmit the virus back to mosquitoes. West Nile virus infection has been documented in many species of wild and domestic animals, but clinical disease is uncommon other than in horses; West Nile disease has been described in cats, dogs, sheep, New World camelids, tree squirrels, and farmed alligators.

Pathogenesis and Pathology

Virulent West Nile virus infection of highly susceptible bird species results in overwhelming infection with very-high-titer viremia and widespread necrosis, hemorrhage, and inflammation in several organs, including heart, skeletal muscle, lungs, spleen, liver, kidney, adrenals, pancreas, intestines, gonads, and nervous system. Brain and heart are characteristically affected in domestic geese. Similar multi-organ involvement has been described in juvenile alligators, and very sporadically in naturally infected dogs. In contrast, horses have only a transient, low-titer viremia and central nervous system lesions occur, with minimal involvement of other organs. Lesions in the brain and spinal cord of affected horses include scattered foci of neuronal necrosis and non-suppurative (predominantly lymphocytic) encephalomyelitis. Similar lesions sporadically have been described in infected New World camelids (llamas and alpacas), sheep, cats, and, with some frequency, tree squirrels.

Diagnosis

The clinical signs of West Nile virus infection of horses are characteristic but not pathognomonic, thus the diagnosis is confirmed by serological testing to detect virus-specific immunoglobulin M (IgM) antibodies that are present in acutely infected horses, typically using IgM capture enzyme-linked immunosorbent assay (ELISA). Virus neutralization assays on paired acute and convalescent sera also are used for serological detection of West Nile virus infection. The virus can be detected at necropsy in the tissues of any affected animal, including birds, by reverse-transcriptase-polymerase chain reaction (RT-PCR), *in-situ* hybridization, or immunohistochemistry, although lesions in the nervous tissues of affected horses frequently are widely scattered and contain sparse viral antigen. West Nile virus can be isolated in Vero or mosquito cells, and identified either by immunohistochemical staining using virus-specific antisera or by RT-PCR.

Immunity, Prevention, and Control

Treatment of horses with neurological disease caused by West Nile virus infection is largely supportive. Animals previously infected with West Nile virus are resistant to reinfection, and several efficacious vaccines have been licensed for protection of horses from West Nile disease, including inactivated, DNA, chimeric, and recombinant canarypox virus vectored vaccines. Vaccines have been effectively used to protect susceptible birds, including geese, and a variety of recombinant potential human vaccines also have been developed.

MURRAY VALLEY ENCEPHALITIS VIRUS

Murray Valley encephalitis virus, another member of the mosquito-borne encephalitis complex, is enzootic in New Guinea and northern Australia, where cases of encephalitis occur very sporadically in humans. The encephalitis and case-fatality rates in humans are similar to those caused by Japanese encephalitis virus, and neurologic sequelae are common in those who recover. Human epidemics occur in the Murray River Valley of southeastern Australia only in occasional summers, following heavy rainfall with extensive flooding. These conditions encourage explosive increases in numbers of wading birds, which are the principal vertebrate reservoirs of the virus, and of its mosquito vectors, notably *Culex annulirostris*.

ST. LOUIS ENCEPHALITIS VIRUS

St. Louis encephalitis virus, a member of the mosquito-borne encephalitis complex, occurs in North, Central, and South America. In North America, although disease now is relatively uncommon, the virus previously caused sporadic human epidemics that manifest as encephalitis or benign febrile illness. Infection of horses has been reported infrequently in enzootic areas. Although encephalomyelitis has been induced experimentally in horses, it is unclear if similar disease occurs after natural infection. The natural cycle of the virus in rural areas of the western regions of the United States involves *Culex tarsalis* and nestling and juvenile passerine birds. In urban regions, *Culex pipiens* and *Culex quinquefasciatus* are the most important vectors in northern and southern latitudes, respectively, although other *Culex* spp. mosquitoes may become important locally.

WESSELSBRON VIRUS

Wesselsbron virus is the cause of an important disease of sheep in many parts of sub-Saharan Africa. The clinical disease and its epidemiology resembles that of Rift Valley fever virus. Disease in sheep is marked by fever, depression, hepatitis with jaundice, and subcutaneous edema. Abortion is common and mortality is high, in pregnant ewes and newborn lambs, respectively. Cattle, horses, and swine are infected subclinically. The virus is transmitted in summer and autumn by freshwater *Aedes* spp. mosquitoes associated with low-lying humid areas, where their density is greatest. Control in sheep involves immunization of lambs with an attenuated virus vaccine that is often combined with Rift Valley fever virus vaccine. Wesselsbron virus is zoonotic, causing a febrile disease in humans, with headache, myalgia, and arthralgia.

DENGUE VIRUSES

Dengue has become the most important arthropod-transmitted viral disease of humans in the world today, with more than two billion people at risk and tens of millions of cases annually. The original natural reservoir of the dengue viruses appears to have been African monkeys, and monkeys may still be virus reservoirs in Southeast Asia. However, the important transmission cycle of the dengue viruses is mosquito–human–mosquito, involving the urban mosquito, *Aedes aegypti*. *Aedes albopictus* also is an efficient vector that has been responsible for smaller outbreaks. Although dengue has been known for over 200 years, before the 1950s, outbreaks were rare because movement of viremic persons between tropical countries was limited, and aggressive campaigns to eradicate *Aedes aegypti* virtually eliminated the vector. Recent advances in transportation and the growth of large cities in the tropics, with ubiquitous breeding sites for *Aedes aegypti*, have led to a global resurgence and major epidemics. The virus has been spread extensively throughout the world, and epidemics recently have occurred in Central America and the Caribbean, South America, the Pacific islands, and China, as well as in Southeast Asia and Africa. Because of the widespread occurrence of *Aedes aegypti*, the recent extensive spread of *Aedes albopictus*, and movement of travelers to and from dengue-endemic areas, this virus is a continuing threat to all regions of the world that have a warm climate.

There are four dengue viruses; infection induces lifelong homologous immunity, but cross-protection between viruses is incomplete. Dengue hemorrhagic fever results from sequential infection of an individual with more than one viral serotype, and this shock syndrome has become a leading cause of hospital admissions and death among children in Southeast Asia; it is increasingly common in the Americas. Control of dengue is focused on the mosquito vector, by killing infected adults or by elimination of larval habitats. Insecticides sprayed from aircraft or trucks are largely ineffective, because *Aedes aegypti* lives inside dwellings and is not reached by spray droplets.

YELLOW FEVER VIRUS

Yellow fever has been one of the great plagues throughout history, being transported, together with its mosquito vector, *Aedes aegypti*, from West Africa to the New World on slave ships. In the 18th and 19th centuries the disease decimated tropical and subtropical coastal cities of the Americas. Thousands of workers died during the construction of the Panama Canal. In its classical form, the human disease begins abruptly with fever, headache, myalgia, and nausea. The disease is biphasic and, after a short period of remission, there is abdominal pain, jaundice, renal failure, and hemorrhage. Approximately 50% of people who progress to this stage die 7–10 days after onset, with progressive hepatic and renal failure, shock, delirium, and convulsions.

In its jungle habitat, yellow fever virus is maintained in a mosquito–monkey–mosquito cycle. Old World monkeys develop only subclinical infections, but New World monkeys often die, reflecting the more recent introduction of the virus to the Americas. Various species of jungle canopy mosquitoes serve as vectors—*Aedes* spp. in Africa and *Haemagogus* spp. in the Americas. These mosquitoes also may transmit the virus to humans entering forested areas; however, it is a mosquito–human–mosquito cycle, involving *Aedes aegypti* in the Western Hemisphere and *Aedes africanus* in Africa, which is responsible for large-scale urban epidemics. Several hundred cases of jungle yellow fever are reported annually in the Western Hemisphere, and a few thousand in Africa, but the true incidence may be higher, as major epidemics that occur in Africa frequently go undocumented. In recent years, populations of *Aedes aegypti* have increased substantially throughout much of the Americas, including southern regions of the United States, and it is now possible that urban epidemics could recur at any time. There are rapid tests for the detection of virus or specific antibody, although their availability is limited. Vaccination is critical to control of yellow fever, traditionally using an attenuated virus vaccine, 17D. New-generation vaccines continue to be developed and evaluated. Prevention also involves *Aedes aegypti* control, but, despite proof of the value of this approach gained early in the 20th century in urban centers of the western hemisphere, such programs have proven difficult to sustain and largely have been abandoned.

OTHER MOSQUITO-BORNE FLAVIVIRUSES

Usutu virus is a mosquito-borne flavivirus, closely related to West Nile virus, that recently emerged in wild and zoo birds in Central Europe (Austria, Hungary). Emergence of this virus has been associated with significant mortality in blackbirds, but apparently not in mammals. Several other flaviviruses from different serocomplexes occur in South America, including Rocio and Ilheus viruses from the Ntaya virus serocomplex, and Bussuquara virus from the Aroa virus serocomplex. The enzootic transmission cycles of these viruses are largely unknown, although they cause human and animal infections. Rocio virus previously has caused extensive epidemics of human encephalitis in Brazil. Israel turkey meningoencephalitis also is a member of the Ntaya serocomplex that may be transmitted by midges (*Culicoides*), and is a sporadic, regional cause of paralysis and mortality in turkeys.

MEMBERS OF THE GENUS *FLAVIVIRUS*: TICK-BORNE ENCEPHALITIS VIRUSES

Tick-borne encephalitis viruses constitute a complex of approximately a dozen flaviviruses, several of which are important zoonotic pathogens, including: tick-borne encephalitis virus (two subtypes, also known as Russian spring-summer encephalitis virus and central European encephalitis virus) and Omsk hemorrhagic fever virus, all in Eurasia; Kyasanur Forest disease virus in India and recently in the Middle East; Powassan/deer tick virus in North America (Table 30.1). Infected dogs and livestock such as cattle, sheep, and goats are important in the spread of these viruses to humans in Europe and eastern and central Asia, where these animals may serve as amplifying hosts for ticks; some may also transmit viruses to humans via raw milk (Figure 30.6). Encephalomyelitis has been described in horses experimentally infected with Powassan virus, but similar disease has not been documented in naturally infected horses in North America.

The epidemiology of tick-borne flaviviruses is more complex than that of their mosquito-borne counterparts, as ticks serve both as reservoirs of infection and as virus vectors. Unlike mosquitoes, ticks can live for several years, often longer than the generational time of their rodent reservoir hosts. Ticks are typically active from spring through to autumn in temperate climates. Ticks develop successively through stages (larva to nymph to adult) and a blood meal is generally required at each stage. Tick-borne flaviviruses are passed from one developmental stage to another (*transstadial transmission*), as well as from one generation of tick to the next (*transovarial transmission*). Some species spend their whole lives on one vertebrate host, whereas others fall off, molt, and seek a different host after each blood meal. Larvae and nymphs generally feed on birds or small mammals such as rodents, whereas adult ticks prefer larger

animals. Although expensive to produce, inactivated-virus vaccines for use in humans are available to prevent tick-borne encephalitis in Europe and eastern Asia.

LOUPING ILL VIRUS

Louping ill is an infectious encephalomyelitis of sheep that occurs in the British Isles and the Iberian Peninsula. It is a typical member of the tick-borne virus complex, with a life cycle that involves transmission to sheep by the tick, *Ixodes ricinus*, with occasional involvement of horses, cattle, deer, and grouse. Horses in enzootic areas sporadically develop encephalomyelitis that resembles that caused by West Nile virus. Louping ill occurs in spring and summer. Infected sheep develop a prolonged viremia and a biphasic febrile response, the second peak of which coincides with the development of nervous system dysfunction, including ataxia, tremors, hyperexcitability, and paralysis. The disease gains its name from the peculiar leaping gait of ataxic sheep. Few animals that develop neurologic signs survive, and most of those that do suffer permanent neurologic deficits. Control of the disease involves immunization of lambs with an inactivated vaccine, use of acaricides on susceptible sheep where allowed, and environmental control of ticks. Louping ill virus is zoonotic, being transmitted to humans by ticks, or occupationally by contact with infected sheep and sheep tissues. The human disease is biphasic: the first phase is influenza-like, and the second phase is characterized by meningoencephalitis that usually resolves, without complications, in 4–10 days.

MEMBERS OF THE GENUS *PESTIVIRUS*

BOVINE VIRAL DIARRHEA VIRUS

Like a number of genetically heterogenic RNA viruses, bovine viral diarrhea virus is best considered, not as a single entity, but rather as a heterogeneous group of related viruses that differ in their antigenicity, cytopathogenicity, and virulence. Two major genotypes (designated types 1 and 2) are recognized, and there are also two distinct biotypes within each genotype: those that induce cytopathic effects in cultured cells (*cytopathic viruses*), and those that induce persistent infection in cells without obvious cytopathology (*non-cytopathic viruses*). Infection of susceptible cattle with different genotypes or biotypes of bovine viral diarrhea virus can result in two clinically dissimilar disease syndromes, respectively designated as bovine viral diarrhea and mucosal disease. Bovine viral diarrhea is an acute, typically epizootic infection of susceptible animals, whereas mucosal disease is a sporadic but fulminant disease syndrome that occurs only in persistently infected cattle, typically in enzootically infected herds. The virus is an important cause of morbidity, mortality, and economic loss worldwide in dairy and beef cattle.

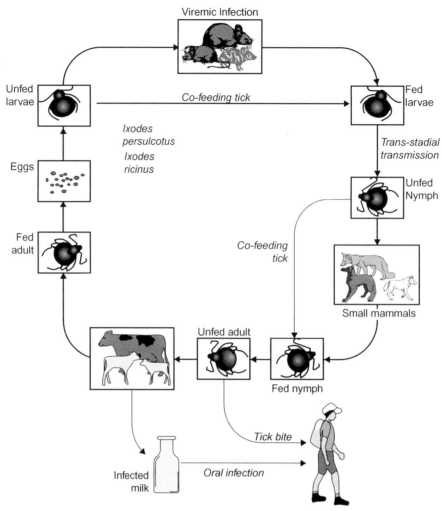

FIGURE 30.6 Transmission cycle of viruses of the tick-borne encephalitis complex, showing hosts for larval, nymphal, and adult ticks. Virus is passed to succeeding tick stages during molting, and is passed transovarially to progeny. Both male and female ticks are involved in transmission. *[From T. P. Monath, F. X. Heinz. Flaviviruses. In:* Field's Virology *(B. N. Fields, D. M. Knipe, P. M. Howley, R. M. Chanock, J. L. Melnick, T. P. Monath, B. Roizman, S. E. Straus, eds.), 3rd ed., pp. 961–1034. Copyright © 1996 Lippincott-Raven, Philadelphia, PA, with permission.]*

In addition to cattle, bovine viral diarrhea virus infects a variety of other species. It has been reported to cause disease in African and Indian buffalo, several species of African antelope, and ill-thrift, respiratory disease, abortion and reproductive failure, diarrhea, and persistent immunotolerant infection all have recently been described in New World camelids (alpacas and llamas).

Vertical transmission of bovine viral diarrhea to the bovine embryo or fetus is a critical aspect of infection that, depending on the infecting virus strain and gestational stage, variously can result in embryonal/fetal death, teratogenesis, persistent infection, or inapparent infection with an immune response.

Clinical Features and Epidemiology

The disease patterns that result from bovine viral diarrhea virus infection may vary substantially within and between herds, depending on herd immunity, including vaccination status, as well as the presence or absence of persistently infected cattle. The clinical and pathologic manifestations of bovine viral diarrhea virus infection in individual cattle also vary with age and pregnancy status. Three situations are considered here: postnatal infection in non-pregnant cattle, infection in pregnant cows, and persistent infection in calves and mucosal disease.

Postnatal Infection in Non-Pregnant Cattle

Cattle of all ages are susceptible, but infection is most common in young animals in herds with enzootic infection. In calves that receive antibodies in colostrum, antibody disappears by 3–8 months of age, and these animals may not show clinical signs after infection until colostral antibodies are lost. A biphasic fever and leukopenia occur in susceptible

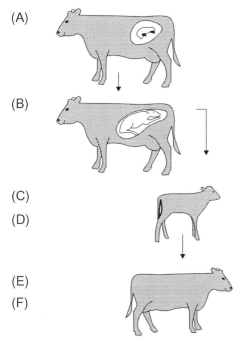

(A)

Cow and fetus infected with non-cytopathic BVDV in early pregnancy

(B)

Cow becomes immune. Fetus becomes tolerant and unable to make antibody

(C)

Calf remains infected with virus for life

(D)

Mutation of virus to cytopathic form may occur

(E)

(F)

Superinfection of this and other viremic animals with cytopathic virus causes fatal mucosal disease

FIGURE 30.7 The pathogenesis of mucosal disease in cattle. (A) *In-utero* infection. (B) Immune tolerance. (C) Persistent viremia. (D) Mutation. (E) Superinfection. (F) Mucosal disease. *[Adapted from J. Brownlie. Pathogenesis of mucosal disease and molecular aspects of bovine viral diarrhea virus. Vet. Microbiol. 23, 371–382 (1990), with permission.]*

animals within an incubation period of 5–7 days after infection, but otherwise the clinical course is usually mild. Some animals in a susceptible herd may develop diarrhea, which can be explosive in character; some may have a nasal and ocular discharge and develop erosions and/or ulcers on the lips, muzzle, and within the oral cavity; in dairy cows there may be a considerable decrease in milk yield. Certain strains of bovine viral diarrhea virus induce profound thrombocytopenia that leads to extensive hemorrhage and high fatality rates in susceptible calves. This was especially characteristic of the initial strains of type 2 bovine viral diarrhea virus that emerged in North America in the mid 1980s. Because of virus-induced immunosuppression, infection in calves frequently results in increased incidence of opportunistic respiratory and intestinal infections and associated increased mortality.

Infection in Pregnant Cows

Transplacental spread of virus to the fetus occurs commonly following infection of susceptible adult cows during pregnancy (Figure 30.7), which may result in any one of several outcomes, depending on the age (immunologic maturity) of the fetus and the strain of virus. Infection very early in pregnancy often results in embryonic death and resorption. Infection before development of immunologic competence at 100–125 days often results in persistent postnatal infection, or in destructive fetal lesions and retardation in growth that result in fetal death or low birth weight ("weak calf syndrome"). Fetal lesions are often manifestations of viral effects on organogenesis that are evident as a spectrum of congenital defects in the eye

(e.g., retinal dysplasia), central nervous system (e.g., cerebellar hypoplasia, hydranencephaly), and other systems (e.g., alopecia). Surviving calves that have been infected *in utero* early in gestation remain as persistently infected virus carriers for the duration of their lives. These infected virus carriers never mount an effective immune response to the virus, and have a persistent, immunotolerant infection. Such cattle, which remain seronegative in all standard tests, may shed large amounts of virus in all body secretions and excretions, and are very efficient in transmitting the virus to susceptible cattle in the herd. Some persistently infected cattle fail to thrive, and some subsequently develop mucosal disease. Others will be apparently healthy throughout their lives and serve as persistent sources of virus. In contrast to the situation just described, fetuses infected after about 125 days of gestation usually survive, whether manifesting tissue injury or not, and usually develop neutralizing antibody and eliminate the virus. Abortion, however, can occur following fetal infection at any stage of gestation.

Persistent Infection in Calves and Mucosal Disease

In susceptible herds in which the virus has been recently introduced, a substantial proportion of calves born in the next calving season are persistently infected. Such calves fail to thrive, and mortality is as high as 50% in the first year of life. Mucosal disease only occurs when two biotypes of bovine viral diarrhea virus are present: the non-cytopathic virus with which the animal originally was persistently infected *in utero*, and a genetically and antigenically homologous cytopathic virus strain. The clinical features of

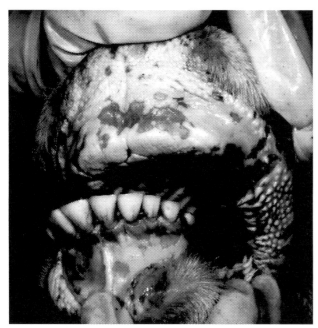

FIGURE 30.8 Mucosal disease in a persistently infected bovine. Extensive and severe oral ulcers. (*Courtesy of M. Anderson, University of California, Davis.*)

mucosal disease mirror bovine viral diarrhea, but with much greater severity, and can even resemble those of rinderpest (Figure 30.8). The onset of mucosal disease may be sudden, or may extend over several weeks or months, with recurrent overt signs. There is fever, anorexia, profuse watery diarrhea, nasal discharge, severe erosive or ulcerative stomatitis, dehydration and emaciation, and, ultimately, death.

Pathogenesis and Pathology

Postnatal Infections

Bovine viral diarrhea is spread amongst calves by the respiratory route. The virus first replicates in the nasal mucosa and tonsils before spreading to the regional lymph nodes, with subsequent widespread dissemination and highest titers of the virus in lymphoid tissues and the intestine. Most infections are subclinical and animals that die of acute bovine viral diarrhea virus infection characteristically have erosive or ulcerative lesions extending from the mouth through the esophagus, forestomachs, abomasum, and intestine. In the intestine, hyperemia and hemorrhage impart a striped appearance to the mucosal surface, with prominent hemorrhagic necrosis of Peyer's patches. Histological changes include necrosis of crypt enterocytes in both the large and small intestine, necrosis of lymphocytes in gut-associated lymphoid tissues, and mucosal and submucosal edema in the affected segments of bowel. Widespread and severe hemorrhage is characteristic of virus strains that induce profound thrombocytopenia, with involvement of the pericardium, epicardium, and serosal and mucosal surfaces

of the entire gastrointestinal tract. Pulmonary involvement also occurs, either as a direct consequence of virus-induced injury to the lung or from secondary bacterial infections.

Prenatal and Persistent Infections

The consequences of vertical transmission are dependent on the virulence of the infecting virus strain and the stage of gestation at infection. Aborted fetuses are typically autolyzed and exhibit few characteristic lesions, although some may show characteristic malformations such as cerebellar hypoplasia, cavitating lesions of the cerebral cortex (hydranencephaly or porencephaly), dysmyelination/hypomyelinogenesis, chorioretinitis or retinal dysplasia, skeletal defects including growth retardation, and abnormalities of the hair coat. Persistently infected calves may appear normal; others are stunted. Many persistently infected calves die in the first year of life from diseases such as pneumonia and enteritis, probably as a consequence of bovine viral diarrhea virus-induced immunosuppression.

Mucosal Disease

Molecular studies have characterized the pathogenesis of mucosal disease. The usual biotype of bovine viral diarrhea virus responsible for initial herd infection is non-cytopathic. The same biotype is regularly isolated from persistently infected, immunologically tolerant cattle in these herds—that is, cattle that were infected *in utero* before the development of immunologic competence. However, cattle with mucosal disease are infected with both non-cytopathic and cytopathic viral biotypes that are genetically homologous. The very close genetic relationship between the two viral biotypes suggests that the cytopathic biotypes arise *de novo* by mutation from non-cytopathic biotypes. Indeed, recent studies have confirmed that cytopathic biotypes are generated during persistent infection from non-cytopathic biotypes by various mutational events, including recombination, insertions of cellular sequences, duplications, deletions, and rearrangements. The mutations all lead to the production of a cytopathic virus and mucosal disease in cattle that are already immunologically tolerant to the non-cytopathic parental biotype. Far less often, superinfection with cytopathogenic virus from an external source is responsible, such as has occurred with some rare vaccine-associated outbreaks of mucosal disease.

It is somewhat uncertain how bovine viral diarrhea virus actually mediates mucosal disease, the course of which can be either rapid (acute mucosal disease) or extended (chronic mucosal disease). It has been proposed that the cytopathic variant of bovine viral diarrhea virus that emerges in persistently infected cattle spreads throughout the intestinal mucosa and lymphoid tissues of affected animals, where it induces extensive apoptosis and the manifestations of mucosal disease. Acute mucosal disease is characterized by striking necrosis throughout the gastrointestinal tract and lymphoid organs, with prominent and characteristic erosions and ulcers in the mucosal epithelium lining the oral and nasal cavities, esophagus, and forestomachs, and in the small intestinal mucosa overlying Peyer's patches (Figure 30.8). Gastrointestinal lesions are not as characteristically present in cattle with chronic mucosal disease; rather, these animals typically present with skin ulcers or areas of hyperkeratosis on the skin of the neck, shoulders, distal extremities, and elsewhere. Microscopic lesions of mucosal disease include necrosis of crypt enterocytes in the small intestine and colon (so-called crypt abscesses), lymphoid necrosis that is especially obvious within the thymus and Peyer's patches, and mononuclear cell infiltration into affected regions of skin and bowel.

Diagnosis

A presumptive diagnosis can be made on the basis of clinical history, examination of herd reproduction records, clinical signs, and gross and microscopic lesions. Laboratory diagnosis is based on virus isolation in cell culture, detection of viral antigen in tissues (such as by immunofluorescent or immunohistochemical staining of ear notch samples, which is especially useful for identification of persistently infected cattle), detection of viral RNA in tissues or blood by RT-PCR assay, and serology. Specimens for virus isolation include nasal exudates, blood, and tissues collected at necropsy of affected cattle or aborted fetuses. Paired acute and convalescent sera may be tested by a neutralization test, but interpretation of negative results must be made with an appreciation of the immunologically tolerant state of persistently infected cattle.

Immunity, Prevention, and Control

Bovine viral diarrhea virus readily is transmitted among cattle and from herd to herd by indirect means, through feed and fomites contaminated with urine, oral and nasal secretions, feces, or amniotic fluid. The virus is usually transmitted rather poorly from acutely affected cattle, but very efficiently from persistently infected animals. Thus identification and elimination of persistently infected cattle are central to the eradication of bovine viral diarrhea infection within herds, as these animals are life-long virus shedders that can facilitate uninterrupted virus transmission in a herd for years if husbandry practices remain unchanged. They also produce persistently infected progeny that further perpetuate the cycle of infection. Where infection has been present in a herd for some time and the majority of cattle are immune, the introduction of susceptible animals, typically heifers, results in sporadic losses. In unvaccinated, virus-free herds, the introduction of a persistently infected animal is often followed by dramatic losses. Because the infection also occurs in sheep and goats, as well as swine, New World camelids, deer, bison, and other domestic and wild ungulates, these species may also rarely be sources of virus for the initiation of infection in cattle herds. Virus can

be introduced in to herds by way of BVDV contaminated biologics such as vaccines and embryo transfer reagents.

The economic importance of bovine viral diarrhea is clear, especially in feedlots and in dairy herds, but control is far from satisfactory. The major objective of control measures is to remove and prevent the further occurrence of persistently infected cattle in the herd. This requires the identification and elimination of such animals and the avoidance of further introductions by quarantine. Immunization is the other major control strategy that is used routinely to reduce clinical disease and prevent fetal infections. Use of inactivated-virus vaccines produced in cell culture has reduced clinical disease, but not fetal infections. Attenuated virus vaccines, also produced in cell culture, are now widely used in enzootic areas, as they provide superior protection against transplacental transmission as compared with inactivated vaccines. Live-attenuated vaccine virus strains theoretically might be transmitted between cattle and in the process undergo genetic variation, but definitive data to support these concerns are lacking.

Regional or national bovine viral diarrhea control or eradication schemes have been introduced in a number of countries, especially in Europe. Most of these campaigns are based on removal of persistently infected cattle, without use of vaccines.

BORDER DISEASE VIRUS

Border disease exists worldwide in sheep, and also is known as "hairy shaker disease" or "fuzzy lamb syndrome." Border disease-like viruses have been isolated from non-domestic sheep and goats, suggesting the possibility of wildlife reservoirs for this virus.

Clinical Features and Epidemiology

Border disease appears as a congenital disorder of lambs and is characterized by low birth weight and poor viability, poor conformation, tremors because of delayed myelination of the central nervous system, and an excessively hairy birth coat. Outcome is dependent on fetal age at infection, and properties of the infecting virus strain. Goat kids may also be affected on occasion.

Transmission of border disease virus is typically by direct contact between sheep, and persistently infected carrier animals are the usual source. Explosive outbreaks can follow the introduction of a persistently infected carrier animal into a susceptible flock, whereas disease is less common in flocks with enzootic infection.

Pathogenesis and Pathology

In adult sheep, the infection is always subclinical, but infection of pregnant ewes results in fetal death or the delivery of dead, deformed, or mummified lambs, depending on the stage of gestation and infection and the virulence of the infecting virus. Neurologic signs reflect defective myelination of nerve fibers in the central nervous system. Infection in early gestation can lead to persistent infection, immunological tolerance, and the birth of lambs that are permanently seronegative or only weakly seropositive. Persistently infected sheep, whether exhibiting clinical signs of infection or not, may become long-term carriers and shed virus continuously in all body secretions and excretions, including semen. Fetuses infected later in gestation typically mount an effective immune response.

Lambs that survive infection at approximately 40–60 days of gestation are born persistently infected, and with a deficiency in myelin throughout the central nervous system. Virus-mediated destruction of oligodendrocytes during differentiation is proposed to be responsible for a deficit in myelin-producing cells, although it also has been shown that infection of the thyroid gland with resultant lack of thyroid hormone contributes to the hypomyelination of congenitally infected lambs. Regardless, the deficiency in myelination is normally resolved within several months of birth if the lamb survives. The characteristic "hairy" fleece of lambs with border disease results from a relative lack of fine wool fibers from secondary follicles, and a disproportionately large number of primary follicles producing large fibers. This change is especially evident in fine-wool sheep breeds, and less apparent in coarse-wool breeds.

Some lambs infected before mid-gestation are born with teratogenic abnormalities, including cavitation of the cerebral hemispheres (hydranencephaly) that results from destruction of neuroblasts and glioblasts before their migration from the subependymal plate to populate the cerebral cortex. Skeletal abnormalities also can occur.

Persistently infected lambs that manifest signs of hairy-shaker disease typically fail to thrive. Persistently infected lambs sometimes develop a mucosal-disease-like syndrome later in life, with the simultaneous presence of the original infecting non-cytopathogenic strain of border disease virus and a closely related cytopathogenic variant.

Diagnosis

As with bovine viral diarrhea virus infection, a presumptive diagnosis can be made on the basis of clinical history and clinical signs. Laboratory diagnosis is based on virus isolation in cell culture, detection of viral antigen in tissues, or detection of virus by RT-PCR assay. Serological findings must be interpreted on the basis that seronegative animals may be persistently infected and immunologically tolerant.

Immunity, Prevention, and Control

In flocks in the first breeding season after the introduction of virus, up to 50% of lambs may be affected; thereafter, the incidence of clinical disease declines precipitously as infection becomes enzootic. This is especially so when clinically recovered lambs are retained for breeding (in surviving lambs neurologic signs often disappear within 3–4 months of age). Control has been attempted using either inactivated or attenuated virus bovine viral diarrhea virus vaccines, but in most practical production settings control measures are not economically worthwhile.

CLASSICAL SWINE FEVER VIRUS

Classical swine fever (*syn.* hog cholera) is an economically important contagious disease of swine worldwide. Infection occurs only in wild and domestic pigs, including wild boar. Enzootic classical swine fever causes severe direct economic losses, and substantial costs are required to maintain immunization or eradication programs. Swine fever is diagnosed regularly in Africa, Asia, and South and Central America. The disease has been eliminated or excluded from the United States, Canada, Australia, New Zealand, the United Kingdom and Ireland, and the Scandinavian countries. Infection still recurs with some regularity in Europe, and, because of quarantines and prohibitions of swine movement and export from affected areas, large numbers of swine have been destroyed in an effort to control recent incursions.

Clinical Features and Epidemiology

Swine fever is highly contagious. The virus most commonly is transmitted between pigs by direct contact, or mechanically by fomites. Contaminated pork and pork products are another important potential source of introduction.

Typical outbreaks of swine fever manifest as acute infection accompanied by high fever, depression, anorexia, and conjunctivitis in affected pigs. These signs appear after an incubation period of 2–4 days and are followed by vomiting, diarrhea and/or constipation, opportunistic bacterial pneumonia, and signs of nervous system dysfunction that include paresis, paralysis, lethargy, circling, tremors, and occasionally convulsions. Light-skinned swine exhibit a diffuse hyperemia and purpura on the abdomen and ears. Severe leukopenia is characteristic. In a susceptible herd, clinical signs are usually seen first in a few pigs; then, over the course of about 10 days, nearly all swine in the herd become sick. Young swine may die without clinical signs, and older pigs may die within a week of onset or later, from opportunistic bacterial infections. Herd mortality may reach 100%.

Less dramatic, subacute and chronic forms of disease have been recognized in which there is a prolonged incubation period, an extended or intermittent course of clinical disease with runting, chronic diarrhea, dermatitis and purpura, secondary bacterial infections, and death occurring after weeks or months. These forms of disease have been associated with virus strains of moderate virulence. Swine infected with virus strains of low virulence exhibit few clinical signs or even remain completely healthy. In immunocompetent swine that survive acute infection, immunity develops quickly. However, virus is shed in all secretions and pigs that develop chronic forms of the disease continue to shed virus continuously or intermittently until their death.

Infection of pregnant sows with virus strains of low virulence leads to fetal infection and embryonic death, abortion, fetal mummification, or stillbirth. Newborn piglets may die or survive with tremors, runting, and progressive disease leading to death weeks or months after birth. Live-born piglets, whether healthy or abnormal, are persistently infected, immunologically tolerant, and life-long virus shedders.

Pathogenesis and Pathology

The most common route of virus entry is oronasal, with the tonsils the site of primary virus replication. The virus quickly disseminates to secondary sites, particularly lymphoid tissues, and later to several parenchymatous organs. The virus has a particular tropism for vascular endothelium, mononuclear phagocytic cells, and other cells of the immune system. In peracute cases there may be no obvious changes at necropsy. In acute cases there are submucosal and subserosal petechial hemorrhages in the gastrointestinal tract, in addition to congestion and highly characteristic multicentric infarction of the spleen, and petechial hemorrhages in lymph nodes and kidney (so-called turkey egg kidney). There is also marked thrombocytopenia, with terminal disseminated intravascular coagulation and thrombosis of small vessels. Encephalitis with perivascular cuffing is frequent. In subacute or chronic cases, there is extensive ulceration of the mucosa of the large intestine (so-called button ulcers) and opportunistic bacterial pneumonia and enteritis, but the hemorrhages and infarction that characterize acute forms of the disease frequently are absent. Perhaps the most prominent lesion in swine dying from chronic swine fever is a general exhaustion of the lymphoid system, with atrophy of the thymus and germinal centers in the spleen and lymph nodes. Immune complexes also form during chronic infections, leading to immune-complex-mediated glomerulonephritis.

Diagnosis

Although the clinical signs and lesions of the acute form of the disease are very characteristic, the diagnosis of classical swine fever is difficult without laboratory confirmation. This is particularly true of the subacute and chronic forms of the disease. Most countries have regulations that require that disease control authorities be notified when the disease is suspected. In such circumstances, tissue specimens (lymph nodes, tonsil, spleen, kidney, ileum, and blood) are submitted to an authorized laboratory. Immunofluorescence or immunoperoxidase staining and antigen-capture ELISA allow rapid detection of viral antigens in tissues, and RT-PCR assays facilitate very rapid identification of viral nucleic acids. Monoclonal antibodies can be used to distinguish swine fever virus from other pestiviruses. Virus isolation and neutralizing antibody assays are performed in swine cell cultures but, because the virus is not cytopathic, such assays require immunological assays to detect the presence of virus. Serologic methods include neutralization and enzyme immunoassay, with reagents chosen, in some cases, to differentiate swine fever virus from bovine viral diarrhea virus. Such differentiation is important in areas where swine fever eradication programs are in place.

Immunity, Prevention, and Control

Classical swine fever virus is transmitted by direct contact between swine or indirectly via virus-laden excretions, secretions, and fomites (such as shoes, clothing, and vehicles). Carriage of virus between herds by inapparently infected swine is also important. Feeding with garbage and kitchen scrap was at one time an important mode of virus transmission between herds; this was especially important because many swine were slaughtered when they showed the first signs of disease, and pork scraps containing high titers of virus were then fed to swine. Garbage-feeding prohibitions and garbage-cooking regulations are now in place in many countries to deal with this risk. Swine fever virus can also survive in frozen pork and pork products for years; the virus can thus be transported over long distances and can reappear in areas otherwise virus free.

Attenuated virus vaccines produced in rabbits or cell culture developed in the 1960s were widely used to eradicate classical swine fever from many countries using a "test and slaughter" program, although problem areas persist. Wild boars in Europe, for example, are infected and represent a potential source of reinfection of domestic swine. New-generation recombinant vaccines have been developed more recently.

OTHER PESTIVIRUSES

A genetically distinct pestivirus (Bungowannah virus) was responsible for an outbreak of stillbirths and sudden death of piglets on a farm in Australia. Lesions in the piglets included non-suppurative myocarditis. Disease also has been described in giraffe infected with an as yet not fully characterized pestivirus.

Chapter 31

Other Viruses: Hepeviruses, *Hepadnaviridae*, Deltaviruses, Anelloviruses, and Unclassified Viruses

Chapter Contents

Inevitably, viruses with distinctive or unique properties are identified that do not readily fit into the existing taxonomic organization of virus families. Some of these agents are identified because of the important disease syndromes with which they are associated, whereas the pathogenic significance of others is uncertain.

MEMBERS OF THE GENUS *HEPEVIRUS*

Viruses in the currently free floating genus *Hepevirus* (proposed family *Hepeviridae*) resemble members of the *Caliciviridae* in their structural morphology, and in their genome organization. Hepevirus virions are non-enveloped, 27–34 nm in diameter, and have icosahedral symmetry. Virions consist of a single capsid protein. The genome is a positive-sense, single-stranded RNA molecule of approximately 7.2 kb that has a 5′ cap and a 3′-poly (A) tail. The genome includes three open reading frames and short 5′ and 3′ non-coding sequences.

The replicative process of human hepatitis E virus (Figure 31.1), the type species of the genus, is similar to that of rubella virus and alphaviruses in the family *Togaviridae*. Phylogenetic analyses of the portions of the genome encoding the helicase and polymerase confirm that hepatitis E viruses from humans and swine segregate in a distinct clade, but are related to members of the *Caliciviridae*, *Togaviridae*, and *Picornaviridae* (Figure 31.2). There are at least four distinct genetic groups (clades) of hepatitis E virus, and strains appear to differ in their virulence.

HEPATITIS E VIRUS

Hepatitis E virus is the cause of outbreaks and individual instances of acute, sometimes fatal hepatitis in humans. The virus is readily transmitted during outbreaks by fecal contamination of water or food, typically because of poor sanitation. Hepatitis E virus appears to have a global distribution, and there is considerable speculation that it is a

HEV (*Hepevirus*) 7.2 kb

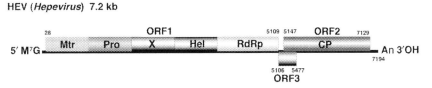

FIGURE 31.1 Geonme organization of hepatitis E virus (HEV) (human strain Burma, M73218). The putative Mtr, Pro, "X", Hel, and RdRp domains are indicated. CP, capsid protein; Hel, helicase; M7G, 7 methyl guanosine; Mtr, methyltransferase; ORF, open reading frame; Pro, protease; RdRp, RNA-dependent RNA polymerase; X, regulatory protein; Anu, poly(A) sequence; number are nucleotide positions. *[From* Virus Taxonomy: Eighth Report of the International Committee on Taxonomy of Viruses *(C. M. Fauquet, M. A. Mayo, J. Maniloff, U. Desselberger, L. A. Ball, eds.), p. 854. Copyright © Elsevier (2005), with permission.]*

Fenner's Veterinary Virology. DOI: 10.1016/B978-0-12-375158-4.00031-6

(A) Helicase region

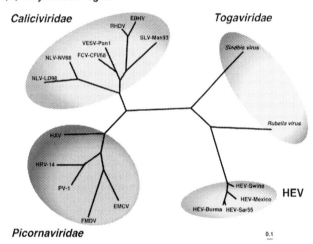

(B) Polymerase region

FIGURE 31.2 Phylogenetic relationships of hepatitis E virus (HEV) with members of the families *Picornaviridae*, *Caliciviridae*, and *Togaviridae*. (A) Helicase region. (B) Polymerase region. EBHV, European brown hare syndrome virus; EMCV, encephalomyocarditis virus; FCV, feline calicivirus; FMDV, foot-and-mouth disease virus; HAV, hepatitis A virus; HEV, hepatitis virus E; HRV, human rhinovirus; PV, poliovirus; NLV, Norwalklike virus; RHDV, rabbit hemorrhagic disease virus; SLV, Sapporo-like virus; VESV, vesicular exanthema of swine virus. [*From* Virus Taxonomy: Eighth Report of the International Committee on Taxonomy of Viruses (C. M. Fauquet, M. A. Mayo, J. Maniloff, U. Desselberger, L. A. Ball, eds.), p. 856. Copyright © Elsevier (2005), with permission.]

zoonotic infection transmitted from an animal reservoir. Similar or identical viruses frequently have been identified in swine, and the virus has experimentally been transmitted from swine to non-human primates. A single serotype of hepatitis E virus has been described, and there is extensive cross-reactivity between virus strains that circulate in humans and pigs. Hepevirus antibodies have been identified in many species of rodents and mammals, although the putative causative viruses have not been characterized.

AVIAN HEPATITIS E VIRUS

A more distantly related but serologically cross-reactive virus (avian hepatitis E virus) that initially was misclassified

as a calicivirus is the cause of hepatitis in chickens, so-called big liver and spleen disease or hepatitis-splenomegaly syndrome. This virus shares approximately 50% nucleic acid homology with the human and swine hepatitis E virus, and tentatively is designated as genotype 5 in the genus *Hepevirus*. The virus only infects chickens. Transmission is via the fecal–oral route, with high levels of virus in feces. Initial virus replication occurs in the gastrointestinal tract, with spread to the liver. Disease has been reported in Leghorn hens, broiler breeders, and dual-purpose hens, and is manifest as increased mortality, decreased egg production, red fluid or clotted blood in the abdomen, enlarged livers and spleens, friable but not fatty livers, and pale combs and wattles. Histologically, lymphocytic periphlebitis and phlebitis with amyloid are prominent within the liver of affected birds. However, some 70% of chicken flocks in the United States have antibodies to this virus, indicating that infection is ubiquitous but usually without clinical disease. A presumptive diagnosis is made on the basis of clinical signs, and gross and microscopic lesions. Definitive diagnosis is made by visualization of 30–35 nm virus particles in bile by negative-stain electron microscopy or isolation of virus in embryonating chicken eggs inoculated intravenously. The avian hepatitis E virus does not replicate in cell culture systems. Virus-specific antibodies can be detected by agarose gel immunodiffusion test or enzyme linked immunosorbent assay.

CUTTHROAT TROUT VIRUS

Cutthroat trout virus was first identified in salmonid fish in California in 1988. Limited sequence data indicate that the putative helicase protein of this virus shares approximately 40% amino acid homology with the helicase of hepatitis E virus. The virus has increasingly been identified in adult salmonid broodstock, including rainbow trout (*Oncorhynchus mykiss*), cutthroat trout (*Oncorhynchus clarki*), brown trout (*Salmo trutta*), and brook trout (*Salvelinus fontinolis*) in several western states of the United States. However, in contrast to other hepeviruses, the salmonid virus has yet to be associated with hepatitis or any other clinical syndrome. Rainbow trout, brown trout, and kokanee salmon (*Oncorhynchus nerka*) are all susceptible to experimental infection with cutthroat trout virus, whereas Chinook (*Oncorhynchus tshawytscha*) and coho (*Oncorhynchus kisutch*) salmon were refractory.

The virus is most readily detected in the fluid surrounding collected eggs (ovarian fluid), or in tissues such as kidney and spleen of adult salmonid broodstocks. The virus replicates in fish (CHSE-214) cells, although cytopathic effects develop very slowly. Control measures are not widely applied for prevention of cutthroat trout virus, because it has not been associated with disease. Interestingly, juvenile rainbow trout exposed to this virus were significantly protected against subsequent experimental challenge infection with the rhabdovirus, infectious hematopoietic necrosis virus. The transient heterologous resistance induced by cutthroat trout virus is proposed to be mediated by interferon induced by the original infection.

MEMBERS OF THE FAMILY *HEPADNAVIRIDAE*

HEPATITIS B VIRUSES

The prototype virus in this group, hepatitis B virus, is an important human pathogen, whereas viruses of the family *Hepadnaviridae* are of limited importance in veterinary medicine. The family has been divided into two genera: *Orthohepadnavirus* includes the mammalian viruses; *Avihepadnavirus* comprises the avian members. The genus *Orthohepadnavirus* includes human hepatitis B and a number of genotypes of related primate hepatitis B virus that infect great apes and woolly monkeys, as well as several viruses that infect members of the squirrel family. The latter include woodchuck hepatitis virus, which infects woodchucks (*Marmata monax*) and chipmunks, and ground squirrel hepatitis virus, which infects ground squirrels (*Spermophilus beecheyi* and *S. parryi*). Avihepadnaviruses include duck B hepatitis, first described in Pekin ducks although it is also found in a variety of ducks and geese; a number of similar viruses occur in other species of birds, including storks, herons, and cranes.

Orthohepadnavirus virions are 42–50 nm in diameter and are composed of an approximately 34 nm icosahedral nucleocapsid (core) surrounded by an envelope. The core protein is the major nucleocapsid protein, and the envelope contains two or three proteins, including a small transmembrane protein (S), an intermediate-sized protein (M), and a large protein (L). The genome consists of a single molecule of circular (via base pairing of cohesive ends), partially double-stranded, partially single-stranded DNA. The complete strand is negative sense and 3.0–3.3 kb in size; the other strand varies between 1.7 and 2.8 kb, leaving 15–50% of the molecule single stranded; the gap is smaller in avian viruses. The complete strand contains a nick at a unique site that is different in the orthohepadnaviruses and avihepadnaviruses. The negative-sense genomic strand has a protein molecule covalently attached to its 5′ end; the positive-sense strand has a 19-nucleotide cap at the 5′ end. Hepadnavirus genomes have three (avihepadnaviruses) or four (orthohepadnaviruses) open reading frames. One major difference between the avian and mammalian hepatitis B viruses is the presence of an open reading frame that encodes the X protein, a regulatory protein involved in virus replication, although its function is not fully understood.

The hepatitis B virus envelope is composed of three viral proteins and some host-cell lipid. These constituents also form non-infectious spherical (22 nm in diameter) or filamentous (22 nm in diameter, varying length) particles called hepatitis B surface antigen particles (that express at least five antigenic specificities). Extraordinary numbers of these particles are formed and circulate in the blood of chronically infected humans or woodchucks, and hepatitis B surface antigen particles produced by recombinant DNA technology are the basis for current hepatitis B vaccines.

Although mammalian hepadnaviruses are extremely difficult to propagate in cell culture, their structure and mode of replication are well characterized. Hepadnaviruses have a unique and complex mode of replication involving a reverse transcriptase (Figure 31.3). In the nucleus of hepatocytes, the viral genome is converted into a complete circular double-stranded DNA by the DNA polymerase carried in the virion nucleocapsid. The negative-sense strand of this DNA is used as the template for the synthesis of a full-length positive-sense RNA transcript, which is packaged in virus core particles in the cytoplasm of the infected cell. The viral reverse transcriptase then transcribes negative-sense DNA from the positive-sense RNA template. As this occurs, the positive-sense template is degraded simultaneously. Next, the viral DNA polymerase utilizes the newly formed negative-sense DNA as the template for the synthesis of positive-sense DNA. Newly synthesized double-stranded DNA is packaged into virions before this last step is complete, which explains why virion DNA is only partially double stranded. Although not part of the normal life cycle, hepadnavirus DNA can be integrated into the DNA of hepatocytes. In woodchucks, integration commonly occurs in or near a retrotransposon, N-myc2. Viral enhancers drive overexpression of N-myc2, and this contributes to neoplastic transformation of hepatocytes in a high proportion of hepatocellular carcinomas in this species. Integration of hepatitis B virus into human hepatocytes is more random, and no consistent association between site of integration and tumor risk has been established.

Hepatitis B virus in humans is a significant health concern. Infection can cause acute hepatitis, but, more importantly, chronic hepatitis can develop into liver cirrhosis, and primary hepatocellular carcinoma. Similarly, woodchucks infected with woodchuck hepatitis virus as neonates develop acute hepatitis and can become chronic carriers. Adult infection is usually self-limiting, as it is in humans. The risk of hepatocellular carcinoma in chronically infected woodchucks is reported to reach 100%, although cirrhosis does not develop. Ground squirrels infected with ground squirrel hepatitis virus develop mild hepatitis, and hepatocellular carcinoma can occur in chronically infected animals. Pekin ducks infected with duck hepatitis B virus show few signs of disease, either acute or chronic, despite high rates of non-cytopathic virus replication in hepatocytes. Unlike mammals, ducks can be infected congenitally with the virus passed through the egg.

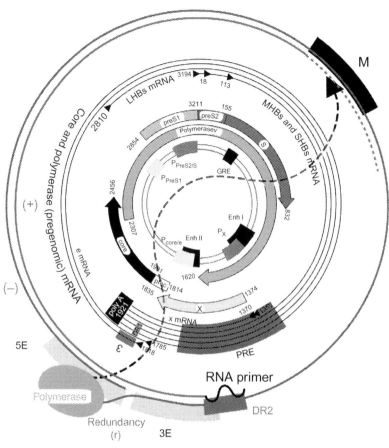

FIGURE 31.3 Genome organization and regulatory elements of orthohepadnaviruses are shown for a typical hepatitis B virus (HBV) isolate of genotype A. The outer circle represents the structure of relaxed circular, viral DNA found within virions, while the inner circle illustrates the structure and regulatory elements on cccDNA, the covalently closed circular DNA from which viral mRNAs are transcribed in the nucleus of the infected cell (red = positive strand; blue = negative strand). Numbering starts at the unique EcoRI restriction site located approximately at the junction of the preS1 and preS2 domains in the open reading frame (ORF) for the viral envelope proteins. The regulatory elements on the DNA are depicted at their approximate position. The promoters (P) are shown as gray boxes, the enhancers (Enh), a glucocorticoid responsive element (GRE), a negative regulatory element (NRE) and a CCAAT element (CCAAT) are depicted as black boxes. Liver-specific promoters are drawn in light gray; non-tissue specific promoters are depicted as medium gray boxes. The ORFs are drawn as arrows with their corresponding start and termination sites. The viral mRNAs are depicted as black circles in the middle region. The black triangles represent their 5'-ends; the 3'-end is common and linked to an approximately 300 nt long polyA. The regulatory elements on the RNAs are depicted as a red box (encapsidation signal ε), a back box (polyadenylation signal), in pink (DR1) and in blue (posttranscriptional regulatory element [PRE]). The genomic DNA is depicted as it is found in the virion. The minus DNA strand is drawn as a blue line with its terminal redundancy (r). The polymerase (green oval) is lined to the 5'-end of the minus strand. The plus strand DNA is shown as a red line. The dotted red line represents the variation of the 3'-end of the plus strand DNA. The 5'-end of the plus strand is bound to its capped RNA primer, depicted as a black wave-line. The dotted black line between the polymerase and the 3'-end of the plus-strand DNA reflects the fact that the polymerase is bound to the 5'-end of the minus-strand DNA, but interacts with the variable 3'-end of the plus-strand DNA for its elongation. The regulatory elements on the minus-strand DNA are the DR2 (red box) and the M, 5E and 3E elements, which are required for circularization of the genome. Note that their position and size are approximate since these elements are not yet completely characterized. (from Kann M. (2002). Structure and molecular virology. In: *Hepatitis B virus Human Virus Guide.* (S. Locarnini and C.L. Lai, eds.) Chapter 2. International Medical Press Ltd., London. with permission). *[From* Virus Taxonomy: Eighth Report of the International Committee on Taxonomy of Viruses *(C. M. Fauquet, M. A. Mayo, J. Maniloff, U. Desselberger, L. A. Ball, eds.), p. 376. Copyright © Elsevier (2005), with permission.]*

MEMBERS OF THE FLOATING GENUS *DELTAVIRUS*

HEPATITIS D VIRUS

Hepatitis D virus, also called hepatitis delta virus, is a satellite virus, in that it requires the simultaneous presence of hepatitis B virus for its replication and assembly in natural infections. This virus is unique among the viruses of

vertebrates. On the basis of its unique biological and molecular properties, the virus has been accorded distinct taxonomic status in the floating genus *Deltavirus*. Hepatitis D virions are 36–43 nm in diameter and consist of a shell made of hepatitis B surface antigen (or woodchuck hepatitis virus surface antigen in experimental infections) surrounding a core containing delta antigen and a circular negative-sense, single-stranded RNA genome,

1.75 kb in size. The genome structure and autocatalytic activities involved in the replication of hepatitis D virus closely resemble those of some viroids and satellite viruses found in plants. Disease is more severe in humans infected simultaneously with hepatitis B and D viruses than in those infected with hepatitis B virus alone, with an increased incidence of cirrhosis and increased mortality. The mechanisms involved in this interaction are unknown. Hepatitis D virus has been transmitted experimentally to woodchucks infected simultaneously with woodchuck hepatitis virus.

MEMBERS OF THE FLOATING GENUS *ANELLOVIRUS*

TORQUE TENO VIRUSES

Torque teno viruses are genetically heterogeneous, single-stranded DNA viruses that are morphologically similar to circoviruses (see Chapter 13), but which are classified in a free-standing genus, *Anellovirus*, because of other distinctive characteristics. In contrast to circoviruses, the torque teno viruses are genomically highly diverse in at least portions of their genomes. Torque teno virus infections have been described in humans, non-human primates, cats, dogs, marine mammals, and farm animals, but their pathogenic significance remains uncertain. The unusual name—torque teno virus—includes the initials (TT) of the human patient in Japan from whom the virus was first identified.

Torque teno virions are variably sized (up to approximately 30 nm), with a genome of negative-sense single-stranded DNA of 2.0–3.9 kb. The inability to culture members of the genus *Anellovirus* has limited their characterization, but at least four messenger RNAs are produced, and it is proposed that complex splicing is necessary for the transcription of some open reading frames (Figure 31.4). Thus replication of torque teno virus is probably unique, but most similar to that of chicken anemia virus (family *Circoviridae*, genus *Gyrovirus*).

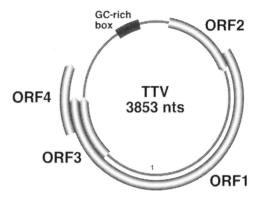

FIGURE 31.4   Genome organization of a torque teno virus (TTV), genus *Anellovirus*. GC, guanosine cytosine; ORF, open reading frame. [*From* Virus Taxonomy: Eighth Report of the International Committee on Taxonomy of Viruses *(C. M. Fauquet, M. A. Mayo, J. Maniloff, U. Desselberger, L. A. Ball, eds.), p. 336. Copyright © Elsevier (2005), with permission.*]

Torque teno viruses replicate to very high titers in infected individuals, and complexes of virus and specific antibody circulate during virus persistence. Torque teno viruses recently have been linked to diseases induced by porcine circovirus.

UNCLASSIFIED ARBOVIRUSES

In the course of arbovirus investigations, dozens of viruses have been isolated that have been characterized only partially; in most cases they have been passaged in mammalian cell cultures and, in some cases, in experimental animals (mice, hamsters). Other viruses have been identified only by molecular methods. In general, little is being done to determine whether any of these viruses may be animal pathogens. Such work is only likely to be done in the wake of substantial disease episodes in domestic or important wild animals in settings where public notice is taken and field investigation is feasible and fundable.

Chapter 32

Prions: Agents of Transmissible Spongiform Encephalopathies

The term "transmissible spongiform encephalopathy" is used for several neurodegenerative diseases: scrapie of sheep and goats, bovine spongiform encephalopathy, feline transmissible encephalopathy, transmissible mink encephalopathy, chronic wasting disease of deer and elk, and four human diseases: kuru, Creutzfeldt–Jakob disease [including variant Creutzfeldt–Jakob disease (vCJD)], Gerstmann-Sträussler–Scheinker syndrome, and fatal familial insomnia. These uniformly fatal diseases are caused by prions—that is, "infectious proteins" or "rogue proteins." The name prion is an acronym from proteinaceous infectious particle. In each of these diseases, the characteristic lesion is spongiform degeneration in the gray matter of the brain, with hypertrophy and proliferation of astrocytes.

The prototype of the prion diseases, scrapie, was first described after the importation of Merino sheep from Spain into England in the 15th century. The name reflects the characteristic scratching behavior of diseased animals. Scrapie is enzootic in sheep in all countries except Australia and New Zealand. In 1963, Dr William Hadlow, a veterinary pathologist, first proposed that the human disease, kuru, was similar to scrapie in sheep, and that it might be transmissible. Kuru, a fatal neurological disease, occurred only in the Fore tribe in the New Guinea highlands, where ritualistic cannibalism was practiced on deceased relatives. Hadlow's idea led to the discovery by Dr Carleton Gajdusek that kuru could be transmitted to chimpanzees, causing a disease indistinguishable from the human counterpart; for this discovery, Gajdusek was awarded the Nobel Prize in Medicine. The importance of this discovery became clear when it was shown that more common human diseases such as Creutzfeldt–Jakob disease, and other animal diseases such as chronic wasting disease of deer and elk, are also transmissible in the same way.

Bovine spongiform encephalopathy ("mad cow disease") was first detected in 1986 in the United Kingdom. Epidemiological observations suggest that the cattle disease originated in the early 1980s and became established in cattle through recycling of rendered bovine meat-and-bone meal in the ruminant food chain. As more and more diseased cattle were slaughtered and rendered to produce meat-and-bone meal, a massive, multiple-point-source epizootic followed. Export of meat-and-bone meal from the United Kingdom introduced the disease into many other European countries, and to Canada. The disease also was introduced into zoo animals and domestic and exotic cats in the United Kingdom through the same source. In 1996, the British government first announced that humans had probably become infected with the bovine spongiform encephalopathy prion through exposure to cattle products. By the end of 2009, the number of human cases of what is now called "variant Creutzfeldt–Jakob disease" (vCJD) had risen to 167 in the United Kingdom and 47 in other countries, although many of these patients had resided in the United Kingdom.

Fenner's Veterinary Virology. DOI: 10.1016/B978-0-12-375158-4.00032-8

Epidemiologic, pathologic, and molecular studies have strengthened the causative association between the bovine prion and the human disease. At the heart of this association were research breakthroughs on the nature of prions and the mechanisms of their pathogenicity; in 1997, for his discovery of the bizarre nature of prions and their exceptional pathogenetic pathways, Stanley Prusiner was awarded the Nobel Prize in Medicine. Exclusion of high-risk bovine materials from the human food chain has resulted in a dramatic decrease in the number of human deaths in the United Kingdom, but inadvertent transmission of vCJD by transfusion of blood products has been reported. The extent and duration of the vCJD outbreak cannot be determined accurately, because of the lack of a suitable blood test for the disorder, and the prolonged incubation period of some prion protein genotypes in individuals.

PROPERTIES OF PRIONS

Classification

Prions have not been classified in the same way as viruses, thus there are no families, genera, or species. They first are identified by their host species and disease association (Table 32.1), and then characterized by their molecular and biological properties. Their primary amino acid sequence mainly reflects the host from which they were isolated, but also registers mutations that define inherited variants—for example, in familial Creutzfeldt–Jakob disease in humans. Full amino acid sequences of virtually all important prion variants have been determined and, as described below, naturally occurring amino acid substitutions are associated with relative susceptibility and incubation time in sheep and cervids (deer and elk).

TABLE 32.1 Prion Diseases of Animals and Humans

Disease	Host	Source of Infection
Scrapie	Sheep, goats	Not certain, most likely by direct contact and contamination of pastures by placentas, blood, and fetal tissues
Bovine spongiform encephalopathy	Cattle	Bovine spongiform encephalopathy prion contamination of meat-and-bone meal
Transmissible mink encephalopathy	Mink	Prion contamination of unknown origin fed to mink
Chronic wasting disease	Mule deer, elk	Unknown source; highly transmissible among deer or elk held in close quarters
Feline spongiform encephalopathy	Cats, felids in zoos	Bovine spongiform encephalopathy prion contamination of meat fed to animals
Exotic ungulate spongiform encephalopathy	Greater kudu, nyala, oryx, and others in zoos	Bovine spongiform encephalopathy prion contamination of meat-and-bone meal
Atypical scrapie and bovine spongiform encephalopathy	Sheep, goats, cattle	Recently reported disorders, possibly sporadic origin
Kuru	Humans	Ritual cannibalism in Fore people
Creutzfeldt–Jakob disease	Humans	Iatrogenic: human prion contamination of dura mater grafts, therapeutic hormones, etc., all derived from cadavers
		Familial: germ line mutation in n gene (*PrP*)
		Sporadic: unknown cause, perhaps somatic mutation in *PrP* gene or spontaneous conversion of PrP^c into PrP^{sc}
Variant Creutzfeld–Jakob disease	Humans	Transmission of bovine spongiform encephalopathy prion to humans, probably by the oral route
Gerstmann–Sträussler–Scheinker syndrome	Humans	Familial: germ line mutation in *PrP* gene
Fatal familial insomnia	Humans	Familial: germ line mutation in *PrP* gene

PrP, prion protein; PrP^c, normal cellular isoform of the prion protein; PrP^{sc}, scrapie isoform of the prion protein.

Certain biological properties are used to distinguish strains of prions, particularly scrapie strains. Following intracerebral injection of prion-containing material into several strains of inbred mice, the following parameters are recorded: (1) incubation period and mortality pattern; (2) distribution and extent of spongiform lesions and prion protein (PrP) plaques in brains (assayed by immunohisto-chemistry using labeled anti-PrP antibodies); (3) (in some cases) titer of infectivity in brains. Prion strains "breed true," giving reproducible results in this kind of biological assay system. For example, prions from cattle, nyala, kudu, and domestic cats behave the same when subjected to this strain characterization protocol, indicating that all have been derived from the same source, namely cattle. Further, mice inoculated in the same way with material from cattle with bovine spongiform encephalopathy and humans with vCJD have behaved the same, yet differently from mice inoculated with material from sporadic cases of Creutzfeldt–Jakob disease or farmers who died of the same disease after working with cattle with bovine spongiform encephalopathy.

Similar results have been recorded by biochemical analysis of prions recovered from various sources; for example, when brain specimens were treated with protein-ase K and their protease-resistant residues were subjected to western blot analysis, four different blot patterns were found. Three patterns represented genetic, sporadic, and iatrogenic Creutzfeldt–Jakob disease in humans; the fourth represented all cases of vCJD, bovine spongiform encephalopathy in cattle, and the similar feline and exotic ungulate diseases.

Prions from animals and humans can also be transmitted to various other animals (hamsters, rats, ferrets, mink, sheep, goats, pigs, cattle, monkeys, and chimpanzees), and again a kind of strain variation is seen. Some donor–recipient pairs lead to short incubation disease, others to longer incubation disease, and yet others no disease even after very long periods of observation or blind passage (the "species barrier").

Prion Properties

Prions are normal cellular proteins that have undergone conformational change as a result of post-translational processing of a normal cellular protein and thereby have become pathogenic. The normal protein, called PrP^c (the term for the normal cellular isoform of the prion protein), is composed of about 208–254 amino acids (M_r 27,000–30,000). It is encoded in the genome of most mammals and is expressed in many tissues, especially in neurons and lymphoreticular cells. The function of PrP^c is unclear; it has been found to bind copper, but knockout mice lacking the gene for the protein appear normal. The amino acid sequence of PrP^c and the abnormal isoform of the protein,

called PrP^{sc} (a term derived from the scrapie isoform of the prion protein, but in general use for all prion diseases) are identical in a given host. Only the conformation of PrP^{sc} is changed, from a structure made up predominantly of α helices to one made up predominantly of β sheets. A monoclonal antibody has been developed that can discriminate between normal and disease-specific forms of PrP. It specifically precipitates bovine, murine, and human PrP^{sc}, but not PrP^c, confirming the presence of an epitope common to prions from different species that is linked to disease but different from the normal isoform of the protein.

When a given animal prion is passaged in mice or hamsters, the amino acid sequence of the recipient PrP^{sc} is that of the PrP^c of the recipient, not the donor. In susceptible host species, there may be many different mutations in the PrP gene, each resulting in a slightly different PrP^{sc} conformation, each in turn resulting in a different lesion pattern and different incubation and mortality patterns. This genetic variability is part of the basis for the differentiation of prion strains. For example, prions from vCJD in humans have characteristics distinct from those in other types of Creutzfeldt–Jakob disease, but similar to prions isolated from cattle, mice, cats, and macaques infected during the bovine spongiform encephalopathy epizootic in the United Kingdom. However, the primary amino acid sequence of PrP^c in the host is not always sufficient to encode a prion strain. Hamsters infected with transmissible mink encephalopathy develop two different prion strains, in spite of a conserved amino acid sequence. Likewise, sheep with a sporadic transmissible spongiform encephalopathy termed "Nor98" have a PrP^{sc} biochemical profile distinct from that observed in genetically matched sheep with classical scrapie.

PrP^{sc} protein is very resistant to many environmental insults, chemicals, and physical conditions that would destroy any virus or microorganism (Table 32.2). PrP^{sc} is also resistant to endogenous proteases, which is the key to its accumulation into aggregates, called scrapie-associated fibrils (SAF; a term derived from scrapie but in general use for all prion diseases), that form neuronal plaques and are associated with spongiform damage and neuronal dysfunction.

Other notable characteristics of prions include: (1) they can reach very high titers in the brains of their hosts—laboratory strains passaged in hamsters can reach titers of 10^{11} ID_{50} per gram of brain tissue (ID_{50} is the dose that will infect 50% of the experimental group); (2) as measured by ultrafiltration, their size seems to be about 30 nm; (3) they are very resistant to ultraviolet and γ-irradiation, having a very small radiation target size; (4) they polymerize, forming helically wound filamentous rods (SAF) 4–6 nm in diameter, which are visible by electron microscopy and which make up the plaques seen in neurons; (5) they evoke no inflammatory or immune response in their host.

TABLE 32.2 Effects of Physical and Chemical Treatments on Scrapie Prion Infectivity[a]

Treatment	Reduction of Infectivity
1 M NaOH	$>10^{6-8}$
Phenol extraction	$>10^6$
0.5% sodium hypochlorite	10^4
Histopathologic processing	$10^{2.6}$
3% formaldehyde	10^2
1% β-propiolactone	10^1
Ether extraction	10^2
Autoclave 132°C for 90 minutes	$>10^{7.4}$
Autoclave 132°C for 60 minutes	$10^{6.5}$
Autoclave 121°C for 90 minutes	$10^{5.6}$
Boiling 100°C for 60 minutes	$10^{3.4}$
Heating 80°C for 60 minutes	10^1

[a] Composite of several studies, therefore no untreated control value given.

There are investigators who do not believe that the etiologic role of prions in the spongiform encephalopathies has been proven. They cite alternate, but unproven, hypotheses to explain experimental findings: (1) the virino theory, suggesting that a nucleic acid genome is present that does not code for any protein but regulates the synthesis of a host-coded protein component of the agent—that is, PrP^{sc}; (2) the virus theory, suggesting that, because there are viruses that have not yet been visualized or cultivated or had their nucleic acid isolated and characterized, it is reasonable that efforts to find a conventional virus may fail, despite intensive research efforts.

Prion Replication

It is the presence of horizontally or perhaps vertically transmitted PrP^{sc} that catalyzes the conversion of normally encoded PrP^c molecules into more PrP^{sc} molecules. Although PrP^{sc} acts as the template, the "seed crystal," for the abnormal folding and polymerization of PrP^c—forming a heterodimer with normal cellular PrP^c—there is evidence that another molecule, called "protein X," is needed for prion replication when transmission occurs between distant host species. In any case, the process cascades exponentially, with newly formed PrP^{sc} in turn serving as a catalyst for the conversion of more and more PrP^c molecules as they are produced in target cells such as neurons (Figure 32.1). Eventually, so much PrP^{sc} builds

up that it polymerizes, forming fibrillar masses that become visible as microscopic plaques; the plaques cause neuronal degeneration and neurological dysfunction via mechanisms that are as yet poorly understood. In a like manner, different isoforms of PrP^{sc} "breed true" and are perpetuated even in mixed infections.

Much of our understanding of the prion replicative process has been confirmed by elegant studies using knockout and transgenic mice—that is, mice lacking the *PrP^c* gene or mice containing only the *PrP^c* gene of another species. For example, mice lacking the *PrP* gene do not develop disease when inoculated with the scrapie prion, and mice expressing reduced levels of the protein have very long incubation periods. Further, when normal brain explants are grafted into the brains of such knockout mice, they develop lesions only in the normal graft tissue. Even more remarkable, transgenic mice, carrying mutated *PrP* genes mimicking those in human familial spongiform encephalopathies, show the neuronal degeneration typical of these diseases even without inoculation of exogenous prions. Finally, transgenic/knockout mice carrying human PrP^c, but not mouse PrP^c, when inoculated with the bovine spongiform encephalopathy prion develop neurologic disease and lesions, starting at about 500 days. This finding is considered a key element in the association of vCJD with the bovine spongiform encephalopathy prion.

SCRAPIE

Although recognized as a distinct disease of sheep and goats in many countries for centuries, scrapie was not understood to be transmissible until an episode in Scotland in 1935. More than 1500 cases of iatrogenic scrapie followed the use of a formalin-inactivated louping ill vaccine prepared from sheep brain. Scrapie is distributed widely in Europe and North America and occurs sporadically in some countries in Africa and Asia. Typically, only a few sheep in a flock are diseased at any given time, but infected flocks suffer losses continuously over many years. In the United Kingdom and the United States, most cases occur in the Suffolk and Hampshire breeds, although most other breeds are affected if genetically susceptible sheep are exposed. Goats seem to be incidental hosts, with infection following commingling with scrapie-infected sheep or exposure to contaminated pastures.

Clinical Features and Epidemiology

The incubation period of scrapie in sheep is 2–5 years and the onset of clinical disease is insidious. Affected sheep may become excitable and develop fine tremors of the head and neck, which may be elicited by sudden noise or movement. Shortly thereafter, animals develop intense pruritus, with wool loss and skin rubbed raw. After 1–6 months of

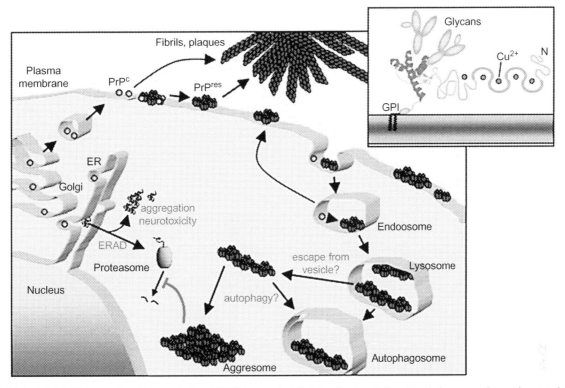

FIGURE 32.1 Model of biogenesis and accumulation of PrP^res in scrapie-infected cells. As a GPI-anchored plasma membrane glycoprotein (inset), PrP^c is first synthesized in the endoplasmic reticulum (ER), then processed in the Golgi apparatus, and transported to the cell surface (main diagram). PrP^res, together with apparent co-factors, directly induces the conversion of GPI-anchored PrP^c on the cell surface and/or in endosomes. PrP^c that is released from the cell may be converted on extracellular deposits such as amyloid fibrils. Once PrP^res is made, it can accumulate on the cell surface, in intracellular vesicles (e.g., lysosomes) and aggresomes, or in extracellular deposits. Under conditions of mild proteasome inhibition, cytotoxic cytoplasmic PrP aggregates (e.g., aggresomes) can be found. Scrapie infection alone can inhibit proteasomes, apparently because of the presence of cytoplasmic PrP oligomers. ERAD, endoplasmic-reticulum-associated protein degradation; GPI, glycophosphatidylinositol; N, N-terminus; PrP^c, normal cellular isoform of the prion protein; PrP^res, proteinase-K-resistant (PrP^Sc) isoform of the prion protein. *[From B. Caughey, G. S. Baron, B. Chesebro, M. Jeffrey. Getting a grip on prions: oligomers, amyloids, and pathological membrane interactions.* Annu. Rev. Biochem. *78, 177–204 (2009), with permission.]*

progressive deterioration, characterized by emaciation, weakness, weaving gait, staring eyes, ataxia, and hindquarter paralysis, animals invariably die. These clinical signs are not invariable however; clinically normal sheep may be found dead or may develop only ataxia in the absence of pruritus.

Genetic susceptibility to scrapie has been evident for decades; the link is so convincing that early reports considered the possibility that scrapie was a familial disease. A large number of studies have demonstrated that, although classical scrapie is an infectious disease, natural variants of the prion gene are associated with relative resistance to disease and differences in incubation time. Genetic testing for the deduced amino acid at residue 171 is now standard in highly affected breeds of sheep such as Suffolk or Hampshire in the United States. In the United Kingdom and some European countries, the polymorphism at residue 136 is the major determinant of susceptibility.

Pathogenesis and Pathology

Although scrapie spreads within flocks, its natural route of infection has not been proven. It is widely considered that sheep acquire the disease by the oral route or from superficial wounds when in pastures contaminated by placental tissue or body fluids. Vertical transmission is still disputed, and transmission from ewes to lambs is most probably the result of postpartum exposure to placenta, blood, birth fluids, and milk of infected dams. Under experimental conditions, peripheral routes of inoculation (intraperitoneal, subcutaneous, or intravenous) produce disease after prolonged incubation periods, whereas intracerebral inoculation leads to disease after a much shorter incubation period.

The first appearance of the scrapie prion in experimentally infected lambs occurs in the intestines, tonsils, spleen, and lymph nodes. Sequential infectivity titrations of organs suggest that, following ingestion of prions, infection is initiated

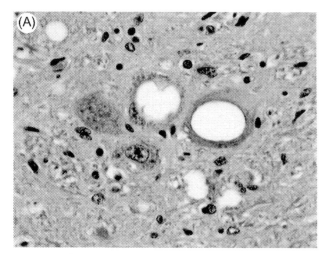

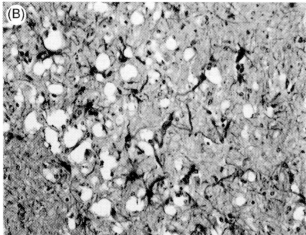

FIGURE 32.2 Lesions in the gray matter of the brain of a sheep with scrapie. (A) Typical spongiform change in neurons. Hematoxylin and eosin stain. (B) Spongiform change and astrocytic hypertrophy and hyperplasia. Glial fibrillary acidic protein stain. Magnifications: ×500. *(Courtesy of R. Higgins, University of California.)*

in gut lymphoid tissues and prions produced in these tissues then move to the central nervous system. At death, lesions in the gray matter of the brain include neuronal vacuolation and degeneration, and astrocytic hypertrophy and hyperplasia (Figure 32.2). There is no inflammatory reaction or evidence of an immune response.

Diagnosis

Diagnosis is based on clinical signs, flock history, and histopathologic examination of the brain of suspect animals. Anti-PrP antibodies are used for immunohistochemical staining of suspect brain and lymphoid tissue specimens, and for western blot assays of solubilized brain extracts. The presence of PrP^{Sc} in any of these target tissues is considered diagnostic. Antemortem testing is based on biopsy sampling of lymphoid tissue from the nictitating membrane,

palatine tonsil, or rectal mucosa. The antemortem tests are generally useful only in sheep older than 14 months.

Immunity, Prevention, and Control

Countries with enzootic scrapie may seek to eradicate the disease. For example, an eradication scheme was established in the United States following the introduction of scrapie into the United States in 1947 and again in 1952. The program has been modified to reflect scientific advances and involves an integrated program of large-scale active and passive surveillance, animal identification to allow trace-back to the farm of origin of diseased sheep, recognition and identification of a prion gene variant associated with nearly absolute resistance to classical scrapie, financial indemnity for removal of genetically susceptible sheep exposed to scrapie, and certification of scrapie-free flocks. This program has resulted in a steady decrease in the prevalence of scrapie.

Given the adverse impact of scrapie and the expenses associated with its eradication, Australia and New Zealand, with their large and scrapie-free sheep populations, have instituted stringent quarantine programs to protect their industries.

SPORADIC SPONGIFORM ENCEPHALOPATHY OF SHEEP AND GOATS

In 1998, Norwegian pathologists described a novel prion-accumulating disorder of sheep (designated Nor98 or atypical scrapie). Lesions and PrP^{Sc} accumulation occur in the cerebellum, rather than in the dorsal motor nucleus of the vagus nerve in the medulla as occurs in scrapie. Further, PrP^{Sc} is apparently absent from lymphoid tissues. The PrP^{Sc} molecules associated with this disease have folding and proteinase cleavage patterns distinct from those of classical scrapie prion. Certain prion gene variants are overrepresented in infected sheep, but no genotype is protective. Most cases are observed in older, clinically normal sheep screened in large-scale slaughter surveillance programs. Epidemiological studies show no evidence of transmission among flock mates, and the disorder is commonly believed to represent a sporadic and non-transmissible spongiform encephalopathy of older sheep and goats. This same disorder has been present in sheep in the United Kingdom since at least 1987, and the disease was also recently described amongst sheep in both the United States and New Zealand, the latter a country free of classical scrapie.

BOVINE SPONGIFORM ENCEPHALOPATHY

Bovine spongiform encephalopathy ("mad cow disease") was first recognized in the United Kingdom in 1986. By 1989, an alarming increase in the number of cases reported led to a ban on the feeding of meat-and-bone meal derived from ruminant meat or offal; however, the ban was only minimally enforced until some years later. The epizootic, as measured by numbers of cases reported and confirmed, peaked in 1993, at which time more than 300 cases were identified per week. By the end of 1997, more than 172,000 cases had been confirmed, involving over 60% of all dairy farms and 14% of beef cow/calf herds. The number of reported and confirmed cases was dwarfed by the actual number of infected animals that entered into the human food chain because of slaughter before the onset of clinical disease.

Initial studies in the United Kingdom indicated a multiple-common-source epizootic. It was soon realized that the epizootic was caused by contamination of meat-and-bone meal with a transmissible spongiform encephalopathy agent. Exclusion of some or all cattle by-products from the ruminant food chain has resulted in a decrease in new cases of bovine spongiform encephalopathy from approximately 6600 per million mature cattle in 1992 to 7.5 per million in 2008. The economic and social impact of this epidemic has been extraordinary, especially in the United Kingdom and, to a lesser extent, other European countries.

Clinical Features and Epidemiology

The bovine spongiform encephalopathy epizootic began simultaneously at many geographic locations and was traced solely to contamination of meat-and-bone meal produced from meat and offal from slaughtered and dead livestock. As the epizootic progressed, it was amplified by the feeding of more and more of the same product produced from infected cattle. The original hypothesis that bovine spongiform encephalopathy originated from inclusion of rendered carcasses from scrapie-infected sheep in the bovine food chain has not been substantiated. The disease may have originated from rendered carcasses of cattle with a sporadic spongiform encephalopathy, or sheep with a novel form of scrapie. The spread of the disease from the United Kingdom to other European countries was via exported meat-and-bone meal and breeding cattle. Between 1986 and 1990, more than 57,900 breeding cattle were exported from the United Kingdom to European Union countries, along with thousands of tons of meat-and-bone meal. The spread of the disease to cats (more than 80 cases) and certain exotic zoo animals (greater kudu, eland, nyala, gemsbok, oryx, puma, cheetah, ocelot, rhesus monkey) was via the same means, with protein supplements derived from rendered cattle products being added to animal feed products, including commercial cat food.

The onset of bovine spongiform encephalopathy is insidious, with tremors, hyperesthesia with kicking during milking, abnormal posture, hind limb ataxia, progressive apprehensive behavior, aggression, and even frenzy, reduced milk yield, and weight loss. The disease is inevitably fatal after a clinical course ranging from 2 to 3 weeks to over a year. Onset is independent of season or stage of lactation. Most cattle affected have been 3–5 years of age; older cattle have been affected and the youngest recorded case was 22 months of age.

Pathogenesis and Pathology

Several lines of evidence indicate that there is a single predominant food-borne strain of the bovine spongiform encephalopathy prion; it is unusually species non-specific, having been shown to cause disease in cats and other ungulates, and to be transmitted easily by oral or intracerebral routes to sheep, goats, mink, marmosets, squirrel monkeys, cynomolgus macaques, mice, and hamsters. There is scant evidence for vertical or horizontal transmission in live cattle.

Characteristic lesions occur only in the brain of cattle with bovine spongiform encephalopathy; they include neuronal vacuolation, degeneration, and loss, and astrocytic hypertrophy and hyperplasia. There is no obvious inflammatory reaction. Lesions are most prominent in the nuclei of the midbrain, brain stem, arid cervical spinal cord, with minimal changes in cerebral cortex, cerebellum, hippocampus, and basal nuclei.

Diagnosis

Diagnosis is based on clinical signs, herd history, histopathologic examination of the brain of suspect animals, and immunoassays (immunohistochemistry or enzyme-linked immunosorbent assay) of the brain for evidence of PrP^{Sc}. Standard coronary sections of the most commonly affected areas—that is, midbrain, brain stem, and cervical spinal cord—are examined for routine diagnosis. Anti-PrP antibodies are used for immunohistochemical staining of suspect brain specimens and for western blot assays of solubilized brain extracts and cerebral spinal fluid. In the absence of PrP^{Sc} accumulation in the lymphoid tissue, as is seen in sheep scrapie, there is currently no established method for use on any practicably obtainable antemortem specimen, neither is there any method useful in animals before the development of frank clinical signs of disease.

Immunology, Prevention, and Control

The control of bovine spongiform encephalopathy in the United Kingdom has rested solely on the exclusion of all meat, offal, and other materials derived from cattle in all cattle feed products. Means to prevent the transfer of the disease into other countries, especially countries of the European Union, have centered on bans against the importation of beef, live bovine animals and embryos, meat-and-bone meal, and other products derived from cattle from the United Kingdom. Beyond this, much of the new international regulation of export/import of beef and other products derived from cattle pertains to concerns over the bovine spongiform encephalopathy prion entering the human food chain.

Biohazard: In 1997, the government of the United Kingdom declared that "the bovine spongiform encephalopathy agent should be considered a human pathogen. Those intentionally working with infected material or preparations should use the same laboratory safety precautions as for Creutzfeldt–Jacob disease."

ATYPICAL BOVINE SPONGIFORM ENCEPHALOPATHY

Novel forms of bovine spongiform encephalopathy distinct from the classical entity have recently been identified in both Europe and North America, through extensive surveillance for bovine spongiform encephalopathy. Because these cases are only found occasionally and usually in clinically normal older animals (at least 8 years), atypical bovine spongiform encephalopathy may represent a sporadic spongiform encephalopathy of older cattle (perhaps analogous to Nor98/atypical scrapie of sheep). The lack of antemortem testing and the low prevalence of the disorder have limited epidemiologic studies of atypical bovine spongiform encephalopathy to date. The stability and pathogenicity of this strain in humans remain to be determined.

TRANSMISSIBLE MINK ENCEPHALOPATHY

Transmissible mink encephalopathy was first recognized on mink ranches in Wisconsin in 1947. Clinical signs included hyper-irritability, ataxia, compulsive biting, somnolence, coma, and death. Histologic lesions in the brains of affected mink were similar to those in scrapie in sheep. The source of transmissible mink encephalopathy appears to be food-borne, but infection by sheep scrapie has not been demonstrated. The biochemical signature of PrP^{Sc} from affected mink shares some characteristics with that of atypical bovine spongiform encephalopathy, suggesting that feeding carcasses from older cows with a sporadic spongiform encephalopathy may have been the source of the rare outbreaks of the disease in mink. Additional studies will clearly be required to define the origin of the mink agent and to determine its epidemiology.

CHRONIC WASTING DISEASE OF DEER AND ELK

Chronic wasting disease is a progressive, fatal neurological disease of captive and/or free-ranging mule deer (*Odocoileus hemionus*), mule deer hybrids, black-tailed deer, white-tailed deer (*Odocoileus virginianus*), Rocky Mountain elk (*Cervus canadensis*), and Shira's moose (*Alces alces*). Chronic wasting disease was first recognized

in captive mule deer in 1980 in Colorado; summaries of harvest survey data published in 2009 varied, from <1–14.3% among mule deer, to <1–2.4% among elk, and to <1% among moose. The disease has since been recognized in extensive portions of western North America. In recent years, the disease has also been found in wild animals that seemingly have lived for many generations far from captive deer and elk facilities. Chronic wasting disease is characterized by abnormal behavior, teeth grinding, polyuria, and polydipsia, and marked loss of weight. Death usually occurs within a few months of the appearance of clinical signs. Histologic lesions include widespread spongiform change of the brain—that is, neuronal vacuolation—as well as astrocytic hypertrophy and hyperplasia. The epidemiology of the disease in deer and elk is unknown.

HUMAN PRION DISEASES

Kuru, Creutzfeldt–Jacob disease, Gerstmann–Sträussler–Scheinker syndrome, and fatal familial insomnia are human prion diseases that are manifested predominantly in middle-aged and older individuals. Usually their onset is indicated by sensory disturbances, confusion, inappropriate behavior, and severe sleeping disorders. Disease progression is marked by myoclonic jerking movements, and, within 6 months to 1 year, progression to frank dementia and, ultimately, a comatose state and death. There are three major classes of these diseases: sporadic, familial, and iatrogenic:

Creutzfeldt–Jakob disease occurs in all three forms: (1) 85% of cases are sporadic, seemingly with quite long incubation periods, cause unknown; (2) 15% of cases are familial, with very long incubation periods, caused by autosomal dominant mutations in the *PrP* gene, more than 18 of which have been mapped; (3) a few hundred cases have been transmitted iatrogenically via contaminated neurosurgical instruments (e.g., implanted stereotactic electroencephalogram electrodes), dura matter and cornea grafts, and hormones, especially growth hormone derived from human cadavers.

Variant Creutzfeldt–Jakob disease (*vCJD*) was first described in the United Kingdom in 1996 amongst individuals who exhibited features not normally associated with Creutzfeldt–Jakob disease: (1) they were between 19 and 45 years of age when diagnosed (as compared with an average age of 63 years for sporadic cases); (2) the course of their disease was longer than usual (mean 14 months, compared with 6 months for sporadic cases); (3) their lesions were different than those seen in sporadic cases (florid neural plaques, rather than spongiform changes); (4) they initially presented with psychiatric problems (personality changes, depression, fearfulness, paranoia), as well as signs of weakness and dementia as seen in sporadic cases; (5) late in the course of their disease, they exhibited cerebellar syndrome, ataxia, cognitive impairment, and myoclonus, in addition to dementia and coma as seen terminally in sporadic cases. As described earlier in this chapter, several lines of molecular evidence have linked vCJD to bovine spongiform encephalopathy, and putatively to exposure to nervous system tissues from infected cattle.

Gerstmann–Sträussler–Scheinker syndrome and fatal familial insomnia are very rare familial diseases caused by autosomal dominant mutations in the *PrP* gene. In the former there is a single point mutation at codon 102 in the *PrP* gene that leads to a single amino acid substitution in the normal PrP protein. When this point mutation is introduced into the *PrP* gene of mice, they develop typical spongiform encephalopathy disease and lesions.

GENERAL REFERENCE LIST

American Fisheries Society Blue Book, **Suggested Procedures for the Detection and Identification of Certain Finfish and Shellfish Pathogens**, 2007 Edition. www.fisheries.org/units/fhs/bb_inspection.php

Boulianne M. **Avian Disease Manual**, 7th ed. American Association Avian Pathologists, 2013.

Charlton, B.R. (ed). **Avian Disease Manual**, 6th ed. American Association of Avian Pathologists, Jacksonville, FL. 2006

Coetzer JA, Tustin RC (eds). **Infectious Diseases of Livestock**. 2nd ed. Oxford University Press, 2004.

Flint SJ, Enquist LW, Racaniello VR, Skalka AM. **Principles of Virology**, 3rd ed. ASM Press 2008.

Fowler ME, Miller RE. **Zoo and Wild Animal Medicine**, 5th ed. Saunders 2003.

Fox JG, Barthold SW, Davisson MT, Newcomer CE, Quimby FW, Smith AL, (eds). **The Mouse in Biomedical Research**, Volume II: Diseases, 2nd ed, Academic Press, 2007.

Greene CE (ed). **Infectious Diseases of the Dog and Cat**. 3rd ed. Saunders Elsevier, 2006.

King AM, Adams MJ, Carstens EB, Lefkowitz. **Virus Taxonomy**. 9th Report. Academic Press Elsevier, 2012.

Knipe DM, Howley PM (eds). **Fields Virology**, 5th ed. Lippincott Williams & Wilkins 2007.

Kumar V, Abbas AK, Fausto N, Aster JC (eds). **Robbins and Cotran Pathologic Basis of Disease**. 8th ed. Saunders Elsevier, 2010.

Mahy BW, Van Regenmortel MHV (eds). **Encyclopedia of Virolgy**, 3rd ed. Academic Press 2008.

Maxie MG (ed). **Jubb, Kennedy and Palmer's Pathology of Domestic Animals**. 5th ed. Elsevier, 2007.

Miller RE, Fowler ME. **Fowler's Zoo and Wild Animal Medicine, Current Therapy**, vol 7, Saunders Elsevier, 2012.

Percy DH, Barthold SW. **Pathology of Laboratory Rodents and Rabbits**. 3rd ed. Blackwell, Ames, 2007.

Saif, YM (ed). **Diseases of Poultry**, 12th ed. Blackwell, 2008.

Sellon DC, Long MT (eds). **Equine Infectious Diseases**. Saunders Elsevier, 2007.

Strauss JH, Strauss EG. **Viruses and Human Diseases**. 2nd ed. Elsevier, 2006.

Straw BE, Zimmerman JJ, D'Allaire S, Taylor DJ. **Diseases of Swine**, 9th ed, Blackwell 2006.

Swayne, D.E. **Avian Influenza**. Wylie-Blackwell Publishing, Ames, Iowa. 628 pp. 2008.

United States Animal Health Association. **Foreign Animal Diseases**, 7th ed. 2008. http://www.usaha.org/Portals/6/Publications/FAD.pdf.

Woo PTK, Bruno DW (eds.). **Fish Diseases and Disorders**, Volume 3: Viral, Bacterial and Fungal Infections, CABI Publishing, 1999.

Zimmerman JJ, Karriker L, Ramirez A, Schwartz KJ. **Diseases of Swine**, 10th ed. Blackwell 2012.

Outbreak information

www.cdc.gov/
www.promedmail.org/
www.eurosurveillance.org/
www.who.int/
www.healthmap.org/en/ (Geographic disease distribution using Google maps)

World Organization for Animal Health (OIE). OIE website provides a wealth of information regarding disease outbreaks, technical reviews on veterinary issues and publications on standards for diagnostic testing for mammals and aquatic animals, www.oie.int/

Vaccine and veterinary infectious diseases

www.AAEP.org
www.AAFP.org
www.AAHA.org
www.WSAVA.org
www.AVMA.org
www.ivis.org
www.vetscite.org
partnersah.vet.cornell.edu/avian-atlas

Viral Taxonomy

www.ictvonline.org/

General Veterinary/Zoonotic Disease

www.inspection.gc.ca/
www.cfsph.iastate.edu/DiseaseInfo/index.php
www.nwhc.usgs.gov/